Advances in Obstructive Jaundice

Diagnosis and Treatment

Advances in Obstructive Jaundice

Diagnosis and Treatment

Chief Editors

McMahon Michael J

Filippou Dimitrios

Skandalakis Panayiotis

Associate Editors

Acalovschi Monica

Vezakis Antonios

PMP

PASCHALIDIS MEDICAL PUBLICATIONS

PMP (Paschalidis Medical Publications, Ltd.).
14th, Tetrapoleos str., Athens, 115 27, Greece
Tel.: 003-210-7789125, 003-210-7793012, Fax: 0030-210-7759421,
e-mail:
orders: Paschalidis@Medical-Books.gr
© information: GP@Medical-Books.gr, CP@Medical-Books.gr

ISBN: 978-960-399-533-3

9 789603 995333

ADVANCES IN OBSTRUCTIVE JAUNDICE. DIAGNOSIS AND TREATMENT

Dedications

To my parents Konstantinos & Niki

and to my new born children

D. K. Filippou
Series Editor

With respect to my teacher Gregorios Skalkeas

Academic and Professor

P. Scandalakis
Series Editor

Al-Bahrani Ahmed, MD, FRCS
Research Fellow, Department of Surgery,
  Manchester Royal Infirmary, Manchester,
  UK
Email: Not Available

Altieri Andrea, MD, PhD
Istituto di Ricerche Farmacologiche "Mario
  Negri", via Eritrea 62, 20157 Milano,
  Italy.
Division of Molecular Genetic Epidemiolo-
  gy, German Cancer Research Centre, Hei-
  delberg, Germany.
E-mail: altieri@marionegri.it;
      a.altieri@dkfz.de;

Ammori Basil, MD, FRCS
Consultant Hepato-Pancreato-Biliary and
  Laparoscopic Surgeon, Manchester Royal
  Infirmary, Oxford Road, Manchester M13
  9WL, UK
Email: Bammori@aol.com,
      Basil.Ammori@CMMC.nhs.uk

Acalovschi Monica, MD, PhD
Professor of Internal Medicine and Gas-
  troenterology, 3rd Medical Clinic, Univer-
  sity of Medicine and Pharmacy, Cluj-
  Napoca, Romania
Email: monacal@umfcluj.ro

Avgerinos Efthimios, MD
First Department of General Surgery,
  Voulas General Hospital "Asclepeion",
  Voula, Athens, Greece
Email: surgmike@hotmail.com

Castro Felipe, MD
Division of Molecular Genetic Epidemiology, German Cancer Research Centre, Heidelberg, Germany
Email: Not available

Consorti Eileen, MD, MS
Assistant Clinical Professor of Surgery,
  University of California San Francisco-
  East Bay Surgery Program and Univer-
  sity of California San Francisco School of
  Medicine Oakland and San Francisco,
  California USA
Email: Not available

Dervenis Christos
First Department of General Surgery, Athens
  General Hospital "Agia Olga", Athens,
  Greece
Email: chrider@otenet.gr

Dwivedi Manisha, MD, DM, FICP, FACG
Professor and Head, Department of Gas-
  troenterology, Moti Lal Nehru Medical
  College, Allahabad, India
Email: manisha_dwivedi@hotmail.com

Ercolani Giorgio, MD
Department of Surgery and Transplantation,
  University of Bologna, Sant'Orsola-
  Malpighi Hospital, Via Massarenti 9,
  40138 Bologna, Italy
Email: gercolani@aosp.bo.it

Filippou Georgios, MD, MSc
First Department of General Surgery, Piraeus
  General Hospital "Tzaneio", Piraeus, Greece
Email: georgiosfilippoumd@hotmail.com

Filippou Dimitrios, MD, PhD
Vis. Professor of Anatomy, Department of
  Nursing, University of Athens, Greece
First Department of General Surgery, Piraeus
  General Hospital "Tzaneio", Piraeus, Greece
Department of Visceral and General Surgery,
  Cantonal Hospital, Fribourg, CH-1708,
  Switzerland
Email: d_filippou@hotmail.com;
      d_filippou@yahoo.gr;
      info@filippou.com

Giampalma Emanuela, MD
Department of Radiology, Sant'Orsola-
  Malpighi Hospital, Via Massarenti 9,
  40138 Bologna, Italy
Email: giampalma@aosp.bp.it

Golfieri Rita, MD
Chairman, Department of Radiology, Sant'
  Orsola-Malpighi Hospital, Via Massaren-
  ti 9, 40138 Bologna, Italy
Email: golfieri@aosp.bo.it

Gulati Gurpreet, MD, PhD
Assistant Professor, Department of Cardiac
  Radiology, Cardiothoracic Sciences Center,
  All India Institute of Medical Sciences,
  New Delhi 110029, India
Email: Not available

Gulati Manpreet, MD, PhD
Associate Professor, Department of Radiodi
  agnosis, All India Institute of Medical
  Sciences, New Delhi - 110029, India
Email: Not available

Jain Tarun, MD
Senior Resident, Department of Radiodiag-
  nosis, All India Institute of Medical Sciences, New Delhi - 110029, India
Email: Not available

Kandpal Harsh, MD
Senior Resident, Department of Radiodiag-
  nosis, All India Institute of Medical Sciences, New Delhi - 110029, India
Email: Not available

Kanematsu Masayuki, MD, PhD
Department of Radiology, Gifu University
  School of Medicine, Gifu, Japan
Email: Not available

Koea Jonathan, MD, FRACS
Assoc Professor, Chief, Hepatobiliary/Upper
  Gastrointestinal Unit, Department of
  Surgery, Auckland City Hospital, Private
  Bag 92024, Auckland, New Zealand
Email: jonathank@adhb.govt.nz

Krahenbuhl Lukas, MD, PhD
Professor of Surgery, Department of Vis-
  ceral and General Surgery, Cantonal
  Hospital, Fribourg, CH-1708, Switzer-
  land
Email: Not available

Leonardou Politimi, MD
Dept. of Radiology, Laiko Athens General
  Hospital, 11527 Goudi, Athens, Greece
Email: Not available

Liu Terrence, MD
Associate Clinical Professor of Surgery,
  University of California San Francisco-
  East Bay Surgery Program and University
  of California San Francisco School of
  Medicine Oakland and San Francisco,
  California USA
Email: Not available

Mairaing Eimorn, MD
Associate Professor of Radiology, Depart-
  ment of Radiology, Faculty of Medicine,
  Khon Kaen University, Khon Kaen 40002,
  Thailand.
Email: eimorn@kku.ac.th

Mairiang Pisaln, MD
Department of Radiology, Faculty of
  Medicine, Khon Kaen University, Khon
  Kaen 40002, Thailand.
E-mail: eimorn@kku.ac.th

Maluf-Filho Fauze, MD
Associate Professor of the Department of
  Gastroenterology, Sao Paulo University,
  Medical School, Sao Paulo, Brazil
Email: Not available

McMahon Michael J, MD, PhD
Professor of Surgery, Director of LIMIT and
  President of ALS
Leeds Institute of LIMIT and Leeds General
  Infirmary
Wellcome Wing, Leeds General Infimary,
  LEEDS, L51 3 EX, United Kingdom
Email: mjm@lapsurg.co.uk

Mimidis Konstantinos, MD, PhD
Ass. Professor, 1st Department of Internal
    Medicine, Medical School, Democretion
    University of Thrace, Alexandroupoli,
    Greece
Email: Not available

**Misra SP, MD, DM, FRCP, FICP,
    FACG, FNASc**
Professor, Department of Gastroenterology,
    Motilal Nehru Medical College, Alla-
    habad 211 001, India
Email: spmisra@sancharnet.in

O'Grady John, MD, PhD
Professor, Institute of Liver Studies, King's
    College Hospital, Denmark Hill, London
Email: Not available

Papadopoulos Vasilios, MD, PhD
Department of Emergencies, Xanthi General
    Hospital, Xanthi, Greece
Email: vaspapmd@hotmail.com

Papas Paris MD, PhD
Dept. of Radiology, Laiko Athens General
    Hospital, 11527 Goudi, Athens, Greece
Email: Not available

Polydorou Andreas, MD, PhD
Associate Professor of Surgery, 3rd Depart-
    ment of Surgery, Medical School, Univer-
    sity of Athens, "Areteion" Hospital, A-
    thens, Greece
Email: Not available

Principe Alfonso, MD
Associate Professor, Department of Surgery
    and Transplantation, University of
    Bologna, Sant'Orsola-Malpighi Hospital,
    Via Massarenti 9, 40138 Bologna, Italy
Email: aprincipe@aosp.bo.it

Qin Lun-Xiu, MD, PhD
Professor, Liver Cancer Institute and
    Zhongshan Hospital, Fudan University,
    136 Yi Xue Yuan Road, Shanghai
    200032, China
Email: lxqin@zshospital.com

**Rawat Saumitra, MD, MS, FRCS (Ed),
    FRCS (Gen.)**
Leeds Institute of LIMIT and Leeds General
    Infirmary
Wellcome Wrug, Leeds General Infirmary
LEEDS, S51 3 EX, United Kingdom
Email: srawatuk@yahoo.com

Richardson Paul, MD
Institute of Liver Studies, King's College
    Hospital, Denmark Hill, London
Email: Not available

Rizos Spiros, MD, FACS
First Department of General Surgery, Pi-
    raeus General Hospital "Tzaneio", Pi-
    raeus, Greece
Email: srizos@otenet.gr

Simopoulos Konstantinos, MD, PhD
Dean and Professor
First Department of Surgery, Medical School,
    Democretion University of Thrace, Alexan-
    droupoli, Greece
Email: Not available

Skandalakis Panayiotis, MD, PhD
Professor of Anatomy, Medical School,
    University of Athens, 11527 Goudi, A-
    thens, Greece
Clinical Professor of Surgical Anatomy, De-
    partment of Anatomy, Emory University,
    Atlanta, USA
Email: tskandalakis@otenet.gr;
    tskandal@parliament.gr

Smailis Dimitris, MD
General Surgeon, Neo Heraklion, Athens,
    Greece
Email: Not available

Solmi Luigi, MD
Department of Internal Medicine and Gas-
    troenterology, Section of Gastroenterology,
    Sant'Orsola-Malpighi Hospital, Via
    Massarenti 9, 40138 Bologna, Italy
Email: solmil@aosp.bo.it

Tantau Marcel, MD,
Lecturer
3rd Medical Clinic, University of Medicine
 and Pharmacy, Cluj-Napoca, Romania
Email: Not available

Triantopoulou Charikleia, MD, Phd
Consultant Radiologist, CT department,
 "Agia Olga" general Hospital, 14233
 N. Ionia, Athens, Greece
Email: chatri@mycosmos.gr

Triga Argiro, MD
Anesthesiologist, Kolonaki, Athens,
 Greece
Email: a_triga@hotmail.com

Tsaroucha Alexandra, MD, PhD
Lecturer, First Department of Surgery,
 Medical School, Democretion University
 of Thrace, Alexandroupoli, Greece
Email: Not available

Vezakis Antonios, MD, PhD
Consultant Surgeon, First Department of
 General Surgery, Piraeus General Hos-
 pital "Tzaneio", Piraeus, Greece
Email: Not available

Zingg Tobias, MD
Chef de Clinique, Department of Visceral
 and General Surgery, Cantonal Hospital,
 Fribourg, CH-1708, Switzerland
Email: Not available

The advances in technology, molecular biology and in pharmacology affect current medical practice. Diagnosis and treatment of several diseases and entities has changes significantly during the last decades. Thus there is an increased need for updated editions of specific topics in order to provide specialists with new diagnostic and therapeutic concepts. Review articles published in well-known and widely accepted scientific journals are not only very common but also very useful. Furthermore we believe that books focused in specific topics covering the current advances and pointing out the future perspectives will contribute to the progression of medical knowledge, also improving the current medical practice.

In many cases the results of clinical and basic research may vary affecting the diagnostic algorithm and the therapeutic strategy. In these cases an edition that will provide a panel for the presentation of possible variations or arguments, as well as a comparison between the different options seems to be essential for the specialists all over the world.

With these thoughts in mind we decided to publish a series of books covering special topics of great interest. Aim of this effort is to provide the recent advances and the new concepts to the physicians all over the world. We decided to use for the series the general title "Advances in", due to the fact that our aim is to present what's new. The present edition is the "Advances in Obstructive Jaundice Diagnosis and Treatment" and is referred to a very interesting and common topic that almost all physicians deal with. The forthcoming editions include: "Advances in Endovascular Aortic Aneursym Repair", "Advances in Obesity", "Advances in Colorectal Cancer Diagnosis and Treatment" and "Advances in Breast Cancer".

We knew how difficult this effort would be and how many problems we had to face. At first we had to form the contents in a way that could assist presentation and understanding, and then to select distinguished researchers, physicians and surgeons with deep knowledge and great experience. We would like to thank all the invited authors who are well-known specialists in their field, they responded to our invitation and worked hard in order that we would be able now to present the first book of the series.

In this edition we made an effort to present the most common and important entities and diseases related with obstructive jaundice and provide the readers not only with the clinical and molecular advances but also to point out we are the future perspectives and what we will have to expect. We think that the presentation of the molecular basis of jaundice, the haemostasis impairment and immune dysfunction induced in obstructive jaundice helps in the deeper understanding of the benign and malignant diseases, their effects in the human body as well as in the value of the diagnostic modalities and the therapeutic strategies. Distinguished authors coming from many countries have contributed to this international edition presenting their experience, their arguments and their perspectives.

We would like to thank all authors who participated in this edition, working hard and timely and contributing to this excellent result. We would also like to thank Professor MacMahon J., leading surgeon and researcher in the field of obstructive jaundice, who agreed to help us in the present edition not only as an author but also as Editor in Chief.

We would also like to thank Pashalidis Medical Publications and in particular the brothers Christos Pashalidis and George Pashalidis, because they believed in our project, worked with us and without their assistance the present edition would not have been possible. We are also grateful to the stuff of Pashalidis Medical Publications who contributed to this excellent edition, especially to Mrs. DeCol Maria, Mrs. Mazaraki Christina, Mrs. Antoniadi Maria, Mrs. Arvanitaki Ioanna, Mrs. Vasilakou Georgia, Mrs. Vourlioti Katerina, Mrs Panopoulou Niki and Mrs. Dimitra Kargadouri.

Finally as Series Editors we would like to thank the Associate Editors Prof. Acalovshi Monica, and Dr. Vezakis Antonios for their considerable effort and time spent as well as for their valuable suggestions.

Panagiotis Scandalakis
Professor of Anatomy,
University of Athens
Series Editor

Dimitrios K. Filippou
General Surgeon, Vis. Professor
of Anatomy, University of Athens
Series Editor

Contents

Obstructive jaundice: An introduction

Dervenis Christos, Rizos Spiros

Biliary obstruction is a common symptom caused by a broad spectrum of benign and malignant diseases. In the western world the most common underline diseases are gallstones, tumors of the liver, biliary tree and pancreas, and benign strictures.

Gallstones produce a variable degree of obstruction, from partial to less likely complete, depending on the size and the number of stones. Is associated with exacerbations and remissions, due to the movement of the stone(s) within the duct lumen, and sometimes leads to the more severe situation of cholangitis, especially due to impaction in the distal part of the duct.

Tumors, produce a progressive obstruction due to its gradual enlarment, until the complete stop flow of the bile. As the complete obstruction separates the sterile bile from the gut lumen tumors is unlikely to be associated with cholangitis.

Benign biliary strictures mainly due to surgical injuries, are most common associated with liver dysfunction because of the long standing obstruction.

Biliary obstruction independently of the aetiology and because of the bilirubin elevation causes a number of pathophysiological changes in the liver and different remote organs (e.g. kidneys) the severity of which depended on the degree, duration and site of obstruction.

EFFECTS ON THE LIVER AND THE DUCTS

Obstruction, either partial or complete, result in an increase of the pressure within the ductal system, which normally is around 10 to 15 cm of water. The increase of intraductal pressure is proportional related to the degree and duration of the obstruction and could reach 25 to 35 cm of water.

There are a number of consequences of these high pressures. It produces dilatation of both the extrahepatic and intrahepatic ducts, changes in the hepatocytic function, bile secretion and bile outflow.

There are differences in the pattern of duct dilatation related to the cause of obstruction. Obstruction to tumor is more markedly in comparison with the stone aetiology. This is mainly because the obstruction in the presence of tumor is more likely to be complete and the duct is generally normal. On the contrary, in the presence of stone(s) the duct wall is usually thick due to the concomitant inflammation that prevents the duct of an extreme dilatation. The presence or absence of the gallbladder also affects the degree of the dilatation. It is known that the gallbladder wall absorbs water from the bile and therefore the intraductal pressure is reduced.

A number of morphological changes also occur because of the obstruction, at both canalicular and cellular level. These changes have been extensively studied in animal experiments and in humans. The most characteristic feature is the formation of plug into the intralobular canaliculi, together with intralobular stasis and periductular extravasation of bile. The later leads to an inflammatory reaction, which might further leads to intralobular fibrosis and probably at a later stage to abscess formation.

At cellular level with the increase of the intraductal pressure and with time specific changes occur from decrease of intracellular membranes (eg. Golgi complex) to the complete loss of the tight junction network. This leads to increased permeability and reflux of bile into the portal sinusoids and increase of plasma serum bilirubin and alkaline phosphatase. The increase of plasma bilirubin, it is not only the result of impaired transportation but of the alteration in its conjugation.

There also differences in the level of bilirubin elevation according to aetiology of the obstruction. In general, tumor obstruction resulted in higher bilirubin values in comparison with lithiasis or post-traumatic strictures. It should be noted here that the increase of serum bilirubin is not unlimited. In patients with normal renal function, in both cases, its values reached a plateau, which for malignant obstruction is 25 to 35 mg/dL, at which point loss in the urine equals the daily production. In benign disease (e.g. common duct stone) the increase of bilirubin is usually transient and ranges from 2 to 4 mg/dL. Obstruction of a single bile duct does not cause jaundice.

Based on those observations the level of both the dilatation and serum bilirubin could be used to differentiate the cause of obstruction between neoplasms and benign conditions.

The rise of alkaline phosphatase in serum caused by obstruction is more sensitive as it raises more rapid, befor bilirubin and it is measured in every case of obstruction, even though the bilirubin is still normal. The increase of the plasma concentrations are not only due to obstructed outflow but also due to de nove increase of its production from the plasma membrane of the hepatocytes. There is no correlation with the level and duration of obstruction but higher values are usually measured with complte obstruction that usually associates malignancy.

SYSTEMIC EFFECTS OF BILLARY OBSTRUCTION

Biliary obstruction has not only local effects on the liver and the ductal system but also, and probably more important, effects the different remote organs. This is why patients with obstructive jaundice should follow closely, especially those individuals with co-morbidities. Organ dysfunctions should always be taking into consideration when the patient become a surgical candidate and should be corrected, if possible, before surgery.

Cardiovascular changes

There are strong evidences from both experiments and human studies that a decrease response of the smooth muscle of the blood vessels is a result of obstructive jaundice. This is most probably because of the alteration in response to different sympathiticomimetic amines. This leads, consequently to decrease of the peripheral vascular resistant and impaired left ventricular function. Clinically this changes expressed by hypotension which become more profound postoperatively as other mechanisms also involved (eg. Endotoxemia) exacerbates vasodilatation and decreased peripheral resistant.

Changes in renal function

Renal dysfunction or failure is common in patients with obstructive jaundice mainly postoperatively. The cause of the increased risk of renal function although has not been fully elucidated, has been attributed to different factors. The most important of these factors are the decrease glomerular filtration rate due to hypovolemia and vasodilatation in the early stage of obstruction, with vasoconstriction because of the loss of response to regulatory mechanisms in later stage, and endotoxemia.

Impairment of the Host defence mechanisms

Endotoxaemia and dysfunction of Kuppfer cells is the main cause of host defence impairment during obstructive jaundice. The absence of bile salts into the gut lumen result in gram negative bacteria overgrowth. This leads to systemic and portal increase in endotoxins which is the main predictor of outcome, especially for those patients who will be candidates for operation. Depression of Kuppfer cell activity, secondary to inraductal pressure, exacerbates the entotoxeamia as these cells represents one of the biggest mass of macrophages in the body. Kuppfer cell are also connected with the production of different cytokines (TNF, IL-6) with a critical role in the immuno- defence mechanism, contributing in further immunosupression.

In conclusion, obstructive jaundice is not only a local phenomenon but has a number of systemic implications which is related to an increase risk of complications and mortality in these patients. As the most of these factors recovers with the relief of obstruction a preoperative temporary drainage (PBD) should be considered. However, although it seems reasonable, preoperative stenting, endoscopically or percoutaneously, have not became a standard practice. Recently, a large meta-analysis published The Netherlands group, included 2,853 patients showed that preoperative drainage with current standards for patients with obstructive jaundice resulting from tumors carries no benefit and should not be performed routinely. We do not know frojm the avalaible evidence the exact role of preoperative drainage in patients with benign diseases cause biliary obstruction. Further studies are needed to establish guidelines together with improvements in instruments and techniques for drainage. We should always keep in mind that in selected cases the policy for PBD should be individualized.

PREOPERATIVE DIAGNOSIS

The questions should be answered initially in patients presenting with jaundice is to differentiate if this is due to extrahepatic obstruction, the so called "surgical" type or to other causes "medical" one. Although in many cases laboratory tests (bilirubin, alkaline phosphatase, γGT) together with medical history of the patient can be helpful to differentiate the type of obstruction there is a substantial gap where this is not possible with accuracy. Imaging is then the most important preoperative tool to give the surgeon the necessary information to design the proper strategy. As in nowadays, a broad spectrum of imaging modalities are available, it is off great important to select this with the highest possible accuracy not only to obtain what we need to know but also to keep the cost low, something which is of a great importance.

In general, surgical demands are accomplished when imaging

- identify the presence of bile duct dilatation,
- define the level of obstruction
- and provide a diagnosis of the nature of the lesion (neoplastic/malignant vs. inflammatoru/postoperative).

Not all imaging modalities have the same accuracy in the different causes of biliary obstruction. Thus, the surgeon should work closely with the radiology to be consulted on the advantages and disadvantages of each imaging technique. Ultrasonography (US), can be the initial examination in almost all the situations, as it is easy to apply, gives useful information about the presence of obstruction in jaundiced patient and it is associated with low cost. Imaging studies should be use quantative signal intensity measurements to provide evidence of lesion type and help in reducing uncertainty and inconsistency associated with visual assessment of brightness, morphology or patterns of contrast medium enhancement

The main disadvantage of US is the fact that it is very much depended with the operator. The CT remains the gold standard modality, especially with the introduction of the new multislice detectors and the modern proocols, as in the most circumstances gives the information the surgeons wants to know with no need of any other preoperative imaging MRI is used as a problem solving modality for lesions considered "intermediate" on other imaging techniques. MRCP can replace accurately ERCP in imaging of the ducts,

with the disadvantage of the inability to perform interventions needed for obstruction relief. Different imaging modalities are complimentary and should be individualized.

MANAGEMENT OF OBSTRUCTIVE JAUNDICE

It is obvious that management of obstructive jaundice is absolute depended on the underlying pathology. However there are a number of issues that the surgeon should be take into consideration before he/she decides about the most proper treatment option.

The knowledge of the pathophysiologic changes produced by the obstruction it is necessary to reduce operative risk. Preoperative evaluation and ASA classification is of great importance as it is important all the consequences to be corrected if possible and the patient should be supported.

As it has been discussed earlier in this chapter preoperative drainage, endoscopicaly or percutaneously it is not always useful. However, in many cases interventional modalities are preferred to surgery, as besides they are more effective, carry less risk for the patient.

It should be mentioned here, that in certain cases, the surgical management of obstructive jaundice, should be performed in specialized centers. There are strong evidence that by treating these patients in a centralized way, the mortality and morbidity is significant lower.

Hilar malignant strictures, complicated post - injury strictures, pancreatic and periampulary tumors are some of the pathologies that patients should always be referred to centers of expertise.

Obstructive jaundice, is a clinical expression of a wide range of pathologies, from those with relative easy management and low risk to those with a number of difficulties and high risk. Therefore, multidisciplinary management is of a great importance. The majority of these patients should be treated in center of excellence and in that way patient will receive the necessary high quality of care.

REFERENCES

Bemelmans MHA, Greve JWM, Guma DJ, Buurman WA. Increased concentrations of tumor necrosis factor (TNF) and soluble TNF receptors in biliary obstruction in mice, soluble TNF receptors as prognostic factors factors for mortality. Gut 1996;38:447-53

Cameron G, Hasan S Disturbances of structures and function in the liver as a result of biliary obstruction J Pathol Bacteriol 1958;75: 333-338

Deitch EA. The realiability and clinical limitations of sonographic scanning ob the biliary ducts. Ann Surg 1981, 193:167-170

Ding JW, Anderson R, Norgren L, Stenram U, Bengmark S: The influence of biliary obstruction and sepsis on reticuloendothelial function in rats. Eur J Surg 1992;158:157-64

Jiang WG, Puntis MCA. Immune dysfunction in patients with obstructive jaundice, mediators and implications for treatments. HPB Surgery 1997;10:129-42

Klein HM, Wein B, Truong S, Pfingsten FP, Gunther RW. Computed tomographic cholangiography using spiral scanning and 3D image processing. Br J Radiol 1993;66(789):762-7.

L. Way and C Pellgrini. Surgery of the Gallbladder and Bile Ducts. Saunders (1987) Philadeplphia USA

Nino-Murcia M, Tamm EP, Charnsangavej C, et al. Multidetector-row helical and advanced post processing techniques for the evaluation of pancreatic neoplasms. Abdom Imaging 2003;28: 366-377.

Sewnath M, Karsten T, Prins M, Rauws E, Obertop H, Gouma D. A meta-analysis on the efficacy of preoperative biliary drainage for tumors causing obstructive jaundice Ann Surg 2002;17-27

Sheen-Chen SM, Chau P, Harris HW. Obstructive jaundice alters Kupffer cell function independent of bacterial translocation. J Surg Res 1998;80: 205-9

Taylor KJW, Rosenfield AT, Spiro HM. Diagnostic accuracy of gray scale ultrasonography for the jaundiced patient. Arch Intern Med 1979, 139:60-63.

van Heek NT, Kuhlmann KF, Scholten RJ, de Castro SM, Busch OR, van Gulik TM, Obertop H, Gouma DJ Hospital volume and mortality after pancreatic resection: a systematic review and an evaluation of intervention in the Netherlands.Ann Surg. 2005 Dec;242(6):781-8

The anatomy of the biliary tree

Filippou Dimitrios, Skandalakis Panayiotis

The knowledge of extrahepatic biliary tract anatomy as well as the anatomy of the main vessels of the area is of great importance in the differential diagnosis and treatment of obstructive jaundice. The knowledge of the causes of obstructive jaundice and the concurrent therapeutic strategies is based of the well and defined understanding of the anatomy of the intra-hepatic and extra-hepatic biliary tract, and the main arteries, vessels and lymphatics of the area. The authors should also have a detailed knowledge of the adjacent organs and structures of the biliary tract, but it is not possible and it isn't also purpose of the present book to describe the anatomy of the upper abdomen. In the present chapter we will present the anatomy of the intra-hepatic and extra-hepatic biliary tree, of the gallbladder and of the main adjacent vessels, which in many cases contribute to the development of obstructive jaundice and the possible therapeutic approaches.

HISTORY

The anatomic and surgical history of the biliary tract begins in the ancient years. First descriptions of the gallbladder can be found in the Ancient Egyptians. The E-gyptians had developed techniques to p-reserve the dead bodies of the Kings by converting them into mummies. Some of these techniques required removal of the viscera, so the Egyptians should be con-sidered the first visceral anatomists.

After the Egyptians in whom medicine and anatomy were mixed with magic, the ancient Greeks were the pioneers who es-tablished the basis for the modern anatomy and surgery. Hippocrates, the fa-ther of modern medicine and his students gave the first descriptions of the biliary diseases, suggesting also the diagnostic and therapeutic approaches. The first de-scription of absence of the gallbladder in animals belongs to Aristotle, who wasn't only one of the greatest philosophers but also distinguished biologist. Four hundred years later Galen (130-200 DC) suggested that the humans have a single bile duct or paired bile ducts. This statement was the first attempt to describe the anatomy of the extra-hepatic biliary tree.

After the Middle Ages the anatomy of

the human body progressed significantly. In 1701 Bergman reported the first case of gallbladder absence in humans. That was also the first description of the gallbladder agenesia, which constitutes a rare congenital abnormality. Morgagni in 1769 described some deformations of the galbadder, Home (1813) the biliary atresia and vonWyss (1870) presented some deformations of the common bile duct.

First, Vater in 1723 described the dilatation of the common bile duct in a patient with obstructive jaundice, and in 1867 Bobbs described the hydrop of the gallbladder due to lithiasis and removed also successfully gallstones. From this point the surgery of the extra-hepatic biliary and the gallbladder developed rapidly, and 30 years later Swain (in 1894) performed the first successful cholecystojejunostomy for cystic dilatation of the bile duct.

In this historical puzzle we must also include Dr Calot, who in 1891 described the cholecysto-hepatic triangle, which is known today as Triangle of Calot and it's very important in surgeons, especially to those who perform laparoscopic cholecystectomy.

Although several descriptions and attempts to explain the possible causes of jaundice development the first who studied the pathophysiology of the c-holestasis was Eppinger 1902. Since then the progress in technology was rapid and several diagnostic and therapeutic advances obtained. The first roentgenography of the biliary tree was achieved by Reich (1918), in a patient with an external fistula, while in 1923 Baker performed the first intraoperative endoscopic visualization of the bile ducts. In 1931 Mirizzi performed the first operative cholangiography and in 1948 reported the syndrome of a long cystic duct with impacted stone which carries his name. During the last century many syndromes and congenital abnormalities of the bile ducts and the

vessels have been described. It's of no use to write down the dates that these abnormalities presented, but just to remember that the anatomy and surgery of the biliary tract posses a history of thousand years.

A. INTRA-HEPATIC BILIARY TRACT

The first part of the biliary system is the intra-hepatic biliary tract, which is originating from the canaliculi. These are small channels that constructed by small portions of the hepatocyte membranes. Both of the right and left lobe of the liver are drained by ducts originating as bile canaliculi in the lobules. The bile ducts in the liver follow the anatomy that is determined by the vascular supply. The canaliculi empty into the canals of Hering in the interlobular triads. The canals of Hering are collected into ducts draining the hepatic areas, the four hepatic segment ducts, and finally, outside the liver, the right and left hepatic ducts. More specifically the left lobar duct is formatted by the union of the ducts of the liver segments II, III and IV and it connected with the right lobar duct in the level of quadrate lobe to form the common hepatic duct, above the right branch of the portal vein. The right lobar duct presents a posterior sectoral duct for segments VI and VII and an anterior sectoral duct for segments V and VIII.

a1. The right hepatic duct

The right hepatic duct, which is shorter, is formed by the union of the anterior and posterior segment ducts at the porta hepatis, and joins the left lobar duct at the base of the right liver lobe. Healey and Schroy refer an incidence of this pattern about in 72%. In the remainder, the posterior segment duct crossed the segmental fissure to empty into the left hepatic duct or one of its tributaries. In these cases, the right hepatic duct is absent. The average length of the right hepatic duct, when present, is 0.9 cm.

a2. The left hepatic duct

The left hepatic duct is usually formed by the union of the medial and lateral segment ducts. The right and left lobar ducts are usually join in the edge of the liver, in line with the left segmental fissure (50%), to the right of the fissure (42%), or to the left of the fissure (8%) to form the common hepatic duct. The average length of the left hepatic duct ranges from 1.7 to 2 cm. In most of the cases the left hepatic duct forms a more anterior and acute angle compared with the right hepatic duct. This anatomic feature is a usual finding during surgical or endoscopical exploration of the common hepatic duct. The right and left hepatic ducts are of equal size, but in patients with chronic biliary obstruction the left hepatic duct is usually larger than the right duct.

The segments of the left liver lobe drain to the left hepatic duct, while those of the right liver lobe to the right hepatic duct. This is a general anatomico-physiological rule although some rare exceptions may occur. The most interesting thing is the drain of the segment I of the liver (or caudate lobe) which presents significant variability. In 80% of the persons may drain both in the right and left liver lobe, in 15% in the left liver lobe and in only 5% of the cases drains to the right liver lobe.

B. EXTRA-HEPATIC BILIARY TRACT

b1. The common hepatic Duct

The common hepatic duct is formed by the union of the right and left hepatic ducts anterior to the portal vein at the transverse fissure of the liver. Its lower end is defined as its junction with the cystic duct and its confluence varies according to the location of this junction. The length of the common hepatic duct ranges 1.0 to 7.5 cm, while the diameter is about 0.4-0.7 cm. The topographical relations of the segments of the biliary tract to the adjacent arteries is of great interest and will be analytically review after finishing the description of the extra-hepatic biliary tree.

b2. Cystic duct

The cystic duct connects the gallbladder with the common bile duct. The junction of the cystic duct with the common hepatic duct is the upper limit of the common bile duct. In the lumen of the cystic duct 5 to 12 crescent shaped folds of the mucosa similar to those in the neck of the gallbladder can be seen. These folds form a spiral valve which is called valve of Heister. The length of the cystic duct and the angle which joins the common hepatic duct to form the upper limit of the common bile duct vary.

Anatomical variations. The extra-hepatic biliray tree presents significant variations. The thorough knowledge of these variations is of great importance for the general surgeons who perform biliary operations, because an intraoperative mistake in the recognition of the anatomy may cause serious problems in the patient, increase the perioperative morbidity and mortality and require re-operations to restore the problem. In 64-75% of the cases the angle that the cystic duct joins the common hepatic duct is 40°. In 17-23%, the cystic duct parallels the hepatic duct for a longer or shorter distance and may even enter the duodenum separately. This is called "absence" of the common bile duct.

In 8-13%, the cystic duct may pass inferior to or superior to the common hepatic duct to enter the latter on the left side. In the parallel type of junction, the common duct is at risk from the surgeon attempting to ligate the cystic duct. If the long parallel portion of the cystic duct is left in place, cystic duct remnant syndrome with various sequelae may result. Less frequently, the gallbladder is sessile with little or no cystic duct. In these cases the cystic duct should be prepared well and ligated not very close to the common bile duct because there is an increased risk of injury during the manipulations. In any case the cystic duct should be recognised, prepared well and ligated appropriately in order to avoid a long cystic duct remnant which may cause postcholecystectomy problems (lithiasis, neuroma or chronic inflammation) or an injury to the common bile duct.

b3. Common bile duct (Ductus choledochus)

The common bile duct is the part of the bile ducts from the union of the cystic and common hepatic ducts to the papilla of Vater in the second part of the duodenum. The length of the common bile duct ranges from 5 cm to 15 cm, depending on the actual position of the ductal union. In about 22%, the common hepatic and cystic ducts may run parallel for 17 mm before they actually join each other.

The average diameter of the common bile duct is about 6 mm. The upper normal limit for the diameter is still controversial. Most of the authors suggest that a normal common bile duct ranges from 6-8 mm, but after cholecystectomy may be dilated to 10-12 mm. The common bile duct lies anterior to portal vein. In their entire route the intra- and extra- hepatic bile ducts lie anteriorly to the corresponding branches of the portal system.

The common bile duct can be divided into four segments: **supraduodenal, retroduodenal, pancreatic,** and **intramural.**

The **supraduodenal segment** of the common bile duct lies between the layers of the hepatoduodenal ligament, and its length ranges from 2 to 5 cm. It is related posteriorly with the minor epiploic foramen of Winslow, anteriorly to the portal vein, while the hepatic artery should lie on the left or right. At its peripheral part is related with the posterior superior pancreaticoduodenal artery which is usually located retroduodenaly. This artery crosses the duct anteriorly at first and then posteriorly. Other arteries that related to the duct are the supraduodenal artery which crosses it anteriorly and the retroportal artery which lies posteriorly. These arteries are of great importance because they can easily injured during common bile duct exploration, especially the posterior superior pancreaticoduodenal artery.

This segment of the common bile duct can easily injured during cholecystectomy, especially in cases with agenesia of the cystic duct, or in cases of acquired absence of the cystic duct secondary to inflammation induced by an impacted gallstone. Although these situations are rather rare the surgeons should always keep them in mind.

The **retroduodenal segment** of the common bile duct is 1 to 3.5 cm long and extends from the upper margin of the first portion of the duodenum to the upper edge of the head of the pancreas. It is related with the gastroduodenal artery to the left, the posterior superior pancreaticoduodenal artery and the middle colic vessels anteriorly. This segment of the duct may be partially fixed to the duodenum.

The **pancreatic segment** of the common bile duct is extending extends from the upper edge of the head of the pancreas to the point of its entrance into the duodenum. Common bile duct which first passes posterior to the first part of the duodenum then courses downward to the right, posterior to the pancreas or within the pancreatic parenchyma, and enters to the wall of the duodenum.

They have been described six patterns that the common bile duct is related to the pancreas.

The **intramural segment** of the common bile duct is the part that extends from the point of its entrance to the wall of the duodenum to the ampulla of Vater on the medial duodenal wall.

C. Ampulla of Vater

In most of the cases, the common bile duct joins the major pancreatic duct near to its peripheral margin and forms the ampulla of Vater. In 90% of the cases the two ducts join each other. In the rest 10% of the cases the ampulla (or papilla) present clearly distinct, separate openings for the common bile and the pancreatic duct.

D. Sphincter of Oddi

In the area of the ampulla of Vater the circular muscle fibers format the sphincter of Oddi. This structure is an anatomic sphincter that regulates the bile flow from the bile ducts and the gallbladder into the duodenum. The sphincter of Oddi constitutes from three major distinct parts: the choledochal sphincter, the pancreatic sphincter and the ampullary sphincter.

The **choledochal sphincter** or sphincter of the choledochus is formed by the circular muscle fibers that surround the intramural and submucosal distal part of the common bile duct.

The **pancreatic sphincter** is consisting of a muscular septum lying between the common bile and the pancreatic duct.

The most important functional part of the sphincter of Oddi is the so-called **ampullary sphincter,** which is formatting of a

layer of longitudinal muscle fibers. The physiological role of this sphincter is to prevent reflux of the intestinal contents into the ampulla of Vater and the bile or pancreatic duct. When the ampullary spincter is absent or insufficient, the patient may presents recurrent cholangitis or/and may develop acute pancreatitis.

E. Gallbladder

The gallbladder is a pear-shaped distensible appendage of the extra-hepatic biliary tract, which is usually 7-10 cm long and holds a capacity of 30-50 ml. It is located on the visceral surface of the liver in a shallow fossa. At this plane a theoretical line that extended from the gallbladder to the inferior vena cava divides the right liver lobe from the medial segment of the left liver lobe. The gallbladder is separated from the liver by the connective tissue of Glisson's capsule. In its anterior surface is covered by peritoneum which continuous and fuses with that of the liver.

Most of the authors, especially the surgeons, suggest that the gallbladder is divided in fundus, body and neck. On the other side most anatomists suggest that the gallbladder should be divided into fundus, body, infundibulum, neck, and cystic duct. However, these divisions are arbitrary and imprecise; some classifications omit the infundibulum. Practically these divisions present only literature interest because from a surgical standpoint it makes no difference which classification you choose. The surgeon should care to recognise correct and safely the cyst bile duct and the cystic artery and not to identify the anatomical regions of the gallbladder. In the following paragraphs we will adopt the division of the gallbladder that adopted from the anatomists and describe the fundus, the body, the infundibulum, and the neck. The cystic duct has been described previously in the extra-hepatic bile ducts.

a. Fundus. The fundus which is usually located at the angle of the ninth costal cartilage is covered completely by peritoneum. The right border is the rectus sheath and the left the hepatic flexure of the colon. When partial folding of the fundus exists the gallbladder is in increased risk of developing lithiasis. This deformity is called "Phrygian cap" and its incidence estimated in 33% of the cases.

b. Body. The body of the gallbladder occupies the gallbladder fossa of the liver. It is not usually covered by peritoneum, except in the cases of the wandering gallbladder, which may lead to gallbladder torsion. It is closely related to the first and second part of the duodenum as well as to the transverse colon.

Usually the body of the gallbladder is not attached to the adjacent structures. In rare cases anomalous folds may be seen due to acute inflammation that may result from large gallstone ulceration from the gallbladder to the intestinal tract. These folds are associated with bilio-intestinal fistulas or gallstone ileus development. The most commonly affected parts of the intestinal tract are duodenum, colon and stomach.

c. Infutibulum. The infundibulum is the angulated posterior part of the body. This part of the gallbladder is located near the neck at the point that the cystic artery enters the gallbladder. In some cases the infundibulum may be dilated presenting an eccentric medial bulging dilation. In these cases is called Hartmann's pouch although that was first described from Broca. The causes of that deformation are still unclear and several hypothesis were developed. He fact is this dilatation is very important especially when the pouch is significantly enlarged in chronic and acute inflammation because in these cases the cystic artery arises from the left aspect than of the apex of the gallbladder.

d. Neck. The terminal part of the gallbladder that leads to cystic duct which is usually lies in the free edge of the hepatoduodenal ligament, is called neck. These part first curves up and forward and then goes back and downward form an S. It is narrowing progressively to form finally the cystic duct. The junction of the neck and the cystic duct is said to be indicated by a constriction. The cystic artery is found in this region coursing in the loose connective tissue that attaches the neck of the gallbladder to the liver. The mucosa lining the neck is a spiral ridge forming a spiral valve. When the neck becomes distended, this spiral gives its surface a spiral groove. The ridges of the valve of Heister, in addition to theneck's spiral valve may stop the passage of gallstones.

After surgical removal of the gallbladder, sometimes bile leakage may be present. Small bile ducts in the liver surface gallbladder bed, which may not enter the gallbladder considered being responsible for this leakage. The small bile ducts may cause postoperative bile leakage if they are injured. These small bile ducts may follow the small veins that drain the gallbladder. The presence of a formal cystic vein suggests an extremely rare phenomenon.

F. HEPATOCYSTIC TRIANGLE, TRIANGLE OF CALOT, AND AREA OF MOOSMAN

In 1891 Calot described the hepatocystic triangle. The right side of this triangle is formed by the proximal part of the gallbladder and cystic duct, the left side from the common hepatic duct, the superior side by the edge of the right liver lobe. In the upper boundary of this triangle the cystic artery can be found.

This area is very important to the surgeons who must recognize correct the cystic artery in order to avoid injury of ligation to one of the hepatic vessels. Although first Calot described the triangle many other anatomists studied the area. Over the years the area of increased interest has enlarged.

In 1951, Moosman and Coller described a larger circular area of about 30 mm diameter, which fits into the hepatocystic duct angle and contains several important structures that must be identified before they are ligated and sectioned: the right hepatic artery, common bile duct, aberrant hepatic artery (if present), and cystic artery.

In 1986 Stemple in a monography explained why the correct identification of the structures in the Calot Triangle or the enlarged Mossman's area is of great importance to avoid injury in the common bile duct or to the hepatic arteries. The deformities or abnormalities in these structures especially in the vessels are very common and may be misdiagnosed. Stremple estimated that 85% of all variations in the hepatic pedicle are found in Moosman's area, and half of them are a potential hazard during cholecystectomy. In 85% of the cases the right hepatic artery after its origin from the proper hepatic artery enters the triangle of Calot and crosses posterior the common hepatic duct. In only few cases (15%) the origin of the right hepatic artery is to the left of the common bile duct, and in these cases it crosses the duct anteriorly, lies parallel to the cystic duct for a short distance, then turns upward and finally enters the liver. The frequency of an aberrant right hepatic artery is about 18%, and gives rise to the cystic artery in about 83% of these cases. The cystic artery is usually found in the triangle of Calot (96%),and in 80% the origin of the artery is inside this area. When the cystic artery origins from the left hepatic artery may cross the common hepatic duct anteriorly and enters the triangle, while in cases that its origin is from the common

hepatic or the gastroduodenal artery it enters the hepatocystic triangle form below. Finally in some cases that are not very rare although the incidence has not been estimated adequately douple or triple cystic arteries should be present. More than 20 patterns of origin of double cystic arteries have been described.

Inadvertent ligation of variant veins or bile ducts may complicate laparoscopic c-holecystectomy. Many rules have been proposed to avoid injury of the hepatic arteries and the common bile duct. As a general rule concerning the vessels we should always keep in mind that no artery more than 0.3 cm in diameter in the triangle will be the cystic artery. On the other side the presence of an epicholodochal venous plexus that helps the surgeon to identify the common bile duct. There is no such venous plexus on the surface of the cystic duct.

G. VARIATIONS AND ANOMALIES OF THE BILIARY DUCTS

The variations and the abnormalities of the biliary system are not rare intraoperative or anatomical findings. These include the extrahepatic biliary atresia, the choledochal cysts and various other variations and duplications of the bile ducts.

Extrahepatic biliary atresia

The most serious and potentially fatal malformation of the bile ducts is the congenital extrahepatic biliary atresia, in which a duct partially or totally, or both ducts are atretic. The atretic duct may be hypoplastic, stenosed, or reduced to a fibrous band that is easily overlooked by the surgeon. They have been decribed seven types of biliary atresia.

Hepatic biliary duct atresias are divided into three groups (Figure 1):
• The first group includes patent proximal hepatic ducts and occluded distal ducts.

Type I.	Normal right and left hepatic ducts, with normal gallbladder and cystic duct and atresia of the common bile duct.
Type II.	Normal right and left hepatic duct with atretic cystic duct and atresia of the common hepatic duct above its union with the cystic duct.
Type III.	Atretic right and left hepatic ducts with normal gallbladder and atretic cystic duct.
Type IV.	Atretic hepatic ducts, with abnormal gallbladder and atretic cystic duct.
Type V.	Normal gallbladder with atretic hepatic ducts and cystic duct.
Type VI.	Normal gallbladder and cystic duct with atretic intra- and extra-hepatic bile ducts.
Type VII.	Normal gallbladder and cystic duct, with atretic intra-hepatic ducts but normal extra-hepatic ducts.

Patency may occur in any portion of the right or left hepatic duct as it emerges from the liver. This group includes the Types I to III and is called "correctable".

- The second group includes occluded proximal ducts, with no portion of the emerging hepatic duct being patent. This group includes the Types IV-VI and is called "noncorrectable".
- The third group includes the presence of intrahepatic atresia, with present or absent extra-hepatic ducts (Type VII). This condition is as yet noncorrectable and requires early liver transplantation.

Surgery is the only therapeutic option for children with extrahepatic biliary atresia. The surgical procedure is usually de-

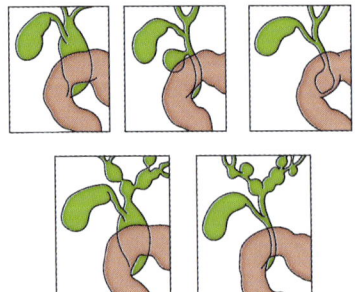

FIGURE 1. The five types of choledochal cyst as they originally described by Todani. (Modified with permission from Skandalakis J, Skandalakis P, et al., Surgical Anatomy, PMP 2005).

cided upon in the operating room y the intraoperative findings. The most known operation is the one reported from Hashimoto recently, which is a modified hepatic portoenterostomy for biliary atresia, using the Cavitron ultrasonic suction aspirator. Persistent biliary drainage resulted in 77% of their cases.

Choledochal cysts (Congenital dilatation of the common bile duct)

The choledochal cysts are local balloon-shaped or cylindrical congenital dilatation of the common bile duct, which are usually presented with symptoms of obstruction. Although several explanations have been proposed, the exact etiology is still obscure. The most possible theories are the following: (a) A congenital abnormal insertion of the pancreatic duct into the common bile duct results in reflux of the pancreatic enzymes into the common bile duct (CBD), or (b) obstruction of the distal CBD which causes primary weakening of the common bile duct.

The diagnosis is difficult to achieved clinically because the classic symptoms of pain, jaundice, and palpable mass are often absent in ductular dilatation. Choledochal cysts are most common in adult females, who complain about biliary tract symptomatology or perhaps pancreatitis. A right upper quadrant mass with pain and jaundice in infants suggests a choledochal cyst. Diagnosis is established by ultrasonography, CT scan, and cholangiography.

The most common used and widely accepted classification of these cysts is the one proposed by Todani, in 1986, which describes five types of choledochal cysts. The classification of choledochal cysts is presented in Figure 2.

- **Type I.** It refers to a solitary fusiform extrahepatic cyst. It's the most frequent congenital dilatation of the common bile duct, accounting for the 80-90% of the reported cases.
- **Type II.** Is the extrahepatic supraduodenal diverticulum. Double gallbladder, with one element sessile without cystic duct.
- **Type III.** Is the intraduodenal diverticulum/choledochocele in which cystic biliary dilatation within the duodenal wall can be found (5%)
- **Type IV.** Multiple cysts in several combinations of types I, II, III (10%)
  - *Type IVA,* Fusiform extra- and intrahepatic cysts, represents a combination of types I and II, and

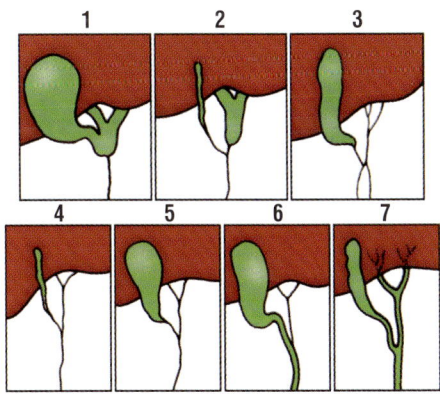

FIGURE 2. Type of atresias of the biliary tree. Note that the first three are correctable, while the last four are not. (Modified with permission from Skandalakis J, Skandalakis P, et al., Surgical Anatomy, PMP 2005).

  - *Type IVB,* Multiple extrahepatic cysts, which is a combination of type I with multiple intrahepatic cysts
- **Type V.** It's a very rare situation with multiple intrahepatic cysts which is also known as Caroli's disease.

The most common type is Type I. The dilatations are usually cylindrical and in most cases the pancreaticocholedochal junction is abnormal. Choledochal cysts of Type III are usually found in the duodenal wall although in many cases may occur in the head of pancreas.

In 1998, O'Neil proposed a presented some histopathological features that characterise the choledochal cysts of the common bile duct: The common bile duct choledochal cysts present a thick-wall of dense connective tissue with bands smooth muscles. The biliary mucosa is acellular. Sparse islands of columnar epithelium with microscopic bile ducts may be a very rare finding. In older patients a chronic inflammatory process may be present, which is usually absent in children. Malignant transformation is rare in children. In adults adenosquamous carcinoma may be present in 5% of the cases.

The incidence of gallbladder carcinoma development is higher in the patients with abnormal pancreatocholedochal junction. The prognosis in these patients is usually poor, so most of the authors suggest prophylactic cholocystectomy even if no malignancy is present in the gallbladder.

The anomalous pancreaticocholedochal junction is also associated with biliary carcinoma even without choledochal cyst. In that cases resection of the extrahepatic biliary tract with cholocystectomy should be performed to prevent bile duct carcinoma. Vitetta et al. suggested that carcinoma of the gallbladder is an age-dependent malignancy, present mostly in females, intimately associated with long term benign gallstone disease, and the choledochal cysts may also increase the risk.

For adult patients with anomalous junction of pancreaticobiliary ductal system (A-JPBDS) without bile duct dilatation, Tanaka *et al.* recommended prophylactic cholecystectomy even if no malignant lesion is found in the gallbladder. They make this recommendation because patients with A-JPBDS have a high incidence of gallbladder cancer as well as poor prognosis.

Miscellaneous asymptomatic anomalies

Numerous variations in the biliary tract have been described. Some of these variations may be more prone to lithiasis than the normal configuration. The surgeons who perform biliary operations should aware of these variations and its possible occurrence, recognise them and preserve the vital structures, than trying to make the findings at operation fit the normal pattern. This is critical especially in laparoscopic surgery and suggests the possible value of the selective cholangiography in a difficult cholecystectomy.

Purpose of this chapter is not to present analytically all the possible variations and abnormalities of the biliary tract. These can be found in detail in anatomical books. For that reason we should not perform a detail description of these variations, but we will just refer the most frequent in order to awaken the biliary surgeons.

- The *variations of the hepatic ducts* include the intrahepatic union of the right and left hepatic duct, the normal proximal extrahepatic union, and the distal union which results in absence of the common hepatic duct. In some cases accessory hepatic ducts can be found as it is presented in Figure 3.
- The *variations of the common bile duct* include the low junction of the cystic duct and the common hepatic duct that results in a short choledochal duct, and the total absence of the common bile duct as in Figure 4.

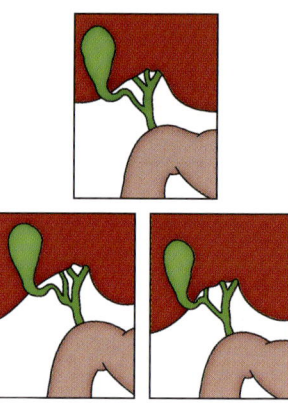

FIGURE 3. Accessory hepatic ducts. (Modified with permission from Skandalakis J, Skandalakis P, et al., Surgical Anatomy, PMP 2005).

- The *variations of the cystic duct* include the absence of the cystic duct with sessile gallbladder, and the cystic duct atresia with normal gallbladder.

Another large category of variations are the duplications.
- Duplications of the common hepatic duct (Figure 5)
  - It can occur immediately below the union of the right and left hepatic

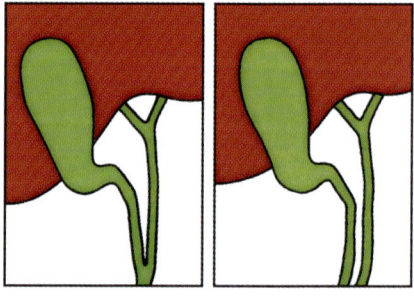

FIGURE 4. Variations of the common bile duct. **A,** Low junction of cystic and common hepatic ducts. **B,** Absence of a common bile duct. (Modified with permission from Skandalakis J, Skandalakis P, et al., Surgical Anatomy, PMP 2005).

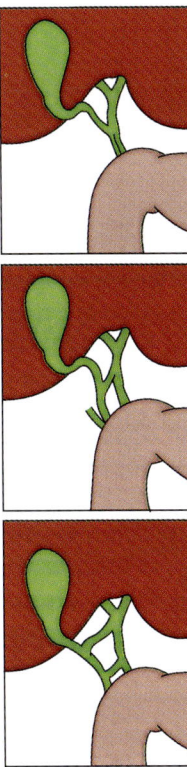

FIGURE 5. Types of duplications of the common bite duct. (Modified with permission from Skandalakis J, Skandalakis P, et al., Surgical Anatomy, PMP 2005).

duct. Both of the common hepatic ducts are patent.
- Duplication of the common hepatic duct at the same pattern, but the normal located duct is atretic, and the duplication is patent.
- Absence of the common bile duct. The right hepatic duct joins the cystic duct and format an unilateral "common bile duct", while the left hepatic duct runs independently.
- The **duplications of the common bile duct** include the double parallel lumina of the duct, the X pattern of anastomosis between the duplicated bile ducts, and the X and H pattern of anastomosis between the two ducts.

- The **duplications of the cystic duct** are divided in two groups. Those of the first group that co-exist with gallbladder duplication are discussed to the gallbladder duplications. The second group includes duplications of the cystic duct without duplication of the gallbladder. In those duplications, either cystic ducts may enter the common hepatic duct, an accessory cystic duct opening into the right hepatic duct may coexist, or a doubled-barrelled duplication of the cystic duct may present.

VARIATIONS AND CONGENITAL ANOMALIES OF THE GALLBLADDER

The variations and the congenital abnormalities of the gallbladder are more frequent than those of the biliary ducts. An ultrasonographic study of 1823 patients revealed morphologic variations and abnormalities in approximately 33% of the cases, topographic variations in 3.5%, and 3 cases of gallbladder duplication.

The most common variations and congenital abnormalities of the gallbladder are the following.

Absence/Agenesis of the Gallbladder. In rare cases the gallbladder and usually the cystic duct is absent or vestigial. The absence must be confirmed by ruling out an intrahepatic gallbladder or a left-sided gallbladder. Wilson and Deitrich suggested that the gallbladder absence may be a familial trait. Agenesis of the gallbladder is usually associated with lithiasis of the common bile duct or other anomalies.

The diagnosis of gallbladder absence can easily achieved by ultrasound. In patients with clinical symptomatology of gallbladder disease the diagnostic modalities include also preoperative cholangiography, exploratory laparoscopy and laparoscopic ultrasound, and in cases where the previous techniques failed to demonstrate a gallbladder an exploratory laparotomy is necessary to establish the diagnosis of gallbladder agenesis and absence.

Multiple Gallbladders. The first case of a double gallbladder in a human described in 1674 by Blasius in 1674, who identified this abnormality in an autopsy, while the first case of intra-operative recognition if this anomaly reported in 1911.

In one of the most important reviews of these rare congenital gallbladder anomalies, 297 cases of double and 8 cases of triple gallbladders were studied. Double gallbladders may have a separate or a common cystic duct, while triple gallbladders may have one, two or three cystic ducts.

Gallbladder duplication is diagnosed more often in women than in men (1.7:1), though to the greater incidence of gallbladder disease in women. The real frequency is the same. When disease is present, both gallbladders are usually affected if they are intimately connected, less frequently if separation is complete. Symptoms of gallbladder disease in a patient who has previously undergone cholecystectomy can suggest the presence of a second organ or of cystic duct remnant syndrome.

The diagnosis of gallbladder duplication can be achieved by ultrasound, which successfully replaces the oral or intravenous cholecystogram. Other radiological exams that may be useful in the diagnosis of this rare anomaly are the nuclear medicine scan, but if cystic duct obstruction is present it will fail to demonstrate one or both organs, and the CT and MRI which present high sensitivity and specificity.

For practical purposes, the anomalies are divided into six types. Three types belong to the split primordium group and three belong to the accessory gallbladder group. All are described below.

(a) Split primordium group

In a split primordium, multiple gallbladders drain to the common bile duct by a single cystic duct. Three types have been described.

- **Septate gallbladder.** A longitudinal septum divides the gallbladder into two chambers. The septum may have external trace, or a cleft extending toward the neck (11.3%) may be present.
- **Bilobate "V" gallbladder.** Two gallbladders which are separated at the fundus joined at the neck by a single normal cystic duct (8.5%).
- **"Y" duplication.** There are two separate gallbladders, and their cystic ducts join to form a common cystic duct before entering the common bile duct (25.3%).

(b) Accessory gallbladder group

The accessory gallbladder group includes the following types.
- **Ductular "H" duplication.** The cystic duct and the accessory cystic duct enter the common bile duct separately (47%).
- **Trabecular duplication.** The accessory cystic duct enters a branch of the right hepatic duct within the liver (2.1%). In rare cases cystic duct duplication without duplication of the gallbladder may be present.
- **Triple gallbladder.** Various combinations may be present (5.6%).

Left-Sided Gallbladder. In rare cases the gallbladder situated on the left lobe of the liver, the cystic duct enters the common bile duct from the left and the function of the organ is absolutely normal.

Intrahepatic Gallbladder. An intrahepatic gallbladder is submerged in the liver and gives the appearance of absence of the gallbladder. This anomaly is associated with a increased occurrence of lithia-sis and can be revealed only by CT scan or ultrasonography.

Mobile Gallbladder. In that rare anomaly the gallbladder is mobile be-cause is attached to the liver by a mesen-tery cord, and can easily be torched or strangulated.

EXTRAHEPATIC TRIAD AND EXTRAHEPATIC HEPATIC VEINS

The extrahepatic triad consists of the hep-atic artery, the hepatic portal vein, and the hepatic duct. In the present chapter the hepatic duct is discussed separately a-long with the extra-hepatic duct. The cystic duct is described with the extra-hepatic ducts, while the cystic artery is discussed in the unit referred to gallblad-der. (Figure 6).

Hepatic artery, common hepatic artery, and proper hepatic artery

The hepatic artery provides 25% of the af-ferent blood supply to the liver and about

50% of the oxygen, while the rest is sup-plied from the portal vein. In 55% the hep-atic arteries arise from the celiac trunk in 55%, while in the rest 45%, the common hepatic artery, the right hepatic, or the left hepatic may arise from vessels other than the celiac trunk (aberrant hepatic arteries). The common hepatic artery origins from the celiac trunk in about 83-86%. More rare it may arise from the superior mesen-teric artery (2.9%), from the aorta (1.1%), from the left gastric artery (0.54%), or oth-er arteries.(Figure 7).

By definition, the normal common hep-atic artery becomes the proper hepatic artery at the point where the gastroduode-nal artery rises. Then the proper hepatic artery divides into a right and a left hepat-ic branch, and according to some authors in some cases a third branch may rise, the middle hepatic vein.

The proper hepatic artery may divide into its right and left hepatic arteries at any point between the liver hilum and its ori-gin. In rare cases the proper hepatic artery may not exist because the right and the left hepatic arteries rise at the site of o-rigin of the gastroduodenal artery. If the normal common hepatic artery bifurcates

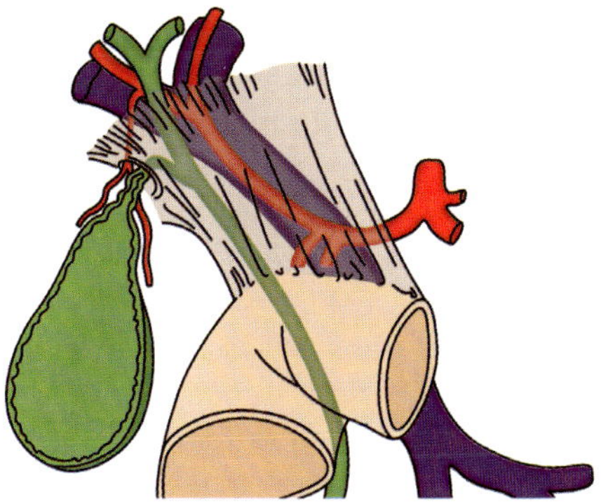

FIGURE 6. The celiac trunk. (Modified with permis-sion from Skandalakis J, Skandalakis P, et al., Surgi-cal Anatomy, PMP 2005).

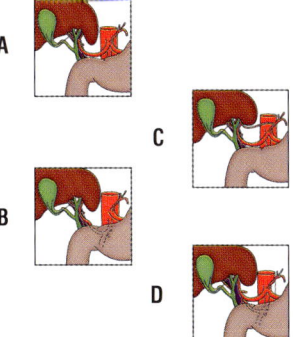

FIGURE 7. **A,** The hepatic artery normally arises from celiac trunk. **B-D,** In some cases may arise from the left gastvic, and the superior mesentenic artery as common hepatic, or from the SMA as right hepatic artery.

early, medial to the portal vein, the right hepatic artery pass behind the portal vein, and its pulsations can be palpated through the hiatus of Winslow.

As we can see the course of the common hepatic artery varies and depends to the arterial anatomy. The typical common hepatic artery passes horizontally along the upper border of the head of the pancreas and then turns upward to ascend between the layers of the lesser omentum. The peritoneum of the posterior wall of the omental bursa covers the horizontal portion of the artery. The ascending part of the artery is enveloped between the hepatoduodenal ligament leafs. In these cases the proper hepatic artery lies in front of the foramen of Winslow to the left of the common bile duct and anteriorly to the portal vein.

Aberrant hepatic arteries (Figure 8)

Many terms, like aberrant, replacing, atypical and accessory, have been used to describe the hepatic arteries that they do not raise normally from the celiac axis, but from other arterial sources. The most widely accepted term is aberrant hepatic arteries. The frequency of these arteries is about 43-46%.

An aberrant artery may supply an entire liver lobe or the entire liver. If these arteries arise from an aberrant source and are additive to lobar branches that derived normally from the celiac axis, they called accessory hepatic arteries.

The common hepatic artery may arise from the superior mesenteric, the aorta, the left gastric, or other sources, as noted above. The left hepatic artery arises in 25-30% of cases from the left gastric artery. The right hepatic artery originates from the superior mesenteric in about 17% of cases. The middle hepatic artery arises with equal frequency from the left or right hepatic artery. The aberrant hepatic

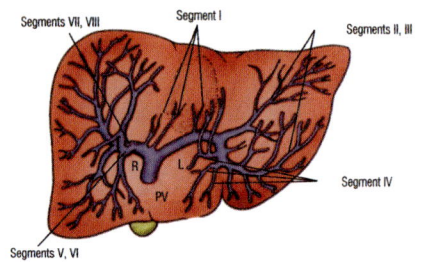

FIGURE 8. Portal venous supply and liver segments.

arteries do not follow a specific pattern of contribution, but various combinations of can occur in the same person. For example a replaced right hepatic may exist together with an accessory left hepatic at the same time.

The main arterial branches that give rise to the aberrant hepatic arteries are the celiac and the superior mesenteric artery. These branches may present various infrequent collateral anastomoses. The most common types are the direct connection, the anastomosis with the hepatic artery, the anastomoses following pre- or postnatal stenosis, and the pancreatic arcades.

The accessory hepatic arteries play a crucial role and the surgeons who perform operations in the upper abdomen should be informed about the anatomic variations of these arteries, because the correct surgical exposure and preservation of these vessels is essential for the survival and the appropriate function of the liver parenchyma. For the general surgeons it is important to know the gross anatomy of the hepatic arteries before an intervention on the liver and pancreas. The origin and course and the right hepatic artery present special interesting for pancreatectomy and hemihepatectomy, while the origin and course of the left hepatic artery in hemihepatectomy. In several other surgical, endoscopical, or minimally invasive techniques the detailed knowledge of the hepatic arteries anatomy is also useful and necessary. These interventions include the ligation or embolization of hepatic arteries in the treatment of liver trauma, hepatic tumor or lesions of the hepatic vessels such as aneurysm, arteriovenous fistula or hemobilia.

Hiatt et al reported the most usual anatomic variations in a large series of liver donors used for transplantation. According to them the most usual arterial patterns are the following: (a) The common hepatic artery arises from the celiac axis, gives the gastroduodenal and proper hepatic artery. The proper hepatic artery is dividing to the right and the left hepatic arteries. This is the normal and the most common arterial pattern. (b) An accessory right hepatic artery may arise from the superior mesenteric artery. (c) An accessory left hepatic artery may arise from the left gastric artery. (d) The common hepatic artery may arise from the superior mesenteric artery. (e) The common hepatic artery may arise from the aorta. (f) Both the hepatic arteries may arise abnormally. The right hepatic artery may arise from the superior mesenteric artery, while at the same time the left hepatic artery arises from the left gastric artery.

Hepatic portal vein

As already referred in the previous unit the hepatic portal vein provides 75% of the blood and about 50% of the oxygen to liver. The length of the portal vein ranges from 7 to 10 m, and the diameter from 0.8 to 1.4 cm. It is a wide vein which lacks of valves. The portal vein is formed by the confluence of the superior mesenteric and the splenic vein which takes place behind the neck of the pancreas. The inferior mesenteric vein may enter the splenic or the superior mesenteric vein before their union and the portal vein formation, or the portal vein in the same frequency. In some cases the inferior mesenteric vein

may contribute directly to the portal vein formation. The course of the portal vein does not present significant variations. Normally the vein lies in front of the inferior vena cava, on the left of the common bile duct and on the right of the proper hepatic artery.(Figure 9) During its course usually receives the coronary gastric vein, the pancreaticoduodenal vein, the pyloric vein, as well as an accessory pancreatic vein.

Hepatic veins (Upper portas)

The liver is drained by the three major dorsal hepatic veins, which are located in the anterior posterior surface of the liver in an area which is called "upper hilum". Usually are recognised three major veins, the right, the middle, and left hepatic vein, and some more smaller veins that drain direct into the inferior vena cava. The number of these smaller veins ranges from 10-50.

The extrahepatic length of the three major veins varies from 0.5 cm to 1.5 cm.

The right hepatic vein lies in the right segmental fissure, draining the entire posterior segment and the anterior superior segment of the right lobe. As well as it

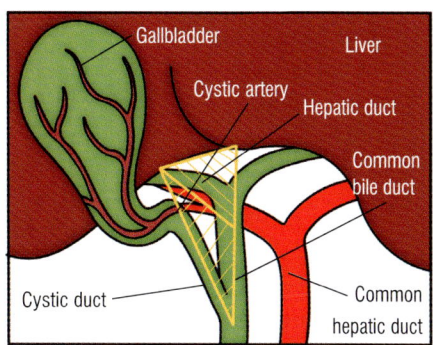

FIGURE 9. Hepatocystic triangle and triangle of Calot. (Modified with permission from Skandalakis J, Skandalakis P, et al., Surgical Anatomy, PMP 2005).

drains most of the liver parenchyma, is the largest of the hepatic veins. The middle hepatic vein lies in the main lobar fissure, and drains the anterior inferior segment of the right lobe and the inferior medial segment of the left lobe. The right and the middle vein can enter the inferior vena cava separately or as single vein. In some other cases the right hepatic vena presents a retrohepatic course, and be vulnerable to posterior incisions, or surgical approaches for posterior abdominal injuries.

The last of the major hepatic veins is the left hepatic vein which lies in the upper part of the left segmental fissure, and usually drains the superior medial segment and the entire left lateral liver segment. The left hepatic vein enters directly to the inferior vena cava. This vein may be injured or torn during manipulations in the gastroesophageal junction when the left triangular ligament is incised. Except the major hepatic veins the liver is also drained by 10-50 smaller veins that enter the inferior vena cava directly. From these veins only 5-10 will have to be ligated or dissected during hepatic resections, especially those which drain the posterior segment of the right liver lobe. The caudate lobe of the liver is drained also by two small veins that enter directly the inferior vena cava on its left side. These veins should always be ligated separately during right hemipatectomies. The exposure and ligation of these veins is difficult and posses an increase risk of intra-operatively bleeding.

VASCULAR ANOMALIES

The vascular congenital abnormalities of the liver vessels are very rare, and they mainly refer to the portal vein and its branches. We refer the most important of them.

Congenital Portocaval Shunt. In that very rare anomaly which was first de-scribed in 1793 the portal vein enters directly the inferior vena cava. This anomaly consists a natural portocaval shunt and it's compatible with life. The exact mechanism of this anomaly is not clear. Most authors consider this anomaly as a result of persisting supracardinal veins. It's likely a congenital anomaly of the inferior vena cava development than of portal vein.

Preduodenal Portal Vein. This rare vascular abnormality first described by Knight in 1921. In this anomaly the portal vein cross the duodenum anteriorly instead of posteriorly and usually compresses it. Most patients develop symptoms of the duodenum compression.

Failure of Portal Vein to Bifurcate. Only one case of this congenital vascular abnormality has been reported. The portal vein failed to bifurcate and only a single portal vein branch provided blood to the entire liver.

Congenital Absence of Portal Vein. Congenital absence of the portal vein is a very rare anomaly. The blood from the intestinal and splenic venous drainage drains directly to the inferior vena cava. Grazioli et al described this congenital absence of the portal vein and suggested that the liver by pass may cause nodular regenerative hyperplasia.

Anomalous Pulmonary Veins. Anomalous pulmonary veins that pierce the diaphragm and enter the portal system have also been reported. These ectopic pulmonary veins compose the 15% of all pulmonary veins anomalies, and they form a natural left to right shunt. Woodwark et al first reported a successful correction of a single case by anastomosing the pulmonary anomalous branch to the left atrium.

REFERENCES

Arias I, Che M, Catmaitan Z, et al, The biology of the bile canaliscus, Hepatology 1993, 17:318.

Bergamaschi R, Ignjatovic D. More than two structures in Calot's triangle: a postmortem study.
Surg Endosc 2000, 14:354-57.

Boles ET Jr, Smith B. Preduodenal portal vein. Pedi-
atrics 1961, 28:805.

Calot JF. De la cholccystectomie. (Thesis) Paris,
1890, No. 25, p. 50.

Caudle SO, Dimler M. The current management of c-
holedochal cyst. Am Surg 1986, 52:76.

Daseler E, Anson B, Hambley W, Reiman A. Cystic
artery and constituents of the hepatic pedicle.
Surg Gynecol Obstet 1947, 85:47.

Davies F, Harding HE. Pouch of Hartmann. Lancet
1942,1:193-195.

Diaz MJ, Fowler W, Hnatow BJ. Congenital gallbladder duplication: preoperative diagnosis by ultrasonography. Gastrointest Radiol 1991, 16:198-
200.

Di Vita G, Sciume C, Lauria Lauria G, Patti R. Agenesis of the gallbladder. G Chir 2000, 21:33-36.

Dorrance HR, Lingam MK, Hair A, Oien K, O'Dwyer
PJ. Acquired abnormalities of the biliary tract from
chronic gallstone disease. J Am Coll Surg 1999,
189:269-273.

Edwards EA. Clinical anatomy of the lesser varieties
of the inferior vena cava. Angiology 1951, 2:85.

Elias H, Petty D, Gross anatomy of blood vessels and
ducts within the liver, Am J Anat 1952, 90:59.

Feigl W, Firbas W, Sinzinger H, Wicke L. Various
forms of the celiac trunk and its anastomoses
with the superior mesenteric artery. Acta Anat
1975, 92:272-284.

Filippou G, Filippou D, Vczakis A, Koilakos K, Rlzos S,
Gallstone ileus. Arch Surg 2005, under publication.

Gotohda N, Itano S, Horiki S, Endo A, Nakao A. Terada N, Tanaka N. Gallbladder agenesis with no other biliary tract abnormality: report of a case and
review of the literature. J Hepato Biliary Pancreatic
Surg 2000, 7:327-330.

Gray SW, Olafson RP, Skandalakis JE, Harlaftis N.
Developmental origin of the double gallbladder.
Contemp Surg 1974, 4:71-76.

Grazioli L, Alberti D, Olivetti L, Rigamonti W, Codazzi
F, Matricardi L, Fugazzola C, Chiesa A. Congenital
absence of portal vein with nodular regenerative
hyperplasia of the liver. Eur Radiol 2000, 10:820-
825.

Hardy KJ, Jones RMcL. Failure of the portal vein to b-
ifurcate. Surgery 1997, 121:226-228.

Harlaftis N, Gray SW, Olafson RP, Skandalakis JE.
Three cases of unsuspected double gallbladder.
Am Surg 1976, 42:178-180.

Harlaftis N, Gray SW, Skandalakis JE. Multiple gallbladders. Surgery 1977, 145:928-934.

Hashimoto T, Otobe Y, Shimizu Y, Suzuki T, Nakamura T, Hayashi S, Matsuo Y, Sato M, Manabe T.
A modification of hepatic portoenterostomy (Kasai
operation) for biliary atresia. J Am Coll Surg 1997,
185:548-553.

Healey JE Jr, Schroy PC. Anatomy of the biliary ducts
within the human liver: analysis of the prevailing
pattern of branchings and the major variations of
the biliary ducts. Arch Surg 1953, 66:599.

Healey JE Jr, Schwartz SI. Surgical anatomy. In:
Schwartz SI (ed) Surgical Diseases of the Liver.
New York McGraw-Hill, 1964.

Hermann RE. Manual of Surgery of the Gallbladder,
Bile Duct and Endocrine Pancreas. New York:
Springer-Verlag, 1979.

Hiatt JR, Gabbay J, Busuttil RW. Surgical anatomy of
the hepatic artery in 1000 cases. Ann Surg 1994,
220:50.

Jones AL, Anatomy of the normal liver, In Zakim D,
Boyer T (ed): Hepatology, WB Saunders Philadelphia 1982, pp. 3-31.

Kennedy PA, Madding GF. Surgical anatomy of the
liver. Surg Clin North Am 1977, 57:233.

Leal del Rosal P, Marquez Monter H, Avila L, Arce
Gomez F. Anomalous entry of the pulmonary
veins into the umbilical vein and the vena portae:
presentation of a case and the autopsy findings.
Rev Med Hosp Gen (Mex) 1962, 25:535.

Lindner HH, Green RB. Embryology and surgical
anatomy of the extrahepatic biliary tract. Surg Clin
North Am 1964, 44:1273.

Lipsett PA, Segev DL, Colombani PM. Biliary atresia
and biliary cysts. Ballieres Clin Gastroenterol
1997, 11:619-641.

Longmire WP. Congenital biliary hypoplasia. Ann
Surg 1964, 159:335.

Manganas D, Filippou D, Tsitsimelis D, Dimoulas K,
Papatheodorou D, Nisiotis A, Rizos S, Highly selective use of intraoperative cholangiography in
laparoscopic cholocystectomy, Minimally Invasive Interventional Techniques: Facing the New

Millenium, edit. Tsigris C, Diamantis T. Athens 2000.

McGregor AL, Du Plessis DJ. A Synopsis of Surgical Anatomy. 10th ed. Baltimore: Williams & Wilkins, 1969, p. 529.

Michels NA. Blood Supply and Anatomy of the Upper Abdominal Organs. Philadelphia: Lippincott, 1955.

Michels NA. Newer anatomy of the liver and variant blood supply and collateral circulation. Am J Surg 1966, 112:337.

Moosman DA, Coller FA. Prevention of traumatic injury to the bile ducts: a study of the structures of the cystohepatic angle encountered in cholecystectomy and supraduodenal choledochostomy. Am J Surg 1951, 32:132.

Nakamura S, Tsuzuki T. Surgical anatomy of the hepatic veins and the inferior vena cava. Surg Gynecol Obstet 1981, 152:43.

Newman HF, Northrup JD. Extrahepatic biliary tract anatomy. West J Surg Obstet Gynecol 1963, 71:59.

O'Neill JA Jr. Choledochal cyst. In: O'Neill JA Jr, Rowe MI, Grosfeld JL, Fonkalsrud EW, Coran AG. Pediatric Surgery (5th ed). St. Louis: Mosby, 1998, pp. 1483-1493.

O'Neill JA Jr. Choledochal cyst. Curr Probl Surg 1992, 29:361-410.

Flannery MG, Caster MP. Congenital abnormalities of the gallbladder: 101 cases. Int Abstr Surg 1956, 103:439.

Saint JH. The epicholedochal venous plexus and its importance as a means of identifying the common duct during perations on the extrahepatic biliary tract. Br J Surg 1961, 48:489.

Sarli L, Violi V, Gobbi S. Laparoscopic diagnosis of gallbladder agenesis. Surg Endosc (Online) 2000, 14:373.

Senecail B, Texier F, Kergastel I, Patin-Philippe L. Anatomic variability and congenital anomalies of the gallbladder: ultrasonographic study of 1823 patients. Morphologie 2000, 84:35-39.

Sherren J. A double gallbladder removed by operation. Ann Surg 1911, 54:204.

Skandalakis J, Branum G, Colborn G, Weidman T, Skandalakis P, Skandalakis LJ, Zoras O, Extrahepatic biliary tract and gallbladder. In Skandalakis JL, Skandalakis LJ, Gray G, Skandalakis P, The

Surgical Anatomy, PM Publications, Athens 2004, pp 1093-1050.

Skandalakis JE, Gray SW. Embryology for Surgeons. 2nd ed. Baltimore: Williams & Wilkins, 1994.

Skandalakis LJ, Gray SW, Colborn GL, Skandalakis JE. Surgical anatomy of the liver and associated extrahepatic structures. Part 4: Surgical anatomy of the hepatic vessels and the extrahepatic biliary tract. Contemp Surg 1987, 31(1):25-36.

Smanio T. Varying relations of the common bile duct with the posterior face of the pancreas in Negroes and white persons. J Int Coll Surg 1954, 22:150.

Stremple JF. The need for careful operative dissection in Moosman's area during cholecystectomy. Surg Gynecol Obstet 1986, 163:169.

Suzuki T, Nakayasu A, Kauabe K, Takeda H, Honjo I. Surgical significance of anatomic variations of the hepatic artery. Am J Surg 1971, 122:505.

Taylor LA, Ross AJ III. Abdominal masses. In Walker WA, Durie PR, Hamilton JR, Walker-Smith JA, Walkins JB (eds). Pediatric Gastrointestinal Disease (2nd ed). St. Louis: Mosby, 1996, 227-240.

Tanaka K, Ikoma A, Hamada N, Nishida S, Kadono J, Taira A. Biliary tract cancer accompanied by anomalous junction of pancreaticobiliary ductal system in adults. Am J Surg 1998, 175:218-220.

Todani T, Watanabe Y, Fujii T, Toki A, Uemura S, Koike Y. Congenital choledochal cyst with intrahepatic involvement. Arch Surg 1984, 119:1038.

Townsend C, Woods J, Sabinston Textbook of Surgery. The biological basis of modern surgery, 16th ed, WB Saunders Philadelphia, London, New York, St Luis, Sydney, Toronto, 2001 pp. 997-1080.

Tuech JJ, Pessaux P, Aube C, Regenet N, Cervi C, Bergamaschi R, Arnaud JP. Cancer of the gallbladder associated with pancreatobiliary maljunction without bile duct dilatation in a European patient. J Hepato Biliary Panc Surg 2000, 7:336-338.

Van Damme JP. Behavioral anatomy of the abdominal arteries. Surg Clin North Am 1993, 73:699-725.

Van Damme JP, Bonte J. The branches of the celiac trunk. Acta Anat 1985, 122:110.

Vitetta L, Sali A, Little P, Mrazek L. Gallstones and gall bladder carcinoma. Aust NZ J Surg 2000, 70:667-673.

Wayson EE, Foster JH. Surgical anatomy of the liver. Surg Clin North Am 1964, 44:1263.

Williams PL. Gray's Anatomy (38th ed). New York: Churchill Livingstone, 1995.

Witzleben CL. Bile duct paucity ("intrahepatic atresia"). Perspect Pediatr Pathol 1982, 7:185.

Wilson JW, Deitrich JE. Agenesis of the gallbladder: case report and familial investigation. Surgery 1986, 99:106.

Woodwark GM, Vince DJ, Ashmore PG. Total anomalous pulmonary venous return to the portal vein. J Thorac Cardiovasc Surg 1963, 445:662.

Biliary and bile physiology, calculous disease & pathophysiology of obstructive jaundice

Avgerinos Efthimios, Filippou Georgios, Filippou Dimitrios, Triga Argiro, Smailis Dimitrios, Acalovschi Monica

BILIARY PHYSIOLOGY

Hepatic bile formation serves two major functions: (1) the promotion of dietary fat absorption in the lumen of the gut through the detergent action of bile salts and (2) elimination of waste products. Bile constitutes the primary pathway for elimination of bilirubin, excess cholesterol and xenobiotics that are insufficiently water soluble to be excreted into urine.

The bililary tree is designed for the transport and storage of bile produced in the liver by hepatocytes and destined for the duodenal lumen to participate in the digestion of food stuffs. Filling of the gallbladder, results from the continuous production of bile, by the liver, in the face of a contracted sphincter of Oddi. As the pressure within the common bile duct exceeds that within the gallbladder lumen, hepatic bile enters the gallbladder via retrograde flow through the cystic duct, wherein it is rapidly concentrated. Within a few hours the gallbladder mucosa, apparently by means of an active sodium-coupled transport mechanism, removes more than 90% of its water content, creating the more highly concentrated gall-bladder bile. Consequently, the amount of electrolytes, lipids, bile salts and pigments in gallbladder bile is significantly more concentrated than that found in hepatic bile (Table 1).

Bile flow differs when a person is in the fasted versus the postprandial state. Under fasting conditions, biliary tree motility and thus bile flow are regulated by the Intermittent Myoelectric Migratory Complex of the intestinal tract and approximated by the cyclical activity of the duodenum The gallbladder follows a phasic activity: gradual filling with bile followed by gallbladder contraction and partial emptying (15%-20%), associated with increased plasma levels of motilin. Along with the gallbladder contraction the sphincter of Oddi relaxes. The gallbladder's phasic activity represents a protective mechanism by which stasis of saturated bile and the increased risk of gall stone formation is avoided.

Following a meal, the gallbladder contracts in response to both a vagally mediated cephalic phase of activity and the release of cholecystokinin (CCK), the major regulator of gallbladder function. During the following 60-120 min, approximately

TABLE 1

BILIARY LIPID COMPOSITION OF GALLBLADDER BILE. SOURCE: THISTLE ET AL AND LAMONT AND CAREY

Lipid Component	Controls	Cholesterol Stones	Change (%)
Biliary lipid (moles %)			
Bile salts	72	70,2	-2,5
Phospholipids	21,1	20,6	-2,4
Cholesterol	6,9	9,0	+30
Cholesterol saturation index	1,00	1,32	+32
Cholesterol: phospholipids ratio	0,34	0,46	+35
Cholesterol: bile salt ratio	0,10	0,13	+30

80-90% of gallbladder bile is steadily emptied into the intestinal tract. CCK is localized to the proximal small intestine where its release is stimulated by intraluminal fat, aminoacids and gastric acid and inhibited by bile. CCK acts directly via smooth muscle receptors in the gall bladder wall, stimulating muscle contraction in direct proportion to its concentration. CCK also acts to functionally inhibit the normal phasic motor activity of the sphincter of Oddi, thus facilitating the delivery of bile into the proximal small intestine. Gallbladder function is also influenced by other hormones, including vasoactive intestinal polypeptide (VIP), somatostatin, substance P and norepinephrine. Both VIP and somatostatin inhibit contraction of the gallbladder. The role of substance P, norepinephrine and other neuropeptides in the regulation of gallbladder function remains to be elucidated.

BILIRUBINE AND BILE SYNTHESIS

Bilirubin is the end product of heme degradation. The majority of daily production (0.2 to 0.3 gm) is derived from breakdown of senescent erythrocytes by the mononuclear phagocyte system, especially in the spleen, liver, and bone marrow. Most of the remainder of bilirubin is derived from the turnover of hepatic hemoproteins (e.g. the P-450 cytochromes) and from premature destruction of newly formed erythrocytes in the bone marrow. The latter pathway is important in hematologic disorders associated with excessive intramedullary hemolysis of defective erythrocytes (ineffective erythropoiesis). Whatever the source, heme oxygenase oxidizes heme to biliverdin (step 1 in Figure 1), which is then reduced to bilirubin by biliverdin reductase. Bilirubin thus formed outside the liver is released and bound to serum albumin (step 2). Albumin binding is necessary since bilirubin is virtually insoluble in aqueous solutions at physiologic pH. The small fraction of unbound bilirubin in plasma may increase in severe hemolytic increase in severe hemolytic disease or when protein binding drugs displace bilirubin from albumin.

[Hemolytic disease of the newborn (erythroblastosis fetalis) may lead to accumulation of unconjugated bilirubin in the brain, which can cause severe neurologic damage, referred to as kernicterus]]

Hepatic processing of bilirubin involves carrier mediated uptake at the sinusoidal membrane (step 3), conjugation with one or two molecules of glucuronic acid by bilirubin uridine diphosphate - glucuronosyltransferase (UGT) in the endoplasmic reticulum (step 4), and excretion of the water-soluble, nontoxic bilirubin glucuronides into bile. Most bilirubin glucuronides are deconjugated by bacterial β-glucuronidases and degraded to colorless urobilinogens (step 5). The urobilinogens, and the residue of intact pigment, are largely excreted in feces. Approximately 20% of the urobilinogens formed are reabsorbed in the ileum and colon returned to the liver, and promptly re-excreted into bile. The small amount that escapes this enterohepatic circulation is excreted in urine.

[In contrast to the unconjugated bilirubin, conjugated bilirubin is water soluble, nontoxic, and only loosely bound to albumin. Because of its solubility and weak association with albumin, excess conjugated bilirubin in plasma can be excreted in urine. With prolonged hyperbilirubinemia, a portion of circulating pigment may become covalently bound to albumin (the delta fraction).]

Bile acids

The brilliant yellow color of bilirubin makes it an easily identified component of hepatic bile formation. However, bilirubin metabolism and excretion is but a minor cog in the hepatic machinery that secretes 12 to 36 gm of bile acids into bile per day. Bile acids are carboxylated steroid molecules derived from cholesterol and are the detergent molecules primarily responsible for promoting bile flow and the secretion of phospholipid and cholesterol. The primary human bile acids are cholic acid and chenodeoxy-cholic acid, which are secreted as taurine and glycine conjugates. 10% to 20% of excreted bile acids is deconjugated in the intestines by bacterial action. Virtually all conjugated and deconjugated bile acids are reabsorbed, primarily through the action of a sodium-bile acid co-transporter in the apical membrane of ileal enterocytes, and are returned to the liver for uptake, reconjugation, and resecretion. Fecal loss of bile acids (0.2 to 0.6 gm/day) is matched by de novo hepatic synthesis of bile acids from cholesterol. The enterohepatic circulation of bile acids provides an efficient mechanism for maintaining a large endogenous pool of bile acids for digestive and excretory purposes. Predominately, the enterohepatic circulation of bile acids regulates the overall production rate of bile by the liver.

JAUNDICE

In the normal adult, total serum bilirubin levels vary between 0,3 and 1,2 mg/dl, and the rate of systemic bilirubin production is equal to the rates of hepatic uptake, conjugation and biliary excretion.

Because bile formation is one of the most sophisticated functions of the liver, it is also one of the most readily disrupted. Both unconjugated bilirubin and bilirubin glucuronides may accumulate systemically and deposit in tissues, clinically evident as jaundice: yellow discoloration of the skin (when bilirubin >5 mg/dl) or sclerae (when bilirubin >2,5 mg/dl), due to retention of pigmented bilirubin.

Jaundice occurs when the equilibrium between bilirubin production and clearance is disturbed by one or more of the following mechanisms: (1) excessive production of bilirubin, (2) reduced hepatocyte uptake, (3) impaired conjugation, (4) decreased hepatocellular excretion, and (5) impaired bile flow (intrahepatic or extrahepatic). The first two mechanisms produce unconjugated hyperbilirubinemia and the last two conjugated hyperbilirubinemia. However, often, more than one mechanisms exist, thus mixed conjugated and unconjugated hyperbilirubinemia is produced.

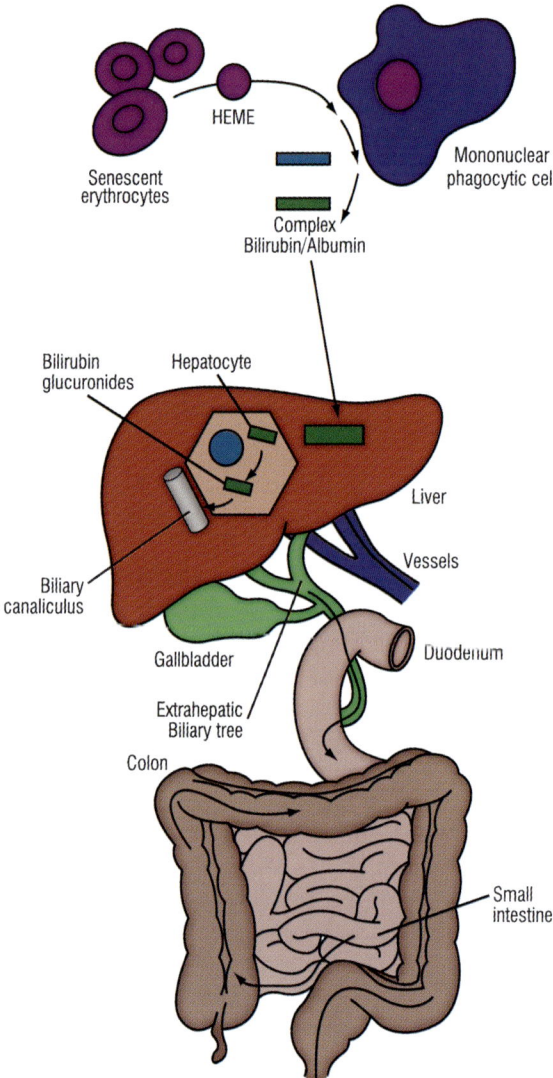

FIGURE 1: The Metabolism of Bilirubin. Bilirubin is formed from the heme that is marnly devired from the enythrocytes breakdown. After bluding to albumin extrahepatic bilirubin is denred from the hypatocytedsm glycuronidated and secreted to intestine via bite where is finally deconjugated and transform toy urobilinogens.

HEME

Senescent
erythrocytes

Mononuclear
phagocytic cell

Complex
Bilirubin/Albumin

Bilirubin
glucuronides

Hepatocyte

Liver

Vessels

Biliary
canaliculus

Gallbladder

Duodenum

Extrahepatic
Biliary tree

Colon

Small
intestine

Rectum

Obstructive Jaundice - Differential Diagnosis

Jaundice resulting from biliary tract obstruction is presumably caused by the reflux of conjugated bilirubin directly across either the basement membrane of the hepatic sinusoids or damaged canaliculi. The rise in conjugated bilirubin (direct reacting) is in contrast to the increased levels of unconjugated bilirubin (indirect reacting) observed with hepatocellular injury. Interestingly significant elevations of the total serum bilirubin level are indicative of common bile duct obstruction.

Thus, once the presence of direct hyperbilirubinemia is confirmed, the next step is to determine whether the jaundice is hepatic or post hepatic. The conjugated hyperbilirubinemia may derive either from a defect in hepatocellular function (nonobstructive jaundice) or from a blockage somewhere in the biliary tree (obstructive jaundice). Tables 2 & 3 list the different causes of hepatic and posthepatic - obstructive jaundice.

Cholestasis

Cholestasis is characterized by systemic retention of not only bilirubin but also other solutes eliminated in bile. The term c-holestasis refers to decreased delivery of bilirubin into the intestine (and subsequent accumulation in the hepatocytes and in the blood), irrespective of the underlying cause. As cholestasis worsens, a conjugated hyperbilirubinemia develops that presents as jaundice.

The syndrome is characterized by signs and symptoms that are related either to the conjugated hyperbilirubinemia

TABLE 2
CAUSES OF HEPATIC JAUNDICE

Hepatitis
Drugs and hormones
Diseases of the intrahepatic bile ducts
Liver infiltration and storage disorders
Systemic Infections
Total parenteral nutrition
Postoperative intrahepatic cholestasis
Cholestasis of pregnancy
Benign recurrent intrahepatic cholestasis
Infantile cholestatic syndromes
Inherited metabolic defects
Idiopathic hepatic jaundice

(e.g. jaundice, dark urine, pale stools, pruritus) or to chronic malabsorption of fat soluble vitamis (A, D, E, K): bruising,

TABLE 3
CAUSES OF POST - HEPATIC JAUNDICE

Causes of Posthepatic Jaundice (other than choledocholithiasis)	Mirizzi syndrome
Upper third obstruction	Extrinsic nodal compression (e.g. from breast cancer or lymphoma)
Polycystic Liver Disease	Iatrogenic bile duct injury
Caroli Disease	Cystic fibrosis
Hepatocellular Carcinoma	Benign idiopathic bile duct stricture
Oriental cholangiohepatitis	
Hepatic Arterial thrombosis (e.g. after transplantation or chemotherapy)	*Lower third obstruction*
Hemobilia	Cholangiocarcinoma
Iatrogenic bile duct injury	Sclerosing cholangitis
Cholangiocarcinoma (Klatskin tumor)	Papillomas of the bile duct
Sclerosing Cholangitis	Pancreatic tumors
Papillomas of the bile duct	Ampullary tumors
	Chronic Pancreatitis
Middle third obstruction	Sphincter of Oddi dysfunction
Cholangiocarcinoma	Papillary stenosis
Sclerosing Cholangitis	Duodenal diverticula
Papillomas of the bile duct	Penetrating duodenal ulcer
Gallbladder cancer	Retroduodenal adenopathy (e.g. lymphoma, carcinoid)
Choledochal cyst	
Intrabilliary parasites	

steatorrhea, night blindness, osteomalacia and neuromuscular weakness.

A characteristic laboratory finding is elevated serum alkaline phospatase an enzyme present in bile duct epithelium and in the canalicular membrane of hepatocytes. An isozyme is normally present in many other tissues such as bone and so the increased levels must be verified as being of hepatic origin.

Pathology of Cholestasis

Cholestatic pathologic features depend somewhat on severity, duration, and underlying cause. Common to both obstructive and hepatocellular cholestasis is the accumulation of bile pigment within the hepatic parenchyma (Figure 2), Elongated grecn-brown plugs of bile are visible in dilated bile canaliculi. Rupture of canaliculi leads to extravasation of bile, which is phagocytosed by Kupffer cells. Droplets of bile pigment also accumulate within hepatocytes, which can take on a wispy appearance (feathery or foamy degeneration).

Obstruction to the biliary tree, either intrahepatic or extrahepatic, induces distention of upstream bile ducts by bile. The bile stasis and back-pressure induce proliferation of the duct epithelial cells and looping and reduplication of ducts, termed bile duct proliferation, The labyrinthine ducts further slow the flow of bile and favor the formation of concrements, which obstruct their lumens. Associated portal tract findings include edema and periductal infiltrates of neutrophils. Prolonged obstructive cholestasis leads not only to foamy changes of hepatocytes but alos to focal destruction of the parenchyma, giving rise to bile lakes filled with cellular debris and pigment. Unrelieved obstruction leads to portal tract fibrosis, which initially extends into and subdivides the parenchdhyma with relative preservation of hepatic architecture.

Ultimately, an end stage, bile stained, cirrhotic liver is created (billiary cirrhosis).

CALCULOUS DISEASE - GALLSTONES, CHOLELITHIASIS, CHOLEDOCHOLITHIASIS

In the United states about 12% of the population has cholelithiasis, while in East Africa and other developing countries the incidence is as low as 2% to 3%.

Children and adolescents rarely have gallstones, by the seventh decade of life 10% of men and 25% of women have documented cholelithiasis.

Choledocholithiasis represents gallbladder stones that have migrated into the common bile duct via the cystic duct, stones which were left in the common duct following biliary tract surgery (retained stones) or stones that originated within the intra or extrahepatic bile ducts primarily (pigment stones only). Cholesterol stones in the common bile duct are always by migration from the gallbladder. The overall incidence of choledocholithiasis is not clear, but up to 15% of patients who undergo gallbladder surgery are found to have common duct stones. 95% of patients with choledocholithiasis have also cholelithiasis.

Classification and pathogenesis of gallstones

The exact pathogenesis of calculous disease is incompletely understood and remains a subject of significant research.

There are three types of gallstones: cholesterol, pigment and mixed stones. Most gallbladder stones developing in industrialized societies are mixed in composition but still cholesterol-rich. Therefore, the remainder of this chapter focuses deeper on the pathogenesis of cholesterol-rich stones forming within the gall-bladder.

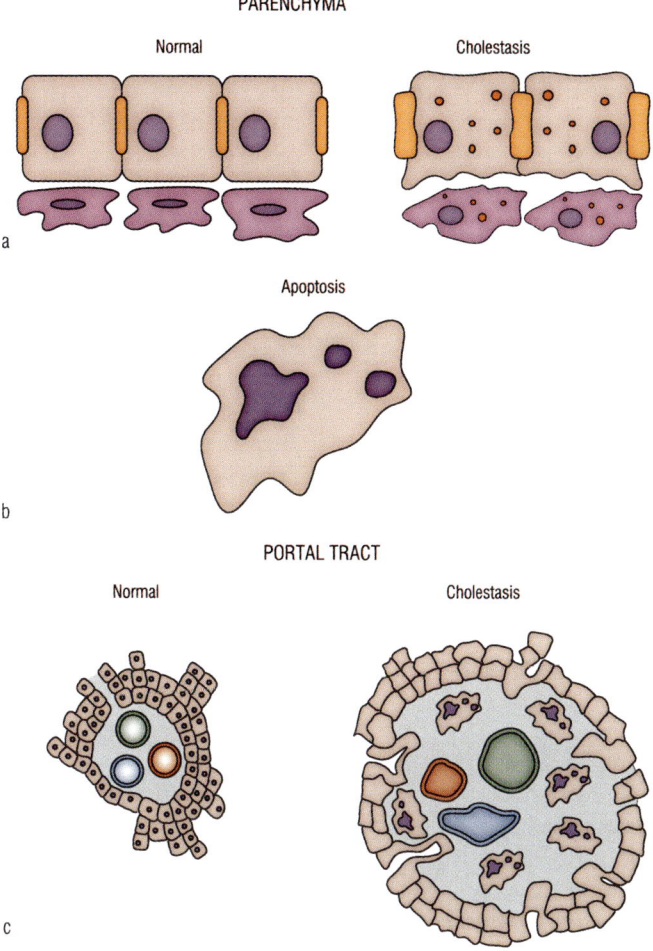

FIGURE 2: Morphological alterations of the hepatocytes and the portal tract induced by cholostasis. The presense of inflammatory changes and apoptotic cells in obvius in Jaundice.

• *Pigment Stones*

Risk Factors for Pigment gallstones formation:

1. Chronic haemolysis (sickle cell anaemia, thalasaemic syndromes etc.)
2. Bile stasis
3. Biliary tract infections
4. Chronic liver disease (e.g. liver cirrhosis)

Pigment stones consist of polymerized bilirubin and varying amounts of calcium salts. They are found, with increased frequency, in patients with haemolysis and in those with hepatic cirrhosis. Under these conditions, an excessive load of bilirubin is delivered to or synthetized within the liver that far exceeds organ capacity to conjugate (and thus render water soluble) this macromolecule. Presumambly the unconjugated, relatively hydrophobic pigment is then directly secreted into bile, where it can precipitate with calcium carbonate.

Pigment stones are classified as black

and brown. Black pigment stones, composed of oxidized polymers of the calcium salts of unconjugated bilirubin, are found in sterile bile. Brown pigment stones, composed of pure calcium salts of unconjugated bilirubin, are found in infected intrahepatic or extrahepatic ducts.

• *Cholesterol Stones*

Risk Factors for cholesterol gallstones formation:

1. Female gender; estrogens increase the uptake of plasma cholesterol by the liver
2. Age >60 years; gallstone formation is a time depended process
3. Contraceptives and pregnancy
4. West type diet and diabetes
5. Quick weight loss in obese
6. Liver cirrhosis
7. Ileum disease
8. Gastric & Duodenal operations
9. Familial reasons

Gallstone formation pathogenetically depends on three components (the 'triple defect'): (i) supersaturated bile; (ii) abnormal nucleation; and (iii) stasis within the gall-bladder.

Cholesterol gallstones are formed depending on the relative concentrations of solutes in bile. Three major components comprise 80-95% of solids that are diluted in bile: bile salts, lecithin (phosphatidylocholine) and cholesterol.

Profoundly, the three bile components should be maintained in adequate relative concentrations so that cholesterol precipitation is not enhanced. Should this relative balance breaks, the excess lipid precipitates and lithogenicity is activated.

The major pathogenetic mechanism of cholesterol gallstone formation is the secretion of bile supersaturated with cholesterol by the hepatocytes. The initial cause is not yet clear. Various mechanisms have been proposed, such as (i) hypersecretion of biliary cholesterol, (ii) hyposecretion of bile acids, (iii) hyposecretion of phospholipids (iv) decreased reabsorption of bile salts in the ileum (disruption of the enterohepatic cycle and reduction of bile salts) or (v) some combined secretory abnormality.

Once bile has become supersaturated with cholesterol, the formation of a cholesterol-enriched gallstone presumably begins with a nucleation event. The precipitation of crystalline cholesterol is thought to occur via either the fusion or implosion of cholesterol-rich vesicles. A variety of different crystal shapes have been identified. These crystals consist the lithogenous nucleous over which the gallstone is formed by deposition of new cholesterol molecules and calcium salts.

Following the nucleation event, different variables are involved in the process of stone formation (see risk factors above). The presence of a nidus is lithogenetic. Nidus could be mucous of the gallbladder epithelium, bacterial, parasite or apoptotic cell aggregates. Stone formation is promoted by the trapping of cholesterol mycrocrystals.

Bile stasis has long been associated with the formation of gallstones. Stasis may be due to impaired gall-bladder emptying (or, more correctly, filling and emptying) or to excess mucus glycoprotein synthesis and secretion by the gall-bladder mucosa. Decreased gallbladder motility promotes nidus formation and lithogenicity. Moreover, various other clinical situations promote bile stasis e.g. vagotomy, Total Parenteral Nutrition, pregnancy, octreotide therapy etc.

Recently, lithogenicity is also attributed to a more widespread motility disorder of the foregut. For example, women with gallbladder stones were found to have significantly longer whole gut transport times with only half the stool output as compared to stone free patients. In addition, many gallstone patients were found to have longer cycles of the intestinal migrating motor complex (MMC) with disruption of motilin release.

In biliary cholesterol secretion, transport and saturation, recent developments include evidence in humans and animals that bile lipid secretion is under genetic control.

Patients with spontaneous gallstone disease also have prolonged Large bowel transit times (LBTTs), more colonic Gram-positive anaerobes, increased bile acid metabolizing enzymes and higher intra-colonic pH values, than stone-free controls. Together, these changes lead to increased deoxycholic acid formation, solubilization and absorption. Thus, in addition to the 'lithogenic liver' and 'guilty gall-bladder' one must now add the 'indolent intestine' to the list of culprits in cholesterol gallstone formation.

REFERENCES

Barkun J., Barkun A. Jaundice. ACS Surgery, Principles and Practice. American College of Surgeons. 2004, pp 289-301

Cahalane MJ, et al: Physical-chemical pathogenesis of pigment gallstones. Semin Liver Dis 8:317-328, 1988

Carey MC, Cahalane MJ: The enterohepatic circulation. In Arias I, et al (eds): The Liver: Biology and Pathobiology, 2nd ed. New York, Raven Press, 1988, pp 573-616

Carey, MC. Formation of cholesterol gallstones: the new paradigms. In: Paumgartner, G Stiehl, A Gerok, W, eds. Trends in Bile Acid Research. Dordrecht/Boston/London: Kluwer Academic Publishers, 1989; 259-81

Carey MC, O'Donovan MA: Gallstone disease: current concepts on the epidemiology, pathogenesis and management. In Harrison's Principles of Internal Medicine, Update V. New York, McGraw-Hill, 1984, pp 139-168

Carey MC, LaMont JT: Cholesterol gallstone formation. 1. Physical chemistry of bile and biliary lipid secretion. Prog LiverDis 10:139-163, 1992

Deleuze, J-F, Jacquemin, E, Dubuisson, C et al. De-fect of multidrug-resistance 3 gene expression in a subgroup of progressive familial intrahepatic cholestasis. Hepatology 1996; 23, 904-8.

de Vree, JML, Jacquemin, E, Sturm, E et al. Mutations in the MDR3 gene cause progressive familial intrahepatic cholestasis. Proc Natl Acad Sci USA 1998; 95, 282-7.

Dowling, RH, Gleeson, D, Ruppin, DC et al. Gallstone recurrence and post-dissolution management. In: Paumgartner, G Stiehl, A Gerok, W, eds. Enterohepatic Circulation of Bile Acids and Sterol Metabolism. Lancaster: MTP Press Ltd, 1985; 361-9

Green RM, Crawford JM: Hepatocellular cholestasis: pathobiology and histological outcome. Semin Liver Dis 15:372-389, 1995

G. P. vanBerge-Henegouwen, N. G. Venneman, P. Portincasa, A. Kosters, K. J. van Erpecum, A. K. Groen. Relevance of Hereditary Defects in Lipid Transport Proteins for the Pathogenesis of Cholesterol Gallstone Disease. Scand J Gastroenterol 2004 (Suppl 241)

Holan, KR, Holzbach, RT, Hermann, RE, Cooperman, AM, Claffey, WJ. Nucleation time; a key factor in the pathogenesis of cholesterol gallstone disease. Gastroenterology 1979; 77

Jazrawi, RP, Pazzi, P, Petroni, ML et al. Postprandial gallbladder motor function: refilling and turnover of bile in health and in cholelithiasis. Gastroenterology 1995; 109

Khanuja, B, Cheah, YC, Hunt, M et al. Lith1, a major gene affecting cholesterol gallstone formation among inbred strains of mice. Proc Natl Acad Sci USA 1995; 92, 7729-33.

Konikoff, FM, Chung, DS, Donovan, JM, Small, DM, Carey, MC. Filamentous, helical and tubular microstructures during cholesterol crystallization from bile. Evidence that biliary cholesterol does not nucleate classic monohydrate plates. J Clin Invest 1992; 90, 1156-61.

LaMont JT, Carey MC: Cholesterol gallstone formation. 2. Pathobiology and pathomechanics. Prog Liver Dis 10:165-191, 1992

Lindberg G, Bjorkman A, Helmers C: A description of diagnostic strategies in jaundice. Scand J Gastroenterol 18:257, 1983

Messing B, Bories C, Kunstlinger F, Bernier JJ. Does Total Parenteral Nutrition induce gallbladder sludge formation and lithiasis? Gastroenterology 1983;84:1012-1019

Norton JA, Bollinger RR, Chang AE, Lowry SF, Mulvihill SJ, Pass HI, Thompson RW. Surgery, Basic Science and Clinical Evidence. Biliary System. Springer - Verlag New York, Inc. 2001, pp 553-584

Patankar, R, Ozmen, MM, Bailey, IS, Johnson, CD. Gallbladder motility, gallstones, and the surgeon. Dig Dis Sci 1995; 40Redfern, JS & Fortuner, Wj II. Octreotide-associated biliary tract dysfunction and gallstone formation: pathophysiology and management. Am J Gastro 1995; 90

Portincasa, P, van Erpecum, KJ, Jansen, A, Renooij, W, Gadellaa, M, vanBerge Henegouwen, GP. Behavior of various cholesterol crystals in bile from patients with gallstones. Hepatology 1996; 23, 738-48.

Robbins. Pathologic Basis of Disease. Ch.19 - The liver and the biliary tract. 6th Edition Saunders. 1999 p.g. 848-852

Salen G., Shefer S. Bile acid synthesis. Annu Rev Physiol 45:679, 1983

Schiff's Diseases of the Liver, 8th ed. Schiff ER, Sorell MF, Maddrey WC, Eds. Lippicott-Raven, Philadelphia, 1999, p 119

Smit, JJ, Schrinkel, AH, Oude Elferink, RP et al. Homozygous disruption of the murine mdr2 P-glycoprotein gene leads to a complete absence of phospholipid from bile and to liver disease. Cell 1993; 75, 451-62.

Strange RC. Hepatic bile flow. Physiol. Rev., 64:1055, 1984

Thistle JL, Cleary PA, Lachin JM, Tyor MP, Hersh T. The natural history of cholelithiasis: the National Cooperative Gallstone Study. Ann Intern Med 1984;101:171-175

Thomas, LA, Veysey, MJ, Murphy, GM, Dowling, RH, King, A, French, GR. Is cholelithiasis an intestinal disease? Gut.; 41 (Suppl.), 1997, 3), A2 (Abstract)

Thomas, LA, Bathgate, T, Veysey, MJ et al. Transit-induced changes in colonic bacteriology, bile acid metabolizing enzymes and luminal pH influence deoxycholic acid metabolism. In: Paumgartner, G Stiehl, A Gerok, W Kepper, D Leuschner, U, eds. Bile Acids and Cholestasis. Dordrecht, Boston, London: Kluwer Academic Publishers, 1999; 284-5.

Wang, DQ, Paigen, B, Carey, MC. Phenotypic characterization of Lith-genes that determine susceptibility to cholesterol cholelithiasis in inbred mice: physical-chemistry of gallbladder bile. J Lipid Res 1997; 38, 1395-411.

Molecular pathogenesis of cholestasis

Acalovschi Monica

"Cholestasis" means decreased bile formation or secretion and may result from a functional defect in bile formation at the level of hepatocytes (hepatocellular cholestasis) or from an impairment in bile secretion and flow at the level of bile ducts (ductular/ductal cholestasis). According to the site, it may be intrahepatic or extrahepatic. Intrahepatic cholestasis is the term used for diseases in which no obstruction of the major bile ducts can be identified by endoscopic retrograde cholangiopancreatography (ERCP).

The research in the physiologic regulation of various transporters and their deregulation in experimental models of cholestasis and in patients with cholestatic disorders has lead to a better understanding of the molecular pathogenesis of cholestasis. It has been demonstrated that decreased or absent expression of hepatocellular transporters may impair transport function resulting in hyperbilirubinemia and cholestasis. Many of the hepatobiliary transporters have recently been cloned from rodents and man.

Some of these transporters are localized at **the basolateral membrane** of the hepatocyte (Figure 1):
– the Na$^+$ taurocholate cotransporter (NTCP) mediates predominantly bile salt uptake in the hepatocyte and is the major Na$^+$ dependent bile salt transporter;
– the organic anion transporter protein (OATP) mediates uptake of unconjugated bile salts such as cholate as well as other organic anions - BSP, estrogen conjugates, xenobiotics;
– the organic cation transporter (OCT) mediates transport of organic cations into the hepatocytes.

The transport across **the canalicular membrane** is the rate-limiting step of bile formation and is driven by unidirectional ATP-dependent transport systems (the "export pumps"). The canalicular membrane transporters belong to the ATP-binding cassette (ABC) transporter superfamily
– the phospholipid export pump (MDR3) is a phospholipid transporter that translocates phosphatidyl-choline from the inner to the outer leaflet of the canalicular membrane (subsequently forming cholesterol-phospholipid vesicles);
– the conjugate export pump (the multidrug resistance associated protein, MRP2)(cMOAT) transports divalent bile salts and anionic conjugates, i.e. glucuronides such as bilirubin. Absence of canalicular MRP2 expression characterizes the Dubin-Johnson syndrome, an

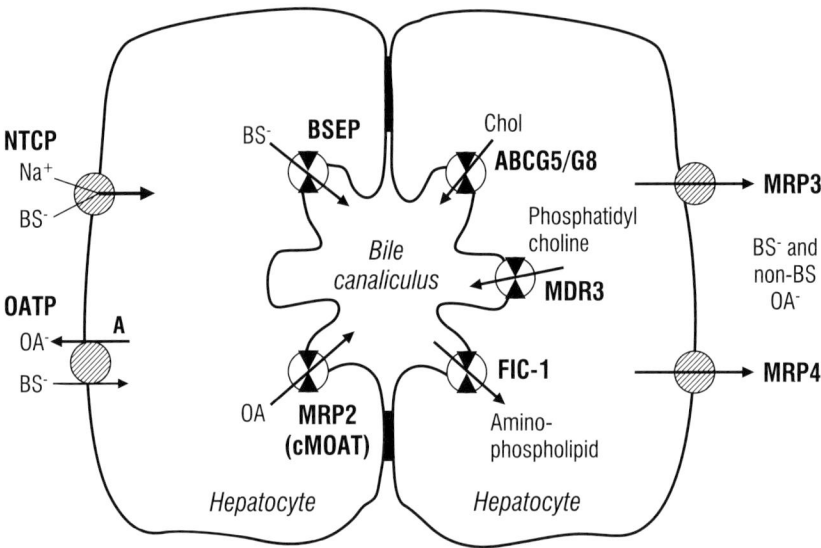

FIGURE 1: Hepatocellular transporters of bile acids and bilirubin (BS = bile salts; OA = organic anions; NTCP = Na+ taurocholate cotransporter; OATP = organic anion transporter protein; BSEP = bile salt export pump; MRP2, 3, 4 = multidrug-resistance proteins 2,3,4; MDR3 = multidrug export pump 3).

inherited form of conjugated hyperbiliru-binemia;

– the bile salt export pump (BSEP) mediates the canalicular efflux of bile acids;

– the multidrug-resistance proteins (MRP3 and 4) mediate sinusoidal efflux of organic anions, including toxic bile acids (being a secondary route to eliminate the organic anions that cannot be eliminated into bile in the absence of MRP2);

– the multidrug export pump (MDR1) exports cationic drugs;

– the anion exchanger (AE) mediates chloride/bicarbonate exchange at the canalicular, as well as apical membrane of the cholangiocyte;

– the two half-transporters ABCG5/ABCG export cholesterol into bile;

– the breast cancer resistance protein (BRCP) mediates excretion of organic anions into bile;

– FIC1 is an aminophospholipid transporter which may play an important role in bile salt reabsorption (cholehepatic and enterohepatic circulation of bile salts). Mutations in *FIC1* gene result in progressive familial intrahepatic cholestasis (PFIC) type 1.

Bile formation being an osmotic process, the impaired function of these pumps decreases bile flow and leads to cholestasis. The function of the hepatobiliary transporters was confirmed by the study of some *inherited* cholestatic diseases, which are caused by mutations in their genes. These molecular defects were subsequently found to have pathological consequences and to be involved also in the pathogenesis of *acquired* cholestatic diseases or syndromes (Table 1).

Bile acids are the major determinant of bile formation, but accumulation of the bile acids in the hepatocyte might become toxic. The hepatic defense against bile acid toxicity implies several mechanisms:

– down-regulation of the baso-lateral Na/taurocholate cotransporter NTCP and or-

TABLE 1

ACQUIRED AND HEREDITARY MOLECULAR CHANGES OF HEPATOCELLULAR TRANSPORT SYSTEMS IN HUMANS

Disease	Molecular change
Acquired	
Primary biliary cirrhosis	AE mRNA and protein reduced: hepatocytes and cholangiocytes are affected.
	MDR3 mRNA levels unchanged
Extrahepatic biliary atresia	NTCP mRNA reduced. Inverse correlation with serum bilirubin level
Primary sclerosing cholangitis	OATP mRNA increased
Biliary obstruction	MDR4 and MDR3 mRNA increased. Direct correlation with serum bilirubin levels
Hereditary	
Progressive familial intrahepatic cholestasis (PFIC)	
PFIC-1	Mutation of FIC1 gene; low γ-GT
PFIC-2	Mutation of BSEP gene; low γ-GT
	Canalicular BSEP protein absent
PFIC-3	Mutation of MDR3 gene; high γ-GT
	Canalicular MDR3 protein absent
Benign recurrent intrahepatic cholestasis (BRIC) type 1	Mutation of FIC1 gene
Benign recurrent intrahepatic cholestasis (BRIC) type 2	Missense mutation in ABCB11
Dubin-Johnson syndrome	Mutation of MRP2 gene
	Canalicular MRP2 protein absent

ganic anion transporting proteins OATP limits bile acid uptake;

– induction of canalicular export pumps such as BSEP for monovalent bile acids and MRP2 for divalent bile acids enhances bile acid excretion;

– induction of alternative baso-lateral efflux pumps MRP3 and 4 reduces hepatocellular bile acid retention;

– down-regulation of bile acid synthetic enzymes reduces synthesis, and

– induction of phase I and II (hydroxylating and conjugating) enzymes results in less toxic bile acids.

Mutations in a gene encoding for a particular transporter may result in the lack of its transporting function and causes cholestasis. For example, mutations in *BSEP*, *MDR3* and *MRP2* genes are implicated in PFIC-2, PFIC-3 and Dubin-Johnson syndrome, respectively. Apart from genetic defects, regulation of transporters at the level of transcription, translation, and post-translation may be altered by chemicals or disease processes leading to decreased bile formation and, hence, cholestasis.

Transport proteins, like other proteins, are synthetised in the endoplasmic reticulum, processed in the Golgi complex, and then translocated to their site of action. Here they are inserted into the membrane and allow the transport of solutes across it. This complex regulated process requires the participation of specific signaling molecules along with vesicles and cytoskeletons.

Pathogenesis of cholestasis involves the following **mechanisms**

a. reduced activity of transporters due to reduced expression of their genes or target proteins on the canalicular membrane;

b. disruption of the cytoskeleton and of the vesicle transport which normally ensure the secretory polarity of the hepatocyte;

c. alteration of the signal transmitting pathways which coordinate the cellular functions in the hepatic lobule and stimulate contraction of the biliary ductules;

d. defects in the tight junctions leading to dissipation of the osmotic gradients via paracellular pathways;

e. biliary ductule/duct dysruption caused by immunologic or toxic mechanisms.

It was very recently discovered that the **nuclear (orphan) receptors** (NR) are transcriptional regulators of the key enzymes in sterol metabolism and of hepatobiliary transporting proteins. The NRs belong to a superfamily of cellular receptors that regulate gene transcription (Table 2). In general, these proteins are activated upon binding ligands, i.e. small hydrophobic molecules like bile salts and steroid hormones. Dimers of the retinoid receptor that binds retinoic acid (RXR) and a specific ligand bind to a responsive element in the promoter region of a gene and thereby regulate transcription. For example, BSEP expression is controlled by the nuclear receptor pair RXR/FXR, in which the farnesoid X receptor (FXR) has high affinity for bile salts. Hence, the binding of bile salts to FXR in the dimer RXR/FXR induces transcription of the *BSEP* gene, leading to enhanced BSEP levels and increased bile salt secretion. FXR activates not only transcription of *BSEP* gene, but also of the small heterodimer partner (SHP). This is a transcriptional repressor of the bile salt uptake systems NTCP and OATP.

MRP2 is activated by the pregnane X receptor/steroid X receptor PXR/SXR, as well as by androstane constitutive receptor (CAR). PXR and SXR accommodate as ligands a large number of xenobiotics, as for example rifampicin and phenobarbital.

TABLE 2

Nuclear Receptors Involved in the Hepatocellular Transport of Bile Acids

Nuclear receptors	Ligand	Gene activated
RXR/FXR	Bile acids	*BSEP,NTCP (via SHP)*
RXR/SXR	Rifampicin	*MRP2,MDR1,OATP...2*
XR/PXR	Lithocholate, xenobiotics	*MRP2,MDR1,OATP2*
RXR/CAR	Fenobarbital, bilirubin	*MRP2*
RXR/PPAR α, γ, δ	Fibrates, statin, fatty acids	*ABCA1*
RXR/HNF4 α	Fatty acids	*CYP7A1*
RXR/LXR α	Oxysterols	*ABCG5/ABCG8, ABCA1*
RXR/RAR	Bile acids	*NTCP*

HEREDITARY (MONOGENIC) CHOLESTATIC DISEASES

Are very rare diseases, occurring mainly in childhood, and will not be described here.

ACQUIRED CHOLESTATIC DISEASES

Intrahepatic (hepatocellular) cholestasis

Hepatocellular cholestasis may be non-inflammatory (drugs, hormones) of inflammatory (drugs, alcohol, sepsis).

- *Intrahepatic cholestasis of pregnancy*

Intrahepatic cholestasis of pregnancy (ICP) is a reversible form of cholestasis that may develop in the third trimester of a normal pregnancy and usually rapidly resolves after delivery. The main symptoms are pruritus, and to a lesser extent, jaundice. Serum bile salt level is increased. Increased incidence of fetal distress, premature birth, and even stillbirth in association with ICP might occur. Jaundice is relatively uncommon, complicating only the most severe and prolonged episodes.

The coexistence of PFIC 3 and ICP in a consanguineous family was reported. *FIC1, MRP2* gene mutations were described in some patients, as well as *MDR3* mutations. This mutation was described in association with cholesterol cholelithiasis, and might explain the higher prevalence of gallstones in ICP patients.

During pregnancy, there is a more or less generalized reduction in bile formation. The mechanism of the reduced bile formation is hypothetized to be related to the high levels of circulating hormones during the last trimester. The most important observation in support of this

hypothesis is that women with a history of ICP are also prone to cholestasis induced by oral contraceptives and vice versa. Estrogen metabolites can be cholestatic, and progesterone metabolites may also play a part as these are produced at high rates during the last phase of pregnancy. These hormones may have an inhibitory effect on canalicular transporters.

The reduction in bile formation combined with a pre-existent subclinical defect in any of these transporters may induce clinical symptoms of cholestasis. In a proportion of patients, ICP is due to a genetic predisposition, but the etiology of ICP is multifactorial, and hormonal factors have important roles.

- *Cholestasis associated with inflammation and sepsis*

The inflammatory cholestasis is characterized by the inhibition of transporter expression and function by the pro-inflammatory cytokines.

Sepsis is associated with impaired biliary secretion. Patients with sepsis often develop a conjugated hyperbilirubinemia, indicating an impaired secretion of bilirubin into bile. Experiments in rodents by injection of lipopolysaccharides (LPS) found that *Mrp2* is strongly downregulated under these conditions.

Members of the NR family play a major part as transcription factors in the regulation of expression of transporter genes, including *MRP2*. MRP is regulated by CAR and PXR/SXR that dimerise with RXR. Expression of RXR is strongly downregulated during endotoxaemia in hamsters and this leads to downregulation of *Mrp2*. Expression of BSEP is also regulated by the nuclear receptor dimer RXR/FXR. Expression of NTCP, which is involved in bile salt uptake by hepatocytes, is regulated by the dimer RXR/RAR. Hence the expression of both BSEP and NTCP might also be downregulated during sepsis.

LPS and LPS-induced cytokines may also contribute to impaired hepatobiliary excretory function in other disorders, such as cholestasis during total parenteral nutrition and viral hepatitis.

In the evolution of liver disease, increased levels of TNFα, IL1β and IL6 are associated with a decrease in mARN coding for certain NR proteins such as RXR, LXRα, PPARα etc. Reduction of RXR levels and of other NR levels in the liver could be a mechanism which down-regulates ABC transporter genes during the acute phase response.

Apart from the metabolic changes induced, the NRs PXR and CAR form heterodimers with RXR and modulate drug metabolism by regulating expression of some CYP450 enzymes.

- *Primary biliary cirrhosis and primary sclerosing cholangitis*

The pathogenesis of primary biliary cirrhosis (PBC) and primary sclerosing cholangitis (PSC) remains unknown, although a dysregulation of the immune system in context with environmental factors and a genetic susceptibility seem to be important. PBC is characterized by destruction or disappearance of small biliary ductules (vanishing bile ducts). *MDR3* mutations in PBC patients without AMA were recently described, but controversies exist whether a genetically determined dysfunction of the canalicular membrane transporters BSEP and MDR3 plays a pathogenetic role in PBC and PSC.

The altered expression of hepatic transport proteins (decreased expression of MRP2, BSEP and NTCP, maintained expression of BSEP and increased expression of MRP3) described in PBC and PSC are rather secondary changes, as adaptive responses in the defense against hepatocyte overloading with cytotoxic bile acids.

Extrahepatic obstructive cholestasis

Common bile duct stones and tumors of the common bile duct and pancreas produce mechanical obstruction of the large, macroscopically visible bile ducts (extrahepatic bile duct obstruction). The experimental rat model for these extrahepatic forms of obstructive cholestasis is represented by ligation of the common bile duct. Under this condition, biliary pressure is increased and the hepatocellular excretion of bile salts and various other organic anions is markedly impaired, leading to the retention of toxic biliary constituents within hepatocytes.

The enterohepatic circulation of bile salts is disrupted in extrahepatic obstructive cholestasis. The cholehepatic shunt is increased. Bile from the bile duct proximal to the obstruction site returns to the liver instead of being excreted in the small intestine, leading to bile acid accumulation in the liver. Bile salts are partially detoxified by phase I and II enzymes in the liver, eliminated into plasma through the basolateral membrane (MRP3 and 4) and then excreted by the kidney. These protective mechanisms might limit cholestatic hepatocyte injury. Similar to PBC or PSC, the expression of the hepatobiliary transporters is changed as an adaptive mechanism to the accumulation of bile salts in the liver.

Translocation of LPS-producing bacteria as a consequence of bacterial overgrowth due to absence of bile salts in the intestinal lumen may also contribute to cholestasis in case of extrahepatic obstruction.

CONCLUSION

Gene polymorphisms causing a reduction in transport protein level or activity are much more frequent than monogenic inherited disorders involving hepatobiliary transporters, and could predispose individuals to cholestasis or to other liver diseases. Mutations of transporter genes may play a role in more common disease phenotypes. An example of this situation is MDR3 deficiency. A complete absence of this phospholipid-translocating protein causes severe liver disease (PFIC type 3). Heterozygous females may develop ICP. Several gallstone patients have mutations of the *MDR3* gene. *MDR3* mutations were also found in patients with anti-mitochondrial antibody-negative PBC.

Changes in the expression of the transporter proteins may also be secondary, developing as adaptive mechanisms to the primary cause of the disease (such as biliary tract obstruction) trying to limit the extension of liver injury. Therapeutic measures targeting these transporters or the NRs which transcriptionally influence their expression are actually in development.

REFERENCES

Boyer JL. Nuclear receptor ligands: rational and effective therapy for chronic cholestatic liver disease? Gastroenterology 2005;129:735-740.

Deitch EA, Sittig K, Li M, Berg R, Specian RD. Obstructive jaundice promotes bacterial translocation from the gut. Am J Surg 1990;159:79-84.

Jacquemin E. Role of multidrug resistance 3 deficiency in pediatric and adult liver disease: one gene for three diseases. Semin Liver Dis 2001; 21:551-562.

Jansen PL, Sturm E. Genetic cholestasis, causes and consequences for hepatobiliary transport. Liver Int 2003;23:315-322.

Kullak-Ublick GA, Meier PJ. Mechanisms of cholestasis. Clin Liver Dis 2000;4:357-385.

Lammert F, Marschall HU, Glantz A, Matern S. Intrahepatic cholestasis of pregnancy: molecular pathogenesis, diagnosis and treatment. J Hepatol 2000;33:1012-1021.

Lammert F, Carey MC, Paigen B. Chromosomal organization of candidate genes involved in cholesterol gallstone formation: a Murine Gallstone Map. Gastroenterology 2001;120:221-238.

Milkiewicz P, Elias E. Obstetric cholestasis. Br Med J 2002;324:123-124.

Oude Elferink R. Cholestasis. Gut 2003;52:ii42-59.

Pauli-Magnus C, Kerb R, Fattinger K, al et. BSEP and MDR3 haplotype structure in healthy Caucasians, primary biliary cirrhosis and primary sclerosing cholangitis. Hepatology 2004;39:604-607.

Rosmorduc O, Hermelin R, Poupon R. MDR3 gene defect in adults with symptomatic intrahepatic and gallbladder cholesterol cholelithiasiss. Gastroenterology 2001;120:1459-1467.

Savander M, Ropponen A, Avela K, et al. Genetic evidence of heterogeneity in intrahepatic cholestasis of pregnancy. Gut 2003;52:1025-1029.

Trauner M, Meier PJ, Boyer JL. Molecular pathogenesis of cholestasis. N Engl J Med 1998;339: 1217-1227.

Trauner M, Meier PJ, Boyer JL. Molecular regulation of hepatocellular transport systems in cholestasis. J Hepatol 1999;31:165-178.

Trauner M, Wagner M, Fickert P, Zollner G. Molecular regulation of hepatobiliary transport systems. Clinical implications for understanding and treating cholestasis. J Clin Gastroenterol 2005; 39:S111-S124.

Wittenburg H, Lyons MA, Li R, Churchill GA, Carey MC, Paigen B. FXR and ABCG5/ABCG8 as determinants of cholesterol gallstone formation from quantitative trait locus mapping in mice. Gastroenterology 2003;125:868-881.

Zanlungo S, Nervi F. Discovery of the hepatic canalicular and intestinal cholesterol transporters. New targets for the treatment of hypercholesterolemia. Eur Rev Pharmacol Sci 2003;7:33-39.

Haemostasis impairment and immune dysfunction in patients with obstructive jaundice

Papadopoulos Vassilios, Mimidis Konstantinos

I. OVERVIEW OF HAEMOSTASIS

Haemostasis is the process of blood clot formation to prevent excessive blood loss in case of vessel injury. When endothelium is injured, the subendothelial matrix is revealed; it thus provides the substrate for two platelet-collagen receptors (glycoproteins, or GP, Ia, IIa and VI) [Watson, 1999]. The activated platelets express the receptor GPIb-IX-V complex that further strengthens their adhesion through linking with von Willebrand factor, which is expressed on the subendothelial matrix [Berndt MC, 2001]. The result of subendothelium/platelet interaction is the formation of a platelet monolayer over the injured area. Additional platelets are triggered and aggregated in order to form a platelet plug through linking to fibrinogen molecules via another receptor, GPIIb/IIIa [Savage B, 1992]. At the same time, the coagulation cascade is activated resulting in formation and deposition of fibrin which stabilize the newly formed platelet plug.

The coagulation cascade, though classicaly described as having three pathways (intrinsic, extrinsic and common), is currently considered under a more unifying aspect, as many cross-linking reactions joining extrinsic and intrinsic pathways have been described. Cleavage of fibrinogen to fibrin is the common result of the sequential activation of inactive precursors. Typical clot formation occurs through the interaction of a small amount of normally circulating activated factor VII with tissue factor, which is exposed on certain cell surfaces only after endothelial damage. The bimolecular complex FVIIa/TF activates factor X through a temporarily formed trimolecular complex ("priming" step). The generation of thrombin, even in small amounts, will activate factors VIII, V and XI and platelets bursting the cascade ("propagation" phase) [Caldwell SH, 2004].

Whether coagulation will start, most usually, from the formation of the extrinsic tenase complex (formed by tissue factor and factors VIIa and X under the presence of Ca^{++} and phospholipids) or the intrinsic tenase complex (formed by factors X, IXa and VIIIa under the presence of Ca^{++} and phospholipids) is indifferent regarding the final result, which is the activation of factor X, the formation of the prothrombinase complex (factors Xa, Va and prothrombin under the presence of Ca^{++} and phospholipids) and the production of active thrombin. By the time the first amounts of thrombin are generated, the whole process is multiplied as thrombin, apart from polymerizing fibrinogen, further enhances the previous described steps by activating factors V and VIII (absolutely necessary cofactors for prothrombinase and intrinsic tenase complex, respectively), factor XI, as well as factor XIII, which serves to cross-link fibrin polymers. Moreover, by the time the extrinsic prothrombinase complex is formed, it serves to the concomitant activation of factor IX, further extending its prothrombinase activity in an indirect way (enabling the formation of the intrinsic prothrombinase complex, whose substantial compound is factor IXa). The role of the so-called "intrinsic cascade", namely the activation of factor XII under the presence of High Molecular Weight Kininogen (HMWK) and prekallikrein (PK), followed by the activation of factor XI and factor IX, serves as a guarding mechanism to ensure the continuous presence of even small amounts of factor IXa.

As the haemostatic process starts, a number of inhibitory mechanisms is activated in order to limit and localize the formation of clot to the injured area. These natural anticoagulants are antithrombin III (which inactivates thrombin and factors IXa, Xa, XIa and XIIa), heparin cofactor II (which inactivates thrombin), a_2-macroglobulin (which is a general serine protease inhibitor, mainly exerting its action against factor Xa and plasmin), protein C (which is activated by thrombin via thrombomodulin binding and inactivates factors Va and VIIIa), protein S (which enhances protein C activity), protein Z-dependent protease inhibitor (which inactivates factor Xa), tissue factor pathway inhibitors (TFPI) 1 and 2 (which inactivate tissue factor and factors VIIa and Xa through a quadruple molecular complex) and platelet inhibitors (prostaglandin I_2 and nitric oxide).

When the formation of clot has been settled, fibrinolysis is activated in order to assure clot removal and vessel patency restoration once injury has been successfully faced. Plasmin, resulting from the activation of plasminogen, is the key enzyme of the fibrinolytic mechanism and serves for cleavage of the polymerized fibrin to fibrin degradation products (FDPs). Plasminogen activation is driven through tissue plasminogen activator (tPA) and urokinase. This process is counterbalanced by the presence of an antifibrinolytic mechanism, including plasminogen activation inhibitor (PAI) 1 and 2, a_2-antiplasmin and thrombin activatable fibrinolysis inhibitor (TAFI).

II. AN INTRODUCTION TO THE PHYSIOLOGY OF THE IMMUNE SYSTEM

The immune system provides a means of recognition of foreign materials and a series of specific responses based upon prior recognition. Invasion of host tissues by microorganisms evokes a complex and highly conserved response that serves to recruit inflammatory cells to the site of challenge and to optimize local defences to kill the invading bacteria, minimize microbial dissemination beyond the site of infection, and initiate the processes of tissue repair. Immunity to pathogens links two effector arms of the immune response: the defences of innate immunity with that of adaptive immunity.

The innate immunity is particularly important in warding off bacterial and viral infections presenting at the mucosal cell surface [Yuan, 2004]. The components of innate immunity are: physical and chemical barriers (epithelia, antimicrobial chemicals), natural killer cells and phagocytes (macrophages, neutrophils), blood proteins (complement) and cytokines. The effective development of the overall immune response depends on careful interplay and regulation between innate and adaptive immunity [Parish, 1997]. Epithelial and immune cells of the innate immunity defence system can recognize pathogen-associated molecular patterns, such as those that occur in the bacterial cell wall, through their Toll-like receptors (TLRs) [Lien, 2002] and then elicit pathogen-specific cellular immune responses.

The adaptive immune system can be divided into humoral and cell-mediated responses. In humoral immunity, B lymphocytes secrete Abs and eliminate extracellular microbes, this process requires the help of activated T cells.

In cell-mediated immunity, T lymphocytes are subdivided due to their membrane-associated glycoproteins into helper T cells (CD4+) and cytotoxic T cells (CD8+). T lymphocytes either activate macrophages to kill phagocytosed microbes (CD4+ T cells) or destroy infected cells (CD8+ T cells). CD4+ T helper lymphocytes may differentiate further into Th1 and Th2 subsets of effector cells, producing distinct sets of cytokines [Romagnani, 1991]. Th1 cells favor the phagocyte-cell mediated functions, producing interleukin (IL)-2 and interferon gamma (IFNγ), thus activating CD8+ cells. Conversely, Th2 cells secrete IL-4, IL-5, IL-6 and IL-10, activate B cells, stimulate immunoglobulin E (IgE) reactions and downregulate Th2 responses. Unlike B cells, which recognize Ag in its native form, T cells recognize the Ag after it has been processed and attached to specific protein complexes, major histocompatibility complex (MHC) class I or II molecules, on the surfaces of Ag presenting cells (APCs) [Braciale, 1991]. MHC is the gene region coding for "transplantation Ag", in humans called the "human leukocyte Ag" (HLA). The contact with the Ag by the specific T cell receptor (TCR) triggers the immune response, through release of cytokines from the activated T cells. T lymphocytes expressing the surface marker CD8 recognize foreign Ag in association with MHC class I, and CD4+ cells recognize Ag in association with MHC class II. MHC class I Ag are expressed on most nucleated cells and MHC class II Ag are expressed on B lymphocytes, APCs, macrophages, activated T lymphocytes, but also on endothelial and epithelial cells.

III. An Introduction to the Pathophysiology of Obstructive Jaundice

Obstructive jaundice, or else posthepatic jaundice, is most commonly attributed to biliary obstruction by a stone in the common bile duct or to a carcinoma of the pancreas. Nevertheless, numerous causes, including pancreatic pseudocyst, chronic pancreatitis, sclerosing cholangitis, bile duct stricture and parasites, may contribute to the etiology of the disease.

Bilirubin is minimally soluble in water at physiologic pH. In plasma, bilirubin is tightly bound to albumin and thus is poorly filtered by the renal glomeruli. The bilirubin-albumin complex is carried to the sinusoidal surface of hepatocytes, passes through the large sinusoidal pores to the perisinusoidal space of Disse, and enters the hepatocyte by active transport. Within the hepatocyte, bilirubin is conjugated by glucuronyl-transferase. The conjugated bilirubin is water soluble and rapidly excreted into the bile canaliculi through a rate-limiting process [Scott-Conner CEH, 1994].

Approximately 0,25-0,3 g of bile acids is synthesized daily in the liver; a similar amount is lost through excretion in the feces. Bile salts are conjugates of bile acids which are produced in the liver through linkage with taurine or glycine. Glycocholate and glycochenodeoxycholate compose approximately 30% of the bile salts each. Secondary bile salts are produced in the gut as bacterial products. Bile salts act as detergent into the gastrointestinal tract and enable fat emulsification. The main site of reabsorption is terminal ileum via an active transport mechanism. Portal vein transport the absorbed salts in the liver, from where they are again excreted into the bile canaliculi. The bile flow continues to the larger intrahepatic ducts, which converge to the left and right hepatic ducts. This transit is called enterohepatic circulation.

Hepatic bile is isotonic with plasma and is composed mainly by water and electrolytes. Organic solutes constitute a small amount (5%) and include bile salts, lipids (mainly cholesterol and phosphatidylcholine) and conjugated bilirubin. The relative rates of excretion of bile salts and lipids determine the lithogenicity of the bile.

Biliary obstruction causes mainly two mechanical problems: First, the enterohepatic circulation is interrupted; thus, substances like bile salts, cannot recirculate and are lost in the feces. Second, the pressure within the ducts is elevated and this may cause bile reflux; the consequence is that total and direct bilirubin and serum alkaline phosphatase are increased and urinary and fecal urobilinogen is absent. High intrabiliary pressure causes a decrease in bile salt synthesis and bile is excreted in the urine; bile salt pool is diminished and redistributed to the systemic circulation and body water. Total hepatic blood flow decreases despite the initial increase of portal vein flow. This change accounts for the main alterations in the reticuloendothelial function as well as the hepatic necrosis, which follows.

Liver function tests are crucial in the differential diagnosis of jaundice. Elevated serum levels of alanine transaminase (ALT) suggest a process of the hepatic parenchyma. Controversially, elevated alkaline phosphatase indicate damage of the epithelial cells of the bile canaliculi and is observed predominantly in patients with intrahepatic cholestasis, cholangitis or extrahepatic obstruction. Serum gamma-glutamyl transferase and 5' nucleotidase along with calcium and phosphorus levels should be measured in case that a bone disease is suspected to account for elevated alkaline phosphatase. In these cases, gamma-glutamyl transferase and 5' nucleotidase remain normal. Occasionally, the enzymatic profile may be suggestive of a combined biliary and hepatic component; this is usual in cholangitis, where obstruction is accompanied by infection [Beckingham IJ, 2001].

Albumin is produced in hepatocytes.

During severe impairment of liver function, serum albumin levels fall below normal after at least 10 days, as the observed half-life of albumin in plasma is about 20 days. Thus, low serum albumin suggests chronic liver disease.

IV. Immune Dysfunction in Patients with Obstructive Jaundice

Endotoxin and the gut barrier

Endotoxin is the lipopolysaccharide constituent of the outer membrane of Gram-negative bacteria. Endotoxaemia is described as an important predictor of outcome in patients undergoing surgery for obstructive jaundice. Portal endotoxaemia has sometimes been found to be higher than systemic endotoxaemia, suggesting that endotoxin originates from the gut. Numerous factors contribute to endotoxaemia in jaundice and can be summarized as disturbances in the homeostasis of the gut-liver-axis [Clements, 1998]. The absence of bile salts leads to an unbalanced intestinal bacterial flora with overgrowth of Gram-negative bacteria [Ding, 1994]. Obstructive jaundice causes bacterial translocation and increased mucosal permeability combined with decreased elimination of endotoxin by Kupffer cells [Osterberg, 2004]. Bacterial translocation was found in about 75% of rats after one week of bile duct ligation [Deitch, 1990], and was further increased by additional surgical trauma. Spontaneous endotoxaemia occurred after three weeks of bile duct ligation in rats, whereas the anti-core glycol-

ipid IgG and IgM concentrations were raised after the first week [Kennedy, 1999]. The occurrence of endotoxaemia and subsequent cytokine induction, and bacterial translocation to mesenteric lymph nodes were significantly reduced by internal biliary drainage, and cellular immunity was restored towards normal.

As the relevance of data obtained in animal models remains unknown, the question arises whether the inflammatory status found in experimental obstructive jaundice also exists in the clinical situation. In addition it remains uncertain whether preoperative drainage by endoscopic insertion of an endoprosthesis influences the inflammatory response. One uncontrolled clinical study reported a reduction in morbidity [Trede, 1988], but recent prospective randomized trials showed no significant reduction of morbidity after preoperative drainage [Lai, 1994][Karsten, 1996]. In the study of Kimmings et al [Kimmings, 2000] was shown that biliary drainage significantly reduced important inflammatory mediators (IL-8 and endotoxin binding proteins) but did not change many of the mediators suggested to be responsible for mortality in animal experiments. This is in agreement with the findings of another study [Padillo 2002] were internal biliary drainage in patients with biliary obstruction induced only a transitory improvement in the acute phase response displayed by obstructive jaundice.

Macrophages and Kupffer cells

Macrophages, the basic unit of the RES, have a central role in immune regulation. In addition to their phagocytic and antigen presenting functions, they can produce numerous substances such as cytokines (interleukins, colony-stimulating factors, tumor necrosis factor (TNF), and interferon), prostaglandins, and oxygen free radicals. The largest numbers of fixed tissue macrophages are the Kupffer cells in the liver [Kennedy, 1999]. The principal role of these cells is to eliminate foreign particles, including endotoxin and bacteria, transported by portal venous blood. However, when the balance of proinflammatory and anti-inflammatory stimuli is lost, Kupffer cells could be involved in further host reactions. Various data have revealed that hyperactive macrophages and the overproduction of macrophage-derived mediators (TNF-α, IL-1, IL-6, IL-8, and prostaglandins) play important roles in the development of multiple organ failure and septic shock [Lazar, 2002]. Additionally, both experimental and clinical observations have indicated that Kupffer cells are involved in the increased cytokine secretion in obstructive jaundice [Bemelmans, 1992] [Puntis, 1996]. Moreover, in the study of Lazar et al. was shown that attenuation of Kupffer cell function by gadolinium chloride, decreases endotoxin-induced lethality and morbidity in rats with obstructive jaundice.

In order to study phagocytic function ^{51}Cr-labelled endotoxin was used. A significant increase in the phagocytic index was found in jaundiced animals compared with controls. A significant increase in PGE$_2$ production was also detected, together with a decrease in IL-2 receptor expression. There was no difference in IL-1 pro-

duction between cells obtained from jaundiced animals and controls. A possible role for the increased PGE$_2$ concentration in IL-1 downregulation and altered IL-2R expression was suggested [Adachi, 1992]. Bile salts given by osmotic pumps prevented an increase in bacterial translocation in bile-duct-ligated rats, but there was no difference in the increased phagocytic activity of harvested Kupffer cells from jaundiced animals, with or without bile salts [Sheen-Chen, 1998].

During cholestasis in rats, constitutive NF-κB is activated in isolated hepatic macrophages, which are resistant to further activation by LPS. The activation was insensitive to the antioxidant α-tocopherol, but dexamethasone modulated constitutive NF-κB activation by inducing IκB expression and reversed the spontaneous TNFα secretion [Fox, 1997]. NF-κB has also been reported to be activated in hepatocytes during obstructive cholestasis and results in a reduction in liver damage [Miyoshi, 2001].

Cytokines

Cytokines are small molecular weight peptides produced by the cells of both innate and adaptive immunity. They act in networks leading to a change in cell proliferation, differentiation and function [Fong Y, 1990]. TNFα is one of the main proinflammatory cytokines and an early central mediator of sepsis. Endotoxins are the most powerful stimulus for release [Ksontini, 1998]. Kupffer cells are the main source of TNFα and IL-6 within the liver [Kennedy, 1999]. Their prolonged stimulation or activation is thought to be a critical factor in the continued and uncontrolled release of inflammatory mediators that may contribute to the pathogenesis of multiple organ dysfunction. In a model of isolated perfused rat liver, bile duct ligation increased the amounts of TNFα produced in the liver in response to endotoxin. Increased serum concentration of TNFα after injection of low doses of endotoxin was thought to be the result of an increased sensitivity to endotoxin in jaundiced animals [O'Neil, 1997].

In animal models of experimental biliary obstruction, the circulating TNF concentration increases and significant levels of circulating TNF are present [Kennedy, 1999]. Two types of soluble TNF receptors have been reported, STNFr-p55 and STNFr-p75, which can be released from the cell membrane by endotoxaemia [Bemelmanns, 1993]. These are natural inhibitors that bind circulating TNF, and turn it into a biologically inactive receptor-TNF complex. Increased concentrations of circulating TNFα were found in rats after bile duct ligation at 8 days, with a peak on day 16, but a biologically active form was not detected by bioassay, suggesting that the circulating TNFα existed in an inactive complex [Bemelmanns, 1996]. A rapid increase in the sTNFr concentration was seen after 12 days of biliary obstruction in rats, while renal function did not seem to be affected.

The presence of inactivated TNF and the increased concentration of sTNFr were indicative of an ongoing inflammatory process. In addition, sTNFr concentrations correlated with mortality. High concentrations of circulating TNF and relatively low concentration of sTNFr were seen in jaundiced patients who had a poor immediate outcome [Puntis, 1997]. Considering that the TNF-sTNFr complex is biologically inactive, the imbalance between TNF production and sTNFr in jaundiced patients may be deleterious. Various types of cells such as macrophages, monocytes, neutrophils, and fibroblasts produce IL-6, which has a major stimulatory effect on the synthesis of hepatic acute phase proteins, but also plays a part in T and B cell activation, and the induction of fever. Increased concentrations of IL-6 are also seen in rats with biliary obstruction [Houdijk AP, 1996].

Many other inflammatory mediators are likely to play a role in obstructive jaundice. Transforming growth factor β (TGFβ) is a growth factor present in platelets and also released by different inflammatory cells, having a role in wound healing, reducing protease activity, but increasing collagen deposition and induction of apoptosis [Miyoshi, 1998]. It is one of the suppressor cytokines. IL-1 is a major proinflammatory cytokine produced by monocytes, macrophages, neutrophils, B-lymphocytes, and endothelial cells. In response to endotoxin, IL-1 contributes to release of inflammatory mediators and procoagulant activity of endothelial cell [Fisher, 1994]. Monocytes from peripheral blood in jaundiced patients produced increased amounts of IL-6 and TNFα but not IL-1β and TGFβ in response to LPS stimuli, despite increased concentrations of TGFβ in serum, implying that other sources were producing the IL-1. Raised plasma concentrations of TNFα and IL-6 are associated with a poor immediate outcome in jaundiced patients [Puntis, 1996]. An exaggerated cytokine response after hepatectomy was reported in jaundiced patients with biliary obstruction, particularly in those who developed postoperative septic complications [Kimura, 1998]. The decreased production of Il-1 and IL-2 by stimulated peripheral monocytes, as reported in jaundiced patients with gastrointestinal carcinomas, improved after percutaneous transhepatic common duct drainage (PTCD), though no beneficial effect on survival could be assigned to the use of external drainage [Haga, 1989].

Interleukin-6 has been demonstrated to have most pro- as well as anti-inflammatory effects. Mononuclear phagocytes from both innate and adaptive immunity mainly produce IL-6. Unlike most cytokines, is more readily detected systemically, and thus may be used as a marker of tissue injury helping to identify patients with systemic inflammation. Significantly higher concentrations of IL-6 have been reported in the bile of jaundiced patients after ineffective as opposed to effective PTCD. As IL-6 concentrations in bile did not correlate with those in serum, it was suggested that biliary IL-6 originated from inflammatory cells or the epithelium of the biliary ducts rather than from Kupffer cells. Subclinical biliary infection, liver dysfunction, and advanced age promoted IL-6 production in jaundiced patients [Kimura, 1999].

Interleukin-12 is produced by monocytes, macrophages, and B cells. It induces interferon γ (IFNγ) production of NK and T cells, improves NK and ADCC activity and has a role in proliferation and differentiation of T-helper cells [Jiang, 1996]. Furthermore, IL-12 has a suppressive effect on tumour growth and on the induction of systemic immunity. A significant increase in production of IL-12 by isolated monocytes from jaundiced patients was seen in response to LPS, suggesting a possible role of IL-12 in the immunological changes that accompany jaundice [Tahara, 1994].

Various types of cells, including macrophages, endothelial cells, neutrophils, hepatocytes, and fibroblasts produce IL-8, which plays a major part in the regulation of transendothelial migration of polymorphonuclear leucocytes and the increase of their chemotactic activity [Hisama, 1995]. Increased IL-8 production in isolated Kupffer cells that were harvested from rats with biliary obstruction after hypoxic and reoxygenation challenge, was reported compared with those from control animals. As obstructive jaundice induces IL-8 production by Kupffer cells during hypoxia and reperfusion, IL-8 inhibition was suggested to be potentially beneficial for the prevention of ischaemia and reperfusion injury [Okamura, 1999].

Neutrophils

Neutrophils play a major role in the first line of host defense against bacteria. Dysfunction of leucocytes may be responsible for the septic complications in cholestatic patients. It has been postulated that cholestasis affects the function of neutrophils by impeding chemotaxis, rolling, adhesion, transmigration, priming, phagocytosis, and reactive oxygen metabolite production. A priming effect of various cytokines has been reported. IL-8 regulates transendothelial migration of polymorphonuclear leucocytes [Edwards JCW, 1981] and an upregulation of the IL-8 receptor by endotoxin has also been reported [Manna SK, 1995]. However, studies of the effects of biliary obstruction on neutrophil function have given controversial results, which can be explained partly by differences in the models that were used. Levy et al. demonstrated enhanced superoxide production, phagocytosis, and chemotaxis [Levy 1993]. The results suggest neutrophil overactivity in obstructive jaundice. The findings were confirmed by other groups [Tsuji, 1999] [Yamamoto, 1998]. On the other hand other studies have shown that the neutrophil function is impaired in obstructive jaundice. Tjandra et al. demonstrated phagocytic dysfunction and impaired bacterial killing by neutrophils, as well as depressed superoxide generation [Tjandra, 1997]. In the study of Li et al. has also been demonstrated that leukocyte count rises sharply after bile duct ligation [Li, 2003]. The increase in leukocyte count is mainly due to an increase in neutrophils and monocytes. Despite an increase in the number of phagocytes, the phagocytic function, as measured by ingestion of microspheres, was depressed. This was consistent with the findings by Roughneen et al. in which leucocytes harvested from the peritoneal cavity of rats with obstructive jaundice showed decreased phagocytosis [Roughneen, 1989]. In the analyses of oxygen metabolism Li et al. found that neutrophils seem to be in an inactivated state for H_2O_2. Hydrogen peroxide production by neutrophils decreased to about 40% in jaundiced rats compared with sham rats, although the difference was not statistically significant. Tjandra et al. also found that neutrophil superoxide production was decreased in obstructive jaundice by 30-50% [Tjandra, 1997]. Together, these findings indicate that the intracellular H_2O_2 generation by polymorphonuclear neutrophils was reduced in c-holestasis. On the contrary, H_2O_2 generation by the mononuclear cells -lymphocytes and monocytes- was increased in obstructive jaundice. These findings suggest that polymorphonuclear cells and mononuclear cells seem to possess different functions of releasing intracellular H_2O_2 in rats with obstructive jaundice. The meaning of these findings is unclear. Cellular immunity alterations in terms of phagocytic dysfunction and deranged intracellular H_2O_2 production by leukocytes may contribute to the high incidence of septic complications associated with obstructive jaundice.

In human neutrophils, the oxidative response of cells obtained from jaundiced patients, stimulated by formyl-methionyl-leucyl-phenylalanine (fmlp), increased compared with controls [Jiang, 1994]. The free radical mediated apoptotic cellular injury is thought to be mediated by a cycle involving activation of nuclear factor kappa B (NFκB) and proinflammatory cytokines [Liu, 2001]. An extremely high oxidative response was detected in patients who died. The priming effect of various cytokines, such as TNFα, IL-1, IL-6, IL-8 and granulocyte macrophage colony stimulating factor (GM-CSF), for the oxidative response of neutrophils under stimulation with fmlp, was measured by chemiluminescence. TNF and IL-8 were intense primers of control neutrophils, while IL-6 and GM-CSF were relatively weak. In neutrophils obtained from jaundiced patients, IL-6, IL-8, and TNFα failed to have a further priming effect, unlike IL-1 and GM-CSF [Jiang, 1994].

Higher plasma concentrations of IL-6, IL-8, and TNFα have been found in patients with biliary obstruction [Puntis, 1996], while GM-CSF and IL-1 concentrations were not raised in jaundiced patients. The accumulation of polymorphonuclear leucocytes in the sinusoidal spaces [Ohtsuka, 2000], impaired microvascular perfusion [Scott-Conner, 1993], and increased neutrophil-endothelium interaction may account for liver damage in patients with obstructive jaundice. High concentrations of IL-8-like chemoattractant (cytokine-induced neutrophil chemoattractant – (CINC) were seen concurrently with the accumulation of neutrophils in the hepatic sinusoids after two weeks of bile duct ligation despite the upregulation absence of intercellular adhesion molecule-1 (ICAM-1). The expression of adhesion receptors (L-selectin) on neutrophils obtained from patients with obstructive jaundice was significantly lower in jaundiced patients than in controls. In response to various concentrations of fmlp or polysaccharide, stimulated neutrophils from jaundiced patients expressed significantly less CD11b. These data imply a defect in neutrophil function in obstructive jaundice in humans [Ohtsuka, 1997]. The expression of adhesion molecules on endothelial cells also contributes to adhesion. ICAM-1 in liver tissue in rats [Koeppel, 1997] and sICAM-1 [Polzien, 1996] expression in humans was upregulated in biliary obstruction, and the expression could be induced by proinflammatory cytokines on the surface of various cell types [Cruick-shank, 1998] [Deitch, 1990]. ICAM-1 on sinusoidal endothelial cells was, however, weakly expressed after two weeks of bile duct ligation [Ohtsuka, 1997], but increased expression was detected after a major operation, suggesting that cytokines and not jaundice participate in the induction of ICAM-1 expression on the surface of the sinusoidal endothelial cells.

The serum purine nucleoside phosphorylase:alanine transaminase ratio, which is a marker of sinusoidal endothelial cell injury, was significantly higher in jaundiced rats, at the same time as the upregulation of ICAM-1. These data suggest a role for neutrophil accumulation in the sinusoidal spaces in sinusoidal cell injury during ICAM-1 overexpression in obstructive jaundice. Platelet activating factor (PAF) increased adhesion to and migration out of postcapillary mesenteric venules and neutrophils in controls, while this was not seen in jaundiced animals. Higher concentrations of PAF, however, induced a similar adhesion in both the jaundiced and control groups [Swain, 1995]. Plasma from animals with biliary obstruction reduced adhesion of neutrophils by phorbol myristate acetate (P-MA) in both control and jaundiced animals, suggesting that there is a plasma factor that is responsible for the antiadhesive effect on neutrophils in jaundice [Swain, 1995]. Numerous studies have investigated the role of toxic agents [Biltzer, 1994] and elastase [Sun, 1999] derived from neutrophils on endothelial cell injury. From *in vitro* studies on human neutrophils elastase was thought to be the major cause of neutrophil-mediated endothelial cell injury. No difference was seen in neutrophil elastase production between jaundiced and control subjects. Biliary decompression resulted in increased elastase production [Shimizu, 1997]. Data obtained from patients with obstructive jaundice undergoing endoscopic biliary drainage showed that obstructive jaundice seems to result in neutrophil overactivity, which is however reduced, by biliary drainage [Takaoka, 2001].

Cellular immunity and humoral immunity

Although lymphocytes are one of the most important parts of the immune system, the changes in the population have been rather less well studied in jaundiced patients. In animal models cellular immunity measured by the effect of the mitogens, concanavalin-A (ConA) and phytohaemagglutinin on the uptake of ^{3}H-thymidine by lymphocytes harvested from the rat spleen was significantly lower in lymphocytes from rats with ligated bile duct, while this suppression of cellular immunity was not found in germ-free rats after bile duct ligation. A low dose of endotoxin resulted in impaired cellular immunity in both conventional and germ-free rats [Jiang, 1997]. These data implied that gut-derived endotoxin might be involved in the suppression of cellular immunity in jaundice.

Patients with obstructive jaundice of either benign or malignant etiology have increased concentrations of circulating IgA that correlate with increased C3 levels [Oshio, 1986]. The role of the decreased concentration of sIgA in gut lumen is uncertain, as only about 1% of it is transported by bile in humans [Brown, 1989]. On the other hand, specific IgA secretion into bile can be seen in response to various antigen challenges in the gut lumen in rats [Reynoso-Paz, 1999]. Increased deposition of IgA in the glomerular basement membrane is seen in a large proportion of jaundiced patients and animal models [Kawaguchi, 1987], which may be explained by the lack of an immune-complex clearing effect by bile during biliary obstruction.

V. HAEMOSTASIS IMPAIRMENT IN PATIENTS WITH OBSTRUCTIVE JAUNDICE

An introduction to the pathophysiology of haemostasis impairment in obstructive jaundice

As part of the multifactorial role of liver in protein synthesis, many coagulation factors (fibrinogen, prothrombin, V, VII, VIII, IX, X, XI, XII, XIII, prekallikrein, HMWK), natural anticoagulants (antithrombin-III, heparin cofactor-II, Protein C, protein S, TFPI-1, TFPI-2), and compounds of the fibrinolytic system (plasminogen, a_2-antiplasmin, TAFI) are produced in the liver. A prolonged liver disease, either biliary obstruction or parenchymal liver disease, is thus accompanied by abnormal clotting, as most usually measured by the prothrombin time and the International Normalized Ratio (INR).

The impaired production of coagulation factors by damaged hepatocytes is superimposed by the poor absorption of vitamin K due to the absence of bile in the gut. Vitamin K is an essential cofactor for a microsomal enzyme that catalyzes the post-translational carboxylation of multiple, specific, peptide-bound glutamic acid residues in inactive hepatic precursors of factors II, VII, IX, and X. The resulting gamma-carboxyglutamic acid residues convert the precursors into active coagulation factors that are subsequently secreted by liver cells into the blood.

Despite oral (along with bile acids) or parenteral vitamin K administration in patients with obstructive jaundice, the surgeon might still face difficulty in overcoming haemostasis impairment in these patients. Bleeding episodes or thrombotic events may further complicate a jaundiced patient. These manifestations need careful clinical and laboratory approach for an accurate diagnosis to be established and an effective treatment to be offered.

Bacterial translocation plays a key role in the pathophysiology of haemostasis impairment in patients obstructive jaundice. Numerous studies have demonstrated that obstructive jaundice significantly promotes bacterial translocation in animal models [Ding JW, 1992] as well as in humans [Kuzu MA, 1999]. In these cases gut derived bacteria and endotoxins can cross the mucosal barrier and reach mesenteric lymph nodes or other distant tissues, thus causing a systemic inflammatory response. As a consequence, septic complications and multiple organ failure evolve in a considerably high percentage of these patients. The triggering of coagulation cascade, mainly via tissue factor pathway, is a key parameter for the final outcome; the extreme and unbalanced production of tissue factor (mainly by tissue factor pathway inhibitor) and the subsequent uncontrolled extrinsic tenase complex activation may lead even to clinically evident thrombotic events and/or disseminated intravascular coagulation.

Systemic inflammation is also present in two chronic liver diseases with cholestasis; primary biliary cirrhosis and primary sclerosing cholangitis, where a hypercoagulable state has been documented [Van Thiel DH, 2004].

Apart from septic/inflammatory complications, which result in hypercoagulability, the underlying pathology is crucial in determining additional pathophysiological pathways of haemostasis impairment in obstructive jaundice. It is well known that malignant diseases, which are presented by obstructive jaundice, and especially adenocarcinomas of the pancreas, may affect coagulation in various ways. Additionally, acute pancreatitis (which may result from choledocholithiasis) has been demonstrated to be accompanied by a prethrombotic state, mainly due to platelet stimulation [Mimidis, 2004 a,b].

Thus, the above mentioned mechanisms that affect haemostasis in obstructive jaundice are discussed in four paragraphs: The first one refers to vitamin K insufficiency in obstructive jaundice, the second describes the effect of ongoing liver fibrosis and cirrhosis on haemostasis, the third analyzes the interlinkage of sepsis and haemostasis and its clinical significance in patients with obstructive jaundice and the fourth focuses on certain entities that manifest with obstructive jaundice and may by themselves interfere with the haemostatic mechanism.

Vitamin K deficiency in obstructive jaundice

Vitamin K is an essential co-factor for synthesis of factors II, VII, IX and X, as well as proteins C, S and Z, as it catalyzes gamma-carboxylation of glutamic acid in their amino-terminal region. The reduction of these proteins in plasma may reflect vitamin K deficiency; this situation is not caused by liver injury *per se* but is frequently associated with liver disease. In fact, the molecular result of severe vitamin K deficiency is the production of decardoxylated precursors, named PIVKA (precursors induced by vitamin K absence), which are of diminished activity [Amitrano, 2002].

Vitamin K is a fat-soluble vitamin requiring bile salts for its absorption from the gut. The intestinal bacterial flora is involved as well, either participating in the biliary salt metabolism or producing small amounts of vitamin K. Thus, reduced intestinal absorption of vitamin K occurs during intra- or extrahepatic cholestasis [Sherlock S, 1970] resulting to vitamin K deficiency in patients with obstructive jaundice; these patients often present haemorrhagic diathesis despite the presence of a merely normal coagulation profile as estimated by prothrombin time [O'Brien DP, 1994]. Apart from prothrom-

bin time, measurement of PIVKA levels (and especially PIVKA-II, or des-gamma-carboxylated prothrombin) has been used for the assessment of the severity of vitamin K deficiency but this procedure is prone to errors if hepatocellular carcinoma has not been carefully excluded. The parenteral administration of 10 mg vitamin K replenishes rerum levels, normalizes prothrombin time and prevents from bleeding episodes.

Progressive hepatic failure and cirrhosis

As liver fibrosis evolves and hepatic failure is settled in a cirrhotic environment, a generalized derangement of haemostasis becomes evident through laboratory tests and, later on, through clinical signs and symptoms. The ongoing proccess toward cirrhosis in a patient with cholestasis is rare in malignant diseases, as the time is too short in most cases. Nevertheless, in other benign models of obstructive jaundice, as primary sclerosing cholangitis, cirrhosis is the inevitable result. The possibility of chirrosis should be evaluated in every patient who has a medical record of chronic cholestatic syndrome of undetermined etiology.

The presence of thrombocytopenia in cirrhosis is profound and is mainly explained by the increased platelet sequestration in the enlarging spleen (congestive splenomegaly) [Aster RH, 1966]. Moreover, a reduction in thrombopoietin levels has been suggested to contribute to this anomaly, as liver transplantation increases thrombopoietin levels and reverses thrombocytopenia independently of the size of spleen [Peck-Radosavljevic M, 2000]. Nevertheless, conflicting results regarding plasma trombopoietin levels in chronic and acute liver failure have been published [Goulis, 1999], [Stockelberg D, 1999], [Koike, 1998]. Other causes for thrombocytopenia as reduced platelet half-life [Stein SF, 1982], presence of autoantibodies, especially in patients with primary biliary cirrhosis or sclerosing cholangitis [Pereira J, 1995], folic acid deficiency and [Lindenbaum J, 1980], ethanol toxicity on megacaryopoiesis [Levine RF, 1986], especially in alcohol abusers have been proposed. Finally, the presence of even low-grade disseminated intravascular coagulation is still debatable [Ben-Ari Z, 1999].

Platelet function defects are often encountered in patients with chronic or acute liver disease. *In vitro* platelet aggregation in response to ADP, arachidonic acid, collagen, and thrombin has been shown to be defective [Escolar G, 1999], [Laffi G, 1988]. Also, platelet-vessel wall interaction studied under flow conditions has been shown to be impaired [Ordinas A, 1996]. Impaired aggregation might be caused by defective platelet signal transduction mechanisms [Laffi G, 1993], an acquired storage pool deficiency [Laffi G, 1992], and decreased levels of arachidonic acid (required for thromboxane A2 production) in the platelet membrane [Owen JS, 1981]. Furthermore, increased production of prostacyclin and nitric oxide (both powerful platelet inhibitors) by endothelial cells may contribute to impaired platelet function *in vivo* [Guarner C, 1992], [Albornoz L, 1999]. Finally, platelet-vessel wall interaction may be defective in patients with liver disease due to proteolysis of platelet receptors by plasmin [Michelson AD, 1990], [Pasche B, 1994], or due to the presence of a reduced haematocrit [Turitto VT, 1975].

Apart from platelet defects, decrased synthesis of coagulation factors is observed in patients with liver impairment. Merely all proteins that constitute coagulation cascade, are synthesized in the liver and for many of them liver is the exclusive site of production. The degree of the reduction of the procoagulants is related to the severity of liver damage, bleeding diathesis and, finally, prognosis. Usual coagulation tests are not affected until plasma levels of the relevant factors fall below 30-40% of normal and the specific tests for each factor, although available, are not very informative in the routine clinical practice. As factor V and especially VII have the shorter half-lives (12 and 4-6 hours, repsectively), their determination might be helpful in acute liver failure. As factor VII and fibrinogen are acute phase proteins, they are initially increased and their substantial decrease might underline the presence of disseminated intravascular coagulation.

The main qualitative disorder that may accompany liver failure is dysfibrinogeanemia, which is characterized by abnormal polymerization of fibrin monomers as a consequence of hypersyalilation of the fibrinogen molecule.

Advanced liver disease is also characterized by the presence of hyperfibrinolysis, which is revealed by the shortened euglobin clot lysis time and elevated levels of D-dimers, FDPs and fibrin and attributed mainly to the reduced clearance of fibrinolytic agents, mainly tPA. Additionally, low levels of α_2-antiplasmin and thrombin activatable fibrinolysis inhibitor (due to the impaired protein production from hepatocytes) may contribute to the progressive enhancement of this phenomenon [Van Thiel DH, 2001]. Whether hyperfibrinolysis is totally a primary procedure or is partly an effect of the continuous triggering of coagulation has not been answered yet [Violi F, 1993], [Car JM, 1989], [Hersch SL, 1987].

In a recent study, an exhaustive analysis of primary and secondary haemostatic mechanism in 32 cirrhotic patients showed that all variables except fibrinogen, factor XIII, plasminogen inhibitor and TFPI were impaired. PFA-100 closure time after ADP stimulation, PT activity, factor X, factor V, fibrin and plasminogen were independently correlated with the severity of cirrhosis and decline from normal mean in the early stages of the disease, suggesting that haemostasis impairment is present even in subclinical cirrhosis [Papadopoulos, 2004].

Despite that the net outcome of the alteration in the haemostatic system in cirrhotic patients is a bleeding diathesis, thrombosis of the portal vein has been frequently observed in these patients; thus, in case of a sudden deterioration of a cirrhotic patient, portal vein thrombosis should be carefully excluded from differential diagnosis [Belli L, 1986]. However, the development of thrombosis might be attributed to local circulation parameters and mainly to the reduced blood flow in the protal vein. This aspect is enhanced by the findings of a recent study, which suggests that the feared coagulopathy in cirrhotics is more a myth than a reality, as these patients generate adequate thrombin when endogenous thrombin potential assay is performed [Tripodi A, 2005], [Bosch J, 2005].

Systemic inflammation/sepsis and haemostasis impairment in patients with obstructive jaundice - the central role of tissue factor

The occurence of disseminated intravascular coagulation in obstructive jaundice and its relation to biliary tract infection has been early recognized [Takeda S, 1977]. Elevated plasma levels of endotoxin, cytokines and C-reactive protein in patients with obstructive jaundice and positive bile cultures were temporarily improved after drainage [Padillo FI, 2002]. Infection enhances the production of the cytokines interleukin-1 (IL-1), IL-6, and tumor necrosis factor that are able to activate clotting and fibrinolysis [Grignani G, 2000] via stimulation of the extrinsic pathway. Endotoxins, produced by bacteria, stimulate tissue factor expression on macrophages

and clotting activation via an oxidative process [Basili S, 1999], [Saliola M, 1998]. A relationship has been demonstrated between tissue factor levels and markers of lipid peroxidation, clotting activation, and fibrinolysis in cirrhotic patients [Ferro D, 1999]. Hyperfibrinolysis delays clotting activation through clotting factor consumption and inhibition of fibrin polymerization and reduces platelet adhesion and aggregation as well [Okajima K, 2000]. Platelet functions are further impaired by increased prostacyclin levels, which are induced by endotoxin and endothelin via nitric oxide formation [Goulis J, 1999]. How these phenomena induced by sepsis can trigger bleeding remains speculative and requires further study.

The relationship between coagulation and inflammation is still poorly understood. Blood clotting, apart from leading to fibrin deposition and platelet activation, results in vascular cell activation, thus contributing to leukocyte activation [Amaral A, 2004]. On the other hand, sepsis and septic shock is well known to provoke activation of the extrinsic coagulation pathway, as has been clinically shown by ELISA measurements of tissue factor in septic patients [Gando S, 1998]. Tissue factor over-expression is normally compromised by tissue factor pathway inhibitor (TFPI) [Doshi SN, 2002]. Nevertheless, septic patients who present insufficient TFPI balancing mechanism, have poor prognosis as the over-production of tissue factor can not be outweighted [Gando S, 2002]. Other anticoagulants, as antithrombin and activated protein C have been found to exert antiinflammatory properties [Amaral A, 2004]. In fact, recombinant activated protein C (drotrecogin-alfa) has demonstrated direct activity in blocking thrombin formation, enhancing fibrinolysis and diminishing the expression of inflammatory molecules; under this profile, the drug is now indicated in severe sepsis (with APACHE II score ≥25 or more or with 2 or more organs with impaired function).

A potent pathway, which explains sepsis and coagulation pathways interference, is the stimulation of *F3* expression in peripheral blood cells and endothelium, which normally lack this mechanism, directly by LPS and peptidoglycans or indirectly by TNF-α, VEGF, IL-1β, IFN-1γ and many other inflammation mediators [Tapper H, 2000], [Lopes-Bezzera LM, 2003].

F3 is the gene coding for tissue factor. Tissue factor is a protein having a large extracellular domain (219 residues), a small transmembrane domain and a small cytoplasmic tail. Its role is to form a trimolecular complex with FVIIa and FX (activating FX) and thus initiating coagulation [McVey JH. 1999], [Riewald M, 2002]. F3 is expressed in normal conditions mainly in brain, lung, placenta and kidney and, after stimulation, in peripheral blood cells and endothelium. Trace amounts are detected in plasma [Giessen PLA, 1999]. The physiological importance of TF was demonstrated in experiments on transgenic mice, to which *F3* knocking-out had been lethal [Bugge TH, 1996].

F3 is also expressed with another splice variant, which includes *F3* exons 1, 2, 3, 4 and 6 and leads to the production of the alternatively spliced Human Tissue Factor (as-HTF). As-HTF is a protein, which lacks the transmembrane and cytoplasmic tail of TF and has a unique termination sequence due to the exons 4/6 fusion. Both TF and as-HTF share the same active catalytic domain and the same procoagulant properties, acting as propagators of the coagulation process in the borders of newly synthesized thrombi. TF is membrane-bound whereas as-HTF circulates freely [Bogdanov VY, 2003].

The role of tissue factor in the systemic inflammatory response accompanying cholestasis has been investigated in the elegant study of Semeraro *et al.* [Semerano, 1989]. These investigators studied the procoagulant activity of peripheral blood monocytes in 41 patients with severe obstructive jaundice and in 27 nonjaundiced control patients using a one-stage clotting assay. Mononuclear cells from jaundiced patients, tested immediately after isolation, expressed low levels of procoagulant activity, which were, however, significantly higher than in cells from controls (p <0.01). In addition, after incubation in short-term cultures with and without endotoxin, these cells generated more procoagulant activity than did the controls (p <0.001). No significant difference in procoagulant activity was found between patients with and without malignancy in either group. The relief of biliary obstruction resulted in the reduction of both serum bilirubin levels and monocyte procoagulant activity. Endotoxin-induced monocyte procoagulant activity was about threefold higher in the jaundiced patients who died than in the survivors (p <0.001). In rabbits made icteric by bile duct ligation and separation (15 days), the endotoxin-induced monocyte procoagulant activity was markedly increased as compared with sham-operated animals (p <0.005). In all instances, procoagulant activity was identified as tissue factor. The increased capacity of mononuclear phagocytes to produce procoagulant activity might explain the activation of blood coagulation in severe obstructive jaundice.

A well determined paradigm of how systemic inflammation, apart from true sepsis, can be interlinked with coagulation in clinical practice is chronic cholestatic liver disease due to primary biliary cirrhosis or primary sclerosing cholangitis. These entities are characterized by a better outcome of variceal bleeding and less blood loss in liver transplantation, suggesting the presence of a hypercoagulable state. During their course, levels of factors VIII and vW are increased, while proteins C, S, Z, antithrombin III, α_2 macroglobulin and heparin cofactor II are all reduced. This imbalance along with the presence of antiphospholipid, anticardiolipin and antineutrophil cytosolic autoantibodies in many patients favour hypercoagulability [Van Thiel DH, 2004]. In a recent study, hypercoagulability in non-cirrhotic patients with primary biliary cirrhosis and primary sclerosing cholangitis has been attributed to the elevated fibrinogen and the hyperactivity of platelets, which is not observed in non-cholestatic liver disease (chronic hepatitis C and alcoholic cirrhosis). These changes are believed to be the result of a marked systemic inflammatory activity; whether this phenomenon involves platelets directly or indirectly (through tissue factor expression) has not been clarified yet [Pihusch R, 2004].

Underlying pathology in patients with obstructive jaundice as an additional mechanism of haemostasis impairment

a. Pancreatic adenocarcinoma

Data from *in vitro* and *in vivo* studies show that coagulation cascade is activated in human pancreatic carcinoma. As a result of the intrinsic hypercoagulable state, pancreatic cancer is associated with a high risk of developing thromboembolic disease. Moreover, proteins that are part of the coagulation cascade have been proved to be important for angiogenesis; thus, induction of coagulation cascade leads also to the induction of angiogenetic signalling pathways. More specifically, tissue factor, apart from being the key molecule in the triggering of the extrinsic pathway of the coagulation cascade, leads to the upregulation of vascular endothelial growth factor (VEGF) and downregulation of thrombospondin, which serves as angiogenesis inhibitor. The role of tissue factor in the angiogenetic control

can explain why expression of tissue factor is associated with poor prognosis.

Hypercoagulability accompanying pancreatic cancer is created by three distinct mechanisms: 1) tumour cells stimulate platelet adhesiveness and aggregation *in situ,* a process which has been evaluated as essencial for the development and metastasis of the tumor, as activation of the coagulation pathway is interlinked with activation of angiogenesis pathway, 2) circulating carcinoma mucins (e.g. Ca 19-9) induce the formation of circulating microthrombi (without the participation of thrombin in that process) and thus contribute to the occlusive/ischaemic microangiopathy often observed in pancreatic cancer and 3) tumour cells produce various procoagulant factors, especially tissue factor and prothrombin.

In an interesting study, the expression of tissue factor was observed immunohistochemically in about one half of pancreatic tumors (29 out of 55 samples), but never in healthy pancreatic tissue (0 out of 18 samples). Moreover, tissue factor expression by tumor cells was found to correlate significantly with histological grade: while 77% of poorly differentiated tumours produced tissue factor, only 20% of well-differentiated tumours presented the same pattern [Kakkar AK, 1995]. In another study, the *in situ* formation of tissue factor, prothrombin and fibrinogen, has been demonstrated in pancreatic tumours; interestingly, both tissue factor pathway inhibitor and plasminogen activators had been found in trace quantities. These data can explain the prothrombotic potential that is generated *in situ* in cases of pancreatic tumours [Wojtukiewicz MZ, 2001].

Platelet aggregation induced by tumour cells is an important process for hematogenous metastasis, apart from contributing to the prothrombotic state. An *in vitro* study has demonstrated that malignant pancreatic cells can induce platelet aggregation with a thrombin-dependent mechanism [Heinmoller E, 1995]. A possible association between the cell-surface sialylation of tumour cells and their ability to aggregate platelets and induce thrombosis has been referred [Scialla SJ, 1979]. This observation is in keeping with newer data suggesting that the circulating carcinoma mucins, such as Ca 19-9, interact with platelet P-selectin and leukocyte L-selectin and that these interactions generate platelet-rich microthrombi without thrombin production. These process may well be inhibited by heparin but not by warfarin; thus, unfractionated or low-molecular-weight heparin is much more effective than oral anticoagulants in treating malignant disease associated with thrombosis [Wahrenbrock M, 2003].

Thrombotic events in portal vein may additionally compromise haemostasis through lowering platelet number as a result of pooling in the enlarging spleen. Portal vein thrombosis is a major complication of pancreatic carcinoma and in some cases it remains subclinical or unsymptomatic. In case of acute or increased abdominal pain, jaundice and progressive ascites in a patient with a medical record of pancreatic cancer, an abdominal CT would be useful to assess the diagnosis of portal vein thrombosis [Khorana AA, 2004].

b. Cholangiocarcinoma

Cholangiocarcinoma is a malignant disease of the biliary duct system, which progresses slowly, infiltrate the duct walls and leads to biliary tract obstruction. It has been reported that prothrombin time and activated partial thromboplastin time are important determinants for survival after surgery for cholangiocarcinoma [Nagorney DM, 1989]. Hui and coworkers found no significant difference in prothrombin time and activated partial thromboplastin time between cholangiocarcinoma patients with and without cirrhosis

[Hui CK, 2003]. In a recent study, a relation between prolongation of the activated partial thromboplastin time and aminotransferases (AST and ALT) was observed. As there were no significant correlation of the APTT anomaly with alkaline phosphatase or serumbilirubin, the investigators formulated the hypothesis that this bleeding tendency might be attributed to the excessive liver parenchymal involvement seen in the majority of patients and be treated as a form of hepatocellular failure [Wiwanitkit V, 2004].

c. Hepatocellular carcinoma

Although hepatocellular carcinoma seldom results in true obstructive jaundice, the cholestasis observed during its course is mainly attributed to damaged hepatocytes and progressive hepatic failure. Nevertheless, as this tumour is accompanied by various haemostatic derangements, it is included in this chapter mainly for differential diagnosis purposes.

Hepatocellular carcinoma results in dysfibrinogenaemia [Drin FG, 1976], an acquired disorder of haemostasis that is characterized by the presence of excessive number of syalic acid residues on the molecule of fibrinogen which interact with the enzymatic activity of thrombin and is caused by an increased activity of the enzyme syalil-transferase. This enzyme is fetal and can be reexpressed in tumour cells [Barr RD, 1978]. The clinical result of dysfibrinogenaemia is the production of abnormally polymerized fibrin, which leads to the disproportionally severe prolongation of thrombin time comparing with the mild prolongation of PT and PTT and the normal amounts of fibrinogen.

Additionally, a posttranslational defect in gamma carboxylation induced by tumour cells [Liebman HA, 1984] is considered to account for the elevated levels of decarboxylated prothrombin that characterize hepatocellular carcinoma [Weitz IC, 1993], [Nakao, 1991]. Decarboxylated prothrombin is antigenically identical to that produced during warfarin therapy. Moreover, elevated D-dimer levels have been detected in hepatocellular carcinoma and reflect the tumour stage and vascular invasion of the malignancy [Tseng CS, 2004]. The relation between haemostasis and tumour growth has been clinically evaluated in terms of heparin administration in patients with malignant diseases; similar trials are proposed for hepatocellular carcinoma [Zacharski LR, 2004].

Another mechanism of haemostasis impairment is the over-production of functionally intact factors of coagulation and fibrinolysis. A case report, which describes the immunohistochemically documented production of antithrombin-III by tumour hepatocellular carcinoma cells, to which haemorrhagic diathesis was attributed, is referred as a paradigm [Akiyama K, 1993].

Controversially, apoptotic hepatocellular carcinoma HepG2 cells have been demonstrated to accelerate blood coagulation through the expression of a phosphatidyl serine-dependent pro-coagulant surface in a recent study [Miyamoto Y, 2004]. These investigators took into consideration that a) intrasinusoidal microthrombosis is considered to be a cause of massive hepatocyte death in fulminant hepatic failure and b) generally, apoptotic cells express phosphatidyl serine outside the plasma membrane, which is also expressed on the surface of activated platelets and accelerates fibrin-thrombus formation; they thus postulated that the acceleration of blood coagulation on the surface of apoptotic hepatocytes may occur because hepatocytes are in direct contact with plasma that passes through fenestrations of the sinusoidal endothelium. The above mentioned hypothesis was tested by investigation of the coagulation activity of apoptotic hepatocytes. This mechanism may well contribute to the prothrombotic potential of acute or chronic hepatic failure and the rate of apoptosis may be a crucial parameter for this phenomenon.

d. Acute pancreatitis

The pathophysiology of acute pancreatitis has not been elucidated. Numerous mechanisms have been proposed to explain the initiation as well as the propagation of pancreatic tissue damage.

One theory is that of "oxidative stress", according to which the overproduction of free radicals, not neutralised by scavenger molecules, plays a crucial role in setting off the initial "spark" initiating pancreatitis. Another theory is the "self-digestion" process, which is claimed to be the result of activation of pancreatic enzymes inside the gland, as a consequence of restricted damage serving as "first hit".

What is intriguing is that, after the initiation of acute pancreatitis the same type of histological and biochemical derangements follow. Nevertheless, the ongoing procedure is characterized by a broad spectrum of manifestations varying from simple oedematous pancreatitis to necrotizing forms of the disease. A common denominator of these manifestations has been an increased thrombogenicity, documented as early as twenty years ago in hypothermic patients who presented intrapancreatic thrombosis. [Mikhailidis DP, 1983].

In a recent paper, a strong prognostic value was reported between extensive coagulation activation and poor outcome in severe necrotizing pancreatitis. Briefly, changes in protein C, antithrombin III (AT III), D-dimer and plasminogen activator inhibitor – 1 (PAI-1) levels indicating exhaustion of fibrinolysis and coagulation inhibitors, predicted a bad prognosis [Radenkovic D, 2004].

The latter is in keeping with the results of another recent article, where it was claimed that the D-dimers levels in plasma reflect the expression of pancreatitis and the extension of systemic involvement [Salomone T, 2003].

Two of our recently published articles assessed platelet activation in mild forms of acute pancreatitis. In the first study [Mimidis K, 2004 a], we focused on two successive end points: (i) the activation of platelets during acute pancreatitis and (ii) the alterations of platelet number and indexes between onset and remission of the disease, which reflect the bone marrow response. In a cohort of 54 patients with acute pancreatitis, activated platelet ratio (APR) was estimated using flow cytometry at onset and remission. The first end-point of the study, was reached at patient 14 as APR was found elevated at onset of acute pancreatitis (p = 0,01). The second endpoint was fulfilled at patient 12 for mean platelet volume (MPV), platelet large cell ratio (P-LCR) and platelet distribution width (PDW), which were found elevated at remission of the disease (p <0,01) but not for platelet number (PLT), until the last patient (p = 0,34). The elevated APR at the onset in combination with the elevation of the platelet indexes at later stages of acute pancreatitis may imply a direct involvement of platelets in the systemic inflammatory process of the disease, which leads to consumption compensated by an immediate bone marrow response.

In our second study [Mimidis K, 2004 b], we evaluated alterations of platelet function by using a recently developed platelet function analyser (PFA-100TM). Sixteen patients with acute edemetous pancreatitis were studied along with 32 normal controls. The hemostatic capacity of platelets was tested in citrated blood and standard cartridges containing collagen-ADP or collagen-epinephrine. A statistically significant shortening of the collagen-ADP closure time, but not of that of the collagen-epinephrine time was noted. These findings confirm an increased platelet adhesiveness and aggregation in the early stages of the inflammatory process of acute pancreatitis, which may underline the prethrombtic potential of the disease.

Evidence supports a role for thrombosis in the ongoing process of pancreatic tissue damage. What remained unclear until recently was the exact mechanism of coagulation initiation. One study evaluated coagulation activation after islet transplantation and the subsequent release of insulin. Even in the absence of signs of intraportal thrombosis, they concluded that the endocrine, but not the exocrine, cells of the pancreas synthesise and secrete active tissue factor (TF). The clotting reaction triggered by pancreatic islets in vitro could be abrogated by blocking the active site of TF with specific antibodies or site-inactivated factor VIIa, a candidate drug for inhibition of TF activity in vivo. Thus, blockade of TF could represent a new therapeutic approach that might increase the success of islet transplantation in patients with type 1 diabetes, in terms of both the risk of intraportal thrombosis and the need for islets from more than one donor [Moberg L, 2002].

These results are supported by the demonstration that pancreatic duct cells can produce TF, possibly explaining graft rejection following islet transplantation when islet preparations are not 100% devoid of any epithelial cells [Beuneu C, 2004]. The destruction of epithelial pancreatic duct cells due to mechanical reasons in pancreatitis, especially of biliary etiology, might account for the enhanced primary heamostasis observed in the latter [Mimidis K, 2004 a].

Therefore, even minimal pancreatic tissue damage, including epithelial components, may trigger TF-dependent coagulation initiation. This may not be limited to local thrombotic events, but can practically initiate a systemic inflammation process (SIRS) involving upregulation of adhesion molecule expression and chemokine production. At this point, the role of platelet activating factor (PAF), together with other proinflammatory cytokines such as IL-1b, IL-6, IL-8, TNF-α and the anti-inflammatory cytokines IL-2 and IL-10, in the pathogenesis of SIRS should not be underestimated [Zhou W, 1993]; PAF increases vascular permeability, induces leukocyte infiltration, oedema and tissue injury, and has a negative inotropic effect [Emanuelli G, 1989]. A propagation phase, through a mechanism of positive feedback loop, might result in systemic manifestations of unpredictable extent [Johnson GB, 2004], [Hirota M, 2004].

What new question that arises is whether SIRS, well known to accompany acute pancreatitis, is a result of the key role of TF in interlinking between coagulation and inflammation. TF is produced in two forms: the first represents a cell-bound molecule having a transmembrane region and the second a soluble molecule lacking this transmembrane domain as a result of alternative splicing (as-HTF) [Bogdanov VY, 2003].

Although TF has been shown to act as an adhesion molecule, cytokine receptor and signal transduction molecule, enhancing the inflammatory process, its splice variant asTF probably lack these attributes, serving only as propagator of coagulation [Versteeg HH. 2004].

Another molecule, TFPI (Tissue Factor Pathway Inhibitor) impedes TF function [Price GC, 2004]. Thus, while the ratio (TF+as-HTF)/TFPI indicates the thrombotic potenitial, the TF/as-HTF ratio is a measure of balance between thrombosis and inflammation. Measuring TF/as-HTF in early stages of acute pancreatitis would enable us to propose whether the interlinkage between thrombosis and inflammation is impaired towards one direction.

What is the real consequence of the thrombosis of the microvasculature during acute pancreatitis? As preventing further complications remains a major therapeutic goal for patients suffering from the disease, the role of antithrombotic agents cannot be underestimated. Indeed, many recent articles focus on the usefulness of low molecular weight heparin during the course of acute pancreatitis. An anti-TF monoclonal antibody, having been clinically tested in sepsis with debatable success, still remains to be evaluated in acute pancreatitis. Moreover, biosynthetic TFPI may be proven useful in controlling the rapid extra-pancreatic tissue damage that can follow an episode of acute pancreatitis.

Treatment of haemostatic abnormalities in patients with obstructive jaundice

Vitamin K deficiency is likely in patients with cholestatic disease. A dose of 10 mg of vitamin K for 3 days is likely to correct prothrombin time prolongation in these patients. The intravenous administration of vitamin K has the risk of anaphylaxis. Subcutaneous administration is characterized by an inconstant rate of absorption and intramascular injection should be avoided because of the risk of hematomas.

Low platelet count is not believed to be threatening when platelet number exceeds 50.000/µl. Whenever platelet number falls beyond this limit during a bleeding episode or before a surgical procedure, platelet transfusion is advisable. One unit of platelet concentrate increases the peripheral platelet count by about 10.000/µl. The increase in platelet count is less in patent with hypersplenism, as the majority of the transfused platelets are sequestrated in the enlarges spleen. Recombinant trhombopoietin for the correction of platelet count in cirrhotics is still under investigation.

Prolonged bleeding time, mainly attributed to low platelet count, may be reversed by the administration of 0.3 µg/kg of 1-deamino-8-D-arginine vasopressin (D-DVAP), especially when surgical procedures should be undertaken. Although D-DVAP increases the plasma levels of factor VIII and vWF, the exact mechanism of DDVAP action remains unknown.

Deficiencies in coagulation factors may be corrected by fresh frozen plasma [Markus M, 2002]; administration of 10 to 20 ml/kg body weight may curtail prothrombin time prolongation to less tnah 3 seconds. Nevertheless, the correction of coagulopathy lasts no more than 12-24 hours (as FVII has a half-life of only 4-6 hours); the lack of correction after adequate fresh frozen plasma transfusion indicates the presence of dysfibrinogenemia or FDPs. Fluid overload is a frequent complication in fresh frozen plasma administration as large quantities (1-1,5 lt) may be needed. Besides, the risk of infection can not be underestimated; solvent detergent-treated plasma reduces this possibility, but is devoid of factor VIII, proteins S and C and $α_2$-antiplasmin.

Instead of fresh frozen plasma infusion, plasma exchange has been used with simiral results regarding the treatment of coagulopathy without the risk of volume overload [Sallah S, 1999].

As an alternatively solution, the infusion of prothrombin concentrates, containing only the vitamin K dependent coagulation factors, may only partly correct the coagulopathy and have the risk of thromboembolic complications and disseminated intravascular coagulation.

Cryoprecipitates contain factors VIII and XIII, fibrinogen, vWF and fibronectin. One unit of cryoprecipitate (20-30 ml) is enough for every 10 kg of body weight. The administration of cryoprecipitates is indicated when plasma fibrinogen levels fall below 100 mg/dl as a consequence of disseminated intravascular coagulation or massive blood transfusion.

A new approach is the administration of recombinant activated factor VII (rFVIIa). In preliminary reports, a dose of 80 µg/kg normalized prothrombin time for more than 12 hours in patients with cirrhosis. However, the prolongation of the prothrombin time induced by the rFVIIa does not necessarily reflect hemostatic efficacy and care must be taken in patients with subclinical disseminated intravascular coagulation [Caldwell SDH, 2004].

In cases of a hyperfibrinolysis syndrome and concomitant bleeding, the need for antifibrinolytic agents as ε-aminocaproic acid, tranexamic acid or aprotinin should be estimated. Again thromboembolic events are a major threat; thus, the use of these agents must stop after the successful managenet of haemostasis. Aprotinin has the lower relative risk for these complications [Parekh, 2001].

Conclusion

The potent haemostatic derangement in a patient with obstructive jaundice is multifactorial and difficult to assess. A general rule is that a doctor has to treat the patient, not the laboratory findings; thus, the information given by the coagulation assays should be carefully studied and interpreted through the clinical practice.

An uncomplicated benign cholestasis which is prolonged will drive to haemorrhagic diathesis; prophylactic administration of vitamin K should be administered in these cases. If septic complications and/or pancreatic involvement is superimposed, the net effect on haemostasis might be a prothrombotic state; thus, low-molecular-weight heparin might be helpful in selected patients.

Unresolved cholestasis may progressively lead to liver dysfunction and evolution of cirrhosis; in these cases, more generalized haemostatic disorders affecting practically all pathways are observed; thrombocytopenia, decreased synthesis and clearance of coagulation factors and inhibitors, dysfibrinogenemia, hyperfibrinolysis and overt disseminated intravascular coagulation along with portal vein stasis and thrombosis may converge to a single patient. The consultation of a haematologist concerning the administration of platelets, fresh frozen plasma, cryoprecipitates, prothrombin complex precipitates, recombinant factor VII, D-DVAP or antifibrinolytic agents is thought to be essential when treating such a patient.

When malignancy has been documented, the situation is more complicated. Mucuous adenocarcinomas (eg. of the pancreas or the colon) and hepatocellular carcinomas can induce activation of haemostasis; thromboembolic events, es-pecially in the former, are usual and serious complicating events resulting in poor prognosis. The use of low-molecular weight heparin fractions in these patients, apart from preventing thrombosis and embolism, may compromise tumour growth through inhibition of a tissue-factor mediated angiogenesis mechanism.

Understanding the pathophysiology of haemostatic changes in patients with cholestasis, and, more generally, liver disease, is the hallmark of accurate diagnosis and treatment. Thus, the combination of good knowledge with close inspection of every patient could lead to the most promising result.

REFERENCES

I. OVERVIEW OF HAEMOSTASIS

Berndt MC, Shen Y, Dopheide AM, *et al.* The vascular biology of the glycoprotein Ib-IX-V complex. Thromb Haemost 2001;86:178-188

Caldwell SH, Chang C, Macik BG. Recombinant activated factor VII (rFVIIa) as a hemostatic agent in liver disease: a break from convention in need of controlled trials. Hepatology 2004;39:592-8

Savage B, Shattil SJ, Ruggeri ZM. Modulation of platelet function through adhesion receptors: a dual role for glycoprotein IIb-IIIa (integrin alpha IIb beta 3) mediated by fibrinogen and glycoprotein Ib-von Willebrand factor. J Biol Chem 1992;267:11300-11306

Watson SP. Collagen receptor signalling in platelets and megakaryocytes. Thromb Haemost 1999; 82:365-376

II. AN INTRODUCTION TO THE PHYSIOLOGY OF IMMUNE SYSTEM

Parish CR, O'Neill ER: Dependence of the adaptive immune response on innate immunity: some questions answered but new paradoxes emerge. Immunol Cell Biol 1997;75:523-7

Yuan Q, Walker WA: Apoptosis and the regulation of cell number in normal and neoplastic tissues: an overview. Cancer Metastasis Rev 1992;11:95-103

III. AN INTRODUCTION TO THE PATHOPHYSIOLOGY OF OBSTRUCTIVE JAUNDICE

Beckingham IJ, Ryder SD. ABC of diseases of liver, pancreas, and biliary system: Investigation of liver and biliary disease. BMJ 2001;322:33-36

Braciale TJ, Braciale VL. Antigen presentation : structural themes and functional variations. Immunol Today 1991;12:124-9

Lien E, Ingalls RR: Toll-like receptors. Crit Care Med 2002;30:1-11

Romagnani S. Type 1 T helper and type 2 T helper cells: functions, regulation and role in protection and disease. Int J Clin Lab Res 1991;21: 152-8

Scott-Conner CEH, Grogan JB. The pathophysiology of biliary obstruction and its effect on phagocytic and immune function. J Surg Res 1994;57: 316-36

IV. IMMUNE DYSFUNCTION IN PATIENTS WITH OBSTRUCTIVE JAUNDICE

Endotoxin and the gut barrier

Clements WDB, McCaigue MD, Halliday I, Barclay GR, Rowlands BJ. Conclusive evidence of endotoxaemia in biliary obstruction. Gut 1998;42: 293-9

Deitch EA, Sitting K, Li M, Berg R, Specian RD. Obstructive jaundice promotes bacterial translocation from the gut. Am J Surg 1990;159:79-84

Ding JW, Andersson R, Soltesz VL et al. Inhibition of bacterial translocation in obstructive jaundice by MTP-PE in the rat. J Hepatol 1994;20:720-8

Karsten TM, Allema JH, Reinders ME, et al. Preoperative biliary drainage, bile colonisation and postoperative complications in patients with pancreatic head tumors: an analysis of 241 consecutive patients. Eur J Surg 1996;162:881-8

Kennedy JA, Clements WDB, Kirk SJ et al. Characterization of the Kupffer cell response to exogenous endotoxin in a rodent model of obstructive jaundice. Br J Surg 1999;86:628-33

Kimmings AN, van Deventer SJH, Obertop H, Rauws EAJ, Huibregtse K, Gouma DJ. Endotoxin, cytokines, and endotoxin binding proteins in obstructive jaundice and after preoperative biliary drainage. Gut 2000;46:725-31

Lai ECS, Mok FPT, Fan ST, et al. Preoperative endoscopic drainage for malignant obstructive jaundice. Br J Surg 1994;81:1195-8

Osterberg J, Ljungdahl M, Lundholm M, Engstrand L, Haglund U. Microbial translocation and inflammatory response in patients with acute peritonitis. Scand J Gastroenterol. 2004 Jul;39(7):657-64.

Padillo FJ, Muntane J, Montero JL, Briceno J, Mino G, Solorzano G, Sitges-Serra A, Pera-Madrazo C. Effect of internal biliary drainage on plasma levels of endotoxin, cytokines, and C-reactive protein in patients with obstructive jaundice. World J Surg 2002;26:1328-32

Trede M, Schwall G. The complications of pancreatectomy. Ann Surg 1988;207:39-41

Macrophages and Kupffer cells

Adachi Y, Arii S, Sasaoki T, et al. Hepatic macrophage malfunction in rats with obstructive jaundice and its biological significance. J Hepatol 1992;16:171-6

Bemelmans MHA, Gouma DJ, Greve JW, Buurman WA. Cytokines tumor necrosis factor and interleukin-6 in experimental biliary obstruction in mice. Hepatology 1992;15:1132-6

Fox ES, Kim JC, Tracy TF. NF-κB activation and modulation in hepatic macrophages during cholestatic injury. J Surg Res 1997;72:129-34

Kennedy JA, Clements WDB, Kirk SJ et al. Characterization of the Kupffer cell response to exogenous endotoxin in a rodent model of obstructive jaundice. Br J Surg 1999;86:628-33

Lazar G, Paszt A, Kaszaki J, Duda E, Szakacs J, Tiszlavicz L, Boros M, Balogh A, Lazar G. Kupffer cell phagocytosis blockade decreases morbidity in endotoxemic rats with obstructive jaundice. Inflamm Res 2002;51:511-8

Miyoshi H, Rust C, Guicciardi ME, Gores GJ. NF-kappa B is activated in cholestasis and functions to reduce liver injury. Am J Pathol 2001;158:967-75

Puntis MCA, Jiang WG. Plasma cytokine levels and monocytes activation in patients with obstructive jaundice. J Gastroenterol Hepatol 1996;11: 7-13

Sheen-Chen SM, Chau P, Harris HW. Obstructive jaundice alters Kupffer cell function independent of bacterial translocation. J Surg Res 1998;80: 205-9

Cytokines

Bemelmans MHA, Guma DJ, Buurman WA. LPS induced sTNFr release in vivo in murine model: investigation of the role of TNF, interleukin-1, LIF and IFNγ. J Immunol 1993;151:5554-62

Bemelmans MHA, Greve JWM, Guma DJ, Buurman WA. Increased concentrations of tumor necrosis factor (TNF) and soluble TNF receptors in biliary obstruction in mice, soluble TNF receptors as prognostic factors factors for mortality. Gut 1996;38:447-53

Fisher CR, Dhainaut JF, Opal SM, et al. Recombinant human interleukin-1 receptor antagonist in the treatment of patients with sepsis syndrome: Results from a randomized, double-blind, placebo-controlled trial. Phase III rhIL-1ra Sepsis Syndrome Study Group. JAMA 1994;271:1836-43.

Fong Y, Moldawer LL, Shires GT, Lowry SF. The biologic characteristics of cytokines and their implication in surgical injury. Surg Gynecol Obstet 1990;170:363-78

Haga Y, Sakamoto K, Egami H, et al. Changes in production of interleukin-1 and interleukin-2 associated with obstructive jaundice and biliary drainage in patients with gastrointestinal cancer. Surgery 1999;106:842-8

Hisama M, Yamaguchi Y, Miyanami N, et al. Ischemia-reperfusion injury: the role of Kupffer cells in the production of cytokine-induced neutrophil hemoattractant, a member of interleukin-8 family. Tranplant Proc 1995;27:1604-6

Houdijk AP, Boermeester MA, Wesdorp RI, Hack CE, van Leeuwen PA. Tumor necrosis factor unresponsiveness after surgery in bile duct-ligated rats. Am J Physiol 1996;271:G980-6

Jiang WG, Puntis MCA. Monocyte and blood interleukin-12 levels in patients with obstructive jaundice. HPB Surg 1996;9:219-21

Jiang WG, Puntis MCA. Immune dysfunction in patients with obstructive jaundice, mediators and implications for treatments. HPB Surgery 1997; 10:129-42

Kimura F, Miyazaki M, Suwa T et al. Hyperactive cytokine response after partial hepatectomy in patients with biliary obstruction. Eur Surg Res 1998;30:259-67

Kimura F, Miyazaki M, Suwa T et al. Serum interleukin-6 levels in patients with biliary obstruction. Hepatogastroenterology 1999;46:1613-7

Ksontini R, MacKay SL, Moldawer LL. Revisiting the role of tumor necrosis factor alpha and the response to surgical injury and inflammation. Arch Surg 1998;133:558-67

Miyoshi H, Gores GJ, Apoptosis and the liver: relevance for the hepato-biliary-pancreatic surgeon. J Hepatobiliary Pancreat Surg 1998;5: 409-15

Okamura K, Noshima S, Esato K. Cytokine release during hypoxia reoxygenation by Kupffer cells in rats with obstructive jaundice. Surg Today 1999; 29:730-4

O'Neil S, Hunt J, Filkins J, Gamelli R. Obstructive jaundice in rats results in exaggerated hepatic production of tumor necrosis factor-alpha and systemic and tissue tumor necrosis factor-alpha levels after endotoxin. Surgery 1997;122:281-7

Tahara H, Zeh HJ, Storkus J, et al. Fibroblasts genetically engineered to secrete interleukin-12 can suppress tumor growth and induce antitumor immunity to a murine melanoma in vivo. Cancer Rec 1994;54:182-9

Neutrophils

Bilzer M, Lautenburg BH. Oxidant stress and potentiation of ischaemia/reperfusion injury to the perfused rat liver by human polymorphonuclear leukocytes. J Hepatol 1994;20:473-77

Cruickshank SM, Southgate J, Selby PJ, Trejdosiewicz LK. Expression and cytokine regulation of immune recognition elements by normal human biliary epithelial and established liver cell lines in vitro. J Hepatol 1998;29:550-58

Edwards JCW, Sedgwick AD, Willoughby DA. The formation of a structure with features of synovial lining by subcutaneous injection of air: an in vivo tissue culture system. J Pathol 1981; 134;147-56

Jiang WG, Puntis MCA, Hallett MB. Neutrophil priming by cytokines in patients with obstructive jaundice. HPB Surg 1994;7:281-9

Koeppel TA, Trauner M, Baas JC, et al. Extrahepatic biliary obstruction impairs microvascular perfusion and increases leukocyte adhesion in rat liver. Hepatology 1997;26:1085-91

Levy R, Schlaeffer F, Keynan A, Nagauker O, Yaari A, Sikuler E. Increased neutrophil function induced by bile duct ligation in a rat model. Hepatology 1993;17:908.

Li W, Sung JJ, Chung SCS. Reversibility of leukocyte

dysfunction in rats with obstructive jaundice. J Surg Res. 2004;116:314-21

Liu TZ, Kee KT, Chern CL, Cheng JT, Stern A, Tsai LY, Free radical-triggered hepatic injury of experimental obstructive jaundice of rats involves overproduction of proinflammatory cytokines and enhanced activation of nuclear factor kappa B. Ann Clin Lab Sci 2001;31:383-90

Manna SK, Bhattacharya C, Gupta SK. Regulation of interleukin-8 receptor expression in human polymorphonuclear neutrophils. Mol Immunol 1995; 32:883-893

Ohtsuka M, Miyazaki M, Kondo Y, Nakajima N. Neutrophil-mediated sinusoidal endothelial cell injury after extensive hepatectomy in cholestatic rats. Hepatology 1997;25:636-41

Ohtsuka M, Miyazaki M, Kubosawa H, et al. Role of neutrophils in sinusoidal endothelial cell injury after extensive hepatectomy in cholestatic rats. J Gastroenterol hepatol 2000;15:880-886

Polzien F, Ramadori G. Increased intracellular adhesion molecule-1 serum concentration in cholestasis. J Hepatol 1996;25:877-86

Puntis MCA, Jiang WG. Plasma cytokine levels and monocytes activation in patients with obstructive jaundice. J Gastroenterol Hepatol 1996;11:7-13

Roughneen PT, Drath DB, Kulkarni AD, Kumar SC, Andrassey RJ, Rowlands BJ. Inflammatory cell function in young rodents with experimental cholestasis: Investigations of functional deficits, their etiology, and their reversibility. J Ped Surg 1989;24:668

Scott-Conner CEH, Grogan JB. The pathophysiology of biliary obstruction and its effect on phagocytic and immune function. J Surg Res 1994;57: 316-36

Shimizu Y, Miyazaki M, Ito H, etal. Enhanced endothelial cell injury by activated neutrophils in patients with obstructive jaundice. J Hepatol 1997;27:803-9

Sun Z, Wang X, Lasson A, et al. Roles of platelet-activating factor, interleukin-1β and interleukin-6 in intestinal barrier dysfunction induced by mesenteric arterial ischemia and reperfusion. J Surg Res 1999;87:90-100

Swain MG, Tjandra K, Kanwar S, Kubes P. Neutrophil adhesion impaired in a rat model of cholestasis. Gastroenterology 1995;109:923-32

Takaoka M, Kubota Y, Tsuji K, et al. Human neutrophil functions in obstructive jaundice. Hepatogastroenterology 2001; 48:71-5

Tjandra K, Woodman RC, Swain MG. Impaired neutrophil microbicidal activity in rat cholestasis. Gastroenterology 1997;112:1692

Tsuji K, Kubota Y, Yamamoto S, Yanagitani K, Amoh Y, Takaoka M, Ogura M, Kin H, Ogura M, Inoue K. Increased neutrophil chemotaxis in obstructive jaundice: an in vitro experiment in rats. J Gastroenterol Hepatol 1999;14:457

Yamamoto S, Kubota Y, Tsuji K, Yanagitani K, Takaoka M, Kin H, Ogura M, Inoue K. Effect of obstructive jaundice on neutrophil chemotactic activity: An in vivo assessment in zymosan-induced peritonitis model in rats. J Gastroenterol Hepatol 1998;13:405

Cellular immunity and humoral immunity

Brown WR, Kloppel TM. Liver and IgA: Immunological, cell biological and clinical implications. Hepatology 1989;9:763-84

Jiang WG, Puntis MCA. Immune dysfunction in patients with obstructive jaundice, mediators and implications for treatments. HPB Surgery 1997; 10:129-42

Kawaguchi K, Koike M. Glomerular arterations associated with obstructive jaundice. Hum Pathol 1987;18:1149-54

Oshio G, Furukawa F, Manabe T, Tobe T, Hamashima Y. Relationship between secretory IgA, IdA-containing (C3-fixing) circulating immune complexes, and complement components (C3, C4) in patients with obstructive jaundice. Scand J Gastroenterol 1986;21:151-7

Reynoso-Paz S, Coppel RL, Mackay IR, Bass NM, Ansari AA, Gershwin ME. The immunobiology of bile and biliary epithelium. Hepatology 1999;30: 351-7

V. HAEMOSTASIS IMPAIRMENT IN OBSTRUCTIVE JAUNDICE

An introduction to the pathophysiology of haemostasis impairment in obstructive jaundice

Ding JW, Anderson R, Norgren L, Stenram U, Bengmark S: The influence of biliary obstruction and sepsis on reticuloendothelial function in rats. Eur J Surg 1992;158:157-64

Kuzu MA, Kale IT, Col C, Tekeli A, Tanik A, Koksoy C: Obstructive jaundice promotes bacterial translocation in humans. Hepatogastroenterology 1999; 46:159-64

Mimidis K, Papadopoulos V, Kotsianidis J, Filippou D, Spanoudakis E, Bourikas G, Dervenis C, Kartalis G. Alterations of platelet function, number and indexes during acute pancreatitis. Pancreatology 2004;4:22-7.

Mimidis K, Papadopoulos V, Kartasis Z, Baka M, Tsatlidis V, Bourikas G, Kartalis G. Assessment of platelet adhesiveness and aggregation in mild acute pancreatitis using the PFA-100 system. JOP 2004;5:132-7

Van Thiel DH, George M, Mindikoglu AL, Baluch MH, Dhillon S. Coagulation and fibrinolysis in individuals with advanced liver disease. Turk J Gastroenterol 2004;15:67-72

Vitamin K deficiency in obstructive jaundice

Amitrano L, Guardascione MA, Brancaccio V, Balzano A. Coagulation Disorders in Liver Diesease. Semin Liv Dis 2002;22:83-96

O'Brien DP, Shearer MJ, Waldron RP, Horgan PG, Given HF. The extent of Vitamin K deficiency in patients with cholestatic jaundice. J R S Med 1994;87:320-2

Sherlock S. Nutritional complications of biliary cirrhosis. Am J Clin Nutr 1970;23:640-4

Progressive hepatic failure and cirrhosis

Albornoz L, Bandi JC, Otaso JC, Laudanno O, Mastai R. Prolonged bleeding time in experimental cirrhosis: role of nitric oxide. J Hepatol 1999; 30:456-460

Aster RH. Pooling of platelets in the spleen: role in the pathogenesis of "hypersplenic" thrombocytopenia. J Clin Invest 1966;45:645-57

Belli L, Romani F., Sansalone CV, Aseni P, Rondinara G. Portal thrombosis in cirrhotics. A retrospective analysis. Ann Surg 1986;203:286-91

Ben Ari Z, Osman E, Hutton RA, Burroughs AK. Disseminated intravascular coagulation in liver cirrhosis: fact or fiction? Am J Gastroenterol 1999; 94:2977-2982.

Bosch J, Reverter JC. The coagulopathy in cirrhosis: Myth or reality? Hepatology 2005;41: 434-5

Car JM. Disseminated intravascular coagulation in cirrhosis. Hepatology 1989;10:103-110

Escolar G, Cases A, Vinas M, Pino M, Calls J, Cirera I, et al. Evaluation of acquired platelet dysfunctions in uremic and cirrhotic patients using the platelet function analyzer (PFA-100): influence of hematocrit elevation. Haematologica 1999;84: 614-619

Goulis J, Chau TN, Jordan S, Mehta AB, Watkinson A, Rolles K, et al. Thrombopoietin concentrations are low in patients with cirrhosis and thrombocytopenia and are restored after orthotopic liver transplantation. Gut 1999;44:754-758

Guarner C, Soriano G, Such J, Teixido M, Ramis I, Bulbena O, et al. Systemic prostacyclin in cirrhotic patients Relationship with portal hypertension and changes after intestinal decontamInation. Gastroenterology 1992;102:303-309

Hersch SL, Kunelis T, Francis RB. The pathogenesis of accelerated fibrinolysis in liver cirrhosis: a critical role for plasminogen activator inhibitor. Blood 1987;69:1315-1319

Koike Y, Yoneyama A, Shirai J, Ishida T, Shoda E, Miyazaki K, et al. Evaluation of thrombopoiesis in thrombocytopenic disorders by simultaneous measurement of reticulated platelets of whole blood and serum thrombopoietin concentrations. Thromb Haemost 1998;79:1106-1110

Laffi G, Cominelli F, Ruggiero M, Fedi S, Chiarugi VP, La Villa G, et al. Altered platelet function in cirrhosis of the liver: impairment of inositol lipid and arachidonic acid metabolism in response to agonists. Hepatology 1988;8:1620-1626

Laffi G, Marra F, Failli P, Ruggiero M, Cecchi E, Carloni V, et al. Defective signal transduction in platelets from cirrhotics is associated with increased cyclic nucleotides. Gastroenterology 1993;105:148-156

Laffi G, Marra F, Gresele P, Romagnoli P, Palermo A, Bartolini O, et al. Evidence for a storage pool defect in platelets from cirrhotic patients with defective aggregation. Gastroenterology 1992;103:641-646.

Levine RF, Spivak JL, Meagher RC, Sieber F. Effect of

ethanol on thrombopoiesis. Br J Haematol 1986; 62:345-354

Lindenbaum J. Folate and vitamin B12 deficiencies in alcoholism. Semin Hematol 1980;17:119-129

Michelson AD, Barnard MR. Plasmin-induced redistribution of platelet glycoprotein Ib. Blood 1990;76: 2005-2010

Ordinas A, Escolar G, Cirera I, Vinas M, Cobo F, Bosch J, et al. Existence of a platelet-adhesion defect in patients with cirrhosis independent of hematocrit: studies under flow conditions. Hepatology 1996;24:1137-1142

Owen JS, Hutton RA, Day RC, Bruckdorfer KR, McIntyre N. Platelet lipid composition and platelet aggregation in human liver disease. J Lipid Res 1981;22:423-430

Papadopoulos V., Kartasis Z., Mimidis K., Papantoniou S., Baka M., Kotsiou S., Bourikas G., Kartalis G. Evaluation of haemostasis impairment in early stages of liver cirrhosis: a clinical study. HAEMA 2004;7(4):471-478

Pasche B, Ouimet H, Francis S, Loscalzo J. Structural changes in platelet glycoprotein IIb/IIIa by plasmin: determinants and functional consequences. Blood 1994;83:404-414

Peck-Radosavljevic M, Wichlas M, Zacherl J, Stiegler G, Stohlawetz P, Fuchsjager M, et al. Thrombopoietin induces rapid resolution of thrombocytopenia after orthotopic liver transplantation through increased platelet production. Blood 2000; 95:795-801

Pereira J, Accatino L, Alfaro J, Brahm J, Hidalgo P, Mezzano D. Platelet autoantibodies in patients with chronic liver disease. Am J Hematol 1995;50:173-178

Stein SF, Harker LA. Kinetic and functional studies of platelets, fibrinogen, and plasminogen in patients with hepatic cirrhosis. J Lab Clin Med 1982;99: 217-230

Stockelberg D, Andersson P, Bjornsson E, Bjork S, Wadenvik H. Plasma thrombopoietin levels in liver cirrhosis and kidney failure. J Intern Med 1999; 246:471-475

Tripodi A, Salerno F, Chantarangkul V, Clerici M, Cazzaniga M, Primignani M, et al. Evidence of normal thrombin generation in cirrhosis despite abnormal conventional coagulation tests. Hepatology 2005;41:553-8

Turitto VT, Baumgartner HR. Platelet interaction with subendotheliumin a perfusion system: physical role of red blood cells. Microvasc Res 1975; 9:335-344

Van Thiel DH, George M, Fareed J. Low levels of thrombin activatable fibrinolysis inhibitor (TAFI) in patients with chronic liver disease. Thromb Haemost 2001;85:667-670

Violi F, Ferro D, Basili S, et al. Hyperfibrinolysis resulting from clotting activation in patients with different degree of cirrhosis. Hepatology 1993; 17:78-83

Sepsis and haemostasis impairment in patients with obstructive jaundice - the central role of tissue factor

Amaral A, Opal SM, Vincent JL. Coagulation in sepsis. Intensive Care Med 2004;30:1032-40

Basili S, Ferro D, Violi F. Endotoxaemia, hyperfibrinolysis and bleeding in cirrhosis. Lancet 1999; 353:1102

Bogdanov VY, Balasubramanian V, Hathcock J, et al: Alternatively spliced human tissue factor: a circulating, soluble, thrombogenic protein. Nature Medicine 2003;9:458-462.

Bugge TH, Xiao Q, Kombrinck KW, et al: Fatal embryonic bleeding events in mice lacking tissue factor, the cell-associated initiator of blood coagulation. Proc Natl Acad Sci U.S.A. 1996; 93:6258-6263.

Doshi SN, Marmur JD: Evolving role of tissue factor and its pathway inhibitor. Crit Care Med 2002;30:

Ferro D, Basili S, Pratico D, et al. Vitamin E reduces monocyte tissue factor expression in cirrhotic patients. Blood 1999;93:2945-2950

Gando S, Kameue T, Morimoto Y, Matsuda N, Hayakawa M, Kemmotsu O: Tissue factor production not balanced by tissue factor pathway inhibitor in septis promotes poor prognosis. Crit Care Med 2002;30:

Gando S, Nanzaki S, Sasaki S, et al: Activation of the extrinsic coagulation pathway in patients with severe sepsis and septic shock. Crit Care Med 1998; 26:2005-9.

Giessen PLA, Rauch U, Bohrmann B, et al: Blood-borne tissue factor: Another view of thrombosis. Proc Natl Acad Sci U.S.A. 1999; 96:2311-2315.

Goulis J, Patch D, Burroughs AK. Bacterial infection in the pathogenesis of variceal bleeding. Lancet 1999;353:139-142

Grignani G, Maiolo A. Cytokines and hemostasis. Haematologica 2000;85:967-972

Lopes-Bezzera LM, Filler SG. Endothelial cells, tissue factor and infectious diseases. Braz J Med Biol Res 2003; 36:987-991.

McVey JH. Tissue Factor Pathway. Baillere's Clinical Haematology 1999; 12:361-372.

Okajima K, Sakamoto Y, Uchiba M. Heterogeneity in the incidence and clinical manifestations of disseminated intravascular coagulation: a study of 204 cases. Am J Hematol 2000;65: 215-222

Padillo FJ, Muntane J, Montero JL, Briceno J, Mino G, Solorzano G, Sitges-Serra A, Pera-Madrazo C. Effect of internal biliary drainage on plasma levels of endotoxin, cytokines and C-reactive protein in patients with obstructive jaundiuce. World J Surg 2002;26:1328-32

Riewald M, Ruf W. Orchestration of Coagulation Protease Signaling by Tissue Factor. TCM 2002; 12:149-154

Saliola M, Lorenzet R, Ferro D, et al. Enhanced expression of monocyte tissue factor in patients with liver cirrhosis. Gut 1998;43:428-432

Semeraro N, Montemurro P, Chetta G, Altomare DF, Giordano D, Colucci M. Increased procoagulant activity of peripheral blood monocytes in human and experimental obstructive jaundice. Gastroenterology 1989;96:892-8

Takeda ST, Takaki A, Ohsato K. occurrence of disseminated intravascular coagulation (DIC) in obstructive jaundice and its relation to biliary tract infection. Jap J Surg 1977;7:82-9

Tapper H, Herwald H. Modulation of hemostatic mechanisms in bacterial infectious diseases. Blood 2000;96:2329-2337.

Underlying pathology in patients with obstructive jaundice as an additional mechanism of haemostasis impairment

a. Pancreatic toumours

Heinmoller E, Schropp T, Kisker O et al. Tumour cell-induced platelet aggregation in vitro by human pancreatic cancer cell lines. Scand J Gastroenterol 1995;30:1008-16

Kakkar AK, Lemoine NR, Scully MF et al. Tissue factor expression correlates with histological grade in human pancreatic cancer. Br J Surg 1995;82: 1101-4

Khorana AA, Fine RL. Pancreatic cancer and thromboembolic disease. Lancet Oncol 2004;5: 655-63

Scialla SJ, Speckart SF, Haut MJ, Kimball DB. Alterations in platelet surface sialyltransferase activity and platelet aggregation in a group of cancer patients with a high incidence of thrombosis. Cancer Res 1979;39:2031-5

Wahrenbrock M, Borsig L, Le D, et al. Selectin-mucin interactions as a probable molecular explanation for the association of Trusseau syndrome with mucinous adenocarcinomas. J Clin Invest 2003; 112:853-62

Wojtukiewicz MZ, Rucinska M, Zacharski LR, et al. Localization of blood coagulation factors in situ in pancreatic carcinoma. Thromb Haemost 2001;86: 1416-20

b. Cholangiocarcinoma

Hui CK, Yuen MF, Tso WK, Ng IO, Chan AO, Lai CL. Cholangiocarcinoma in liver cirrhosis. J Gastroenterol Hepatol 2003;18:337.

Nagornay DM, van Heerden JA, Ilstrup DM, Adson MA. Primary hepatic malignancy: surgical management and determinants of survival. Surgery 1989;106:740.

Wiwanitkit V. Activated partial thromboplastin time abnormality in patients with cholangiocarcinoma. Clin Appl Thromb Haemost 2004;10:69-71

c. Hepatocellular carcinoma

Akiyama K, Nakamura K, Makino I, Takeda Y, Kubota K, Tazawa S, Hayashi T, Niiya K, Sakuragawa N. Antithrombin III producing hepatocellular carcinoma. Thromb Res 1993;72:193-201

Barr RD, et al. Dysfibrinogenemia and liver cell growth. J Clin Pathol 1978;31:89-92

Blanchard RA, Furie BC, Jorgensen M, et al. Acquired vitamin K dependent carboxylation deficiency in liver disease. N Engl J Med 1981;305:242-248

Drin FG, Thomson JM, Dymock IW, et al. Abnormal fibrin polymerisation in liver disease. Br J Haematol 1976;34:427-437

Liebman HA, Furie B, Tong M, et al. Des-gamma-carboxy (abnormal) prothrombin as a serum marker of primary hepatocellular carcinoma. N Engl J Med 1984;310:1427-1431

Nakao A, Virji A, Karr B, et al. Abnormal prothrombin (des-gamma-carboxy prothrombin) in hepatocellular carcinoma. Hepatogastroenterology 1991; 38:450-453

Tseng CS, Lo HW, Chuang WL, Juan CC, Ker CG. Clinical significance of plasma D-dimer levels and serum VEGF levels in patients with hepatocellular carcinoma. Hepatogastroenterology 2004;51: 1454-8

Weitz IC, Liebman HA. Des-γ-carboxy (abnormal) prothrombin and hepatocellular carcinoma: a critical review. Hepatology 1993;18:990-997

Yasuhiro Miyamoto, Yasuhiro Takikawa, Shi De Lin, Shinichiro Sato, Kazuyuki Suzuki. Apoptotic hepatocellular carcinoma HepG2 cells accelerate blood coagulation. Hepatol Res 2004;29:167-72

Zacharski LR, Hommann M, Kaufmann R. Rationale for clinical trials of coagulation: reactive drugs in hepatocellular carcinoma. Expert Rev Cardiovasc Ther 2004;2:777-84

d. Acute pancreatitis

Beuneu C, Vosters O, Movahedi B, Remmelink M, Salmon I, Pipeleers D, Pradier O, Goldman M, Verhasselt V. Human Pancreatic Duct Cells Exert Tissue Factor-Dependent Procoagulant Activity. Diabetes 2004;53:1407-1411.

Bogdanov VY, Balasubramanian V, Hathcock J, Vele O, Lieb M, Nemerson Y. Alternatively spliced human tissue factor: a circulating, soluble, thrombogeneic protein. Nature Med 2003; 9:458-462.

Emanuelli G, Montrucchio G, Gaia E, Dughera L, Corvetti G, Gubetta L. Experimental acute pancreatitis induced by platelet activating factor in rabbits. Am J Pathol 1989; 134:315-26.

Hirota M, Sugita H, Maeda K, Ichibara A, Ogawa M. The concept of SIRS and severe acute pancreatitis. Nippon Rinsho 2004 Nov;62(11):2128-36.

Johnson GB, Brunn GJ, Platt JL. Cutting edge: an endogenous pathway to systemic inflammatory response syndrome (SIRS) - like reactions through Toll-like receptor 4. J Immunol 2004 Jan 1;172(1):20-4.

Mikhailidis DP, Hutton RA, Jeremy JY, Dandona P. Hypothermia and parcreatitis. J Clin Pathol 1983; 36:483-4.

Mimidis K, Papadopoulos V, Kotsianidis J, Filippou D, Spanoudakis E, Bourikas G, Dervenis C, Kartalis G. Alterations of platelet function, number and indexes during acute pancreatitis. Pancreatology 2004;4:22-7.

Mimidis K, Papadopoulos V, Kartasis Z, Baka M, Tsatlidis V, Bourikas G, Kartalis G. Assessment of platelet adhesiveness and aggregation in mild acute pancreatitis using the PFA-100 system. JOP 2004;5:132-7.

Moberg L, Johansson H, Lukinius A, Berne C, Foss A, Kallen R, Ostraat G, Salmela K, Tibell A, Tufveson G, Elgue G, Nilsson Ekdahl K, Korsgren O, Nilsson B. Production of tissue factor by pancreatic islet cells as a trigger of detrimental thrombotic reactions in clinical islet transplantation. Lancet 2002;360:2039-45.

Price GC, Thompson SA, Kam PCA. Tissue factor and tissue factor pathway inhibitor. Anaesthesia 2004;59:483-492.

Radenkovic D, Bajec D, Karamarkovic A, Stefanovic B, Milic N, Ignjatovic S, Gregoric P, Milicevic M. Disorders of hemostasis during the surgical management of severe necrotizing pancreatitis. Pancreas 2004 Aug;29(2):152-6.

Salomone T, Tosi P, Palareti G, Tomassetti P, Migliori M, Guariento A, Saieva C, Raiti C, Romboli M, Gullo L. Coagulative disorders in human acute pancreatitis: role for the D-dimer. Pancreas 2003 Mar;26(2):111-6.

Versteeg HH. Tissue Factor as an Evolutionary Conserved Cytokine Receptor: Implications for Inflammation and Signal Transduction. Semin Hematol 2004;1(Suppl.1):168-172.

Zhou W, Levine BA, Olson MS. Platelet-activating factor: a mediator of pancreatic inflammation during cerulein hyperstimulation. Am J Pathol 1993; 142:1504-12.

Treatment of haemostatic abnormalities in patients with obstructive jaundice

Caldwell SH, Chang C, Macik BG. Recombinant activated factor VII (rFVIIa) as a hemostatic agent in liver disease: a break from convention in need of controlled trials. Hepatology 2004;39: 592-8

Mueller MM, Bomke B, Seifried E. Fresh frozen plasma in patients with disseminated intravascular coagulation or in patients with liver diseases. Thrombosis Res 2002;107:9-17

Parekh SJ. Surgery in patients with liver disease: hematological management. Ind J Gastroenterol 2001;20:104-7

Sallah S, Bobzien W. Bleeding problems in patients with liver disease. Postgrad Med 1999;106:187-190.

Constitutive Reviews for Further Reading

Amitrano L, Guardascione MA, Brancaccio V, Balzano A. Coagulation disorders in liver disease. Semin Liv Dis 2002,22:83-96

Jiang WG, Puntis MCA. Immune dysfunction in patients with obstructive jaundice, mediators and implications for treatments. HPB Surgery 1997; 10:129-42

Kimmings AN, van Deventer SJ, Obertop H, Rauws EAJ, Gouma DJ. Inflammatory and immunologic effects of obstructive jaundice: pathogenesis and treatment. J Am Coll Surg 1995;181:567-81

Lisman T, Leebeek FWG, de Groot PG. Haemostatic abnormalities in patients with liver disease. J Hepatol 2002;37:280-7

Nehez L, Andersson R. Compromise of immune function in obstructive jaundice. Eur J Surg 2002; 168:315-28

Oldenburg J, Schwaab R. Molecular biology of blood coagulation. Semin Thromb Haemost 2001; 27:313-24

Scott-Conner CEH, Grogan JB. The pathophysiology of biliary obstruction and its effect on phagocytic and immune function. J Surg Res 1994;57:316-36

Violi F, Ferro D, Quintarelli C, Saliola M, Cordova C, Balsano F. Clotting abnormalities in chronic liver disease. Dig Dis 1992;10:162-72

Cholelithiasis and choledocholethiasis

Simopoulos Konstantinos, Tsaroucha Alexandra

INTRODUCTION

The cause, the prevention of recurrence and the treatment of common bile duct lithiasis remain very attractive issues in biliary surgery. The common bile duct stones are classified as primary and secondary. However, the majority of them are secondary calculi, which migrate from the gallbladder through the cystic duct. Indeed, 10 to 15% of patients with cholelithiasis have also stones in the common bile duct. Gallbladder lithiasis is a multifactorial phenomenon which depends on nutrition habits, and genetic and environmental factors. Hypersecretion of cholesterol of the liver, cholesterol crystal formation, bile concentration, state of the gallbladder mucosa, and mobility of the gallbladder wall are among the factors that play a role in lithogenesis. Early in the 1970s, new information become available, regarding lith gallstone genes, attributing cholesterol gallstone formation to a response to interactions between various genes and environmental stimuli. Lith genes control gallstone formation, a finding that may lead to new therapeutic strategies. Megalin, which is a protein, multiple-ligand receptor expressed on the apical surface of epithelial tissues of several organs, including the gallbladder, seems to play a role in the pathophysiology of gallbladder stone formation.

On the other hand, primary common bile duct lithiasis is rare and associated with infections and bile stasis, which may include biliary stricture, papillary stenosis or sphincter dysfunction. The incidence of primary common bile duct stones is still under discussion and varies from 4% to 56% of diagnosed common bile duct stones.

The time interval between cholecystectomy and the diagnosis of primary common duct stones can be up to several years. Primary common bile duct stones develop more often in patients with a long period of symptoms of the disease, who have had previous biliary surgical treatment. Primary stones are an index of existent biliary stasis, and have to be taken into serious consideration in treatment of these patients. The following criteria for identifying primary common bile duct lithiasis have been proposed: 1. previous cholecystectomy; 2. a two-year symptoms-free period after cholecystectomy; 3. presence of soft, light brown stones with bile duct shape or sludge in the common duct; and 4. absence of stenosis from the previous surgery. Madden defined primary common bile duct stones as solitary, ovoid, light brown in color, soft and easily crushable. Brown pigment stones predominate in primary common duct lithiasis, while cholesterol stones do in gallbladder and secondary common duct lithiasis. Stones formed in the gallbladder generally show linear, radial growths of cholesterol crystals, while those fromed in the common duct present a polystratified, concentric deposition of microgranules composed mainly of pigmentary salts. There is also a relationship between patient age and the diamcter of the primary common bile duct stones.

Several times residual common duct stones may exist after cholecystectomy, which were most likely present at the time of surgery. These stones may remain asymptomatic for years or may cause cholangitis and sepsis. Approximately 5 to 10% of patients treated with cholecystectomy and having an exploration of the common bile duct present after the cholecystectomy with retained stones. Finally, there is the question if simultaneous formation of stones in the gallbladder and the common bile duct is possible. Although stone formation mechanisms are not fully understood yet, and it is still difficult to distinguish between primary and secondary bile duct lithiasis, it would be very useful and of practical significance to know the real cause of choledocholithiasis in order to decide on the best treatment method.

CLINICAL ASPECTS

Choledocholithiasis may be silent and symptoms-free for years or may be symp-

tomatic as a result of complications. Small stones may pass spontaneously into the duodenum without causing symptoms or may temporarily obstruct the pancreatic duct causing pancreatitis. The diagnosis in asymptomatic patients can be given only by routine US imaging or may be discovered at the time of routine cholecystectomy for chronic lithiasic cholecystitis. Common bile duct stones may cause bile duct obstruction, partial or total, cholangitis, or acute or chronic pancreatitis. Stones wedged in or passing through the ampulla of Vater are the ones that can cause pancreatitis.

Generaly, choledocholithiasis symptoms may include one or more of the following: 1. acute pain in the epigasrtium which reflects to the right hypochondrium; 2. general discomfort; 3. biliary colic; 4. jaundice; 5. fever and chills; 6. itching; 7. cholangitis and sepsis. Symptoms and laboratory abnormalities depend on the degree of the obstruction, i.e., total or partial. Symptoms in total biliary obstruction include biliary colic, jaundice (with high serum bilirubin levels), lightening of the color of stools and darkening of the urine, and in presence of cholangitis, fever and chills. If a stone obstructs the common bile duct in the absence of an infected bile, jaundice and pain are present.

The symptoms in patients with residual bile duct stones may also be silent for many years or may cause cholangitis. Symptoms for this kind of stones follow the complications.

TREATMENT

The treatment of choledocholithiasis is not simple, and depends on the clinical situation (emergency or elective), on the age and general condition of the patient, and on the facilities and clinical expertise available. Treatment may be conservative, endoscopic or surgical. Conservative treatment includes systematic control of fluid and electrolyte balance and parenteral administration of antibiotics and vitamin K. However, conservative treatment may be only temporarily effective if the bile duct is completely obstructed.

.

ENDOSCOPIC TREATMENT

Endoscopic retrograde cholangiopancreatography with sphincterotomy and stone extraction were introduced early in the 1970s. Before then the treatment was only surgical, and before the laparoscopic era, open common bile duct exploration was the only choice.

Endoscopic sphincterotomy was initially considered justifiable only in elderly post-cholecystectomy patients with recurrent or retained common bile duct stones, who were at high risk of serious complications from conventional surgical common bile duct exploration or re-exploration, at a time when only few endoscopy centers could offer the technique.

Indications for endoscopic sphincterotomy are the following: 1. retained stones after cholecystectomy with T-tube in situ; 2. retained stones without T-tube; 3. diagnosed common bile duct lithiasis with gallbladder in situ; 4. acute gallstone-associated pancreatitis irrespective of gallbladder status.

Many questions have been asked for the best timing of the endoscopic retrograde cholangiopancreatography, including if the treatment of the common bile duct lithiasis should be preoperative or postoperative? Preoperative endoscopic retrograde cholangiopancreatography has been performed in patients; however, almost half of them had no choledocholithiasis. Successful endoscopic treatment of bile duct stones requires an endoscopic sphincterotomy, and this is now achieved in over 90% of attempts in most reported series. However, there is noticeable im-

provement as experience increases. Complications of endoscopic therapy are acute hemorrhage from the sphincterotomy, acute pancreatitis, cholangitis retroperitoneal perforation, gallstone ileus and acute cholecystitis. Emergency surgery is required in 1% to 2,5% of cases.

Integrated endoscopic therapy for biliary disease is now successful in those centers where surgical and endoscopic clinicians work closely together, and where each provides the other with a suitable forum for critical evaluation of alternative therapeutic techniques. Nevertheless, there is need for clinical studies evaluating relative morbidity and mortality risks, as different groups of patients can be treated by either preoperative endoscopy or postoperative endoscopy. Today endoscopic sphincterotomy is the treatment of choice in common bile duct lithiasis.

SURGICAL TREATMENT

The purpose of common bile duct exploration for choledocholithiasis is to detect and remove all stones within the bile duct system as safely as possible. It includes, however, significant risk. While cholecystectomy alone may be performed with little morbidity, and a mortality of less than 0.5%, the addition of an exploration of the bile duct increases the morbidity, and mortality may rise by three to seven times.

If the gallbladder is in situ and there is gallbladder and common bile duct lithiasis, the treatment is cholecystectomy with bile duct exploration or endoscopic sphincterotomy. The absolute indications for common bile duct exploration are: 1. palpable stones in the common bile duct; 2. jaundice with cholangitis; 3. a stone visualized at intra-operative cholangiography; and 4. preoperative radio-graphic demonstration of choledocholithiasis.

In patients with post-cholecystectomy choledocholithiasis and absence of biliary obstruction or infection, no treatment should be attempted for four to six weeks. During this period the retained stones can be expected to pass spontaneously into the duodenum and no further treatment will be required. If after four to six weeks the stone persists, active treatment should be instituted. Because of low morbidity and mortality, non-operative mechanical extraction is the treatment of choice, and in these patients only 0.2% require surgery. Before the endoscopic era, patients underwent reoperation in 8 to 10 weeks after initial surgery.

For patients without a T-tube in place and retained or recurrent stones, the choice of therapy lies between reoperation and stone extraction by means of endoscopic sphincterotomy. Earlier, the most common surgical procedure for treatment of retained stones was choledocholithotomy, choledochoscopy, placement of a T-tube and completion cholangiography.

Partial or complete obstruction of the pancreatic duct outflow, would possibly explain episodes of acute pancreatitis following operative or endoscopic instrumentation; a similar mechanism may explain the acute pancreatitis which may occur if a long limb surgical T-tube is allowed to pass through the lower common bile duct and on into the duodenum. Of the many patients who suffer from biliary associated pancreatitis it is quite rare to find a stone truly impacted at the ampulla of Vater.

The timing of surgical or endoscopic intervention in acute gallstone pangreatitis is very important. Patients can be subdivided into three categories: The first category includes those who had immediate surgical intervention within 48 hours of hospital admission, because it has been suggested that immediate endoscopic sphincterotomy may be effective. The sec-ond category includes early intervention, which gives more time to have the patient checked (two to seven days). And the traditional approach, delayed intervention, allows the patient to completely recover from the episode of pancreatitis and a subsequent admission for elective biliary surgery can be planed. However, the proper timing of treatment is not clear yet, no matter if pancreatitis is mild, moderate or severe. It is also still under discussion, whether surgery or endoscopic management is the preferred as primary treatment in symptomatic patients with suspected common bile duct stones, because the additional cholecystectomy after endoscopic management is of high risk for complications.

Laparoscopic bile duct exploration after routine laparoscopic cholecystectomy is another alternative for the treatment of choledocholithiasis, although the treatment of choledocholithiasis discovered incidentally during laparoscopic cholecystectomy is not yet standardized. Laparoscopic bile duct exploration can successfully treat common bile duct stones, with minimal to no morbidity.

The combination of laparoscopic cholecystectomy and endoscopic sphincterotomy is a possible treatment for patients suffered of cholelithiasis and choledocholithiasis. However, patients with symptomatic common bile duct stones that undergo laparoscopic cholecystectomy after endoscopic sphincterotomy have higher complication and conversion rates than patients undergoing laparoscopic cholecystectomy without endoscopic sphincterotomy.

Another treatment alternative is laparoscopic cholecystectomy combined with intraoperative endoscopic sphincterotomy. This treatment option, compared with laparoscopic exploration of the common bile duct, because of the minimum invasion has been shown to be a safe and effective treatment for cholecystocholedocholithiasis. The long-term prognosis after treatment of patients with common bile duct lithiasis, using the traditional choledocholithotomy and T-tube drainage, including open and laparoscopic surgery, has shown recurrence of the disease.

In conclusion, the management of stones in the common bile duct in the laparoscopic era was changed. The three major options are preoperative endoscopic retrograde cholangiography, laparoscopic exploration of the common bile duct, or postoperative endoscopic retrograde cholangiopancreatography. The treatment of choice of common bile duct lithiasis is today the endoscopic treatment.

REFERENCES

Admirand WH, and Small DM. The physiochemical basis of cholesterol gallstone formation in man. J Clin Invest. 1968;47:1043-1052.

Akopian G, Blitz J, Vander Laan T. Positive intraoperative cholangiography during laparoscopic cholecystectomy: is laparoscopic common bile duct exploration necessary? Am Surg. 2005 Sep;71(9): 750-3.

Allen NL, Leeth RR, Finan KR, Tishler DS, Vickers SM, Wilcox CM, Hawn MT. Outcomes of Cholecystectomy After Endoscopic Sphincterotomy for Choledocholithiasis. J Gastrointest Surg. 2006 Feb;10(2):292-296.

Blumgard LH. Surgery of the liver and biliary tract. Churchill livingstone 1990 Ch.Endoscopic approaches p593.

Cuevas A, Miquel JF, Reyes MS, Zanlungo S, Nervi F. Diet as a risk factor for cholesterol gallstone disease. J Am Coll Nutr. 2004;23:187-96.

Dowling R H. Review: Pathogenesis of gallstones. Aliment Pharmacol Ther. 2000;14S:39-47.

Erranz B, Miquel JF, Argraves WS, Bath JL, Pimentel F, Marzolo MP. Megalin and cubilin expression in gallbladder epithelium and regulation by bile acids. J Lipid Res. 2004;16.

Garcia Ontiveros A, Cantero Hinojosa J, Gil Extremera

B, Minarro del Moral J. Differences in gallstone structure in primary common bile duct lithiasis and gallbladder lithiasis. Klin Wochenschr. 1990 May 17;68(10):496-502.

Gilat T, Feldman C, Halpen Z, Dan M, Bar-Meir S. An increased familial frequency of gallstones. Gastroenterology.1983;84:242-246.

Hong DF, Xin Y, Chen DW. Comparison of laparoscopic cholecystectomy combined with intraoperative endoscopic sphincterotomy and laparoscopic exploration of the common bile duct for cholecystocholedocholithiasis. Surg Endosc. 2006 Mar;20(3):424-7. Epub 2006 Jan 4.

Lammert F, Wang DQH, Paigen B, Carey MC. Phenotypic characterization of Lith genes that determine susceptibility to cholesterol cholelithiasis in inbred mice: integrated activities of hepatic lipid regulatory enzymes. J Lipid Res. 1999;40:2080-2090.

Lyons MA, Wittenburg H, Li R, Walsh KA, Leonard MR, Churchill GA, Carey MC, Paigen B. New quantitative trait loci that contribude to cholesterol gallstone formation detected in an intercross of CAST/Ei and 129S1/SvlmJ inbred mice. Physiol Genomic. 2003;14:225-239.

Madden JL. Common duct stones: their origin and surgical management. Surg Clin Nort A. 1973 53: 1095-1113.

Mazzariello r. Review of 220 cases of the residual biliary tract calculi treated without reoperatio: an eight year study. Surgery 73: 299-306.

Rhodes M, Sussman L, Cohen L, Lewis MP. Randomised trial of laparoscopic exploration of common bile duct versus postoperative endoscopic retrograde cholangiography for common bile duct stones. Lancet. 1998 Jan 17;351 (9097): 159-61.

Saharia PC, Zuidema GD, Cameron JL. Primary common duct stones. Ann Surg. 1977 May;185(5): 598-604.

Sgourakis G, Dedemadi G, Stamatelopoulos A, Leandros E, Voros D, Karaliotas K. Predictors of common bile duct lithiasis in laparoscopic era. World J Gastroenterol. 2005 Jun 7;11(21):3267-72.

Sherlock S, Dooley J. Diseases of the liver and biliary system, 9th Ed., Blackwell scientific Publication 1993 p. 580.

Suc B, Escat J, Cherqui D, Fourtanier G, Hay JM, Fingerhut A, Millat B. Surgery vs endoscopy as primary treatment in symptomatic patients with suspected common bile duct stones: a multicenter randomized trial. Arch Surg. 1998 Jul;133(7): 702-8.

Uchiyama K, Onishi H, Tani M, Kinoshita H, Kawai M, Ueno M, Yamaue H. Long-term prognosis after treatment of patients with choledocholithiasis. Ann Surg. 2003 Jul;238(1):97-102.

Villacorta Patino J, Medina Nunez JA, Ruiz de Aguiar A. Primary lithiasis of the choledochus: etiologic factors and structural characteristics] Rev Esp Enferm Dig. 1993 Jul;84(1):26-32.

Wang DQH, Lammert F, Paigen B, Carey MC. Phenotypic characterization of Lith genes that determine susceptibility to cholesterol cholelithiasis in inbred mice: pathophysiology of biliary lipid secretion. J Lipid Res. 1999;40:2066-2079.

Cholelithiasis, cholecystectomy and the risk of colorectal cancer

Altieri Andrea, Castro Felipe

ABSTRACT

Cholelithiasis in western countries affects 10-20% of the population, and approximately 35% of untreated cholelithiasis will eventually undergo cholecystectomy. Cholelithiasis is a complex disorder where both environmental and genetic factors contribute towards susceptibility to the disease. Major risk factors include obesity, aging, female gender, family history and more recently lifestyle and dietary habits, including physical activity, high saturated fats consumption and metabolic impairments such as insulin resistance. The evidence from both cohort and case-control studies from different geographical areas and populations suggests that individuals with a history of cholecystectomy have a modest increased risk of colorectal cancer of about 30%. Most, but not all studies, show a persistence of the excess risk over time since a higher risk for women and for the proximal portion of the colon. Increased exposure to secondary bile acids might be the underlying biological explanation. However, animal studies generally show that bile acids are not carcinogenic *per se*, but may act as promoters. We conclude that cholecystectomy or the underlying gallstone disease weakly related to the risk of colorectal cancer. Thus, at a public health level, the overall evidence does not point to the need for increased surveillance for colorectal cancer in subjects that underwent cholecystectomy.

EPIDEMIOLOGY OF CHOLELITHIASIS AND CHOLECYSTECTOMY

Gallstones are solid crystalline precipitates usually formed in the gallbladder. More than 80% of gallbladder stones are cholesterol crystals, deriving from supersaturation of major biliary lipids, namely cholesterol, bile acids, and phospholipids. The remaining stones are black pigment stones, composed predominantly of calcium bilirubinate (Cuevas et al., 2004, Acalovschi, 2001). Cholelithiasis (or gallstone disease), that is the presence or formation of gallstones in the biliary tract, is relatively common in western countries and in some areas of South America, affecting approximately 10-20% of the population, and is one of the most common medical problem leading to surgical intervention (Schirmer et al., 2005, Shaffer, 2005). The available data on cholelithiasis, historically based on necropsy data and more recently on ultrasonography, revealed major differences between different countries (Figure 1). Chile has been reported to be one of the countries with the highest prevalence worldwide, intermediate rates were found in Europe and United States, whereas the lowest cholelithiasis rates were found in Asia (Jorgensen, 1987, Attili et al., 1995, Berndt et al., 1989, Glambek et al., 1987, Everhart et al., 1999, Covarrubias et al., 1984, Moro et al., 2000, Chen et al., 1998, Khuroo et al., 1989, Nomura et al., 1988, Prathnadi et al., 1992, Zhao et al., 1990). In most populations cholelithiasis was approximately twice more common in women compared to men. The incidence time trends of cholelithiasis rates have been reported to increase in the last decades in different geographical areas, reflecting somehow the increasing prevalence of major known risk factors, including population aging overweight and obesity (Schirmer et al., 2005, Acalovschi, 2001).

Cholecystectomy (i.e. the surgical removal of the gallbladder) is rarely performed in individuals with no history of cholelithiasis. Approximately 35% of patients initially diagnosed with cholelithiasis, if not treated, will eventually develop complications or recurrent symptoms leading to cholecystectomy (Schirmer et al., 2005). It has been estimated than every year at least 500,000 cholecystectomies are performed in the United States, and the frequency has been reported to be increased by about 25% after the introduction of modern surgical techniques, mainly laparoscopic cholecystectomy, in the early 1990s (Schirmer et al., 2005, Urbach and Stukel, 2005,Legorreta et al., 1993,

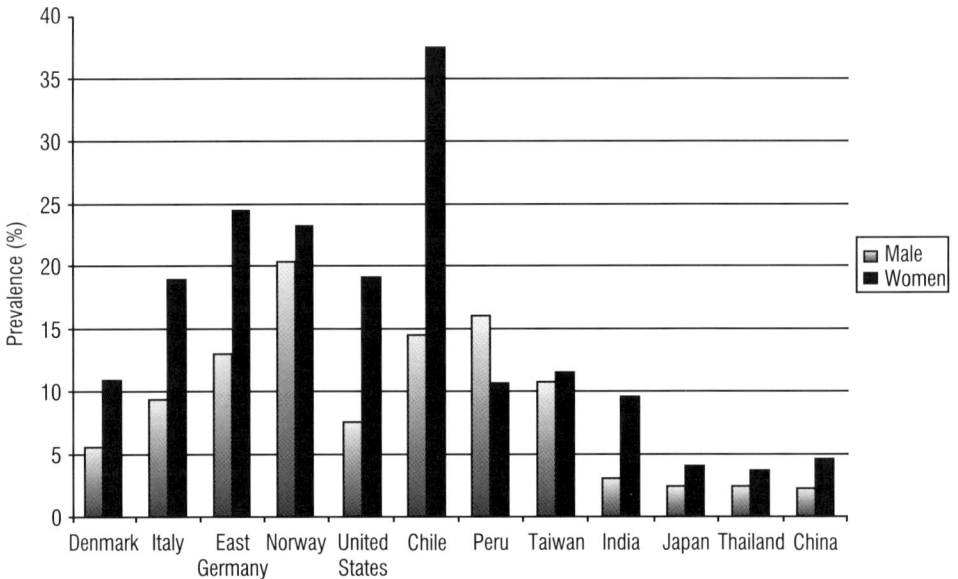

FIGURE 1: Prevalence of gallstones in some areas of Europe, Americas and Asia from selected studies*, according to sex. (* Denmark: Jorgensen et al, 1987; Italy: Attili et al, 1995; East Germany: Berndt et al, 1989; Norway: Glambek et al, 1987; United States: Everhart et al, 1999; Chile: Covarrubias et al, 1995; Peru: Moro et al, 2000; Taiwan: Chen et al, 1998; India: Khuroo et al, 1989; Japan: Nomura et al, 1988; Thailand: Prathnadi et al, 1992; China: Zhao et al, 1990).

Lam et al., 1996, Shaffer, 2005). One for this increase is that severe complications of cholelithiasis, such as acute cholecystitis, acute biliary pancreatitis and acute cholangitis, are potentially life-threatening conditions that require hospital care, and the greater use of elective cholecystectomy in people at risk of severe gallstone complications should result in a lower incidence of such complications (Urbach and Stukel, 2005, Cohen et al., 1996, Legorreta et al., 1993). The international rates of cholecystectomy fluctuate considerably between countries and calendar periods, probably reflecting the delaying in the introduction of new surgical techniques in time, economic disparities and availability of medical care practices (Bateson, 1991, Legorreta et al., 1993).

Risk factors for cholelithiasis and cholecystectomy

Cholelithiasis is a complex disorder where both environmental and genetic factors contribute towards susceptibility to the disease. Obesity, aging, female gender, multiparity and family history are well known risk factors for lithiogenesis, whereas relatively new are the findings that the diagnosis of cholelithiasis is correlated with high and frequent variations in weight, with intake of estrogen treatment and with specific alimentary and lifestyle habits, including total energy intake, high consumption of simple sugars and saturated fats, and with insulin resistance and physical activity (Cuevas et al., 2004, Shaffer, 2005).

Obesity is one of the most established risk factor for cholelithiasis and the evidence has been more compelling for women compared to men (Cuevas et al., 2004, Maclure et al., 1989). A case-control study from Italy including nearly 200 cases reported a consistent positive association between body mass index and the risk of cholelithiasis, even after adjustment for several known or potential confounding factors (La Vecchia et al., 1991). Relative to leaner individuals, the odds ratios (OR) were 1.2, 2.1 and 2.4 for subsequent levels of body mass. These trends in risk were statistically significant and consistent in the two sexes. The biological explanation refers to the fact that obese persons bile appears to be more lithogenetic. The primary reasons is that in individuals with a high body mass index ($\geq$30) present increasing levels in total endogenous synthesis of cholesterol, due to an increased activity of 3-hydroxy-3-methylglutarylcoenzyme A, and a higher ratio of cholesterol to solubilizing lipids (bile acids and phospholipids). This high ratio predisposes to crystallization of cholesterol and gallstones formation.

Physical activity has more recently emerged to have a relevant role in the prevention of symptomatic gallstone disease. A report from the Health Professional Study indicates that 34% of cases of symptomatic gallstone disease in men could be prevented by increasing exercise to 30 minutes of endurance-type training five times per week, and similar results come from the Nurses Health Study for women (Leitzmann et al., 1998, Leitzmann et al., 1999).

The epidemiological evidence shows that cholelithiasis is rare before adolescence, and that the incidence increases with age, being 5 to 10 times higher in elderly compared to young adults. This is probably due to the fact that in the elderly the physiologic metabolism of bile acids is reduced, and in turn the biliary cholesterol saturation is increased (Acalovschi, 2001).

In populations women are 2 to 4-fold as likely as men to experience cholelithiasis, reflecting the prevalence of gallstones in females in their fertile years compared to men (Schirmer et al., 2005). Moreover, women with gallstones are more likely to have had cholecystectomy than men with gallstones (Schirmer et al., 2005). The sex difference could be explained by specific risk factors that apply only to women, mainly pregnancies, but possibly also exposure to hormones and duration of the fertile period. A case-control study reported no consistent pattern of risk of cholelithiasis up to four births, but women with five or more births had an OR of 2.9 (95% CI, 1.1-7.3) (La Vecchia et al., 1991). In that study, the risk decreased with increasing age at first and last birth, both trends being statistically significant. A plausible biological explanation refers to the fact that pregnancy hormonal pattern influences bile composition, increasing biliary cholesterol secretion. Moreover, estrogens up-regulate low density lipoprotein receptor, inducing an increased input of hepatic free cholesterol. Several epidemiological studies showed an increased risk of gallstones in users of oral contraceptives and hormone replacement therapy, in particular for the old high dose formulations, and an increase risk of cholecystectomy and gallbladder malignancies (Gallus et al., 2002,Royal College of General Practitioners' oral contraception study, 1982). However, updated findings from the Royal College Study on low doses formulations appear to be reassuring with reference to gallbladder disorders (Kay, 1984).

Family studies suggest a strong genetic component in the causation of gallbladder disorders, that is corroborated by population studies showing evident racial differences (Gilat et al., 1983, Acalovschi, 2001). Worldwide, one of the highest prevalence of gallbladder disease was registered in the Pima tribe of Arizona, where more than 70% of adult women reported a history of gallstones or cholecystectomy. High rates have also been reported in different ethnic groups in North America and in native populations from South America, such as the Mapuches in Chile. Familial and community clusters are usually explained by shared genetic background or common environmental exposures. These populations are characterized by different lifestyle and exposure to several heterogeneous environmental factors, which suggests a genetic etiologic component of the disease (Urbach and Stukel, 2005). Analysis of the many enzymatic pathways involved in biliary cholesterol secretion reveals many potential susceptibility candidates genes. However, despite the fact that genetic factors clearly play a role, the disease is likely to be polygenic with multifactorial genetic backgrounds and identification and isolation of key role genes still remains an unaccomplished challenging task. Several genetically derived phenotypes in the population are responsible for variations in lipoprotein types, which in turn affect the amount of cholesterol available in the gall bladder. The genetic polymorphisms in various genes for apo E, apo B, apo A1, LDL receptor, cholesteryl ester transfer and LDL receptor-associated protein have been implicated in gallstone formation. However, presently available information on genetic differences is not able to account for a large number of gallstone patients.

Smoking and abstinence from alcohol appear also to be related to cholelithiasis while the significance of diet and other lifestyle factors has been only partially elucidated (La Vecchia et al., 2003,Kameda et al., 1984,Randi et al., 2004). In a case-control study from Italy, the risk of cholelithiasis decreased with increasing alcohol consumption: compared with nondrinkers, the OR was 0.8 for one to three drinks per day and 0.5 for over three (La Vecchia et al., 1991). In a large cohort study from the United States including 7831 female cases of cholecystectomy, relative to subjects who never consumed alcohol, subjects who consumed alcohol 1-2, 3-4, 5-6, and 7 drinks per week had relative risks of cholecystectomy of 0.94, 0.88, 0.87, and 0.73 (0.63, 0.84), respectively that remained unchanged even after adjustment for sever confounders. All alcoholic beverage types were inversely associated with cholecystectomy risk, independent of consumption patterns (Leitzmann et al., 2003).

The recent increase in incidence rates of gallstones in Japan, following lifestyle and dietary westernization, and the shift of prevalence from men to women has been attributed to the increased fat intake and a decreased consumption of fibers and vegetables. The investigation of the role of animal fats and high proteins consumption has lead so far to inconsistent results (La Vecchia et al., 2003,Kameda et al., 1984,Tsai et al., 2004). One large cohort study from the United States including overall 5771 incident cases of cholecystectomy, found that a higher intake of carbohydrate, dietary glycemic load, and glycemic index may enhance risk of cholecystectomy (Tsai et al., 2005). The relative risk (RR) for the highest compared with the lowest quintile of dietary carbohydrate was 1.35 (95% CI: 1.17-1.55, P for trend <.0001). The relative risks for the highest compared with the lowest quintile were 1.50 for glycemic load (95% CI: 1.32-1.71, P for trend <.0001) and 1.32 for glycemic index (95% CI: 1.20-1.45, P for trend <.0001). Independent positive associations were also seen for intakes of starch and sucrose. With reference to specific micronutrients, only calcium and vitamin C have been reported to show a protective effect with gallstone prevalence, but the epidemiological evidence remains scanty (Moerman et al., 1994,Simon and Hudes, 2000).

CHOLECYSTECTOMY AND COLORECTAL CANCER RISK

The geographical distribution of colorectal cancer rates has a similar pattern compared to those of cholelithiasis, suggesting similar risk factors or common etiologic pathways (Figure 2) (Ferlay et al.,

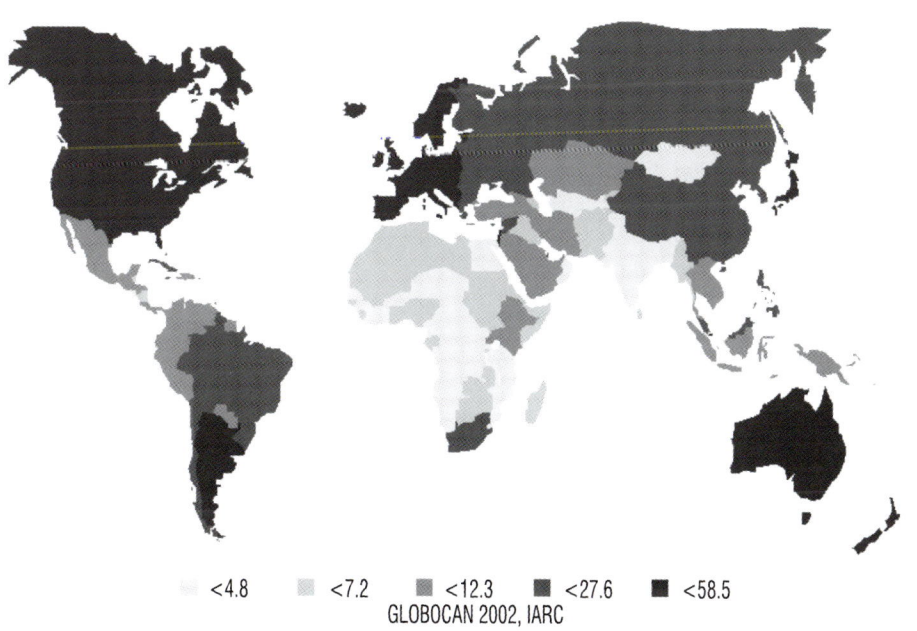

| <4.8 | <7.2 | <12.3 | <27.6 | <58.5 |

GLOBOCAN 2002, IARC

FIGURE 2: Age standardized incidence rates of colorectal cancer in males (rates are per 100,000).

2004). In recent years the attention on colorectal cancer has been focusing on the heritable risk and on familial clustering (Hemminki and Chen, 2005). However, several environmental exposures, mainly dietary items, have been reported to affect colorectal cancer risk. Coffee consumption, for example, has been generally reported to decrease colorectal cancer risk. The biological mechanism refers to reductions of cholesterol, bile acids and neutral sterol secretion in the colon, antimutagenic properties of selected coffee components, including phenolic compounds, and by increasing colonic motility (Tavani and La Vecchia, 2004, Nehlig and Debry, 1994, Leitzmann et al., 2002). The joint effect of environmental risk factors (*i.e.* high education level, low occupational physical activity, high daily meal frequency, low intake of fiber, selected micronutrients such as calcium and beta-carotene) and family history on the subsequent risk of colon cancer has been recently investigated in one of the largest case-control study on colorectal cancer. The higher risk was found for subjects with a family history of colorectal cancer and high risk factor score, the OR being 7.08 (95% CI = 4.68-10.71) compared to those with the lowest score and with no family history.

In the following paragraphs we review the published evidence from selected animal studies, and from most recent epidemiological studies conducted on humans, on the association between cholecystectomy and the subsequent risk of a diagnosis of colorectal cancer, covering also the possible biological mechanisms, plausible explanations of the associations reported and public health implications.

Animal studies

The first evidence of a carcinogenic activity of bile acids, namely deoxycholic acid, comes from animal studies conducted in the 1930-1940s, on subcutaneous fibrosarcomas induced in rats and mice by Cook and colleagues (Cook et al., 1940). In several animal experiments published subsequently conducted mainly on rats and mice, several bile acids were shown to be cancer promoters, increasing tumorigenesis by known carcinogens (Bernstein et al., 2005, Narisawa et al., 1974). However, bile acids, by themselves, were not found to be. Secondary bile acids have been found to promote strongly carcinogenesis in the colon of rats, and animal studies suggest that cholecystectomy may increase the incidence of chemically induced colon cancer (Kuniyasu et al., 1986, Narisawa et al., 1985, Narisawa et al., 1978). One study from Japan investigated the relationship between cholecystectomy and large-bowel cancer in rats (Narisawa et al., 1985). The authors concluded that cholecystectomy enhanced the development of dimethylhydrazine (DMH)-induced, large-bowel carcinomas along with the change of fecal bile acid composition, suggesting that changes of bile acid metabolism after cholecystectomy may enhance or promote large-bowel carcinogenesis (Narisawa et al., 1985). In particular, in rats, the bile acids lithocholic, taurodeoxycholic and deoxycholic acids had a promoting effect on colon carcinogenesis after intrarectal instillation of N-methyl-N0-nitro-N-nitrosoguanidine (MNNG). The bile acid, cholic acid, also had a promoting effect on colon tumour formation in rats after intrarectal instillation of N-methyl-N-nitrosourea (MNU) or subcutaneous injection of azoxymethane (Narisawa et al., 1985).

Previous study promoting effect of sodium deoxycholate (DC) on colon carcinogenesis was studied in rats, after intrarectal instillations of N-methyl-N'-nitro-N-nitrosoguanidine (MNNG) for 4 weeks. It was concluded that DC (present in high concentrations in human stools) had a promoting effect on colon carcinogenesis in rats (Reddy et al., 1976). Another study showed the promoting effect of cholic acid ingestion on methylazoxymethanol acetate [(MAM) CAS: 592-62-1]-treated germfree rats (Weidema et al., 1985). These and several other animal studies where recently reviewed by Bernstein and colleagues. The authors concluded that experiments in non-mutated rat model systems have lead to the evidence that bile acids act as promoters, but not as carcinogens.

Studies on humans

In humans, the potential association between cholecystectomy and colorectal cancer risk was firstly suggested by a clinical report published in 1978 (Capron et al, 1978). Subsequently, the potential association between cholecystectomy and colorectal cancer in humans has been investigated by at least 80 epidemiological studies of different design in different populations. In the assessment of the quantification of the association between cholecystectomy and subsequent risk of cancer the latency interval between cholecystectomy and cancer diagnosis also needs to be carefully taken into account. In fact, as carcinogenesis is a multistage process with a long latency of time, an increased risk of colorectal cancer following cholecystectomy is likely to be most apparent at long time intervals after operation. Conversely, increased risk for cholecystectomy in the short-term after surgery is more prone to be due to chance or unaccounted confounding factors. Another potential relevant issue is whether there is a different risk for proximal (or right-sided) compared to distal colon cancer. In fact, it has been postulated that since proximal (i.e. cecum through transverse colon) compared to distal (i.e. splenic flexure through sigmoid colon) colon sites is closer to the releasing site of bile acids, a higher risk should be found for proximal portion of the colon.

Cohort studies are epidemiological studies in which subjects are selected on the basis of their exposure status (for example history of cholecystectomy) and followed in time. After an adequate follow-up period, the incidence of colorectal cancer in those exposed (i.e. individuals with a history of cholecystectomy) is compared with the incidence in those not exposed (i.e. individuals with no history of cholecystectomy). A meta-analysis is an epidemiological quantitative method of combining the results of independent studies (usually drawn from the published literature) and synthesizing summaries and conclusions in one single risk estimate. In 1993, Giovannucci and colleagues published a meta-analysis including 6 cohort studies (Giovannucci et al., 1993). Overall, the authors found no significant association between cholecystectomy and colon cancer. The RR was 0.97 (95% CI, 0.82-1.14). Another meta-analysis conducted subsequently reported very similar results (Reid et al., 1996). In that study, the pooled OR for colorectal cancer in individuals with a history of cholecystectomy was 1.11 (95% CI, 1.02 to 1.21). For women the OR was 1.14 (95 % confidence interval, CI, 1.01 to 1.28) and for right-sided cancer 1.86 (95% CI, 1.31 to 2.65) (Reid et al., 1996). A few other cohort studies have been published subsequently. A large study from Denmark on more than 40,000 gall stone patients showed a modest increase in the number of cancers at all sites combined (RR, 1.07; 95% CI, 1.0 to 1.1) (Johansen et al., 1996). A weak association was found for cancer of the colon (RR, 1.09; 95% CI 1.0 to 1.2), based on 360 cases, which remained unchanged when analysed by sex, anatomical subsite, and duration of follow up. Multivariate analysis with adjustment for cholecystectomy and clinically defined obesity did not change these estimates to any significant extent.

No association was found in another large population-based cohort study from Sweden, including 150 colorectal cancer cases (Adami et al., 1987). A study from Sweden (Lagergren et al., 2001) updating previous Swedish studies (Adami et al., 1987, Ekbom et al., 1993) reported a significant but small increase in risk of intestinal cancer after cholecystectomy. That study included in total more than 270,000 cholecystectomized patients followed up for a maximum of 33 years after surgery. Cholecystectomized patients had an increased risk of proximal intestinal adenocarcinoma, which gradually declined with increasing distance from the common bile duct. The risk was significantly increased for adenocarcinoma (standardized incidence ratio, SIR = 1.77, 95% CI, 1.37-2.24) and carcinoids of the small bowel (SIR = 1.71, 95% CI, 1.39-2.08), and right-sided colon cancer (SIR = 1.16, 95% CI, 1.08-1.24). No association was found with more distal bowel cancer. The increased up to 33 years after cholecystectomy. No differences between sexes were found. The authors concluded that cholecystectomy increased the risk of intestinal cancer and that the risk declined with increasing distance from the common bile duct (Lagergren et al., 2001).

In a report from the Nurses' Health Study, including 877 women diagnosed with cancer of the colorectum, Schernhammer et al. (Schernhammer et al., 2003) found an increased risk for colorectal cancer (RR = 1.21, 95% CI 1.01-1.46) in relation to history of gallstones or cholecystectomy (reported by 133 colorectal cancer cases), after adjusting for potential confounding factors. A higher risk was reported for the proximal colon (RR 1.34, 95% CI 0.97-1.88) and for the rectum (RR 1.58, 95% CI 1.05-2.36).

Another cohort study was conducted in the United Kingdom and included almost 40,000 individuals that underwent c-holecystectomy. The authors reported a short-term significant elevation of rates of cancer at different sites, including the colon. However, the increased risk was limited to the subjects that were recently admitted to the hospital. After excluding colon cancers within two years of admission to hospital, the rate ratio for colon cancer after cholecystectomy, compared to the subjects that never underwent c-holecystectomy was 1.01 (95% CI, 0.90-1.12) and after 10 years or more of follow-up it was 0.94 (95% CI, 0.79-1.10) (Goldacre et al., 2005).

A recent population-based cohort study from the General Practice Research Database from the United Kingdom included nearly 56,000 cholecystectomy patients and 575,000 controls (Shao and Yang, 2005). The incidence rate of colorectal cancer among cholecystectomy patients was 119 (95% CI: 106-133) per 100,000 person-years, compared to 86 (95% CI: 83-90) per 100,000 person-years among patients without a cholecystectomy. The adjusted incidence rate ratio (IRR) of colorectal cancer associated with cholecystectomy was 1.32 (95% CI: 1.16-1.48, p<0.001). The positive association was present for colon cancer (IRR = 1.51, 95% CI: 1.30-1.74, p<0.001), but not for rectal cancer (IRR = 1.00, 95% CI: 0.85-1.17, p=0.99). The pattern of association was similar in men women.

In case-control studies a group of people with disease (cases) and a group of people without that disease (controls) are identified and the prevalence of the exposure (for example cholecystectomy) is measured in the two groups and compared. Case-control studies are particularly useful for analysis of relatively uncommon or delayed outcomes (such as cancer and cholecystectomy), and they allow to collect a much higher number of cases in a much shorter time compared to cohort studies. In addition, they are particularly useful in populations with a well established and uniform medical surveillance system.

The meta-analysis by Giovannucci in 1993 (Giovannucci et al., 1993) included 33 case-control studies. The pooled result from these studies was that an increased risk of colon cancer after cholecystectomy (RR = 1.34, 95% CI, 1.14-1.57), particularly when limited to the proximal colon (RR = 1.88; 95% CI = 1.54-2.30).

The largest case-control study was conducted in Italy (Altieri et al., 2004). The study was based on data from two different multicentric studies conducted from 1985 to 1996 include overall 3533 incident cases of colorectal cancer and 7062 hospital controls. One of the major strengths of the study was the large sample size and the availability of detailed information on known or potential confounding factors, including different measures of body size at different ages and a comprehensive food consumption questionnaire. Table 1 shows the distribution of colorectal cancer cases and controls, and the corresponding ORs, according to the history and time since cholelithiasis. Subjects with a history of cholelithiasis showed no appreciable increased risk of colorectal cancer (OR 1.04, 95% CI 0.90-1.21). Similar results were found for colon (OR 1.08, 95% CI 0.91-1.28) and for rectal (OR 1.03, 95% CI 0.83-1.27) cancer. The OR was 1.03 (95% CI 0.72-1.47) for proximal colon and 1.17 (95% CI 0.93-1.47) for distal colon cancer. The ORs for men were 1.21 for colorectal, 1.24 for colon and 1.22 for rectal cancer, and for women were 0.95, 1.01 and 0.93 respectively. With reference to time since cholelithiasis ORs for less than 10 years were 1.13 for colorectal, 1.16 for colon and 1.12 for rectal cancer. No association was found for 10 or more years before interview.

Another large case-control study was conducted in the US and included overall almost 2000 cases and similar number of controls randomly selected from the population of the same geographic area as cases (Todoroki et al., 1999). After adjustment for age, gender, family history of colorectal cancer, body mass index, dietary energy intake, fiber intake and use of nonsteroidal anti-inflammatory medications and physical activity, no association was found between cholecystectomy and colorectal cancer (OR=1.0, 95% CI, 0.9-1.2). A weak positive association for proximal colon cancer was observed (OR=1.3, 95% CI, 1.0-1.6) in that study. The association with proximal colon cancer disappeared after 14 years since the surgery. The association did not differ by gender.

Carcinogenic activity of bile acids

The biological mechanism that has long been suggested to explain the potential associations is that cholecystectomy increases the exposure to colon to bile acids. In the absence of a gallbladder, instead of periodic release of bile acids from the gallbladder at mealtimes, there is a constant flow of bile leading to increased dehydroxylation and dehydrogenation of primary bile acids to form more secondary bile acids (Malagelada et al., 1973). Primary bile acids, cholic acid and chenodeoxycholic acid, are products of the metabolism of cholesterol in the liver and are stored in the gallbladder. Primary bile acids play a key role in fat emulsion and digestion after meals. Secondary bile acids, *i.e.* deoxycholic acid and lithocholic acid, are produced in the colon by the action of bacteria on primary bile acids. Bile acids, in particular secondary bile acids, i.e. deoxycholic acid and lithocholic acid, have been found to have a carcinogenic activity. Several epidemiological studies found that fecal bile acid concentrations are elevated in populations with a high incidence of colon cancer (Hill, 1990, Cheah and Bernstein, 1990, Hill et al., 1971, Domellof et al., 1982, Red-

TABLE 1

Relation Between History and Time Since Diagnosis of Cholelithiasis and Colorectal Cancer among 3,533 Cases and 7,062 Controls (After Altieri et al, 2004).

Factors	Men		Women		Total	
	Cases: Controls	OR (95% CI)[a]	Cases:Controls	OR (95% CI)[a]	Cases:Controls	OR (95% CI)[a]
Colorectal cancer						
History of cholelithiasis						
No	1858:3761	1[b]	1325:2696	1[b]	3183:6457	1[b]
Yes	139:191	1.21 (0.95-1.54)	211:414	0.95 (0.79-1.15)	350:605	1.04 (0.90-1.21)
Time Since diagnosis (years)[c]						
<10	65:83	1.35 (0.95-1.92)	74:144	0.97 (0.72-1.32)	139:227	1.13 (0.90-1.42)
≥10	72:107	1.11 (0.81-1.52)	137:270	0.96 (0.77-1.21)	209:377	0.99 (0.82-1.19)
Colon cancer						
History of cholelithiasis						
No	1103:3761	1[b]	854:2696	1[b]	1957:6457	1[b]
Yes	83:191	1.24 (0.93-1.64)	140:414	1.01 (0.81-1.26)	223:605	1.08 (0.91-1.28)
Time since diagnosis (years)[c]						
<10	41:83	1.47 (0.98-2.20)	47:144	0.95 (0.67-1.36)	88:227	1.16 (0.89-1.51)
≥10	40:107	1.03 (0.70-1.52)	93:270	1.05 (0.80-1.36)	133:377	1.02 (0.82-1.26)
Rectal cancer						
History of cholelithiasis						
No	755:3761	1[b]	471:2696	1[b]	1226:6457	1[b]
Yes	56:191	1.22 (0.88-1.69)	71:414	0.93 (0.70-1.23)	127:605	1.03 (0.83-1.27)
Time since diagnosis (years)[c]						
<10	24:83	1.21 (0.75-1.97)	27:144	1.03 (0.66-1.59)	51:227	1.12 (0.81-1.54)
≥10	32:107	1.25 (0.82-1.90)	44:270	0.88 (0.62-1.25)	76:377	0.98 (0.75-1.28)

[a] Estimates from unconditional multiple logistic regression models, including terms for age, sex, study center, education, cigarette smoking, alcohol drinking, body mass index, meat consumption, total energy intake, history of diabetes, history of colorectal cancer in parents and siblings, menopausal status, use of oral contraceptives or hormone replacement therapy.
[b] Reference category.
[c] The sum does not correspond to the total number of cases because of some missing values.

dy et al., 1983). The most important bile acids in the etiology of colon cancer in humans appear to be the secondary bile acids, (Hill, 1990). Deoxycholate is also higher in the serum of patients with colorectal adenomas than in individuals without adenomas (Bayerdorffer et al., 1995). Moreover, the fact that the risk appears to be stronger for proximal right colon, where the bile acids are directly secreted, supports the hypothesis of a causal association. Thus, the overall evidence indicates that bile acids may play an etiologic role in gastrointestinal cancers (Bernstein et al., 2005, Shao and Yang, 2005).

Animal experiments indicate that bile acids are not *per se* carcinogenic (Bernstein et al., 2005). However, secondary bile acids have been shown to promote carcinogenesis in the colon of rats (Koga et al., 1982, Narisawa et al., 1974). However, the rodent experiments do not preclude the possibility that bile acids act as carcinogens in humans, considering the great difference in time of tumour development in rodent models compared to humans. Many different studies indicate that bile acids cause DNA damage, strongly suggesting mutagenic and carcinogenic potential. The DNA damaging mechanism seems to be indirect, involving production of reactive oxygen/nitrogen species (Bernstein et al., 2005).

Genetic polymorphism, secondary bile acids and colorectal cancer risk

The large amount of epidemiological literature that has been accumulating in the last decades with the aim to unravel the potential association between cholecystectomy and the subsequent risk of colorectal cancer suggests that one of the major problems in the quantification of the association is the accurate measurement of the exposure to secondary bile acids in the colonic lumen. The association be-

tween cholecystectomy and colorectal cancer is causal, the most plausible biological mechanism appears to proceed through the increased exposure to bile acids. In particularly, by secondary bile acids have the potential to damage cell membranes of the colonic mucosa and might thereby stimulate epithelial proliferation, increasing the risk of adenomas and cancers. The metabolism of secondary bile acids includes the entero-hepathic circulation, by which secondary bile acids are reabsorbed in the liver through the portal vein circulation. Only a small proportion of secondary bile acids is not recaptured and is found in the faeces. This reabsorption of the bile acids occurs at the terminal ileum, and is completely mediated by an active transmembrane protein, the ileal sodium-dependant bile acid transporter (encoded by the SLC10A2 gene), located on the cellular membrane surface in the intestinal lumen (Wang et al., 2001). Genetic polymorphic variations in the ileal sodium-dependant bile acid transporter gene may result in differences in the efficacy of the entero-hepathic reabsorption of bile acids (Davey and Ebrahim, 2003).

In addition, many potential confounding factors, such as age, intestine transit time, selected dietary items, as well as overweight and obesity and hepatic disorders were often under-reported in many previous studies and should be accounted for in the risk estimates of the association between cholecystectomy and colorectal cancer. Moreover, it has been pointed out that in case-control studies the diet modification that may result from the disease would make it hard to assess the levels of secondary bile acids prior to the onset of the disease (Davey and Ebrahim, 2003). In the recent literature an alternative epidemiological approach has been suggested that could help to asses an unbiased and unconfounded estimate of the association between lifetime exposure to secondary bile acids and colon cancer risk (Davey and E-brahim, 2003). The hypothesis is to test the causal association between carcinogenic activity of secondary bile acids and colorectal cancer risk by comparing the risk of cancer in individuals with and without polymorphic variants of the ileal sodium-dependent bile acid transporter gene. In principle, individuals with the null variant, non functional, of the transporter would experience a higher exposure to secondary bile acids (since they are not reabsorbed), and an increased risk of colorectal cancer. A case-control study including 458 cases and a similar number of controls, reported an increased risk of 2.06 (95% CI, 1.10-3.83), for carriers of non functional variants compared to individuals with the fully functional variant (Wang et al., 2001). However, even though this preliminary results seems encouraging, a more compelling evidence of functional polymorphic variants of the ileal sodium-dependent bile acid transporter gene is necessary to allow meaningful interpretations (Davey and Ebrahim, 2003, Wang et al., 2001).

CONCLUSIONS

A large amount of epidemiological evidence has accumulated in the last decades on the potential association between cholelithiasis, cholecystectomy and the subsequent risk of developing cancers of the colon and rectum. Two comprehensive meta-analyses published one in 1993 (Giovannucci et al., 1993) and one in 1996 (Reid et al., 1996) lead to the conclusion, that the strength of the association between cholecystectomy and colorectal cancer is generally modest, and in most cases negligible. The overall evidence from studies published subsequently, which were able to account more carefully for confounding factors, including different measures of body weight, total energy intake as well as other lifestyle and dietary factors, confirm

that, overall, cholelithiasis is not materially associated with colorectal cancer risk. The excess risks reported by most studies did not generally reach statistical significance, confirming that if any association exists, is unlikely to be causal. Some studies reported higher, but still modest excess risks, in the short-term after the operation. Such a time-risk relation is inconsistent with a causal relation of cholelithiasis with colorectal cancer risk. In other studies, however, the excess risk persisted and occasionally increased over time.

However, the strength of the association appears to vary by study design, colorectal subsites, and sex (being somewhat stronger in case-control studies compared to cohort, for proximal colon and for women). Some of the inconsistencies between studies may be due to the fact that different potential confounding factors and time since cholecystectomy were not always adequately taken into account, in particular for early studies. The apparent association reported from some case-control studies may at least in part be due to a more accurate recall of gallbladder disease by colorectal cancer patients and by the inadequate adjustment for other potential risk factors for colorectal cancer, including diet. Overweight and obesity are relevant risk factors for both gallbladder (Lew and Garfinkel, 1979, La Vecchia et al., 1991) and colorectal cancer (Lew and Garfinkel, 1979) and may therefore represent both an underlying pathogenetic mechanism and a potential confounding factor. The higher risk reported for women in several studies remains poorly understood.

A modest increased risk has been consistently reported for proximal, or right-sided, portion of the colon, which is physically closer to the releasing site of bile acids. The finding appears to support the hypothesis that an increased exposure to lithogenic secondary bile acids is the underlying biological mechanism.

In conclusion, a large body of epidemiological studies has accumulated giving reassuring evidence that cholecystectomy does not meaningfully increase the risk of colorectal cancer. Thus at a public health level, these findings lead to the conclusion that an increased medical surveillance of individuals that underwent cholecystectomy is not warrant.

REFERENCES

Acalovschi M. Cholesterol gallstones: from epidemiology to prevention. Postgrad Med J 2001; (77):221-229.

Adami H O, Krusemo U B, Meirik O. Unaltered risk of colorectal cancer within 14-17 years of cholecystectomy: updating of a population-based cohort study. Br J Surg 1987; (74):675-678.

Altieri A, Pelucchi C, Talamini R, Bosetti C, Franceschi S, La Vecchia C. Cholecystectomy and the risk of colorectal cancer in Italy. Br J Cancer 2004; (90):1753-1755.

Attili A F, Carulli N, Roda E, Barbara B, Capocaccia L, Menotti A, Okoliksanyi L, Ricci G, Capocaccia R, Festi D, . Epidemiology of gallstone disease in Italy: prevalence data of the Multicenter Italian Study on Cholelithiasis (M.I.COL.). Am J Epidemiol 1995; (141):158-165.

Bateson M C. Gallbladder disease prevalence and cholecystectomy rates. In: Recent advances in the epidemiology and prevention of gallstone disease. (Fds.Capocaccia L, Ricci G, Angelico F, et al). Dordrecht: Kluwer Academic Publisher, 1991; 13-22.

Bayerdorffer E, Mannes G A, Ochsenkuhn T, Dirschedl P, Wiebecke B, Paumgartner G. Unconjugated secondary bile acids in the serum of patients with colorectal adenomas. Gut 1995; (36):268-273.

Berndt H, Nurnberg D, Pannwitz H. [Prevalence of cholelithiasis. Results of an epidemiologic study using sonography in East Germany]. Z Gastroenterol 1989; (27):662-666.

Bernstein H, Bernstein C, Payne C M, Dvorakova K, Garewal H. Bile acids as carcinogens in human gastrointestinal cancers. Mutat Res 2005; (589):47-65.

Cheah P Y, Bernstein H. Modification of DNA by bile acids: a possible factor in the etiology of colon cancer. Cancer Lett 1990; (49):207-210.

Chen C Y, Lu C L, Huang Y S, Tam T N, Chao Y, Chang F Y, Lee S D. Age is one of the risk factors in developing gallstone disease in Taiwan. Age Ageing 1998; (27):437-441.

Cohen M M, Young W, Theriault M E, Hernandez R. Has laparoscopic cholecystectomy changed patterns of practice and patient outcome in Ontario? CMAJ 1996; (154):491-500.

Cook J W, Kennaway E L, Kennaway N M. Production of tumours in mice by deoxycholic acid. Nature 1940; 627.

Covarrubias C, Valdivieso V, Nervi F. Epidemiology of gallstone disease in Chile. In: *Epidemiology and prevention of gallstone disease.* (Eds.Capocaccia L, Ricci G, Angelico F). Lancaster:MTP Inc, 1984; 26-30.

Cuevas A, Miquel J F, Reyes M S, Zanlungo S, Nervi F. Diet as a risk factor for cholesterol gallstone disease. J Am Coll Nutr 2004; (23):187-196.

Davey S G, Ebrahim S. 'Mendelian randomization': can genetic epidemiology contribute to understanding environmental determinants of disease? Int J Epidemiol 2003; (32):1-22.

Domellof L, Darby L, Hanson D, Mathews L, Simi B, Reddy B S. Fecal sterols and bacterial beta-glucuronidase activity: a preliminary metabolic epidemiology study of healthy volunteers from Umea, Sweden, and metropolitan New York. Nutr Cancer 1982; (4):120-127.

Ekbom A, Yuen J, Adami H O, McLaughlin J K, Chow W H, Persson I, Fraumeni J F, Jr. Cholecystectomy and colorectal cancer. Gastroenterology 1993; (105):142-147.

Everhart J E, Khare M, Hill M, Maurer K R. Prevalence and ethnic differences in gallbladder disease in the United States. Gastroenterology 1999; (117):632-639.

Ferlay J, Bray F, Pisani P, Parkin D M. GLOBOCAN 2002: Cancer Incidence, Mortality and Prevalence Worldwide IARC CancerBase No. 5. version 2.0. Lyon 2004.

Fernandez E, Gallus S, La Vecchia C, Talamini R, Negri E, Franceschi S. Family history and environmental risk factors for colon cancer. Cancer Epidemiol Biomarkers Prev 2004; (13):658-661.

Gallus S, Negri E, Chatenoud L, Bosetti C, Franceschi S, La Vecchia C. Post-menopausal hormonal therapy and gallbladder cancer risk. Int J Cancer 2002; (99):762-763.

Gilat T, Feldman C, Halpern Z, Dan M, Bar-Meir S. An increased familial frequency of gallstones. Gastroenterology 1983; (84):242-246.

Giovannucci E, Colditz G A, Stampfer M J. A meta-analysis of cholecystectomy and risk of colorectal cancer. Gastroenterology 1993; (105): 130-141.

Glambek I, Kvaale G, Arnesjo B, Soreide O. Prevalence of gallstones in a Norwegian population. Scand J Gastroenterol 1987; (22):1089-1094.

Goldacre M J, Abisgold J D, Seagroatt V, Yeates D. Cancer after cholecystectomy: record-linkage cohort study. Br J Cancer 2005; (92):1307-1309.

Hemminki K, Chen B. Familial risks for colorectal cancer show evidence on recessive inheritance. Int J Cancer 2005; (115):835-838.

Hill M J. Bile flow and colon cancer. Mutat Res 1990; (238):313-320.

Hill M J, Drasar B S, Hawksworth G, Aries V, Crowther J S, Williams R E. Bacteria and aetiology of cancer of large bowel. Lancet 1971; (1): 95-100.

Johansen C, Chow W H, Jorgensen T, Mellemkjaer L, Engholm G, Olsen J H. Risk of colorectal cancer and other cancers in patients with gall stones. Gut 1996; (39):439-443.

Jorgensen T. Prevalence of gallstones in a Danish population. Am J Epidemiol 1987; (126):912-921.

Kameda H, Ishihara F, Shibata K, Tsukie E. Clinical and nutritional study on gallstone disease in Japan. Jpn J Med 1984; (23):109-113.

Kay C R. The Royal College of General Practitioners' Oral Contraception Study: some recent observations. Clin Obstet Gynaecol 1984; (11): 759-786.

Khuroo M S, Mahajan R, Zargar S A, Javid G, Sapru S. Prevalence of biliary tract disease in India: a sonographic study in adult population in Kashmir. Gut 1989; (30):201-205.

Koga S, Kaibara N, Takeda R. Effect of bile acids on 1,2-dimethylhydrazine-induced colon cancer in rats. Cancer 1982; (50):543-547.

Kuniyasu T, Tanaka T, Shima H, Sugie S, Mori H, Takahashi M. Enhancing effect of cholecystectomy on colon carcinogenesis induced by methyla-zoxymethanol acetate in hamsters. Dis Colon Rectum 1986; (29):492-494.

La Vecchia C, Chatenoud L, Negri E, Franceschi S. Session: whole cereal grains, fibre and human cancer wholegrain cereals and cancer in Italy. Proc Nutr Soc 2003; (62):45-49.

La Vecchia C, Negri E, D'Avanzo B, Franceschi S, Boyle P. Risk factors for gallstone disease requiring surgery. Int J Epidemiol 1991; (20):209-215.

Lagergren J, Ye W, Ekbom A. Intestinal cancer after cholecystectomy: is bile involved in carcinogenesis? Gastroenterology 2001; (121):542-547.

Lam C M, Murray F E, Cuschieri A. Increased cholecystectomy rate after the introduction of laparoscopic cholecystectomy in Scotland. Gut 1996; (38):282-284.

Legorreta A P, Silber J H, Costantino G N, Kobylinski R W, Zatz S L. Increased cholecystectomy rate after the introduction of laparoscopic cholecystectomy. JAMA 1993; (270):1429-1432.

Leitzmann M F, Giovannucci E L, Rimm E B, Stampfer M J, Spiegelman D, Wing A L, Willctt W C. The relation of physical activity to risk for symptomatic gallstone disease in men. Ann Intern Med 1998; (128):417-425.

Leitzmann M F, Rimm E B, Willett W C, Spiegelman D, Grodstein F, Stampfer M J, Colditz G A, Giovannucci E. Recreational physical activity and the risk of cholecystectomy in women. N Engl J Med 1999; (341):777-784.

Leitzmann M F, Stampfer M J, Willett W C, Spiegelman D, Colditz G A, Giovannucci E L. Coffee intake is associated with lower risk of symptomatic gallstone disease in women. Gastroenterology 2002; (123):1823-1830.

Leitzmann M F, Tsai C J, Stampfer M J, Rimm E B, Colditz G A, Willett W C, Giovannucci E L. Alcohol consumption in relation to risk of cholecystectomy in women. Am J Clin Nutr 2003; (78):339-347.

Lew E A, Garfinkel L. Variations in mortality by weight among 750,000 men and women. J Chronic Dis 1979; (32):563-576.

Maclure K M, Hayes K C, Colditz G A, Stampfer M J, Speizer F E, Willett W C. Weight, diet, and the risk of symptomatic gallstones in middle-aged women. N Engl J Med 1989; (321):563-569.

Malagelada J R, Go V L, Summerskill W H, Gamble

W S. Bile acid secretion and biliary bile acid composition altered by cholecystectomy. Am J Dig Dis 1973; (18):455-459.

Moerman C J, Smeets F W, Kromhout D. Dietary risk factors for clinically diagnosed gallstones in middle-aged men. A 25-year follow-up study (the Zutphen Study). Ann Epidemiol 1994; (4):248-254.

Moro P L, Checkley W, Gilman R H, Cabrera L, Lescano A G, Bonilla J J, Silva B. Gallstone disease in Peruvian coastal natives and highland migrants. Gut 2000; (46):569-573.

Narisawa T, Magadia N E, Weisburger J H, Wynder E L. Promoting effect of bile acids on colon carcinogenesis after intrarectal instillation of N-methyl-N'-nitro-N-nitrosoguanidine in rats. J Natl Cancer Inst 1974; (53):1093-1097.

Narisawa T, Reddy B S, Weisburger J H. Effect of bile acids and dietary fat on large bowel carcinogenesis in animal models. Gastroenterol Jpn 1978; (13):206-212.

Narisawa T, Sano M, Sato M, Takahashi T, Tanida N, Shimoyama T. The correlation between cholecystectomy and fecal bile acids, and large-bowel cancer induced with 1,2-dimethylhydrazine in mice. Dis Colon Rectum 1985; (28):27-30.

Nehlig A, Debry G. Potential genotoxic, mutagenic and antimutagenic effects of coffee: a review. Mutat Res 1994; (317):145-162.

Nomura H, Kashiwagi S, Hayashi J, Kajiyama W, Ikematsu H, Noguchi A, Tani S, Goto M. Prevalence of gallstone disease in a general population of Okinawa, Japan. Am J Epidemiol 1988; (128): 598-605.

Prathnadi P, Miki M, Suprasert S. Incidence of cholelithiasis in the northern part of Thailand. J Med Assoc Thai 1992; (75):462-470.

Randi G, Altieri A, Gallus S, Chatenoud L, Montella M, Franceschi S, Negri E, Talamini R, La Vecchia C. Marital status and cancer risk in Italy. Prev Med 2004; (38):523-528.

Reddy B S, Ekelund G, Bohe M, Engle A, Domellof L. Metabolic epidemiology of colon cancer: dietary pattern and fecal sterol concentrations of three populations. Nutr Cancer 1983; (5):34-40.

Reddy B S, Narasawa T, Weisburger J H, Wynder E L. Promoting effect of sodium deoxycholate on colon adenocarcinomas in germfree rats. J Natl Cancer Inst 1976; (56):441-442.

Reid F D, Mercer P M, harrison M, Bates T. Cholecystectomy as a risk factor for colorectal cancer: a meta-analysis. Scand J Gastroenterol 1996; (31):160-169.

Royal College of General Practitioners' oral contraception study. Oral contraceptives and gallbladder disease. Lancet 1982; (2):957-959.

Schernhammer E S, Leitzmann M F, Michaud D S, Speizer F E, Giovannucci E, Colditz G A, Fuchs C S. Cholecystectomy and the risk for developing colorectal cancer and distal colorectal adenomas. Br J Cancer 2003; (88):79-83.

Schirmer B D, Winters K L, Edlich R F. Cholelithiasis and cholecystitis. J Long Term Eff Med Implants 2005; (15):329-338.

Shaffer E A. Epidemiology and risk factors for gallstone disease: has the paradigm changed in the 21st century? Curr Gastroenterol Rep 2005; (7):132-140.

Shao T, Yang Y X. Cholecystectomy and the risk of colorectal cancer. Am J Gastroenterol 2005; (100):1813-1820.

Simon J A, Hudes E S. Serum ascorbic acid and gallbladder disease prevalence among US adults: the Third National Health and Nutrition Examination Survey (NHANES III). Arch Intern Med 2000; (160): 931-936.

Tavani A, La Vecchia C. Coffee, decaffeinated coffee, tea and cancer of the colon and rectum: a review of epidemiological studies, 1990-2003. Cancer Causes Control 2004; (15):743-757.

Todoroki I, Friedman G D, Slattery M L, Potter J D, Samowitz W. Cholecystectomy and the risk of colon cancer. Am J Gastroenterol 1999; (94): 41-46.

Tsai C J, Leitzmann M F, Willett W C, Giovannucci E L. Long-term intake of dietary fiber and decreased risk of cholecystectomy in women. Am J Gastroenterol 2004; (99):1364-1370.

Tsai C J, Leitzmann M F, Willett W C, Giovannucci E L. Glycemic load, glycemic index, and carbohydrate intake in relation to risk of cholecystectomy in women. Gastroenterology 2005; (129): 105-112.

Urbach D R, Stukel T A. Rate of elective cholecystectomy and the incidence of severe gallstone disease. CMAJ 2005; (172):1015-1019.

Wang W, Xue S, Ingles S A, Chen Q, Diep A T, Frankl H D, Stolz A, Haile R W. An association between genetic polymorphisms in the ileal sodium-dependent bile acid transporter gene and the risk of colorectal adenomas. Cancer Epidemiol Biomarkers Prev 2001; (10):931-936.

Weidema W F, Deschner E E, Cohen B I, DeCosse J J. Acute effects of dietary cholic acid and methylazoxymethanol acetate on colon epithelial cell proliferation; metabolism of bile salts and neutral sterols in conventional and germfree SD rats. J Natl Cancer Inst 1985; (74):665-670.

Zhao Y, Zhang R, Hu Y, Li R, Liang L, Gang Y. [An epidemiological survey of gallstones with gray-scale ultrasound]. Hua Xi Yi Ke Da Xue Xue Bao 1990; (21):217-220.

Advances in diagnosis and treatment of biliary strictures and stenoses

Principe Alfonso, Ercolani Giorgio, Solmi Luigi, Golfieri Rita, Giampalma Emanuela

ABSTRACT

Benign stenoses and strictures of the biliary tract are uncommon and usually result from iatrogenic injuries of the bile duct occurred during surgical procedures like cholecystectomy, hepatic resection or biliary-enteric anastomosis. They may also complicate liver transplantation. Other causes are chronic inflammation like chronic pancreatitis, choledocholithiasis, parasitic infection and primary sclerosing cholangitis. Rarely benign bile duct stenosis may be congenital (for example biliary atresia), develop as a complication of an acute cholecystitis (Mirizzi's syndrome) or be secondary to trauma or spontaneous biliary rupture which is an exceptional event. Benign strictures can sometimes mimic a malignant disease that has to be ruled out.

Cholestasis is usually the clinical feature that leads to the diagnosis. Once a biliary damage is suspected at surgery, intraoperative cholangiography allows an early detection of the lesion and is therefore advisable. Biliary damages that go unnoticed at surgery can be diagnosed through a percutaneous on endoscopic cholangiography.

An inadequate experience of the surgeon is often the underlying cause of the biliary damage; cholecystectomy should be performed by fully-trained surgeons.

Treatment of biliary stenoses can be non-surgical (percutaneous or endoscopic balloon catheter dilation) or surgical. In this latter case the choice of the surgical strategy will depend on the site and the length of the stenosis.

After resection of the stenotic tract, the biliary-enteric anastomosis should be as wide as possible, which is best achieved by performing a hepatico-jejunostomy proximal to the liver.

In all benign strictures of the biliary tract, the outcome depends on the experience and competence of all the teams involved (surgeons, radiologists and endoscopists) in selecting and performing the most suitable corrective procedure.

IATROGENIC LESIONS OF THE BILIARY TRACT

Iatrogenic lesions of the biliary tract during the course of surgical intervention are always a serious event.

The majority of bile duct lesions are caused by accidental surgical trauma during cholecystectomy (more than 80%)

and, to a lesser degree, during other types of procedures, as a consequence of improperly performed choledochorraphy or bilio-digestive anastomosis (BDA) or hepatic resection.

The advent of Laparoscopic Cholecystectomy (LC) has provoked an increased incidence of iatrogenic biliary lesions with values from 0.3-0.7% versus the low incidence of 0.1-0.2% seen in the last years with Open Cholecystectomy (OC). Thanks to the learning curve in laparoscopic surgery in the last 20 years, the risk of bile duct injuries after LC has been significantly reduced, even if it remains two or three time superior than the risk in OC.

A recent Italian survey reported that between 1998 and 2000 among 56.591 LC the incidence of iatrogenic biliary injuries was 0.41%; the accidental transection of bile duct was reported in 0.31% of cases, while in the other cases minor biliary injuries was found (such as Luschka duct).

Independently of the method adopted for cholecystectomy, the principal surgical causes of biliary lesions are:
– incorrect indication for surgery in cases of acute cholecystitis;
– the presence of congenital anomalies of the bile ducts and/or the arteries, which often run with anomalous course;
– insufficient pre- or intra-operative morphological studies;
– lack of experience of the surgeon; it is well known that the incidence of iatrogenic biliary injuries significantly decreases as the number of performed cholecystectomies by the surgeon increases.

The types of iatrogenic biliary injuries include: partial or total section of the bile duct (with or without loss of substance), ligation of the bile duct, extensive dissection which damages the delicate hepatic microcirculation of the common bile duct causing ischaemic necrosis with formation of scar tissue and retraction of the proxi-

mal stricture toward and into the hilus which may be more frequent in cases of chronic cholecystitis.

In almost 25% of cases, there are technical problems:
– the excessive use of diatermo-coagulation within the Calot's triangle cause an ischaemic scar which may lead to a perforation few days after operation causing a biliary peritonitis; or it may cause a late biliary stenosis due to the chronic inflammatory reaction (careful must be taken in using the diatermo-coagulation close to surgical clip);
– intra-operative bleeding since in order to stop bleeding from cystic artery or pericholedocus vessels the use of surgical clip in a dirty surgical field may cause accidental damage of bile duct.

There are some recommendations which may be suggested to reduce the incidence of lesions during cholecystectomy. First of all, a meticulous dissection to visualize the biliary anatomy. In this regard, most surgeons perform routinely intra-operative cholangiography to define the biliary anatomy, to detect unsuspected CBD stones, and to control the integrity of the biliary duct during OC. Similarly, 50% of Centres in Europe and U.S.A. performed routine intra-operative cholangiography during LC.[20-22] However, some Authors have pointed out that the incidence of biliary lesions is similar between those centres which advocate systematic intra-operative cholangiography and those where it is done selectively. It can be accepted that intra-operative cholangiography is not able to reduce the incidence of biliary injuries but it is useful to recognize them immediately and to treat them in the best way.

Classification of iatrogenic biliary lesions

The classification proposed by Bismuth (Figure 1) is still now the most used and accepted world wide, even if other classifications have been proposed after the introduction of LC.

Other causes of biliary strictures: whenever an hepato-jejunum anastomosis has been performed, it may be complicated by early fistula or late stricture. This reconstruction is usually required in case of tumor of the head of the pancreas or of the bile duct, or after resection of choledochal cysts. Late stenosis are more common when the hepato-jejunostomy is performed with a normal-caliber duct; on the

contrary is less frequent if the anastomosis is performed after long-standing biliary obstruction with a dilated duct.

Even liver resections may be complicated by biliary damage. In cases of suspected biliary injuries an intra-operative cholangiography should be performed and a T-tube eventual leaved in place. Usually postoperative fistula solves spontaneously. However, an aggressive approach may be required in case of persistent fistula after long period of observation or late strictures.

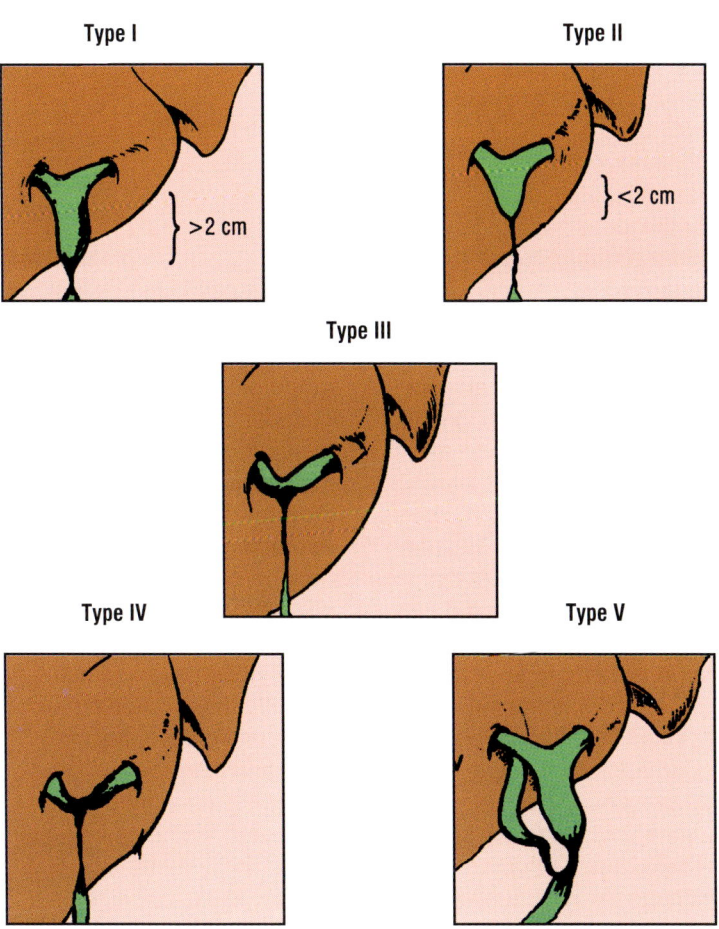

FIGURE 1: Bismuth's classification of iatrogenic biliary strictures.

Diagnosis

Today, the most frequently used imaging procedures in diagnosing biliary tract diseases are ultrasound and magnetic resonance cholangiography (MRCP). Computed Tomography (CT) is more useful in diagnosing malignant diseases, but it is also used in patients with unclear ultrasound findings, especially since the advent of multislice CT, which may in time become a valid alternative to Magnetic Resonance techniques in the diagnosis of biliary diseases. Invasive examinations, such as endoscopic retrograde cholangio-pancreatography (ERCP) and percutaneous transhepatic cholangiography (PTC) are only necessary in solving unclear diagnostic findings or whenever biliary interventional procedures have to be performed.

Ultrasonography (US) is useful in a large percentage of cases (80-90%), being able to identify both segmentary and estensive dilation of biliary ducts. The US findings are different depending on the causes of the benign stenosis of the biliary tree. In iatrogenic lesions after cholecystectomy (laparatomic and laparascopic), the stenosis does not appear on US, which shows only indirect signs represented by upper biliary duct dilation, present in the early postoperative period. After approximately 7% of cases of laparascopic cholecystectomy, US shows an anechoic lesion (biloma), caused by the perforation of common bile duct, in the gallbladder bed or in parahilar site. If the biliary perforation is associated with minimum bleeding, then the fluid collections, represented by haematoma, are larger and appear more echogenic at US examination. In those cases, the first step in treatment will be US or CT-guided percutaneous drainage. In patients with biliary-enteric anastomosis (choledocojejunostomy, choledoco-duodenostomy, hepatico-jejunostomy) as well as in

patients who have undergone orthotopic liver transplantation (OLT), scar strictures are not directly shown by US due to the presence of air in the biliary tree. In such cases, CT is more useful in the evaluation of the diameter of biliary ducts. When an anastomotic stenosis is suspected, the hepatobiliary radionuclide scintigraphy with 99Tc-HIDA represents a useful diagnostic functional examination, because it is able to evaluate the bile flow delayed in the enteric loops.

Computed Tomography, with multi-slice technique of the biliary tract is commonly part of an upper abdominal examination, performed before and after contrast media injection in biphasic acquisition. Portal phase scan is best for showing the intrahepatic bile ducts, providing an optimum contrast between the hypoattenuating bile and the liver parenchyma. The examination may be completed by performing CT cholangiography (CTC). Contrast-enhanced CT cholangiography without cholangiographic contrast media is performed using multiplanar (MPR) and minimum intensity projection (MinIP) reconstructions, while Virtual CT cholangiography (Virtual-CTC) and CT cholangiography with cholangiographic contrast media require the oral or intravenous administration of cholangiographic contrast medium to opacify the biliary tract prior to scanning. CTC with reconstructions provide a panoramic, cholangiographic-like view of the bile ducts, useful in complex situations (Figure 2).

CT scan is also useful in postoperative complications after laparoscopic or laparotomic cholecystectomy. For example, during surgery the common bile duct or a hepatic duct may be mistaken for the cystic duct and may be ligated. Strictures occasionally result from cautery injuries, and bile leaks may also occur. In the postoperative setting, CT is often preferred to US and MRI in diagnosing laparoscopic-related complications, such as bilomas,

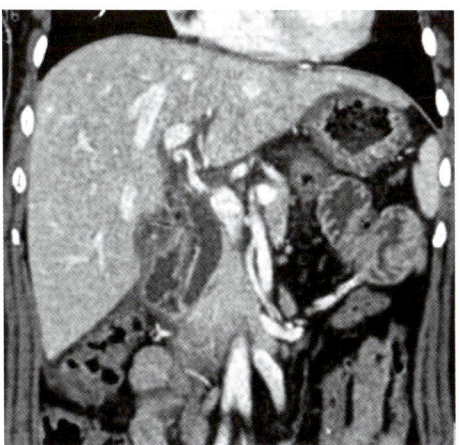

FIGURE 2: CT Multiplanar Reconstruction in coronal projection shows dilated common bile duct.

compared, as some of them, especially VRT, could overestimate stenosis in approximately 40% of cases.

Magnetic resonance cholangio-pancreatography

In patients with benign stenosis of the biliary tract, after US and CT examinations, a cholangiography ought to be performed prior to the therapeutic decision. ERCP and PTC are traditionally the reference standards, but both methods are invasive, time-consuming and associated with 5%-7% morbidity and less than 1% mortality. By MRCP, accurate imaging of the biliary system is possible and that technique has gained recognition as an accurate and non-invasive alternative method for evaluating pancreaticobiliary ductal abnormalities and is gradually replacing direct cholangiography. Several studies demonstrated that the non invasive MRCP have a comparable accuracy with that of ERCP for the differentiation of benign from malignant bile duct strictures: therefore, at present, MRCP is the first choice as non-invasive direct cholangiography for the diagnosis of bile duct disorders, both in patients with normal anatomy and in those with biliary-enteric-anastomoses, with nearly 100% diagnostic accuracy in detecting bile duct strictures. The high sensibility of MRCP relies on its ability to completely visualize both the ductal system proximal to the obstruction and the extent of biliary involvement, without injecting contrast material that sometimes cannot pass beyond a high-grade obstruction and is consequently unable to visualize ducts and strictures beyond an obstruction (Figure 3). However, MRCP have a tendency to overestimate strictures, especially in length, because the duct immediately distal to the stenosis may have collapsed. Moreover, while direct cholangiography (ERCP or PTC) provides functional information and has a higher sensibility in

haematomas, peritoneal haemorrhage or bile peritonitis, due its lower rate of interference from the perihepatic fluids. In these cases, CT detects focal fluid collections in gallbladder fossa and liver hilum, or free fluid in the abdomen. To obtain a specific demonstration of a biliary leak, CTC or ERCP/PTC should be performed.

The ligation or stricture of a normal bile duct leads to marked cholestasis, followed by the atrophy of the drained liver segment, which appears on CT as volume reduction of the parenchyma with marked dilatation of bile segmental ducts.

When accompanied by stenosis or occlusion of the right hepatic artery, arterial phase images (CT angiography) help to demonstrate the absence of intrahepatic arterial visualization, with an increased caliber of extrahepatic systemic arteries and peripheral Transient Hepatic Attenuation Differences (THAD). CT angiography is also indicated in OLT patients with ischemic intrahepatic biliary stenosis in order to identify the level and the severity of the arterial damage. In any case the CT reconstruction algorithms should be integrated (MPR, MIP, VRT) and the results

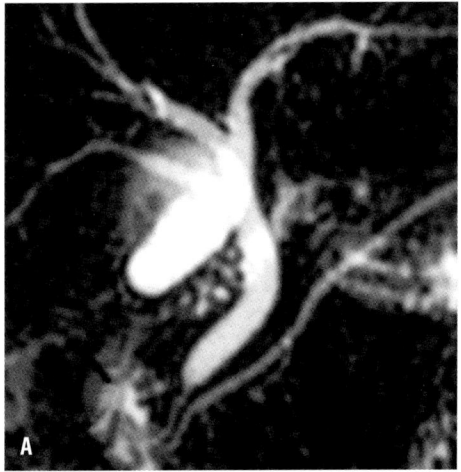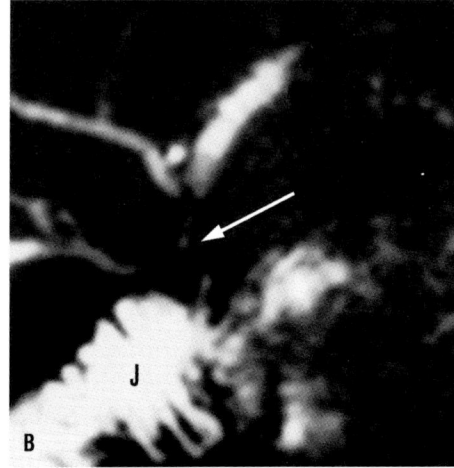

FIGURE 3: MRCP shows entire biliary tract either in normal anatomy **(A)**. Either in hepaticojejunostomy **(B)**. With good visualization of biliary stenosis (b, arrow).

detecting stones, bile leaks and collections, MRC is a static imaging study unable to distinguish strictures from other causes of obstruction (e.g. stones, sludge, compression by a fluid collection). Conventional MRCP can also be limited by conflicting signals from ascites, perihepatic fluid collections and biloma. Recently, to overcome these difficulties, a new contrast agent (Mangafodipir trisodium) primarily excreted in the bile after intravenous injection, has been introduced to increase the quality of the MRC image, compared to the conventional technique, while obtaining functional findings. In fact, mangafodipir trisodium-enhanced MRCP performs better than conventional MRCP in visualizing intra- and extrahepatic ducts and biliary anastomosis, even when intraabdominal fluid or perihepatic edema are present. Moreover, this technique detects biliary leaks and accurately evaluates the delay of excretion into the distal duct and bowel, thus obtaining functional information regarding the presence of biliary strictures: distal excretion within 15 minutes indicates the absence of any significant ductal stenosis.

Percutaneous transhepatic cholangiography and endoscopic retrograde-cholangiopancreatography

Cholangiography with direct injection of contrast media into the biliary system can be performed either after the puncture of an intrahepatic bile duct using a 22-gauge needle under US or fluoroscopic guidance (in PTC), or after the endoscopic cannulation of the common bile duct via the ampulla of Vater (in ERCP). In post-operative bile duct strictures, PTC should be preferred to ERCP as it better defines the anatomy of the proximal biliary tree to be used in surgical reconstruction; yet, in experienced hands, a complete diagnostic cholangiogram can be achieved in nearly all cases of ERCP.

After PTC, a biliary drainage must be inserted to reduce the risk of complications, such as cholangitis, pancreatitis or peritonitis due to bile leakage, and to maintain a bile duct access in case percutaneous treatments become necessary. On the other hand, after ERCP, if sphincterotomy is performed, there is a 5% to

6% risk of pancreatitis and a smaller risk of bleeding, infection or perforation.

At present, the diagnostic role of these standards of reference is limited because both procedures are invasive and associated with morbidity and mortality. Moreover, the direct injection of contrast material may lead to low-grade biliary strictures being overestimated because of the overdistension of ducts, while, because a contrast medium cannot pass beyond a high-grade stricture, any additional stenoses beyond this point would not be detected. Consequently, ERCP or PTC are only necessary when non-invasive procedure findings are not diagnostic or when they are the first step in biliary interventions. When bile ducts are dilated, PTC has a 100% success rate, when they are not, the success rate is lower (80%), while ERCP is unsuccessful in approximately 18% of patients, irregardless of the grade of bile duct diameter.

Direct cholangiography (by ERCP or PTC) is able to define the level of biliary stenosis or obstruction, identify the presence of bile duct stones, and determine the etiology of cholangitis. It can also evaluate suspected bile duct inflammatory disorders and identify the site of a bile leak. In the case of biliary stenosis, it may be difficult to interpret lesion morphology, especially when strictures occur months to years after surgery. Hence, particular caution must be used in putting forward judgements of benign or malignant steno-obstructive alterations. In fact, although benign lesions typically produce harmonic, linear strictures while malignancies produce irregular stenoses with signs of parietal infiltration, morphological pictures do not always fit with that distinction. Consequently, the cholangiography appearance must be integrated with clinical information and with data provided by US and CT in order to obtain the correct diagnosis in patients with biliary stenosis.

Tissue sampling: brushing, biopsy

In some cases of suspected biliary strictures a pathologic examination should be performed in order to obtain the correct differential diagnosis between benign or malignant stenosis (i.e. a differential diagnosis between sclerosing cholangitis and cholangiocarcinoma), before making a therapeutic decision. Endobiliary fluid can be aspirated through the drainage catheter to obtain a specimen for cytology, while tissue sampling can be performed endoscopically or percutaneously under fluoroscopic control. Both during ERCP and PTC is possible to obtain tissue sample in biliary strictures for increasing the rate of correct diagnosis particularly differentiating benign from malignant strictures. Ideally, a tissue sampling technique should have a high sensitivity for detection of cancer, with absolute specificity: unfortunately, none of the currently used PTC-ERCP tissue sampling methods have all these characteristics. All current methods have relatively low to moderate sensitivity but almost 100% specificity. The sensitivity of the individual tissue sampling techniques ranges from approximately 20% to 60%. The detection rate at PTC and ERCP may be increased by combining at least two sampling methods, with the highest sensitivity having been demonstrated for the combination of endoscopic fine-needle aspiration, biopsy and brush cytology. A brush or a forceps device is introduced at site of the obstruction and a specimen for cytology (brushing) or histology (forceps) is obtained (Figure 4). The results of the biopsy can be improved by direct endoscopic vision or percutaneous choledoscopy; both methods allow to provide more precise sampling with forceps. Small calibre endoscopes are now available and can be introduced through standard biliary drainage catheters. While

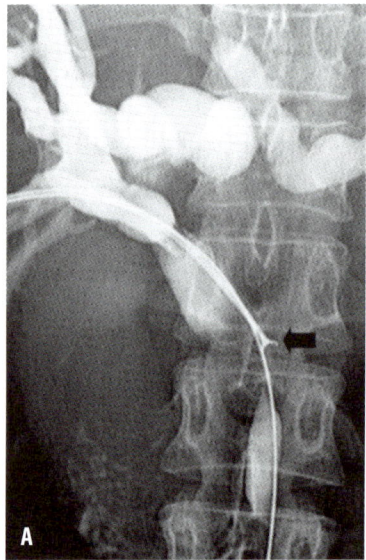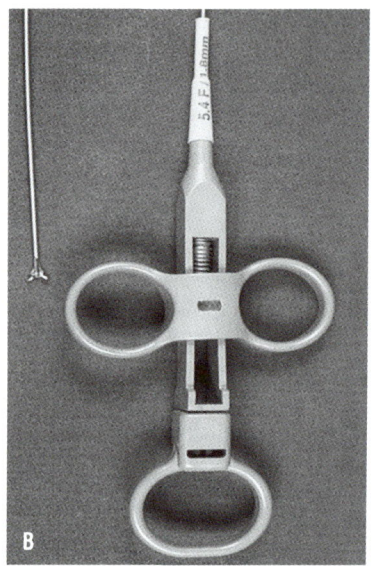

FIGURE 4: Forceps biopsy by percutaneous approach in severe stricture in the common bile duct (**A** - arrow). Thin diameter of device (**B**) allows to introduce it through standard biliary catheters.

histological results by forceps biopsy are quite good (78% sensitivity, 100% specificity, 79% accuracy), the endobiliary cytology obtained by brushing provides poor results in terms of sensitivity (9-24%), specificity (61-100%) and accuracy (43-51%). Therefore, in order to reduce the incidence of false-negative diagnoses, brushing must always be combined with forceps biopsy: the accuracy of these combined methods is high and surgical confirmation is unnecessary in the majority of cases.

TREATMENT

The treatment should be based on the type of lesion, time of recognition, surgical experience in hepato-biliary surgery and non-surgical treatment available. If improperly managed, life-treating complications such as biliary cirrhosis, portal hypertension and cholangitis may be developed.

The goal standard is to select the best treatment for the best long-term result. Moreover the prognosis is strictly correlated with the moment of discovery of the lesion. Regardless of which method is adopted, OC or LC, the lesions can become evident immediately or, they may not appear until later. Unfortunately only a small number of the lesions are immediately recognized at the time of surgery (11-23%); it is not improbable that the extent of the problem may be underestimated and the fibrosis process tends to spread upwards causing retraction of the proximal biliary fragment up to the biliary convergence where the mucosa is uninvolved during the follow up.

Injury recognized at the time of operation

The first description of a surgical approach to repair the biliary tract, injured during an open cholecystectomy, was performed by Kehr in 1899. When the injury of bile duct is recognized at the time of operation, the surgeon should evaluate his experience and competence to solve the problem, the eventual presence of an expert surgeon, or decide to close the abdomen and refer the patient to a specialized centre. Bile duct should be dissected widely to evaluate the damage and intraoperative cholangiography should be performed to study the anatomy. In the case of laparoscopic approach, conversion to laparotomy is mandatory. The aims of immediate repair should be the maintenance of the entire bile duct as long as possible, and the prevention of postoperative bile leakage which can be obtained providing an external drainage by a tube (eventually a T-tube) inserted in the bile duct.

It should be emphasized that the initial repair may not be the definitive solution.

In case of complete transection, if the lesion is minimal and there is no loss of substance, repair is effected by an accurate end-to-end anastomosis on a guide T-tube with re-absorbable suture (to reduce the tension, a complete mobilization of duodenum and pancreatic head should be performed). If there is loss of substance greater than 2 cm. and/or the lesion is near the convergence of the hepatic duct, it is best to effect a wide bilio-digestive anastomosis to the hilar plate (Figure 5).

In case of lateral injuries, again direct suture with re absorbable filament can be applied with an interposition of drainage to drain the bile and to check bile duct integrity postoperatively. Some authors have proposed to a Roux-en-Y loop of jejunum as a serosal patch to prevent stenosis and to maintain the length of bile duct.

Choledocho-duodenostomy can find justification only in lower lesions and in older and weaker patients.

Injury recognized in the postoperative course

It may present as bile leakage through the

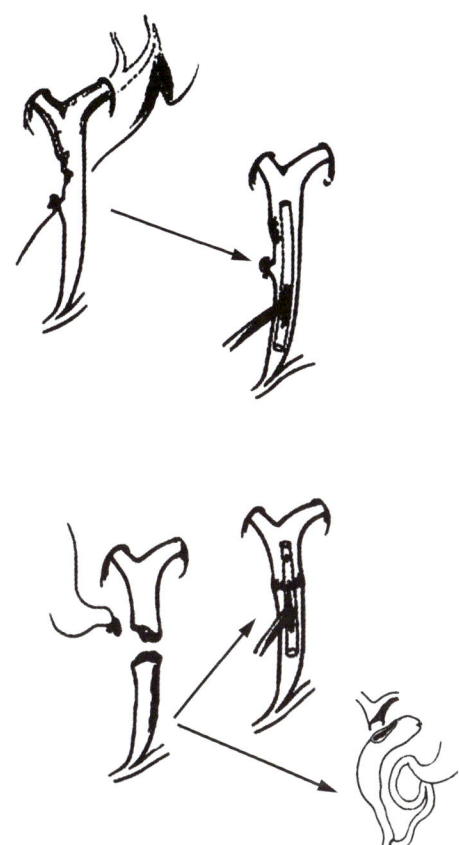

FIGURE 5: Biliary reconstruction in case of lateral injuries of the bile duct and complete transection; when the lesion is near the convergence of the hepatic duct, the suitable reconstruction must be a hepatojejunostomy according to the Hepp-Couinaud technique.

drain or the wound, or with progressive jaundice. A delayed approach is preferable: non-operative closure of the fistula is often associated with dilation of proximal duct with a subsequent easier repair. In order to postpone the operation, a conservative manage of the fistula by endoscopic or percutaneous biliary drainage is advisable to prevent intra-abdominal bile collection and peritonitis; it may control sepsis and allow most biliary fistulae to be closed without early interventional surgery. Early sphincterotomy to reduce intraduct pressure and facilitate transpapillary bile drainage has been reported.

Injury presenting late after operation

The management of postoperative bile duct strictures has also traditionally been surgically, by repair over a T-tube, choledocho-duodenostomy or Roux-en-Y hepatico-jejunostomy. However, during long-term follow-up after surgical repair, 12% to 45% of patients will experience relapsing symptoms because of recurrent stricture formation at the anastomotic site. ERCP and percutaneous transhepatic cholangiography (PTC) have been described as alternatives to surgery (Figure 6).

• *Endoscopic treatment*
The feasibility and success of endoscopic therapy is dependent on several factors;

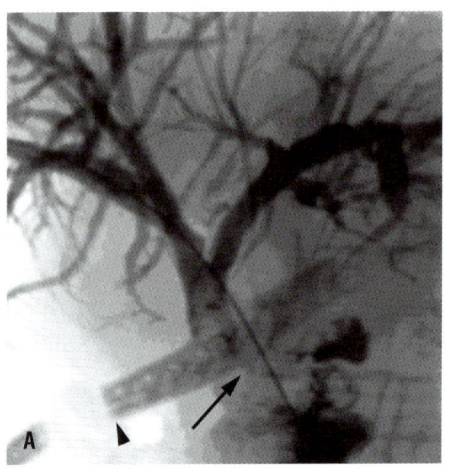

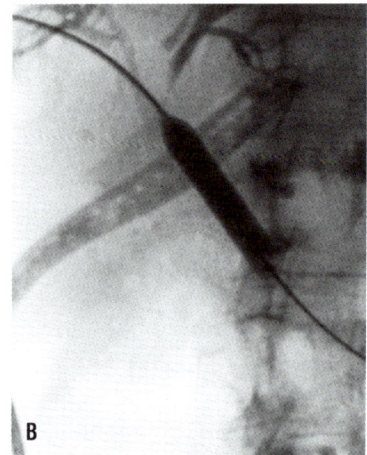

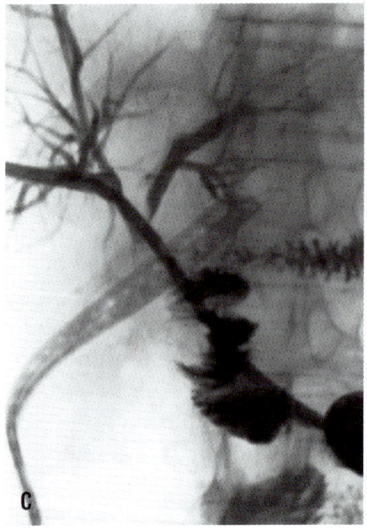

FIGURE 6: PTC in patient with biliary-enteric-anastomosis after laparoscopic cholecystectomy complicated by injury in the common bile duct **(A)**. A bile leak along the surgical drainage (arrow head) appeared some weeks after initial surgery and cholangiographic study demonstrated an associated anastomotic stricture (arrow). The combination of balloon dilation **(B)** and transhepatic catheter placement **(C)** allowed treatment of the stenosis and closure of the fistula without further surgery.

anatomical aspects such as altered anatomy (Billroth I or II) make endoscopic therapy more difficult but feasible. Other anatomical conditions (Roux-en-Y) but also total clip or suture occlusion, total transection or disconnected missing segments make endoscopic therapy by definition impossible. In such cases PTC is the non surgical first step procedure.

At the first ERCP, a sphincterotomy is done to facilitate further instrumentation; after diagnostic cholangiography and imaging of the bile duct stricture, a guide wire is passed. Over this guide wire a hydrostatic balloon (4 up to 8 mm when inflated) is advanced; the balloon is inflated under fluoroscopic control up to 12-14 atmospheres. Balloon dilation only, without subsequent stenting, has not been shown to be effective due to high recurrence rates; thus after dilation, stents need to be inserted. At the first ERCP at least one, but preferably two 10 French stents are inserted; if only one stent can be inserted, six weeks later elective stent exchange is planned with insertion of two or if at all possible, more 10 French stents. From the moment that at least two stents are inserted, elective stent exchange every 3 to 4 months is advise, if clinically indicated earlier, for at least one year. Thus every patient requires multiple (3 to 5) endoscopic management sessions during this period of time; if after one year an inflated balloon with a diameter of 10 mm cannot be passed easily, probably the endoscopic therapy is to be considered a failure. There are no data regarding the optimal duration of stenting, but after one year, or earlier when non progress in dilating is observed, surgery should be considered. The success rate of endoscopic dilation ranges from 80% to 100% in the different series, but during long-term follow-up a 10-15% of patients, similar to that of surgical repair, experience recurrence of strictures. Recently, two retrospective different series suggested a more aggressive approach to endoscopic therapy inserting as many stents as possible at each elective stent exchange; endoscopic treatment was discontinued only if the strictures had completely disappeared on occlusion cholangiogram. All stenosis resolved and none or low percentage of patients developed re-stenosis during long term follow-up.

There are no randomized studies available comparing endoscopic treatment with surgical repair for patients with postoperative bile duct strictures.

ERCP presents some incidence of complications; early complications (5% to 15%) are usually directly procedure related and consist of low grade fever, acute cholangitis, pancreatitis and post sphincterotomy bleeding. Late complications during stenting (11% to 60%) are stent dysfunction due to clogging with or without jaundice and overt cholangitis or stent dislodgement. Late complications are higher in those patients who are not adhering to the planned elective stent exchanges; after stent exchanges however, symptoms resolve quickly and generally complications are of mild severity.

• *Percutaneous treatment*
A transhepatic procedure can be performed with a combination of local anesthesia and intravenous sedation and consists, using the right midline transaxillary approach, in the direct puncture of a right posterior segmental bile duct under fluoroscopic or ultrasound guidance; cholangiogram allows to identify the stenosis that is transversed with a guidewire and dilated using angioplasty-type balloon catheters, chosen on the basis of the location of the stricture and the diameter of the normal bile duct (range from 6 to 12 mm). Usually, the balloon is inflated two or three consecutive times at high pressure for 1-3 minutes (Figures 7, 8). This procedure should be repeated in successive sessions until no residual stric-

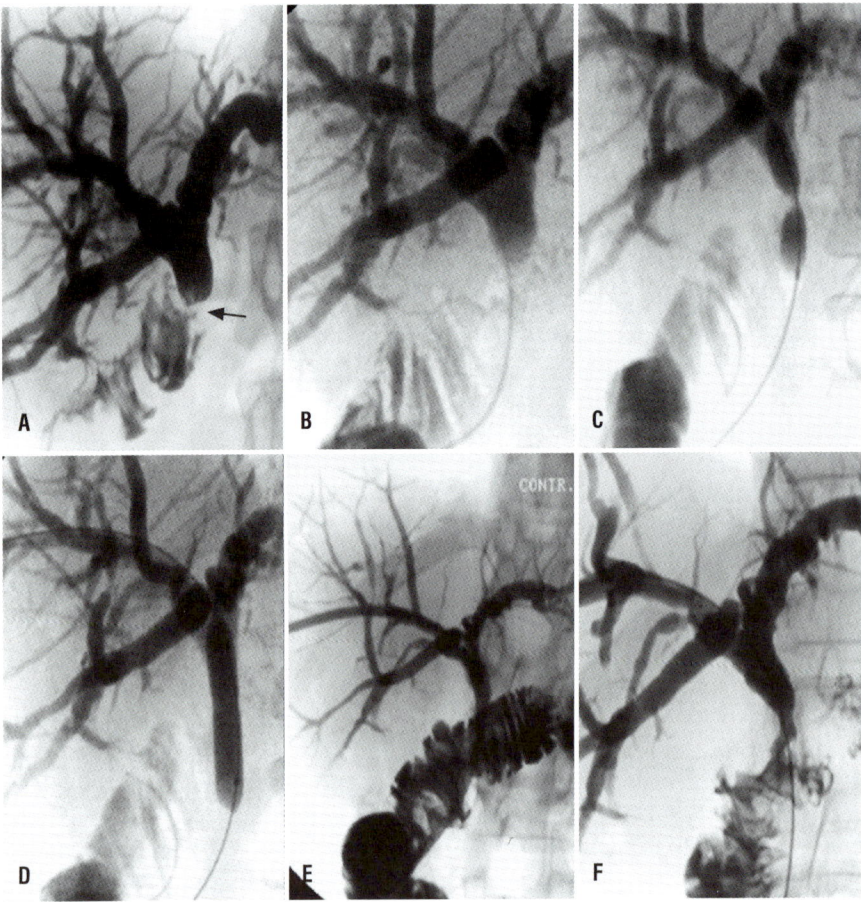

FIGURE 7: PTC **(A)** Shows a tight anastomotic stricture in patient with hepaticojejunostomy (arrow), complication resulting from laparoscopic cholecystectomy. The first step of the percutaneous treatment is to transverse the stenosis with a guidewire; **(B)** then the balloon is inserted and inflated with high pressure until the disappearance of the balloon waist **(C-D)**. At the end of the dilation, a transhepatic biliary drainage **(E)** is left in place for some months to obtain a satisfactory anastomotic diameter **(F)**.

ture can be seen, and the success of dilation is defined as the disappearance of a balloon waist during inflation.

After dilation, a transhepatic biliary catheter of adequate calibre (8 to 12 French) is left in place across the stenosis to gravitate drainage. Subsequently, the catheter is capped off and internalised to preserve the lumen during the healing process. The patient is then discharged with an internalised stent and returns as an outpatient for follow-up cholangiogra-phy, repeated dilation and to replace the biliary catheter at 2- to 3-month intervals. In most cases, numerous balloon dilations are required before the results become stabilised, while the biliary catheter has to remain in place for several weeks or months. In the presence of complex (Bismuth III, IV or V) injuries or strictures, multiple access may be required to place two or more catheters.

In some cases of laparoscopic bile duct injuries in which the bile duct has

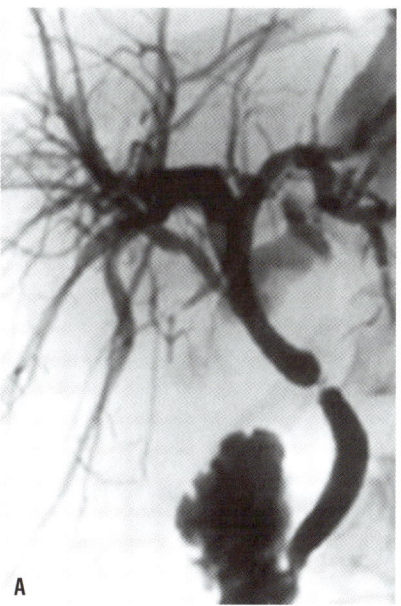

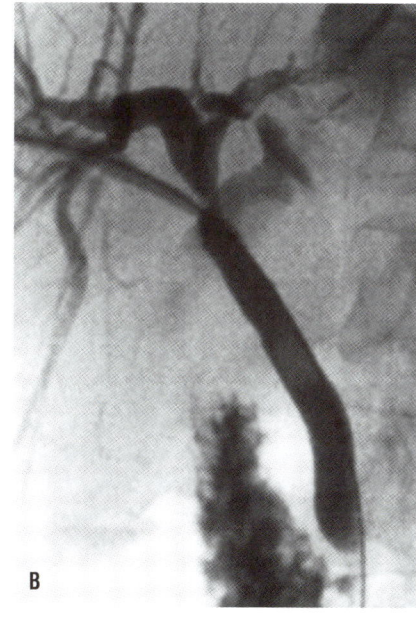

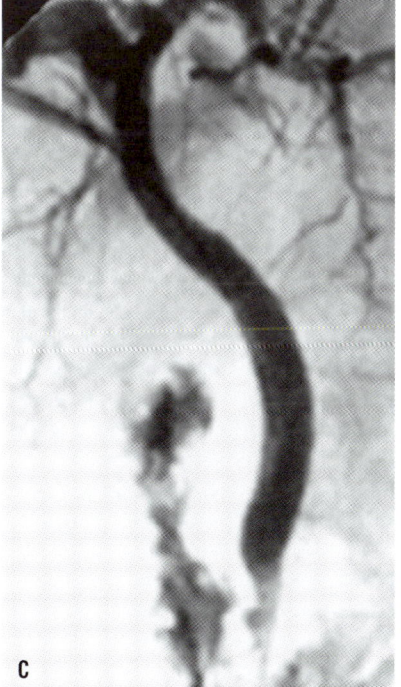

FIGURE 8. PTC **(A)** demonstrates a tight stenosis at the level of the choledococholedocostomy in OLT patient. The one shot balloon dilation **(B)** determines a satisfactory result **(C)** without any recurrence after 3 months.

been transected, percutaneous management is limited to the diagnostic phase, because the presence of biliary-enteric continuity is needed in order to attempt non-operative definitive percutaneous management (Figure 9).

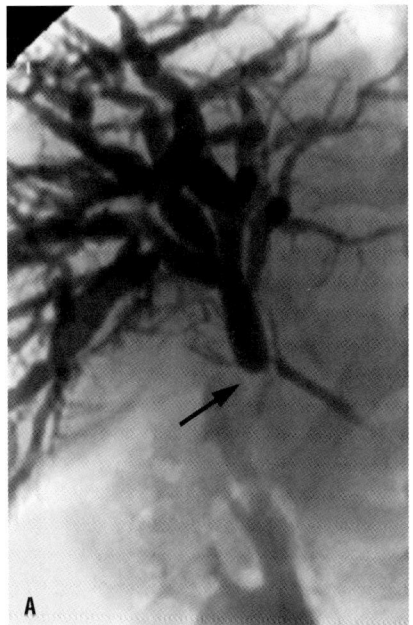

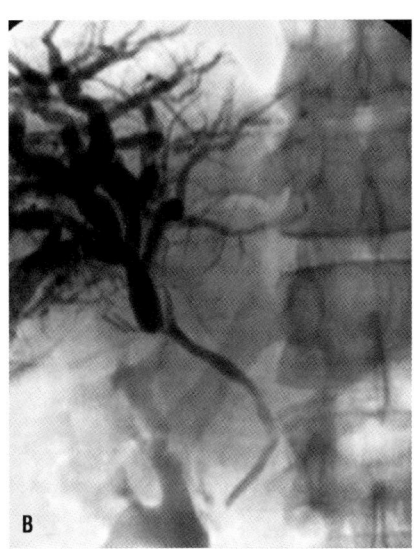

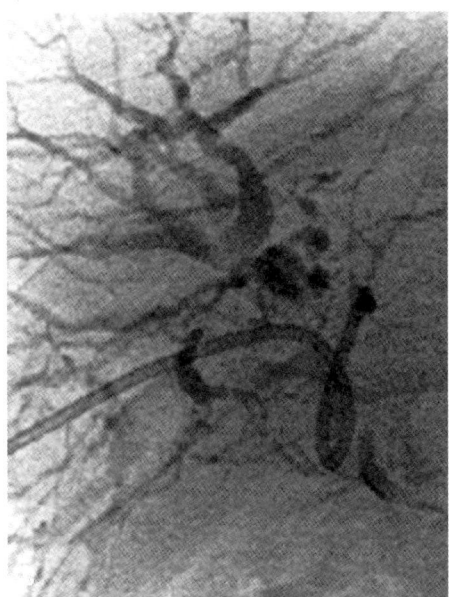

FIGURE 9: PTC post-laparascopic cholecystectomy shows a complete transection of the common bile duct (arrow) with dilation of the right biliary system **(A)** and without evidence of the left one **(B)**. An external preoperative biliary drainage has been left in place **(C)** before performing surgery (left lobectomy and hepaticojejunostomy).

Complications of balloon dilation are frequent but usually mild and recovery is spontaneous. Cholangitis, haemobilia and bile leaks can occur in up to 20% of the patients, while severe bleeding and sepsis are rare. The main cause of morbidity is the result of transversing the hepatic parenchyma by the large percutaneously placed catheters.

Many series during pre-laparoscopic c-holecystectomy report excellent results during a 3-year follow-up, with an overall success rate of 70% to 78%. The patency rate in iatrogenic primary bile duct strictures (range from 76% to 88%) is better than in biliary-enteric anastomotic strictures (range from 67% to 73%).

Several short-term series[70,76,77] that examined the percutaneous management of bile duct injuries following laparoscopic cholecystectomy report good results with a success rate of 64% after a mean follow-up of 28 months, while a recent study, regarding long-term results in a large population of patients undergoing percutaneous balloon dilation, provides an overall primary success rate of 58.8% during a mean follow-up of more than 6 years.

These data demonstrate that the majority of recurrent strictures develop within 3 years following percutaneous treatment. The most significant causes of failure are the presence of more complex injuries (Bismuth III, IV, V, or isolated right hepatic duct) and/or too little time for stenting (less than 4 months), with most strictures recurring within the first 6 months after initial stenting.

It is difficult to compare the results of non-operative dilation with those of surgery as no prospective randomized studies have been published to date. The only exception are three retrospective comparative studies, reporting an overall success rate of 83% to 94% after surgery against a 52% to 72% rate after non-operative treatment, with better results following endoscopic stenting.

In the case of refractory intrahepatic biliary strictures with recurrence after balloon dilation or surgical repair, it is possible to place metallic stent. They are widely used in case of malignant obstructions, but its role in case of benign strictures is still controversial. However, self-expanding stainless steel stents represent a solution because they exert continuous outward radial pressure on the bile duct and prevent the elastic recoil of the wall. The metallic stent is inserted percutaneously and generally placed with its lower end immediately above the papilla (ampulla of Vater) and relaxed with the mid-portion placed at the narrowest point of the stricture. The only exception is a distal common bile duct lesion, in which the stent should abut into the duodenum. Subsequently, an angioplasty balloon catheter may be used to expand the stent until it achieves its maximum internal diameter. If the dilation causes haemobilia, a biliary drain should be left in place for a few days to prevent blood clots from creating a possible occlusion of the lumen.

The initial results of three early trials using self-expanding metallic stents in benign strictures (secondary to chronic pancreatitis) appear promising, with an occlusion rate of 7-13% after a short follow-up (mean 7 months). The long-term patency rate and the effects on the bile duct wall have not yet been documented and further studies are needed.

• *Surgical approach*

Surgery for bile duct strictures should be afforded after full investigation and patients should be operated on in elective set and brought to optimal condition.

In the presence of cholangitis, administration of antibiotics is important preliminarly to surgical treatment. In fact, percutaneous decompression is the only way to treat severe episodes of recurrent cholangitis, but preoperative antibiotics are fundamental to manage mild recurrent attack and in the prevention of perioperative infectious complications. It is usually recommended to continue antibiotics from 2 up to 5 days postoperatively.

The nutritional status of patients with bile duct strictures is usually compromised; preoperative nutritional support is often necessary (in a few cases by enteral feeding via nasogastric tube or parenteral nutrition), in order to improve general clinical conditions, to re-enstablish fluid and electrolyte balance. Coagulation defects secondary to prolong hyper-bilirubinemia may managed by administration of vitamin K or fresh frozen plasma.

First of all to expose proximal bile ducts which drain all hepatic segments. Often, a preoperative evaluation by percutaneous biliary drainage is mandatory to study biliary anatomy and to release jaundice. Then a suitable segment of biliary duct must be prepared to perform the anastomosis with a jejunum loop. Biliary enteric anastomosis using a Roux-en-Y reconstruction is superior to end-to-end anastomosis and should be the treatment of choice for late biliary strictures.

In case of proximal stricture involving common hepatic duct up to the confluence (Type I or II of Bismuth classification), the preparation of a hepatic duct stump suitable for anastomosis is not difficult. However, in case of stenosis involving right or left hepatic duct (Type II or IV), the preparation of a suitable stump is much more difficult. The height and extension of the stricture should guide the type of surgery.

Technique: division of the falciform ligament and freeing the liver from adhesions. Mobilization of the hepatic flexure of the colon. Duodenum should be exposed and mobilize. The essential step is identification and careful approach to the hepatic duct proximal to the stenosis.

At the exploration of the hilus, the bile duct is usually found laterally to the pulse of the hepatic laterally. Then, it is isolated cranially, up to incision at the base of quadrate lobe to lower the hilar plate. This maneuver makes longer the hepatic duct proximal to the stenosis. In some cases, dissection of the hepatic duct is necessary to expose better the biliary confluence, and the anatomy in order to perform a safe and effective anastomosis.

In order to expose the bile duct for repair, it is sometimes necessary to open the liver as a hepatotomy. The most frequent situation is to open the umbilical fis-

sure to access the segment III duct; otherwise, the hepatotomy in the scar of gallbladder fossa may be necessary to visualise the right hepatic duct. It is also possible to do an intrahepatic cholangiojejunostomy (IHCJ), with access to the left hepatic duct according to the Hepp-Couinaud technique, or provide for separate anastomosis between segmental hepatic ducts with or without trans anastomotic tubes. (Figure10).

Liver resection is necessary very rarely in the treatment of late stenosis after cholecystectomy. Usually, it requires the resection of the anterior portion of quadrate lobe to expose the hepatic duct.

In few cases a separate anastomosis on the right and on the left hepatic duct is necessary.

Hepato-jejunostomy is ususaly performed with one layer interrupted suture or continuous suture using a reabsorbable filament. A jejuno-jejunostomy is performed on a 60-70 cm loop jejunum with readsorbable suture material.

Only very rarely, secondary biliary fibrosis due to the strictures progress to cirrhosis. In such cases, liver transplantation may be considered as a valid option. However, in transplant centre, hepato-jejunostomy is the preferred treatment in most cases of benign strictures.

Operative mortality is reported as being 5%. Cause of death may be uncontrolled haemorrhage, or hepatic failure. Morbidity rate can be up to 20%. The most common complications are subphrenic or sub-hepatic abscess, pulmonary complications, biliary fistula, cholangitis.

Factors affecting operative morbidity and mortality are the number of preoperative procedures, level of strictures, hypoalbuminemia, hyper-bilirubinemia, presence of liver disease.

To evaluate long term results, 3 factors should be analysed: presence or absence of symptoms, presence or absence of al-

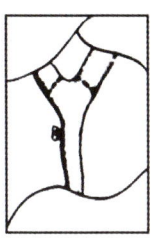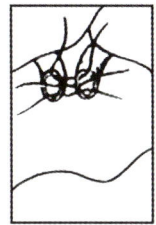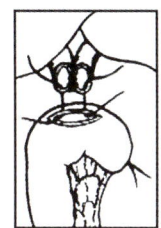

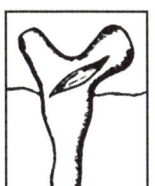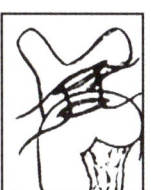

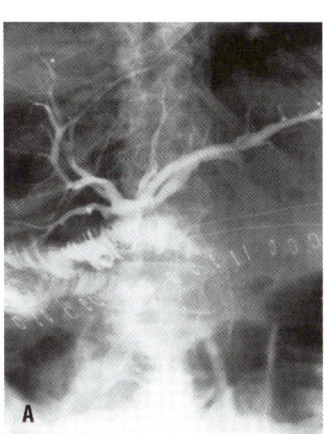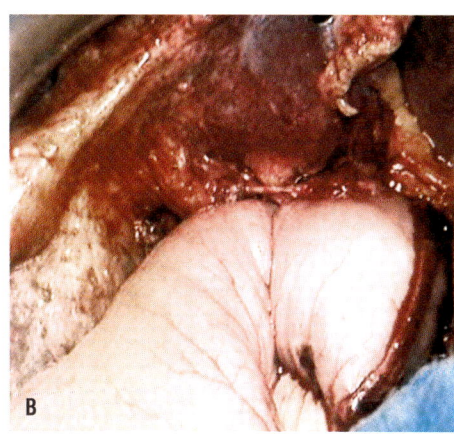

FIGURE 10: Different modalities of technique to perform an intrahepatic cholangiojejunostomy. Percutaneous cholangiography showing hepato-jejunostomy at the biliary confluence **(A)** Intrahepatic cholangiojejunostomy, with access to the left hepatic duct according to the Hepp-Couinaud technique **(B).**

terations of biochemical tests (in particular alkaline phosphatase, presence or absence of abnormal radiologic finding). A 10% of recurrent episodes of cholangitis with transient alterations of biochemical tests should be usually expected. In few cases of anastomotic stenosis, it is possible to perform again an hepato-jejunostomy which is usually associated with higher morbidity rate.

To date, the optimal management of patients with iatrogenic bile duct injury re-

quires a multidisciplinary team with experienced hepatobiliary surgeons, interventional radiologists and endoscopists to decide the most appropriate treatment in each case. In fact non-operative procedures are important options in complex patients when surgical reconstruction has failed and biliary-enteric continuity is intact. On the other hand, if non-operative therapies fail, surgical revision is possible, with a combined overall success rate of 98%.

BILIARY TRACT COMPLICATIONS AFTER OLT

Biliary complications appear in 10-20% of patients after orthotopic liver transplantation and are a significantly source of morbidity and mortality. The spectrum of biliary complications has changed in the last 10 years, because of the more extensive use of split liver, reduced-size, and living donor complications. In these cases, the incidence of complications were about 30% and, just recently with the learning curve being overcome, they decreased to approximately 22%.

A variety of biliary complications after OLT exists: anastomotic leakage, non-anastomotic leakage (T-tube related), bile collection, bile duct stenosis, hemobilia, etc. However, leaks and strictures are the most frequent. Early complications occur within the first three months after OLT; late biliary complications usually follow T-tube removal. Early complications are usually more frequent than late complications.

Anastomotic leaks are caused by ischemic necrosis or unsatisfactory technical suture. Non-anastomotic leaks often result from vascular insufficiency like hepatic artery trombosis. Other cause of biliary leaks is related to the removal of T-tube and the insertion of the T-tube is still now debated.

Anastomotic leakage can be managed conservatively. Endoscopic or percutaneous stenting can solve the majority of problems. In case of a major leaks, or persistent episodes of cholangitis or abdominal bile collection, re-operation is required. In these cases, conversion to a bilio-enteric anastomosis is the safest approach, while primary end-to-end repair should be applied only in ideal situations.

Strictures of the bile duct are the most frequent cause of late biliary complications. They appear in 3-14% of performed liver transplants. Causes of strictures are usually considered technical, if it appears in the early phase, or can be ischemic (injury to the vascular supply, which may be related to the effect of cold ischemia) or due to intensive inflammatory process of fibrosis, or to the size discrepancy between donor and recipient bile duct. It should be emphasized that the etiology of non-anastomotic strictures is poorly understood and probably multifactorial. In these cases, intrahepatic ducts are usually involved. These strictures are more frequent in the cases of prolonged cold ischemic times or with delayed re-arterialization of the graft.[7,9,10] Other factors which may be related to late non-anastomotic biliary strictures are donor age, CMV infection, ABO blood type mis-matched grafts chronic rejection.

DIAGNOSIS

Jaundice with elevation of laboratory tests (transaminases, alkaline phosphatase, gamma-glutamyl transferase) revealing cholestasis, pruritus, pale stools and, in a few patients, episodes of cholangitis are the common presentation of biliary strictures (in few cases asymptomatic elevation of laboratory tests may be the initial presentation). Diagnosis can be suspected by dilatation of intrahepatic ducts visualized at the ultrasonography; this preliminary examination has shown a low sensitivity after liver transplantation, therefore absence of bile duct dilatation should not preclude further evaluation in symptomatic patients.

Ultrasonography study In patients who have undergone OLT, biliary strictures may arise from post-surgical scar tissue in the anastomoses, or from ischemic damage located proximally (intrahepatic or hepatic ducts) or it may occur where T-tube enters the common bile duct. When the biliary stenosis is thought to arise from an ischemic lesion, Doppler examination usually shows the arterial stenosis. The accuracy of US-Doppler study in the diagnosis of hepatic artery stenosis is approximately 85% showing the increase of flow rate associated with turbulence distal to the stenosis. The presence of a flow greater than 2-3 m/sec is highly indicative of significant stenosis. However, in clinical practice, this criteria proves to be a poor indicator as most arterial stenoses occur in extrahepatic sites, which are poorly demostrated by US study. The intrahepatic flow may sometimes show a tardus-parvus waveform. A complete analysis of the components of Doppler examination is more accurate diagnostically. In fact, a resistive index less than 0.5, associated with prolonged systolic acceleration time (greater than 80 msec), have a sensitivity of 85 to 97% for significant hepatic artery complications. On the other hand, there is poor specificity (82-86%) because these findings are also present in patients with arterial-venous fistulas and thrombosis with collateral vessels. When an ischemic lesion is suspected after US, angio-CT or hepatic angiography should be performed. In patients with a stricture at the T-tube insertion site in the common bile duct, US may demonstrate the presence of fluid collections. When fluid collections are not present, the examination is negative and direct cholangiography with contrast media injection through the T-tube should be performed.

Magnetic resonance cholangio-pancreatography

Is presently considered to be the primary imaging modality, following US, especially in OLT patients suspected of having biliary complications, with a 90% accuracy rate in the detection of steno-obstructive biliary disease, 87.5% sensitivity and 92.3% specificity.

Percutaneous transhepatic cholangiography and endoscopic retrograde-cholangiopancreatography

Are commonly considered the gold standard diagnostic methods, due to their higher accuracy in defining the level of biliary stenosis or obstruction, in identifying the presence of bile duct stones or simple inflammatory disorders and precisely defining the site of a post-surgical bile leak: during the same diagnostic session, both techniques could provide the first treatment of these diseases, as previously described, positioning a drainage or a stent.

TREATMENT

Endoscopic treatment

Various endoscopical treatment methods are reported in the literature since some authors place just one stent with or without dilation, others used several stents with increasing number per session generally with associated hydropneumatic dilation (Figure 11). As a relapse of 30-40% has been reported, it is stressed the role of endoscopic stenting with the need of repeated procedure and endoscopic reassessment.

The results of several studies of endoscopic management of biliary strictures after OLT have been reported; endoscopic treatment of anastomotic strictures has been highly successful with a rate from 85% to 100%. Any-away, it may be useful as a bridge treatment until the most appropriate surgical approach can be carried out. Compared to anastomotic strictures, the success rate for non-surgical management of non-anastomotic strictures is lower, with a rate from 50% to 70%.

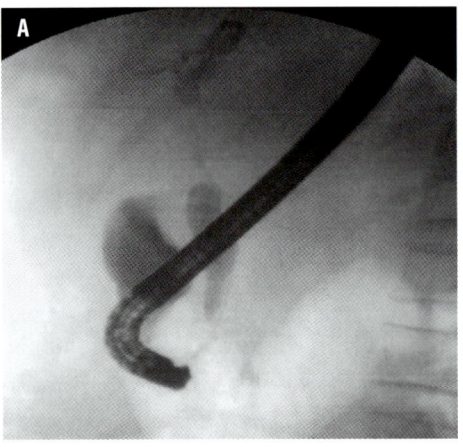

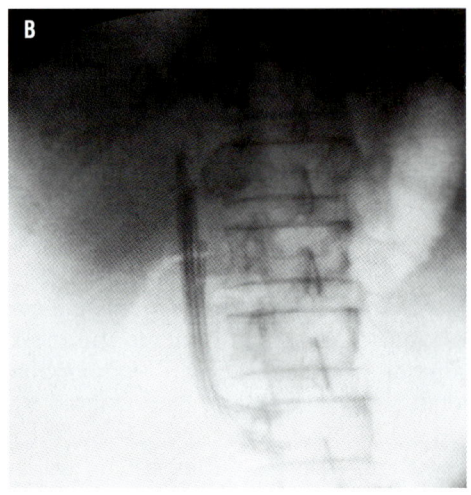

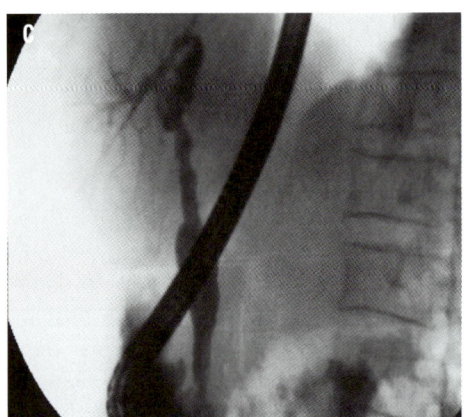

FIGURE 11: ERCP: biliary stricture after OLT, secondary to ischemia **(A)** Plastic stents (4) endoscopically positioned after dilation **(B)** Resolution of the stricture at the end of treatment **(C)**.

Percutaneous treatment

The anastomotic biliary strictures can be treated successfully by either endoscopic (choledocus-choledocus end-to-end anastomosis) or percutaneous (in cases of Roux-en-Y hepato-jejunostomy) dilation together with stent placement.

Repeated percutaneous balloon dilation, which leaves a biliary catheter across the anastomosis, demonstrated a long-term success rate of 66%. Anastomotic stenosis may often recur, requiring repeated interventions, with a success rate of 70% at 6 years and 20% of recurrences within the first year. Since non-anastomotic biliary strictures are frequently located above the hilum, the percutaneous approach plays a major role in their treatment, which consists of using balloon dilation followed by the placement of a biliary catheter or a plastic endoprosthesis, with persistent bile duct patency in as many as 88% of patients (Figure12). Some authors, especially in recurrent stenosis, suggest using metallic stents, which tend to remain patent longer than plastic stents. The primary patency of metallic stents is estimated at 85% at 6 months, 58% at 12 months and 0% at 5 years. When metallic stents are blocked by biliary s-ludge or hyperplasia ingrowth, a percuta-

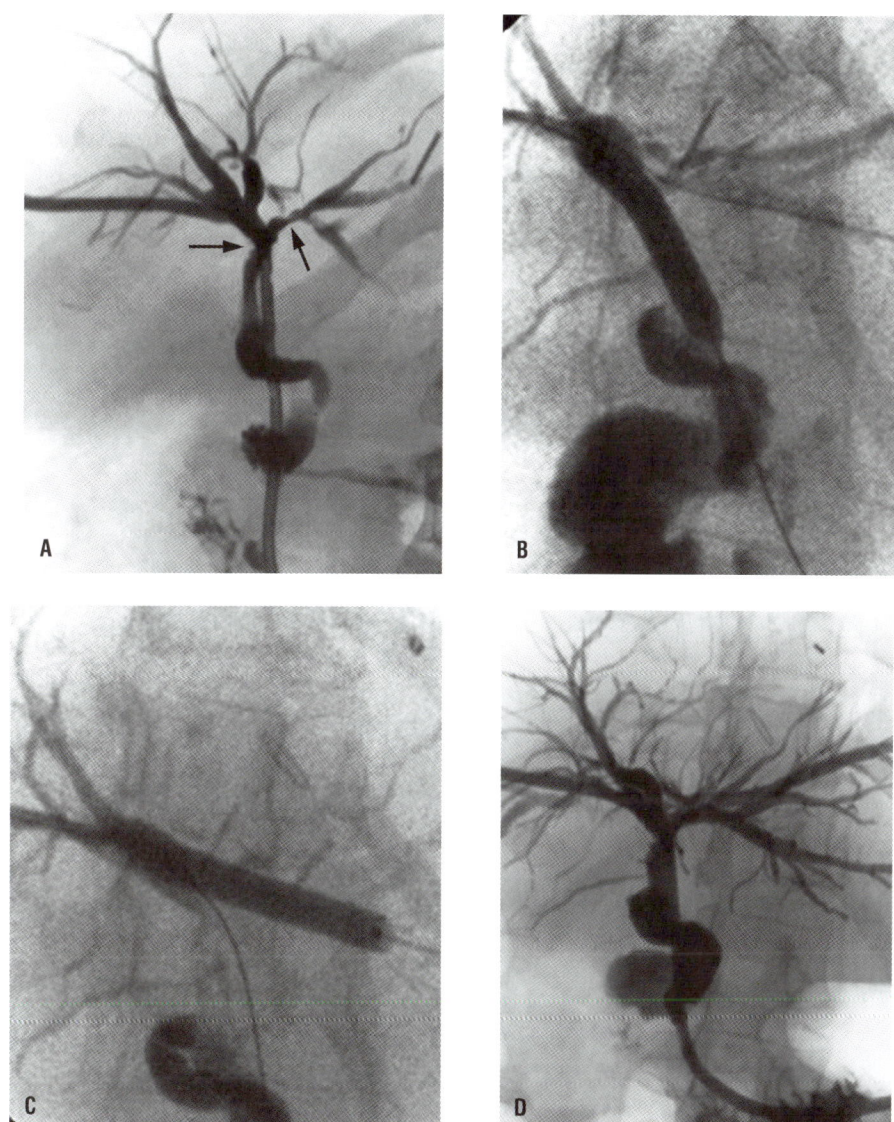

FIGURE 12: PTC in OLT patient with choledococholedocostomy shows the presence of stenosis in the right and left biliary ducts (**A.** arrows). Balloon dilation by transhepatic approach **(B-C)** followed by biliary catheter placement determines a satifactory result at colangiographic control after 3 months **(D)**.

neous reintervention is necessary in order to place a second metallic stent within the first to relieve the obstruction, with a secondary patency of 88% at 5 years (Figure13).

Surgical treatment

An hepato-jejunostomy with a Roux-en-y jejunum loop interposition is required whenever endoscopic treatments fail; this

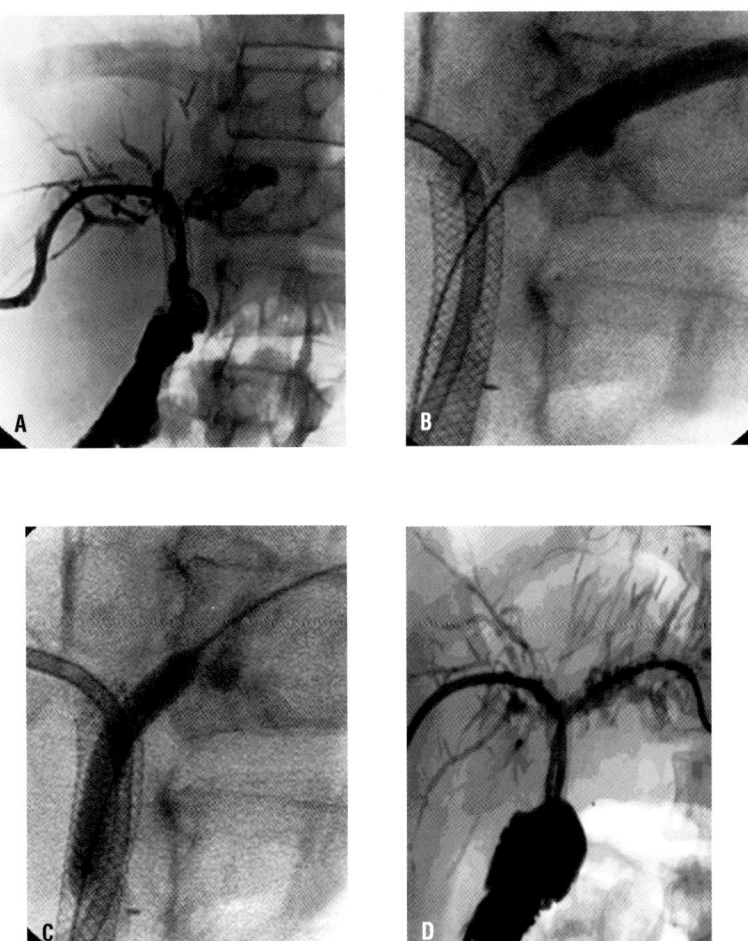

FIGURE 13: OLT patient suffering from recurrent episodes of cholangitis, 1 year after undergoing anastomotic stent placement for fibrotic stricture. PTC demonstrated stent obstruction due to hyperplastic ingrowth, associated with biliary sludge in the left system **(A)** By direct left approach, balloon dilation with stones removal has been performed **(B-C)** and two biliary catheters (right and left side) have been placed **(D)** to allow further percutaneous treatments.

approach is effective in more than 90% of cases (surgical technique has been reported in the previous chapter regarding iatrogenic biliary strictures). Even a redo-hepatojejunostomy is possible in cases of stenotic bilio-enteric anastomosis. Non-anastomotic strictures have been primarily treated by endoscopic or percutaneous approach; however, successful rate is much inferior compare to the approach of the anastomotic stenosis. The surgical approach should be reserved to those patients with recurrent cholangitis and not responsive to repeated endoscopic stenting. If these lesions are combined with unfavourable graft histology (showing severe fibrosis, lack of biliary features) surgical approach may be uneffective and retransplantation may be required to solve definitively biliary strictures.

MIRIZZI SYNDROME

Gallstones can produce complications by erosion into adjacent structures with the formation of fistulas. Duodenum, colon, and stomach are the common sites for fistulization. However, in a small portion of patients with gallstones, the stones may cause erosion directly into the common hepatic duct and provoke the formation of cholecysto-choledochal fistulas (Mirizzi syndrome type II), which may present with obstructive jaundice and cholangitis. Cholecysto-choledochal fistulas are often not recognized until cholecystectomy and are associated with a high risk of intraoperative damage to the common hepatic duct. It remains a major challenge to the surgeon to diagnose the condition before surgery so that operative strategy can be carefully formulated.

Background and classification

In 1948 Doctor Pablo Mirizzi described a syndrome of hepatic duct obstruction in the setting of cholelithiasis and cholecystitis. This syndrome is caused by an impacted gallstone in the cystic duct or the neck of the gallbladder compressing the adjacent bile duct and resulting in complete or partial obstruction of the common hepatic duct. Jaundice and recurrent cholangitis are the two main clinical manifestations. Anatomically, a cystic duct parallel to the bile duct is one of the main features of this syndrome. In 1982 McSherry suggested a subclassification of Mirizzi syndrome into two types: type I was associated with compression ab-estrinseco of the common hepatic duct by a stone impacted in the cystic duct, and type II was associated to a cholecysto-choledocal fistula caused by stone migration into the common hepatic duct. A further modification was introduced considering the type II

when a cholecysto-choledochal fistula involves less than one third of the circumference of the bile duct.

In 1997, Nagakawa developed a new classification of Mirizzi syndrome from diagnostic and therapeutic viewpoints in which type II was characterized by fistulization of the common hepatic duct as a result of a stone lodged in the cystic duct or the neck of the gallbladder.

The incidence of Mirizzi syndrome in patients undergoing biliary surgery usually varies from 0.7% to 1.4%; it can be up to 2.7% in high-risk populations such as Native Americans.

The incidence of cholecysto-choledochal fistulas is reported to be 1.1%. In the largest cohort of patients undergoing surgery for gallstone disease (17.395 patients), 219 (1.3%) had Mirizzi syndrome and/or cholecystobiliary fistulas.

Diagnosis

Preoperative diagnosis of the Mirizzi syndrome is important in order to avoid complications of unrecognized cholecystobiliary or cholecystoenteric fistulas. The symptoms of Mirizzi syndrome are nonspecific and include those of obstructive jaundice. For this reason, the preoperative diagnosis often requires the use of ultrasound, CT and ERCP.

The significant features of the Mirizzi syndrome on ultrasound are 1) dilation of the biliary system above the level of the gallbladder neck, 2) the presence of an impacted stone in the gallbladder neck and 3) an abrupt change in the normal width of the common duct below the level of the stone.

A typical US finding of the Mirizzi syndrome is the presence of three contiguous channels at the hilum, represented by the portal vein running parallel to the enlarged common hepatic and cystic ducts. The US study is not able to demonstrate the presence of cholecysto-choledochal fistulas, a rare complication of the Mirizzi syndrome, which, however, can usually be detected by direct cholangiography (ERCP or PTC).

Preoperative fistula demonstration is only possible by ERCP, from which can be determined the obstruction of the common hepatic duct due to either compression by the stone or the presence of an eroded stone in the common hepatic duct. However, this technique does not reveal the presence of fistulas in all cases. The role of CT in the diagnosis of Mirizzi syndrome is to exclude the presence of malignancy, usually defined by a mass in the porta hepatis or by the presence of liver metastasis. Thin-section helical CT scan can reveal both dilation of intra and extrahepatic bile duct proximal to the compression site, and eventual gallstone impacted in the gallbladder neck or cystic duct. The relationship of the stone with the common bile duct is demonstrated by helical CT or MRP (Figure14). When the stenosis is associated to ascending cholangitis, CT may show the p-

resence of gas in some intrahepatic ducts, and/or intrahepatic abseess which appears as a multiple hypoattenuating lesions with ill-defined margins often containing gas.

Surgical treatment

Cholecysto-choledochal fistulas poses certain technical difficulties for the surgeon during cholecystectomy. When the gallbladder is shrunken and fibrotic and there is a presence of inflammatory adhesions at the junction between the gallbladder and the common duct, the dissection of the Calot's triangle may be difficult. The common duct is prone to operative injuries because it can be easily mistaken for the cystic duct and divided. Even with careful dissection of the Calot's triangle, the problem may remain unsolved because the biliary anatomy is often greatly distorted. The situation may be further aggravated because continual dissection results in the division of the fistula, thereby leaving insufficient tissue

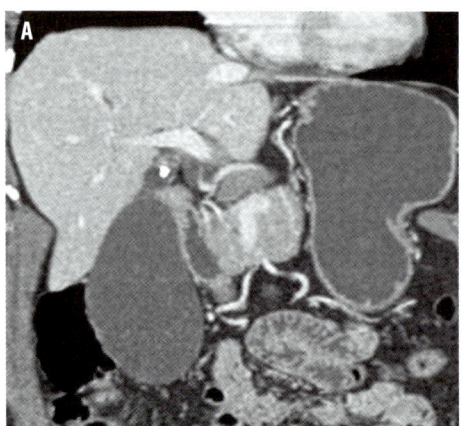 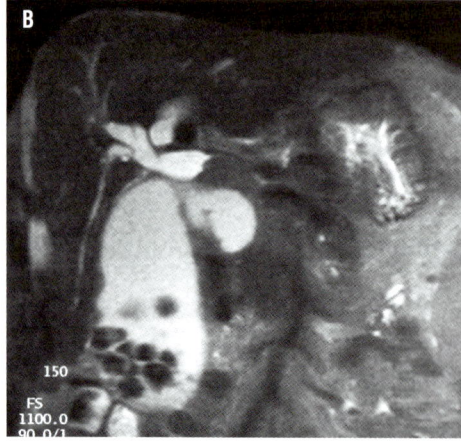

FIGURE 14: Spiral-CT after iv contrast media administration in patient with Mirizzi syndrome shows a gallstone impacted in the cystic duct **(A)** MRP in another case shows a gallstone **(B).**

REFERENCES

Advances in diagnosis and treatment of biliary strictures and stenoses

Andriulli A, Solmi L, Loperfido S, et al. Prophylaxis of ERCP-related pancreatitis: a randomized controlled trial of somatostatin and gabexate mesylate. Clin Gastroenterol Hepatol 2004;2:713-718.

Archer SB, Brown DW, Smith D, et al. Bile duct injury during laparoscopic cholecystectomy.Ann Surg 2001;234:549-559.

Berci GB, Sackier JM, Paz-Partlow M. Routine or selective intraoperative cholangiography during laparoscopic cholecystectomy? Am J Surg, 1991; 161:355-60.

Bergman JJ, van der Brink GR, Rauws EAJ, et al. Treatment of bile duct lesions after laparoscopic cholecystectomy. Gut 1996;38:141-147.

Bergman JJGHM, van den Brink GR, Rauws EA, de-Wit L, Obertop H, Huibregtse K, Tytgat GNJ. Treatment of bile duct lesions after laparoscopic cholecystectomy. Gut 1996;38:141-147.

Bismuth H., Lazorthes F. Les traumatismes operatoires de la voie biliaire principale. Masson Ed. Paris, 1981.

Bismuth H. Postoperative strictures of the bile duct. In The biliary tract. Clinical surgery international (Blumgart ed. - Churchill Livingstone - London 1982;209-218.

Blumgart LH. Surgery of the liver and biliary tract. Second edition - Churchill Livingstone - London 1984.

Boland GW, Mueller PR, Lee MJ. Laparoscopic cholecystectomy with bile duct injury: percutaneous management of biliary stricture and associated complications. AJR Am J Roentgenol 1996; 166:603-607.

Botger T, Junginger T. Long-term results after surgical treatment of iatrogenic injury of the bile ducts. Eur J Surg 1991;157:477-480.

Chaudhary A, Negi SS, Puri SK, et al. Comparison of magnetic resonance cholangiography and percutaneous transhepatic cholangiography in the evaluation of bile duct strictures after cholecystectomy. Br J Surg 2002;89:433-436.

Chen MF, Jan YY, Lee TY. Percutaneous transhepatic cholangioscopy. Br J Surg 1987;74:728-730.

Cohen SM, Kurtz AB. Biliary sonography. Radiol Clin of North Am 1991;29:1171-1198.

Coons HG. Self-expanding stainless steel biliary stents. Radiology 1989;170:979-983.

Corder AP, Scott SD, Johnson CD. Place of routine operative cholangiography at cholecystectomy. Br J Surg, 1992;79:945-7.

Costamagna G, Pandolfi M, Mutignani M, Spada C, Perri V. Long-term results of endoscopic management of postoperative bile duct strictures with increasing numbers of stents. Gastrointest Endosc 2001;54:162-168.

Davidoff AM, Pappas TN, Murray EA, Hillern DJ, Johnson RD, Baker ME, et al. Mechanisms of major injury during laparoscopic cholecystectomy. Ann. Surg., 1992;215:196-202.

Davids PHP, Ringers J, Rauws EAJ, De Wit LTH, Huibregste K, Van Der Heyde, Tytgat GNJ. Bile duct injury after laparoscopic cholecystectomy: the value of endoscopic retrograde cholangio-pancreatography. Gut, 1993;34:1250-1254.

Davids PHP, Tanka AK, Rauws EAJ, van Gulik TM, van Leeuwen DJ, deWit L. Benign biliary strictures. Surgery or endoscopy? Ann Surg 1993; 217:237-243.

Deziel DJ, Millikan KW, Economou SG, et al. Complications of laparoscopic cholecystectomy: a national survey of 4292 hospitals and an analysis of 77,604 cases. Am J surg, 1993;161:9-14.

de Bellis M, Sherman S, Fogel EL, et al. Tissue sampling at ERCP in suspected malignant biliary strictures. Gastrointest Endosc 2002;56:552-561.

Dumonceau JM, Deviere J, Delhaye M, Baize M, Cremer M. Plastic and metal stents for postoperative benign bile duct strictures: the best and the worst. Gastrointest Endosc 1998;47:8-17.

Fiddian-Green RG, Siviski PR, Karol SV. Median hepatotomy using ultrasonic dissection for complex hepatobiliary problems. Arch Surg 1988;123: 901-907.

Flum DR, Koepsel T, Heagerty P, et al. Common bile duct injury during laparoscopic cholecystectomy and the use of intraoperative cholangiography: adverse outcome or preventable error? Arch Surg 2001;136:1287-1292.

Frattaroli FM, Reggio D, Guadalaxara A, Illomei G, Pappalardo G. Benign biliary strictures: a review of 21 years of experience. J Am Coll Surg 1996; 183:506-513.

Fuente SG, Bannura GC. Radiological anatomy of the biliary variations and congenital abnormalities. World J Surg, 1983;7:271.

Gazzaniga GM, Filauro M, Mori L. Surgical treatment of iatrogenic lesions of the proximal common bile duct. World J Surg 2001;25:1254-59.

Gordon RL, Ring EJ, LaBerg JM, et al. Malignant biliary obstruction: treatment with expandable metallic stents: follow-up of 50 consecutive patients. Radiology 1992;182:697-701.

Harewood GC, Baron TH, Stadheim LM, et al. Prospective, blinded assessment of factors influencing the accuracy of biliary cytology interpretation. Am J Gastroenterol 2004;99:1464-1469.

Hausegger KA, Kugler C, Uggowitzer M, et al. Benign biliary obstruction: is treatment with Wallstent advisable? Radiology 1996; 200: 437-441.

Hepp J, Pernod R, HautefeilleP. Contribution de la cholangiographie operatoire r reparatrice des traumatismes biliaires. Ann Chir, 1963, 17:1121, 1963.

Irving JD, Adam A, Dick R et al. Gianturco expandable metallic biliary stents: results of a European clinical trial. Radiology 1989;172:321-326.

Jailwala J, Fogel EL, Sherman S, et al. Triple tissue sampling at ERCP in malignant biliary obstruction. Gastrointest Endosc 2000;51:383-390.

Jeng KS, Sheen IS, Yang FS. Percutaneous transhepatic cholangioscopy in the treatment of complicated intrahepatic biliary strictures and hepatolithiasis with internal metallic stent. Surg Laparosc Endosc Percutan Tech 2000;10:278-283.

Katyal S, Oliver JH 3rd, Buch DG et al. Detection of vascular complications after liver transplantation: early experience in multislice CT angiography with volume rendering. Am J Roentgenol 2000; 175:1735-1739.

Kehr A. Ueber Zwei Seltene Operationen en den Gallangangen. Munch Med. Wschr. 1905; 52: 1097.

Khalid TR, Casillas VJ, Montalvo BM, et al. Using MR cholangiopancreatography to evaluate iatrogenic bile duct injury. Am J Roentgenol 2001;177: 1347-1352.

Kim MJ, Mitchell DG, Ito K, et al. Biliary dilatation. differentiation of benign from malignant causes-

value of adding conventional MR imaging to MR cholangiopancreatography. Radiology 2000;214: 171-181.

Labadie M, Bouvet P, Berger F, et al. Diagnostic contribution of the cytology and histologic examination of endobiliary tissue specimens obtained by brush: a preliminary study in 29 patients. Acta Endoscopica 1985;15:113-114.

Lee MJ, Mueller PR, Saini S, et al. Percutaneous dilatation of benign strictures: single session therapy with general anesthesia. AJR Am J Roentgenol 1991;157:1263-1266.

Liguory C, Bitole GC, Lefebre JF, Bonnel D, Corand F. Endoscopic treatment of postoperative biliary fistulae. Surgery 1991;110:779-783.

Lillemoe KD, Martin SA, Cameron JL, et al. Major bile duct injuries during laparoscopic cholecystectomy. Follow-up after combined surgical and radiologic management. Ann Surg 1997;225:459-471.

Loperfido S, Angelini G, Benedetti G, et al. Major early complications from diagnostic and therapeutic ERCP: a prospective multicenter study. Gastrointest Endosc 1998;48:1-10.

Lorimer JW, Fairfull-Smith RJ. Intraoperative cholangiography is not essential to avoid duct injuries during laparoscopic cholecystectomy. Am J Surg 1995;169:344-347.

Lygidakis N, Matsakis GN, Tepetes KN et al. Intrahepatic cholangiojejunostomy in biliary stricture following resectional liver surgery. Hepato-Gastroenterology 1994; 41:1-3.

Maccioni F, Rossi M, Salvatori FM, et at. Metallic stents in benign biliary strictures: three-year follow-up. Cardiovasc Intervent Radiol 1992;15: 360-366.

MacFadyen BV, Vecchio R, Ricardo AE, et al. Bile duct injury after laparoscopic cholecystectomy. Surg Endosc 1998;12:315-321.

Matthews, JB, Gertsch P, Baer HN, Schweizer WP, Blumgart LH. Biliary stricture following hepatic resection. World J Hepato-Bilio-Pancreatic Surg 1991;3:181-190.

Moore AV Jr, Illescas FF, Mills SR, et al. Percutaneous dilation of benign biliary strictures. Radiology 1987;163:625-628.

Moossa AR, Easter DW, Van Sonnenberg E, et al. Laparoscopic injuries to the bile duct: a cause of concern. Ann Surg 1992;215:203-208.

Morris JB, Margolis R, Rosato EF. Safe laparoscopic cholecystectomy without intraoperative cholangiography. Surg Laparosc Endosc, 1993;3:17-20.

Mueller PR, VanSonnenberg E, Ferrucci JT Jr, et al. Biliary stricture dilatation: multicenter review of clinical management in 73 patients. Radiology 1986;160:17-22.

Muhletaler CA, Gerlock AJ Jr, Fleischer AC, et al. Diagnosis of obstructive jaundice with nondilated bile ducts. AJR Am J Roentgenol 1980;134: 1149-1152.

Nuzzo G. Le lesioni iatrogene della via biliare principale. Collana Monografica della Societa Italiana di Chirurgia, 2002.

Park MS, Kim TK, Kim KW, et al. Differentiation of extrahepatic bile duct cholangiocarcinoma from benign stricture: findings at MRCP versus ERCP Radiology 2004;233:234-240.

Pavone P, Laghi A, Catalano C, et al. MR cholangiography in the examination of patients with biliaryenteric anastomoses. AJR Am J Roentgenol 1997;169:807-811.

Phillips EH. Routine versus selective intraoperative cholangiography. Am J Surg 1993;165:505-507.

Pitt HA, Kaufman SL, Coleman J, et al. Benign postoperative biliary strictures: operate or dilate? Ann Surg 1989;210:417-427.

Raute M, Podlech P, Jaschke W, Manegold BC, et al. Management of bile duct injuries and strictures following cholecystectomy. World J Surg 1993; 17:553-562,1993.

Richardson MC, Bell G, Fullarton GM. Incidence and nature of bile duct injuries following laparoscopic cholecystectomy: an audit of 5913 cases. Br J Surg 1996;83:1356-1360.

Rosch T, Meining A, Fruhmorgen S, et al. A prospective comparison of the diagnostic accuracy of ERCP, MRCP, CT and EUS in biliary strictures. Gastroeintest Endosc 2002;55:870-876.

Rossi P, Bezzi M, Salvatori FM, et al. Recurrent benign biliary strictures: management with self-expanding metallic stents. Radiology 1990;175: 661-665.

Smith M, Sherman S, Lehman GA. Endoscopic management of benign strictures of the biliary tree. Endoscopy 1995;27:523-266.

Soper NJ, Dunnegan DL. Routine versus selective intraoperative cholangiography during laparoscopic cholecystectomy. World J Surg,1992;16:1133-1140.

Stabile Ianora AA, Memeo M, Scardapane A, et al. Oral contrast-enhanced three-dimensional helical-CT cholangiography: clinical applications. Eur Radiol 2003;13(4):867-73.

Stockberger SM Jr, Johnson MS. Spiral CT cholangiography in complex bile duct injuries after laparoscopic cholecystectomy. J Vasc Interv Radiol 1997;8:249-252.

Strasberg SM, Hertl M, Soper JN. An analysis of the problem of biliary injury during laparoscopic cholecystectomy. J Am Coll Surg 1995;180:101-125.

Strasberg SM, Hertl M, Soper JN. An analysis of the problem of biliary injury during laparoscopic cholecystectomy. J Am Coll Surg 1995;180:101-125.

Strasberg SM, Soper NJ. Laparoscopic cholecystectomy: current opinion. Gastroenterology, 1993; 9: 829-834.

Strasberg SM, Soper NJ. Laparoscopic cholecystectomy. Current opinion. Gastrenterology, 1993;9: 829-834.

Taylor TV, Sumerling MD, Carter DC, et al. An evaluation of 99-Tcm-labelled HIDA in hepatobiliary scanning. Br J Surg 1980;67:325-328.

Terblanche J, Allison HF, Northover JMA. An ischaemic basis for biliary strictures. Surgery, 1983, 94: 52-7.

Terblanche J, Allison HF, Northover JMA. An ischaemic basis for biliary strictures. Surgery, 1983,94:52-7.

Trerotola SO, Savader SJ, Lund GB, et al. Biliary tract complications following laparoscopic cholecystectomy: imaging and intervention. Radiology 1992;184:195-200.

Van Sonnenberg E, D'Agostino HB, Easter DW, et al. Complications of laparoscopic cholecystectomy: coordinated radiologic and surgical management in 21 patients. Radiology 188:399-404, 1993.

Vignali C, Bargellini I, Cioni R et al. Diagnosis and treatment of hepatic artery stenosis after orthotopic liver transplantation. Transplant Proc 2004;36(9):2771-3.

Vitellas KM, El-Dieb A, Vaswani KK, et al. Using contrast-enhanced MR cholangiography with IV mangafodipir trisodium (Teslascan. to evaluate bile duct leaks after cholecystectomy: a prospective study of 11 patients. AJR Am J Roentgenol 2002; 179:409-416.

Vogel SB, Howard RJ, Caridi J, et al. Evaluation of percutaneous transhepatic balloon dilatation of benign biliary strictures in high-risk patients. Am J Surg 1985;149:73-79.

Vos PM, van Beek EJ, Smits NJ, et al. Percutaneous balloon dilatation for benign hepaticojejunostomy strictures. Abdom Imaging 2000;25:134-138.

Ward J, Sheridan MB, Guthrie JA, et al. Bile duct strictures after hepatobiliary surgery: assessment with MR cholangiography. Radiology 2004;231: 101-108.

Warren KW, Mountain JC, Midell AI. Management of strictures of the biliary tract. Surg Clin N Am 1971;51:711-731

Warren KW jr, Jefferson MF. Prevention and repair of strictures of the extrahepatic bile ducts. Surg Clin N Am 1973;53:1169-1190.

Way LW, Stewart L, Ganter W, Liu K, Lee CM, Whang K, Hunter JG. Causes and prevention of laparoscopic bile duct injuries: analysis of 252 cases from a human factors a cognitive psychology perspective. Ann Surg 2003;237:460-469.

Williams HJ Jr, Bender CE, May GR. Benign post-operative biliary strictures: dilation with fluoroscopic guidance. Radiology 1987;163:629-634.

Yoon HK, Sung KB, Song HY, et al. Benign biliary strictures associated with recurrent pyogenic cholangitis: treatment with expandable metallic stents. AJR Am J Roentgenol 1997;169:1523-1527.

Zandrino F, Benzi L, Ferretti ML, et al. Multislice CT colangiography without biliary contrast agent: technique and initial clinical results in the assessment of patients with biliary obstruction. Eur Radiol 2002;12:1155-1161.

Z'graggen K, Wehrli H, Metzger A, et al. Complications of laparoscopic cholecystectomy in Switzerland. A prospective 3-year study of 10,174 patients. Swiss Association of Laparoscopic and Thoracoscopic Surgery. Surg Endosc 1998;12: 1303-1310.

Biliary Tract Complications After OLT

Bridges MD, May G, Harnois DM. Diagnosing biliary complications of orthotopic liver transplantation with mangafodipir trisodium-enhanced MR cholangiography: comparison with conventional MR cholangiography. AJR Am J Roentgenol 2004;182:1497-1504.

Campbell WL, Sheng R, Zajko AB, et al. Intrahepatic biliary strictures after liver transplantation. Radiology 1994;191:735.

Civelli EM, Meroni R, Cozzi G et al: The role of interventional radiology in biliary complications after orthotopic liver transplantation: a single-center experience. Eur Radiol 2004;14:579-582.

Colonna Jo, Shaked, Gomes AS, et al. Biliary strictures complicating liver transplantation. Incidence, pathogenesis, management and outcome. Ann Surg 1992;216:344-350.

Crossin JD, Muradali D, Wilson SR. US of liver transplants: normal and abnormal. Radiographics 2003;23:1093-1114.

Culp WC, McCowan TC, Lieberman RP et al: Biliary strictures in liver transplant recipients: treatment with metal stents. Radiology 1996;199:339-346.

Dodd GD 3rd, Memel DS, Zajko AB et al. Hepatic artery stenosis and thrombosis in transplant recipients: Doppler diagnosis with resistive index and systolic acceleration time. Radiology 1994; 192:657-661.

Fischer A, Miller CM. Ischemic-type biliary strictures in liver allografts: the Achilles heel revisited?. Hepatology 1995;21:589.

Grief, F, Bronsther OL, Van Thiel DH, et al. The incidence, timing and management of biliary tract complications after orthotopic liver transplantation. Ann Surg 1994;219:40.

Lerut J, Gordon RD, Iwatsuki S, Starzl TE. Biliary tract complications in human orthotopic liver transplantation. Transplantation 1987;43:47-51.

Linhares MM, Gonzalez AM, Goldman SM et al. Magnetic resonance cholangiography in the diagnosis of biliary complications after orthotopic liver transplantation. Transplant Proc 2004;36(4): 947-8.

Morelli J, Mulchany HE, Willner IR, Cunningham JT, Draganov P: Long-term outcomes for patients with post-liver transplant anastomotic biliary strictures treated by endoscopic stent placement. Gastrointest Endosc 2003;58:374-379.

Moser MA, Wall WJ. Management of biliary problems

after liver transplantation. Liver Transpl 2001;7 (Suppl)2.: S46.

Orons PD, Sheng R, Zajko AB. Hepatic artery stenosis in liver transplant recipients: prevalence and cholangiographic appearance of associated biliary complication. AJR Am J Roentgenol 1995; 165:1145-1149.

Park JS, Kim MH, Lee SK, Seo DW, Lee SS, Han J, Min YI, Hwang S, Park KM, Lee YJ, Lee SG, Sung KB: Efficacy of endoscopic and percutaneous treatments for biliary complications after cadaveric and living donor liver transplantation. Gastrointest Endosc 2003;57:78-85.

Pascher A, Neuhaus P. Bile duct complications after liver transplantation (review Transpl International 2005;18:627-642.

Quiroga S, Sebastia MC, Margarit C et al. Complications of orthotopic liver transplantation: spectrum of appearance with helical CT. Radiographics 2001;21:1085-1102.

Rerknimitr R, Sherman S, Fogel EL, Kalayci C, Lumeng L, Chalasani N, Kwuo P, Lehman GA: Biliary tract complications after orthotopic liver transplantation with choledochocholedochostomy anastomosis: endoscopic findings and results of therapy. Gastrointest Endosc 2002;55:224-231.

Roumilhac D, Poyet G, Sergent G et al: Long-term results of percutaneous management for anastomotic biliary stricture after orthotopic liver transplantation. Liver Transpl 2003;9(4):394-400.

Sanchez-Urdazpal L, orcs GJ, Ward EM, et al. Ischemic type biliary complications after orthotopic liver transplantation. Hepatology 1992;16: 49.

Schlitt HJ, Meier PN, Nashan B, et al. Reconstructive surgery for ischemic type lesions at the bile duct bifurcation after liver transplantation. Ann Surg 1999;229:137.

Scotte M, Dousset B, almus Y, Conti F, Houssin D, Chapius Y. The influence of cold ischemia time on biliary complications following liver transplantation. J Hepatol 1994;21:340-346.

Sutcliffe R, Maguire D, Mroz A, et al. Bile duct stricture after adult liver transplantation: a role for biliary reconstructive surgery? Liver Transpl 2004; 10:928-934.

Torras J, Llado L, Figueras J, Ramos E, Lama C, Fabregat J, et al. Biliary tract complications after liver transplantation: type, management, and outcome. Transpl Proc 1999;31:2406.

Zajko AB, Sheng R, Zetti GM, et al: Transhepatic balloon dilation of biliary strictures in liver transplant patients: a 10-year experience. J Vasc Interv Radiol 1995;6:79-83.

Mirizzi syndrome

Albert MB, Steinberg WM, Henry JP. Elevated serum levels of tumor marker CA 19-9 in acute cholangitis. Dig. Dis. Sci. 1988;33:1223-5.

Becker CD, Hassler H, Terrier F. Preoperative diagnosis of the Mirizzi syndrome: limitations of sonography and computed tomography. AJR Am J. Roentgenol 1984; 142:591-6 Joseph S, Carvajal S, Odwin C. Sonographic diagnosis of Mirizzi's syndrome. J Clin Ultrasound 1985;13:199-201.

Corlette MB, Bismuth H. Biliobiliary fistula. Arch. Surg. 1975;110:377-83.

Csendes A, Carlos Diaz J, Burdiles P. Mirizzi syndrome and cholecystobiliary fistula : a unifying classification. Br. J. Surg. 1989;76:1139-43.

Curet MJ, Rosendale DE, Congilosi S. Mirizzi syndrome in a native american population. Am. J. Surg. 1994 ;168 :616-21.

Glenn F, Reed C, Grafe WR. Biliary enteric fistula. Surg. Gynecol Obstet 1981;153:527-31.

Gupta MK, Arciaga R, Bocci L. Measurement of a monoclonal antibody-defined antigen CA 19-9 in the serum of patients with malignant and non-malignant diseases. Cancer 1985;56:277-83.

Joseph S, Carvajal S, Odwin C. Sonographic diagnosis of Mirizzi's syndrome. J Clin Ultrasound 1985; 13:199-201.

Karakoyunlar O, Sivrel E, Koc O. Mirizzi's syndrome must be ruled out in the differential diagnosis of any patients with obstructive jaundice. Hepatogastroenterology 1999;46:2178-2182.

McSherry CK, Ferstenberg H, Virshup M. The Mirizzi syndrome: suggested classification and surgical therapy. Surg. Gastroenterol. 1982; 1:219-25.

Mirizzi PL. Sindrome del conducto hepatico. J. Int. Chir. 1948;8:731-77.

Nagakawa T, Ohta T, Kayahara M. A new classification of Mirizzi syndrome from diagnostic and therapeutic viewpoints. Hepatogastroenterology 1997;44:63-67.

Nishio H, Kamiya J, Nagino M. Biliobiliary fistula associated with gallbladder carcinoma. Br. J. Surg. 2000;87(12):1656-57.

Principe A, Del Gaudio M, Grazi GL, Paolucci U, Cavallari A. Mirizzi syndrome with cholecysto-choledochal fistula with a high CA 19-9 level mimicking biliary malignancies: a case report. Hepato-Gastroenterology 2003;50:1259-1262.

Redaelli CA, Buchler MW, Schilling MK. High coincidence of Mirizzi syndrome and gallbladder carcinoma. Surgery 1997;121(1):58-63.

Steinberg WM. The clinical utility of the CA 19-9 tumor associated antigen. Am J. Gastroenterol 1990;85:350-5.

Inflammatory stricture mimicking cholangiocarcinoma

Andersson R, Andren-Sandberg A, Lundstedt C and Tranberg KG. Implantation metastases from gastrointestinal cancer after percutaneous puncture or biliary drainage. Eur J Surg 1996;162:551-4.

Blumgart LH, Thomson JN. The management of malignant strictures of the bile duct. Curr Probl Surg 1987;24:69-127.

Cameron JL, Pitt HA, Zinner MJ et al. Management of proximal cholangiocarcinoma by surgical resection and radiotherapy. Am J Surg 1990;159:91-98.

Campbell WL, Ferris JV, Holbert BL, Thaete FL, Baron RL. Biliary tract carcinoma complicating primary sclerosing cholangitis: evaluation with CT, Cholangiography, US, and MR imaging Radiology 1998;207:41-50.

Davidson B, Varsamidakis N. Dooley J, et al.. Value of exfoliative cytology for investigating bile duct strictures. Gut 1992; 33:1408-1411.

Gerhards MF, Vos P, van Gulik TM, Rauws EAJ, Bosma A, and Gouma DJ. Incidence of benign lesions in patients resected for suspicious hilar obstruction. Br J Surg 2001;88:48-51.

Kehagias D, Metafa A, Hatziioannou A, Mourikis D, Vourtsi A, Prahalias A, Smyrniotis V, Gouliamos A, Vlahos L. Comparison of CT, MRI and CT during arterial portography in the detection of malignant hepatic lesions. Hepatogastroenterology 2000;47 (35):1399-403.

Kim M-J, Mitchell DG, Ito K, Outwater EK. Biliary dilatation: differentation of benign from malignant causes- value of adding conventional MR Imaging to MR Cholangiopancreatography Radiology 2000;214:173-181.

Kurzawinski TR, Deery A, Dooley J, et al. A prospective study of biliary cytology in 100 patients with bile duct strictures. Hepatology 1993;18:1399-1403.

Lauffer J.M., Baer H.U., Schajor M., Halter F., Buchler M.W. Choledocholithiasis at the hepatic confluence mimicking a hilar cholangiocarcinoma. Hepatogastroenterology 1998; 45 (24):2339-43.

Lee WF, Lim HK, Fang KM, Kim SH, Lee SF, Lim FH, Choo IW. Radiologic spectrum of cholangiocarcinoma: emphasis on unusual manifestations and differential diagnoses. Radiographics 2001;21: S97-S116.

Manfredi R, Brizi MG, Masselli G, Vecchioli A, Marano P. Malignant biliary hilary stenosis: MR cholangiography compared with direct cholangiography Radiol Med 2001;102 (1-2):48 54.

Mansfield JC, Griffin SM, Wadehra V, Matthewson K. A prospective evaluation of cytology from biliary strictures. Gut 1997;40:671-677.

Nimura Y, Kamiya J, Hayakawa N, and Shionoya S. Cholangioscopic differentiation of biliary strictures and polyps. Endoscopy 1989;21:351-356.

Nimura Y. Staging of biliary carcinoma: cholangiography and cholangioscopy. Endoscopy 1993;25: 76-80.

Pasanen PA, Partanen KP, Pikkarainen PH, Alhava EM, Janatuinen EK, and Pirinen AE. A comparison of ultrasound, computed tomography and endoscopic retrograde cholangiopancreatography in the differential diagnosis of benign and malignant jaundice and cholestasis Eur J Surg 1993;159:23-29.

Principe A, Ercolani G, Bassi F, Paolucci U, Raspadori A, Turi P, Beltempo P, Grazi GL, Cavallari A. Diagnostic dilemmas in biliary strictures mimicking cholangiocarcinoma. Hepato-Gastroenterology 2003;50:1246-1249.

Seo DW, Kim MH, Lee SK, Myung SJ, Kang GH, Ha HK, Suh DJ, Min YI. Usefulness of cholangioscopy in patients with focal stricture of the intrahepatic duct unrelated to intrahepatic stones. Gastrointest Endosc 1999;49 (2):204-9.

Vitellas KM, Enns RA, Keogan MT, Freed KS, Spritzer CE, Billie J, Nelson RC. Comparison of MR cholangiopancreatographic techniques with contrast-enhanced cholangiography in the evaluation of sclerosing cholangitis AJR 2002;178 (2):327-34.

Wetter LA, Ring EJ, Pellegrini CA and Way LW. Differential diagnosis of sclerosing cholangiocarcinomas of the common hepatic duct (Klatskin tumors. Am J Surg 1991;161:57-62.

Biliary atresia

Hays D, Kimura K. Biliary atresia: the Japanese experience. Harvard University Press, Cambridge, 1980.

Hays DM, Snyder WH. Life-span in untreated biliary atresia. Surgery 1963; 64: 373-375.

Kasai M, Ohi R, Chiba T. Intra-hepatic bile ducts in biliary atresia. In: Cholestasis in infancy. Baltimore, 1980.

Kasai M, Suzuki S. A new operation for "non-correctable" biliary atresia: hepatic portoenterostomy. Shujitsu 1959, 13: 733-739.

Primary sclerosing cholangitis

Richardson Paul, O'Grady John

INTRODUCTION

Primary sclerosing cholangitis (PSC) is a chronic cholestatic liver disease of unknown aetiology. In many cases it is a progressive disease that may lead to liver failure and the need for liver transplantation. PSC is a disease that may affect either or both the intra- and extra-hepatic biliary system. It is characterized by diffuse inflammation and obliterative fibrosis leading to progressive stricturing of the biliary system. A secondary impact of the structuring may be parenchymal fibrosis and cirrhosis, which in turn may precipitate portal hypertension and liver failure. PSC patients have a high risk of developing cholangiocarcinoma (CCA), with an incidence of around 15-30%, and those with cirrhosis are also at risk of developing hepatocellular carcinoma.

PSC is strongly associated with inflammatory bowel disease (IBD) and in excess of 70% of cases have this association, principally with chronic ulcerative colitis (CUC). However, the aetiology of the disorder remains obscure although there is a growing body of evidence to suggest an underlying dysregulation of the immune system and many authorities consider it to be an autoimmune disease despite not totally conforming to the classical definition of such diseases. There is also a close association of PSC with other autoimmune disorders and the finding of positive autoantibodies and hypergammaglobulinaemia support an immune basis for this disorder. Further evidence supporting an immune basis is the recent identification of polymorphisms in candidate genes, involved in immune regulation that may render a patient susceptible to developing PSC.

Despite the putative autoimmune aetiology, there is limited evidence that immunosuppression modifies the natural history of PSC with the possible exception of cases diagnosed in childhood. Apart from ursodeoxycholic acid (UDCA), there is no treatment that has been convincingly demonstrated to delay the progression of and reduce the incidence of end stage liver disease or the need for liver transplantation.

EPIDEMIOLOGY

There is a general paucity of data on the epidemiology of PSC in a general population. Most studies to date have been performed in academic centers with an emphasis on patients with co-existing CUC. An early Spanish survey of gastroenterologists and hepatologists reported an annual incidence of 0.07 cases per 100,000 person years and a prevalence of 0.22 cases per 100,000 population. The first population-based study was reported from Norway and this reported a mean annual incidence of 1.3 cases/100,000-person years, with a prevalence of 8.5 cases per 100,000 population. It was postulated that the reason for this order of magnitude of difference was related to differences in the prevalence of CUC in the two populations.

A more recent population based study from Olmsted County Minnesota USA reported an overall incidence of PSC of 0.9 per100,000 person years. The incidence was higher in men at 1.25 per 100,000 person years as compared with 0.54 per 100,000 person years in women, with a prevalence of 20.9 and 6.3 per 100,000 population respectively. IBD was present in 73% of cases with the majority having CUC. Survival for the PSC population was significantly reduced in comparison to the population as a whole with a ten-year survival of 65% versus 94%. Despite a perceived increase in the incidence of PSC over the study period, it is likely that this represents improvement in diagnosis particularly of patients in the early stage of the disease rather than a true increase in incidence.

PATHOPHYSIOLOGY

Genetic susceptibility

The overall influence of genetics on the pathopysiology of PSC has not yet delineated but it is likely to involve a constellation of genetic polymorphisms that increases susceptibility. Polymorphisms in genes important in the regulation of the human immune system have been postulated as candidates for susceptibility to PSC. The main candidates have included the genes of the major histocombatability complex (MHC). Early studies identified an increased frequency of HLA B8 and DR3 and DR2 in PSC patients compared to normal controls. It is notable that these earlier studies were based on serological sub-typing. Molecular genetic techniques brought a greater degree of sophistication to the characterisation of these genes and recent studies have highlighted the strong association of the haplotypes DRB3*0101- DRB1*1301 and DRB3*0101-DRB1*0301 with susceptibility to PSC. Positive associations with MMP-3 and disease progression and a possible link with CTLA-4 have recently been reported.[12-15] Genetic studies that failed to establish a link include those of the cytokines IL-1 and IL-10, FAS, TGFb-1 and CCR5.

Chronic portal bacteraemia

The close association of PSC and CUC generated the hypothesis that PSC was a consequence of either direct portal bacteraemia or absorption of bacterial toxins through an inflamed and permeable bowel mucosa. The lack of evidence of portal vein bacteraemia or histological evidence of ongoing bacterial associated portal vein phlebitis undermines this hypothesis. If central to the development of PSC, uptake of bacterial products by liver based macrophages would be expected to lead to a localised immune response, producing inflammation and fibrosis as witnessed in PSC. Against this attractive hypothesis is the ability of PSC to present years before the onset of CUC, together with the absence of a correlation between the severity of the colitis, and thus permeability of the bowel, and either the risk of developing P-SC or the severity of liver disease. It is also noteworthy that PSC may develop after a pan-proctocolectomy for CUC.

DIAGNOSIS

The diagnosis of PSC is usually precipitated by the detection of cholestatic liver function tests or jaundice. Improvements in diagnostic techniques have eased investigation and facilitated the diagnosis of PSC, particularly in the early stages of the disease. The diagnosis of PSC is principally based on appearances at direct or indirect cholangiography in the absence of alternative disorders associated with abnormal cholangiograms. Supporting diagnostic data may be determined from liver histology, which is also important in staging the severity of the disease.

Diagnostic criteria include:
- cholestatic liver biochemistry present for over 6 months,
- cholangiography demonstrating strictures in either or both the intra and extrahepatic biliary system,
- liver histology showing chronic inflammation and fibrosis centered on the intralobular and septal bile ducts and fibrous obliteration of bile ducts - "onion skin fibrosis",
- exclusion of other causes of secondary biliary sclerosis.

Biochemical and immunological abnormalities

Peristant cholestatic abnormal liver biochemistry is characteristic of, but by no means specific to, PSC. Liver biochemistry commonly fluctuates during the course of the disease. The majority of patients have a cholestatic liver profile with at least a twofold increase in the serum alkaline phosphatase (ALP) and gamma-glutamyl-transpeptidase (GGT). The serum aminotransferase (ALT) may also be raised but rarely to more than three times the upper limit of normal. Higher increases in the AST may indicate a PSC/autoimmune hepatitis crossover syndrome and histology in these cases demonstrates

characteristics of both autoimmune hepatitis and PSC. This dual pathology occurs in 2-8% of patients. Serum bilirubin levels may vary greatly over time and rise in association with dominant stricture formation and bouts of cholangitis. More protracted elevations in serum bilirubin are observed with malignant transformation and end-stage liver disease. Deterioration in hepatic synthetic function is also seen with end-stage disease with a reduction in serum albumin and a prolongation of the prothrombin time.

A range of autoantibodies may be detected in patients with PSC but there is no pattern specific for the disease. Anti-nuclear antibodies and anti-smooth muscle antibodies are present in 55-77% and 13-35% of patients respectively. Antimitochondrial antibodies are present in around 5% of cases and may be useful to differentiate from primary biliary cirrhosis. Atypical perinuclear antineutrophil cytoplasmic antibodies (p-ANCA) are present in 33-88% of patients. This auto antibody is different from the classical p-ANCA and c-ANCA found in Wegner's granulomatosis and the vasculitides and is generally only detected in patients with PSC, CUC and autoimmune hepatitis. Antibodies to biliary epithelial cells have been studied in patients with different autoimmune-based liver disorders. Compared with controls, 63% of PSC patients had detectable antibodies and these antibodies were found to be capabable of inducing biliary epithelial cells to express the proinflamatory cytokine Il-6.

Otherwise, there is little evidence directly link antibodies to disease pathogenesis and they are more likely to be indicative of a general dysregulation of the immune system. A non-specific increase in the immunoglobulin fraction is often present.

Radiological abnormalities

The finding of typical cholangiographic

abnormalities is essential for the diagnosis of PSC. Endoscopic retrograde cholangiopancreatography (ERCP) was considered the gold standard but serious complications occur in 3-8% of patients, including severe pancreatitis, small bowel perforation and death. As a result, there is increasing reliance on indirect cholangiography using magnetic resonance cholangiography (MRP). Recent studies have suggested comparable efficacy in diagnosing biliary tract disorders including PSC for both MRC and ERCP. A further study not only demonstrated comparable accuracy in diagnosis for MRC but also a cost benefit when used as the initial diagnostic tool. Percutaneous cholangiography is now rarely indicated for purposes of diagnosis, as opposed to therapeutic intervention. Typically cholangiopathic findings include random multi-focal areas of stricturing and dilatation ('beading') of the intra- and extra-hepatic biliary system and this is observed in >80% of cases (Figure 1). The findings may be localized

to either the intra-hepatic bile ducts or the extra-hepatic ducts alone.

There may be some evidence of duct dilatation on ultrasound of the liver. Axial imaging of the liver frequently shows areas of hypertrophy or atrophy resulting in unusual shapes. Focal lesions may be present and the differentiation of inflammatory processes from complicating malignancy can be a challenge. Evidence of portal hypertension may exist as splenomegaly or ascites. Additional common observations include enlargement of the gallbladder and abdominal lymphadenopathy.

Histology

The histological appearances of the liver in PSC are variable and depend on the duration of the disease and the presence or absence of intrahepatic disease. Liver biopsies may be relatively normal or show non-diagnostic changes. The more typical changes include a mixed portal tract inflammatory infiltrate, periportal oedema or fibrosis, interface hepatitis, ductopenia, and copper deposition. Apart from 'onion skin fibrosis', these changes lack specificity and are variably observed in large bile duct obstruction, primary biliary cirrhosis and autoimmune hepatitis. It is not uncommon to find patients with classical PSC who had previously been diagnosed with either autoimmune hepatitis or PBC on the basis of a liver biopsy

Despite not being diagnostic, histology is important to stage the disease. Staging is useful for predicting potential complications and to determine the prognosis. There are four histological stages:
- stage 1 demonstrates portal tract oedema, ductular proliferation, and abnormalities that are restricted to the portal tract (Figure 2),
- stage 2 is characterized by periportal fibrosis and inflammation spreading into the surrounding liver parenchyma with interface hepatitis,

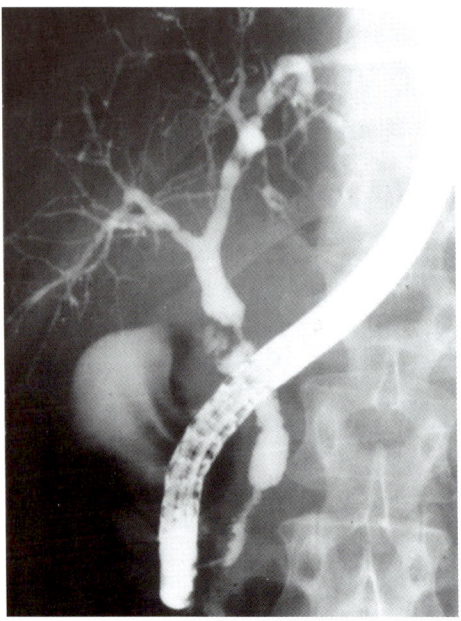

FIGURE 1: Radiological appearances of PSC.

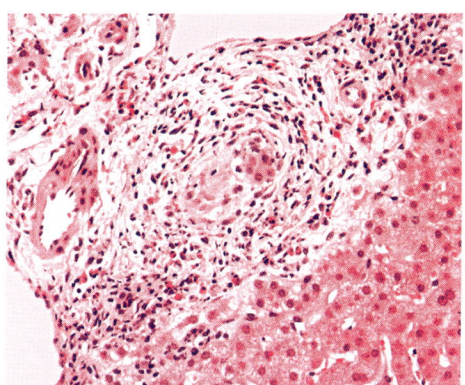

FIGURE 2: Histological appearances of a portal tract in PSC.

– stage 3 demonstrates the formation of fibrous septa and bridging necrosis, and
– stage 4 is characterized by established biliary cirrhosis.

Histological progression has been studied in 107 patients with stage 2 disease progressing in 42%, 66% and 93% in 1, 2 and 5 years, respectively. For stage 3 disease the rates of progression in the same time frame were 14%, 25% and 52%, respectively. A clinical entity with histological and biochemical changes consistent with PSC but normal cholangiography has been described by Wee and Ludwig in 1985 termed small duct PSC. These cases demonstrate normal cholangiographic findings but liver histology consistant with PSC.

NATURAL HISTORY

Observational cohort studies have shown that PSC is generally a progressive disease but it is well recognized that subsets of patients, particularly those with small duct PSC, progress at different rates. Asymptomatic patients make up about 20-40% of cohorts studied The majority of patients who are asymptomatic at the time of diagnosis and have stage 1-2 fibrosis on biopsy will eventually develop symp-

toms. The Kaplan-Meier median estimated survival for such a cohort was 75% at 7 years compared to 96% for a healthy matched group. A study of 174 patients reported from the Mayo clinic contained a subgroup of 45 asymptomatic patients and 31 (76%) of these showed evidence of progression of liver disease within the follow-up period of 6.25 years, with liver failure leading to death or transplantation developing in 31% of patients. In a smaller study from Norway the degree of progression in asymptomatic patients was less pronounced with 11 of 13 remaining asymptomatic over a mean duration of 37 months. The reasons for these apparent discrepancies are unclear though there may be different criteria for categorizing patients as asymptomatic.

Early reports of follow-up of symptomatic patients revealed mortality rates of 14-18% over median intervals of 51-56 months. Larger studies have described a more aggressive clinical deterioration and lower survival rates in symptomatic patients. The Mayo clinic followed up a cohort of 174 consecutive patients and the overall median survival was 11.9 year with 41% developing either liver failure or cholangiocarcinoma, or requiring liver transplantation. For patients who were symptomatic at presentation the median survival was approximately 9 years. A similar median survival of 12 years was also reported in a study cohort of 126 patients from Kings College Hospital London.

A study of 305 Swedish patients (44% were asymptomatic at presentation) showed that the median time to death or transplantation was 12 years. Of note median survival was significantly higher in the asymptomatic group with 22% of these patients developing symptoms during the follow up period.

174 Dutch patients were followed up for a median of 76 months and the median survival from time of diagnosis was 18 years, the incidence of cholangiocarcino-

ma was 10%, and 8% underwent transplantation. In that study cholangiographic scoring was inversely related to survival. The longer life expectancy in the Dutch cohort may be explained partly by differences in the percentage of asymptomatic patients and but also by the fact that it was mainly conducted in the 1990's as opposed to 1970-1980's as in the earlier reports.

A small retrospective study of 6 patients with small duct disease followed up for 7-84 months identified no progression of the disease. In a larger study of 32 Swedish patients followed up for a median of 63 months no patients developed cholangiocarcinoma, one required transplantation for end stage liver disease and only 4/27 patients who underwent repeat cholangiography developed features of classical PSC.

Prognostic models

The use of Cox multivariable regression methodology using independent clinical variables enabled the development of mathematical models to predict disease progression. These models have enabled prediction of survival of individual patients. The Mayo model is the most established, and the independent predictors of survival were serum bilirubin, haemoglobin concentration, patient's age, liver histological stage at biopsy and the presence of inflammatory bowel disease. Three risk groups were identified low, intermediate and high and these predicted survival rates comparable to real patients. The Kings College Hospital model used the patient's age, presence of hepatomegaly and splenomegaly, histological stage and serum alkaline phosphatase as its independent variables predictive of survival.

In order to refine the model concept, data from five centers were combined and analysed. This multi-centre study used data from 426 patients followed up for a median of 3 years. In total 100 deaths (23%) were recorded allowing assessment of the models predictive ability. Predictive variables identified were patient's age, serum bilirubin, histological stage and presence or absence of splenomegaly. This model was flexible to predict survival with different stages of disease but was limited by the need for liver histology and complex mathematical formulae.

To overcome these limitations a study of the predictive value of the CPT scoring was reported from the Cleveland clinic. 208 patients were studied and survival after 7 years for Child's class A, B and C was 89.8%, 68% and 24% respectively. Of this cohort, 140 patients had liver histology available enabling comparison with the multi-centre prognostic models and this suggested the two approaches were comparable but the CPT score was easier to use. The Mayo risk score was refined by including a history of variceal bleeding instead of histological grade to obviate the need for liver biopsy. When comparison to the CPT score, the new Mayo risk score demonstrated overlapping survival curves in CPT B and C class patients. Further analysis demonstrated the superiority of the Mayo risk score over CPT scoring. The new Mayo risk model is calculated with the following formula R = 00.3 x (age in years) + 0.54 x log (serum bilirubin in mg/dl) + 0.54 x log (serum AST) + 1.24 x (history of variceal bleed) - (albumin g/dl).

One difficulty in utilizing these models in general clinical settings is the complexity of the calculations. It must also be noted that these models do not take into account the impact of cholangiocarcinoma. Prognostic models have been used to predict optimal time for liver transplantation and survival after transplantation. 216 patients transplanted for end stage PSC were studied retrospectively and significantly improved survival in favour of transplantation was noted when compared to the predicted survival using the

Mayo risk score (73% versus 28% at five years), demonstrating a positive impact of liver transplantation. Prognostic models have been less reliable in predicting outcome after liver transplantation. Prognostic models have enabled a degree of accuracy in predicting expected survival for individual patients and identify an optimal time for liver transplantation.

DIFFERENTIAL DIAGNOSIS

The differential diagnosis of PSC generally centres around other hepatobiliary diseases that may present with cholestasis. Conditions to be considered include, primary biliary cirrhosis, sarcoidosis, extrahepatic biliary obstruction, drug induced liver injury, viral hepatitis and autoimmune hepatitis. In general an accurate clinical history, biochemistry, serology, histology and cholangiography can secure the diagnosis. A recent addition to the differential diagnosis is the recognition of a PSC like disorder found in patients infected with the HIV virus. This "AIDS related cholangiopathy" was usually observed in patients with a low CD4 count. This condition generally presents with right upper quadrant pain and fever and a cholangiogram indistinguishable from PSC. Culture of the bile from these patients revealed that infection with cryptosporidim species was the infective cause of this disorder. With the use of highly active antiretroviral treatments (HAART) AIDS related cholangiopathy is now rapidly declining in prevalence.

CLINICAL FEATURES

As previously discussed up to 45% of patients are asymptomatic at the time of diagnosis. However, close questioning may reveal fatigue, vague right upper quadrant pain, mild pruritus or sweating episodes (Table 1). The more overt symptoms include jaundice, dark urine, pale stools, fever, rigors, and abdominal pain. On examination patients may be jaundiced or have detectable hepatomegaly or splenomegaly. Cirrhosis is present in 17% of patients at the time of diagnosis and in addition these patients may have ascites, pedal oedema or a history of variceal bleeding. There may be excoriations as a consequence of severe pruritus. Chronic cholesatic liver disorders are associated with hyperlipidaemia with possible cutaneous manifestations such as xanthelasma, corneal arcus and tendon xanthomas being observed.

Associated diseases

The main disease association of PSC is inflammatory bowel disease. Chronic ulcerative colitis is found in approximately 70% of patients but a minority of patients have Crohn's disease. Conversely, the prevalence of PSC in CUC patients is up to 15%. Generally the inflammatory bowel disease presents earlier than the PSC but this is not universal and it has been reported that CUC has even developed after successful liver transplantation. Typically the CUC is relatively quiescent in patients

TABLE 1 SYMPTOMS AND SIGNS AT DIAGNOSIS IN PSC PATIENTS

Signs/symptoms	Frequency at diagnosis
Asymptomatic	15-45%
Fatigue	75%
Pruritus	16-37%
Cholangitis	28%
Jaundice	30-69%
Weight loss	10-34%
Hepatomegaly	34-62%
Splenomegaly	34%
Ascites	7%
Variceal bleed	6%

co-existing CUC. There is an increased risk of colorectal carcinoma in patients with PSC and CUC and these patients require regular colonoscopic surveillance. Given the dysregulation of the immune system in PSC it is not surprising that PSC is associated with a variety of other autoimmune based diseases such as autoimmune thyroid disease, coeliac disease, Sjogren's disease amongst others. Osteopenia is observed in patients with prolonged cholestasis.

Recently autoimmune sclerosing pancreatitis has been demonstrated in assossiation with PSC. It is associated with raised serum IgG4 subclass levels and characteristic lymphoctic infiltration on pancreatic histology. Clinically there are symptoms of chronic central abdominal pain and persistant hyperamylasaemia. Sclerosing pancreatitis is responsive to corticosteroid therapy.

COMPLICATIONS OF PSC

Cholangiocarcinoma

Cholangiocarcinoma (CCA) is a feared complication of PSC with a prevalence of between 5-36%. The variability in prevalence is accounted for on the populations studied and the length of follow up. The overall prognosis is very poor for CCA due to a general lack of effective therapies and the difficulty in securing an early diagnosis. PSC may be perceived as a pre-malignant condition, with an increased relative risk of developing a CCA compared to the general population in excess of 150 times. There is some disparity in the incidence and prevalence of cholangiocarcinoma in patients with PSC being assessed for liver transplantation and non-transplant PSC patients. In the liver transplant patients the reported prevalence was 17.1-36.4%, where as in population-based studies the prevalence was 6.8-

13%. These divergent findings were reproduced in a population-based study from London with 6.3% of patients developing a cholangiocarcinoma as compared with an incidence of 23.1% in the liver transplant candidates. The higher incidence of CCA in transplant candidates suggests that the risk of CCA development increases with more advanced PSC. The association of CCA with more advanced disease is supported by studies showing higher incidences of CCA complicating PSC in patients with high Mayo risk scores, variceal bleeding, and raised bilirubin.

The most common presentation for a CCA is biliary obstruction due to the development of a dominant stricture, with progressive jaundice, abdominal pain and weight loss. It is unusual for patients to present with ascending cholangitis. Occasionally CCA may be asymptomatic and in this instance is generally due to a peripheral intrahepatic tumour. The clinical diagnosis of CCA on a background of PSC remains problematic. Serum CA19-9 is a high molecular weight glycoprotein with sialylated Lewis blood group epitopes. Lewis -ve patients (7% of the population) do not secrete CA19-9. CA19-9 is not specific for CCA and can be increased in pancreatic and stomach cancers and also in cholangitis. In the absence of ascending cholangitis the presence of a dominant stricture with a CA19-9 greater than 100 the sensitivity and specificity for CCA diagnosis is 75-89% and 80-85% respectively.

The mainstay of diagnosis is a combination of imaging and biliary cytology/histology. Cholangiography, either indirect with MRC or direct with ERCP or percutaneous transhepatic cholangiography (PTC), is the most important diagnostic tool. ERCP has the advantage over MRC in being able to obtain biliary brushings or biopsies during the procedure. Cholangiography will generally demonstrate a dominant stricture with possible upstream biliary dilatation. Due to the infiltrative nature of CCA a mass lesion may not be demonstrated on axial imaging.

The diagnostic accuracy of biliary cytology is less than 50% in many series. The combination biliary brush cytology and bile-duct biopsy increases the pick-up rate to 70%. More recently attempts to improve the diagnostic assessment of biliary cytology have included florescent in situ hybridization (FISH) and digitalized image analysis (DIA). In the former bile cytology samples were probed with florescent-labeled DNA probes designed to detect specific chromosomal abnormalities. A comparison of FISH and standard cytology reported a sensitivity of 35%v15% and specificity of 91%v98% respectively. DIA allows a detailed assessment of the cell nucleus in particular chromatin distribution and nucleolar morphology. In comparison to standard cytology DIA had a sensitivity of 39% compared to 18% but a reduced specificity of 77% as opposed to 97%. At present these improved cytological techniques are not in routine clinical practice.

TREATMENT

Therapies have been primarily aimed at delaying the progression of the disease process to end stage liver disease. The approaches may be simplistically divided into medical (Table 2), radiological and surgical.

Medical management

• Ursodeoxycholic acid (UDCA)

UDCA, a hydrophilic bile acid is the 7b-epimer of chenodeoxycholic acid, has been shown to have beneficial hepatic effects. Multiple potential methods of action have been postulated, but it most likely has separate overlapping actions producing a beneficial effect. During treatment

with UDCA the bile acid pool shifts to a more hydrophilic profile. This hydrophilic bile is less cell toxic to the biliary epithelial cells and cholangiocytes. Interestingly it has been demonstrated that UDCA may improve liver biochemistry without a corresponding hydrophilic enrichment of bile. UDCA increases expression of bile acid transporters in the biliary canuliculi; this has a two-fold effect both encouraging bile flow preventing stasis and stimulation of excretion of toxic bile acids. UDCA is also thought to have a direct cytoprotective effect, this effect probably works down two separate pathways; stabilization of the mitochondrial membrane and prevention of membrane permeability via the mitochondria transition permeability pore. UDCA is also a direct inhibitor of apopto-

TABLE 2	SUMMARY OF MEDICAL TREATMENTS IN PSC
Ursodeoxycholic acid(UDCA) (Low dose 10-15mg/kg High dose 20-30 mg/day)	
Immunosuppressive Agents Corticosteroids Budesonide Methotrexate Azathioprine Mycophenolate Mofetil Tacrolimus Cyclosporin	
Antifibrotics Colchicine Perfenidone	
Anti TNF-alpha agents Pentoxifylline Entanercept	
Miscellaneous Penicillamine Nicotine Metronidazole	

sis. It has been demonstrated to induce cell survival via activation of the epidermal growth factor receptor, and mitogen activated protein kinases. UDCA has also been demonstrated to exert a direct immunomodulatory effect. Reduction of class 1 and 2 MHC expression on hepatocytes and cholangiocytes has been observed. UDCA also effects monocyte secretion of cytokines in the in vitro setting.

The rationale for the use of UDCA in PSC was the positive effects on liver biochemistry and disease progression in patients with primary biliary cirrhosis (PBC). To date there have been a number of trials attempting to reciprocate the positive effect of UDCA in a PSC population (Table 3). The majority of trials have been hampered by relatively small patient numbers, short follow up periods and possibly inadequate dosage of UDCA to exert a positive effect. Initial favorable effects on liver biochemistry in PSC were reported in a small open labeled study. However a subsequent randomized double blind study using UDCA (13-15 mg/kg) in 105 patients followed up for a medium of 2.2 years, confirmed the improvement of liver biochemistry but showed no improvement in disease progression, symptoms or improvement in the Mayo risk score. More recently use of higher doses of UDCA (25-30 mg/kg) in 30 patients treated for one year has been reported. These data demonstrated an improvement in both biochemistry and Mayo risk score at 1 year in comparison to both placebo and low dose (13-15 mg/kg) UDCA therapy.

TABLE 3

SUMMARY OF THE TRIALS OF BOTH LOW AND HIGH DOSE URSODEOXYCHOLIC ACID (UDCA) IN PSC

	Size	Study Design	Dose of UDCA	Study period	↓ liver bioche- mistry	Histological improvement	Symptomatic improvement
Low dose UDCA Studies							
O' Brian 1992	12	O L	10 mg/kg	30	Yes	NA	Yes
Lo 1999	23	DBPC	10 mg/kg	24	Yes	No	No
Stiehl 1994	20	DBPC	750 mg	48	Yes	Yes	No
Lindor 1997	105	DBPC	13-15 mg/Kg	34	Yes	No	No
Van Hoogstraten 2001	48	DB	10 mg/kg	24	Yes	NA	No
Okolicsanyi 2003	86	DBPC	8-13 mg/Kg	36	Yes	No	Yes
High Dose UDCA Studies							
Mitchell 2001	26	DBPC	20-25 mg/Kg	24	Yes	Yes	No
Harnois 2001	30	O L	25-30 mg/Kg	12	Yes	NA	NA
Olsson 2004	110	DBPC	17-23 mg/Kg	60	Yes	NA	No

O L: Open Labeled
DBPC: Double blind placebo controlled
NA: Not available

The expected 4-year survival was also significantly different between placebo and high dose UDCA but not between placebo and low dose UDCA. The significance of this study is difficult to assess as it was an open labeled study with small numbers and no liver histology. More recently, a study from Oxford recorded an improvement in both cholangiographic findings and liver histology, but again in a relatively small number of patients. The largest study to date followed up 110 patients treated with UDCA 17-23 mg/kg for 60 months. This study demonstrated an improvement in liver biochemistry and a non-significant trend towards improved survival, there was no improvement in symptoms and no histological assessment. Additional well-designed studies are required to confirm a benefit for UDCA treatment and to identify the optimal dose of UDCA. Recent data has suggested a possible role of UDCA in reduction of the risk of colorectal carcinoma in patients with PSC and CUC. If confirmed in larger studies this would provide further recommendation for UDCA treatment for PSC.

Corticosteroids

Corticosteroids have been used both systemically and locally. Local steroid therapy via nasobiliary infusion had been demonstrated to have some beneficial effects in small studies but a subsequent randomized controlled study failed to show any advantage. There have been small non-randomized studies of oral corticosteroids that have shown improvement in liver biochemistry but no improvement in survival or histology in adults. Concern surrounds the use of long-term steroid treatment due to their potential to exacerbate osteoporosis. However, there is some enthusiasm for the use of long-term corticosteroid therapy in patients diagnosed in childhood.

In an attempt to reduce the systemic side effects of corticosteroids, oral budesonide, a steroid with extensive first pass metabolism, has been evaluated. In one such study patients were treated for 1 year with budesonide 9 mg/day, but with no significant overall benefit and a significant deterioration in osteoporosis. In a further study, budesonide 9 mg or 3 mg or prednisone 10 mg was combined with low dose UDCA in patients who had had no improvement in liver biochemistry when treated with UDCA alone. Patients were treated for 8 weeks. There was a minor symptomatic and biochemical improvement in patients treated with prednisone in comparison to budesonide but these were short lived.

Corticosteroids have also been in combination with colcicine, UDCA and azathioprine with no overall benefit.

• *Other immunosupressive agents*
Azathioprine has been used in small numbers of patients, either alone or in combination with corticosteroids or UDCA. There was no benefit for azathioprine monotherapy. A recent study demonstrated an improvement in liver biochemistry in all 15 patients treated with low dose UDCA, prednisone 1 mg/kg and azathioprine 1-1.5 mg/day and followed-up for a period of 3.5 years. Improvement in liver histology was noted in 6 out of 10 patients with paired liver biopsies.

Methotrexate, in an open labeled study of 10 patients, resulted in an improvement in liver biochemistry but a subsequent placebo controlled trial demonstrated only a modest reduction in serum alkaline phosphatase levels with no benefit in terms of disease progression, liver histology or cholangiographic appearances. Low dose UDCA in combination with methotrexate has been studied in a pilot study in comparison to patients treated with UDCA alone. There was no benefit in the combination group but significant toxicity was noted.

In a study of 30 patients treated with Mycophenolate mofetil, there was a non-clinically relevant improvement in his alkaline phosphatase but no improvement in Mayo risk score. The calcineurin inhibitors, tacrolimus and cyclosporin, have been assessed in small non-controlled studies. In a study of 10 patients treated with tacrolimus for a year, the drug was well tolerated and produced significant improvements in liver biochemistry but again this study was hampered by the lack of liver histology. Cyclosporin has been noted to be of no benefit in small-uncontrolled studies.

• *Antifibrotic agents*
In an attempt to reduce fibrosis progression colchicines, an antifibrotic agent, was studied in a placebo controlled trial with 84 patients randomized to either colchicine 1 mg/day or placebo. Patients were followed up for 3 years. No benefit was noted in survival or histological and biochemical parameters. A small study of 12 patients treated with combination of colchicine and prednisone demonstrated a trend towards reduced rate of clinical deterioration in the treated group in comparison to historical controls but there was no significant difference in histological progression or liver biochemistry. More recently a pilot study of oral pirfenidone in 24 patients for one year was reported. Pirfenidone was associated with a high incidence of side effects but no benefit in histology or Mayo risk score.

Other agents

Pentoxifylline has anti TNF-alpha properties and has been shown to be of benefit in a rat model of PSC. Twenty patients with PSC were treated with pentoxyfilline for 1 year. 4 patients were withdrawn due to side effects and there was no improvement in clinical or biochemical parameters. More recently the anti TNF-alpha

monoclonal antibody entanercept has been studied in 10 patients and despite being well tolerated there was no improvement in liver biochemistry or decrease in disease progression.

Due to the observation that PSC livers had increased levels of copper the cupuretic agent penicillimine was studied in a randomized double-blind placebo controlled study. Patients were followed up for 3 years but there was no improvement in survival or disease progression. Penicillimine was associated with a withdrawal rate of 21%. The antibiotic metronidazole, in combination with low dose UDCA, was compared with UDCA alone. After 3 years there was a significant improvement in serum alkaline phosphatase and Mayo risk score but no improvement in histology or ERCP findings was noted. The recognised inverse association between smoking and UC and PSC led to the study of nicotine in 2 studies. There was a high incidence of side effects and no benefit from treatment.

Ascending cholangitis

Intravenous broad-spectrum antibiotics covering the most common organisms namely E. coli and enterococcus feacalis is the first line treatment. Appropriate imaging should be for evidence of a dominant stricture that may require endoscopic intervention. It must be recognized that any invasive intervention on the biliary system increases the risk of cholangitis and must be covered with prophylactic antibiotics. In patients with recurrent septic episodes, consideration should be given to the use of continuous rotating oral antibiotics although the value of this strategy is unproven and there is an increased risk of antibiotic resistance.

Pruritus

Pruritus is a common symptom of PSC

that impacts negatively on the quality of life and, if severe enough, may be an indication for liver transplantation. The pathophysiology of pruritus is poorly understood but is unlikely to be simply related to the accumulation of toxic bile salts. Recently a central nervous system aetiology centering around endogenous opioid receptors has been postulated.

Cholestyramine, a non-absorbable bile-acid binding anion exchange resin, binds bile acids preventing absorption in the terminal ileum and entering the entrohepatic bile acid circulation. There have been no randomized controlled trials but there is extensive clinical experience to support its use. Initial studies in cholestatic liver disorders recorded a response rate in excess of 80%.

Rifampacin a semi-synthetic antibiotic primarily used in the treatment of tuberculosis has been studied in the treatment of pruritis in cholestatic liver disease, primarily in patients with PBC. Three out of 4 small studies using rifampacin 300-600 mg/day reported a significant improvement in the pruritus. However, the incidence of rifampacin hepatitis was as high as 12% and liver function tests should be monitored closely for at least 2 months when rifampicin is used. It may also be prudent to start at an initial dose of 150 mg/day and Increase to 600 mg/day if tolerated.

Opioid antagonists function by prevention of binding of endogenous opioid agonists to opioid receptors that are increased in cholestatic liver disease. Most studies have used naloxone, naltrexone or nalmafene, but generally in small studies of patients with PBC. A significant improvement has been recorded in all trials. Two small studies with a variety of cholestatic liver diseases including PSC have studied the effect of ondansetron on pruritus. Both studies demonstrated a significant improvement with few side effects.

The molecular absorbent recirculation system (MARS) has been demonstrated to markedly reduce albumin bound molecules including bile acids and can be very effective in ameliorating pruritus. It is invasive, time-consuming and expensive and should be reserved for patients with intractable pruitus unresponsive to conventional medical treatment. However, there are at present no studies specifically in patients with PSC.

Fatigue

Fatigue is a well-recognized symptom in patients with cholestatic liver disorders effecting >80% of patients and reported as the most disabling symptom in over half. The underlying cause is obscure and is not related directly to the severity of the underlying liver disease and may include abnormalities in central neurotransmitter pathways and neuroendocrine causes. Potential associated disorders should be sought including hypothyroidism, active inflammatory bowel disease and anemia. Potential side effects of drugs should also be considered particularly beta-blockers used for management of portal hypertension. Depression may also contribute to fatigue and if suspected a trial of antidepressants is warranted although a recent study using fluvoxamine in patients with either PBC or PSC demonstrated no positive benefit.

Metabolic bone disease

Osteomalacia due to impaired Vitiman D absorption in advanced cholestasis is now rarely seen. Osteoporosis is less common in PSC than in PBC and is related to age and the presence of IBD and more advanced liver disease. Osteopenia has been observed in up to 30% of PSC patients. The management strategies for osteopenia have largely been extrapolated from studies performed in patients with PBC. General life style advice should be given such as avoidance of alcohol, cessation of smoking and regular exercise. If there is evidence of severe cholestasis or Vitamin D malabsorbtion, supplementation with calcium is recommended. Postmenopausal women maybe treated with HRT but liver biochemistry must be monitored for deterioration in cholestasis. The use of biphosphoanates in cholestatic liver disease is controversial despite being of benefit in postmenopausal patients in the general population. Studies in PBC patients are inconclusive. However, the case for using biphosphonates is more apparent In patients with co-existent IBD and especially in those needing steroid treatment.

Steatorrhoea

Fat malabsorbtion is a consequence of advanced cholestatic liver disease. Associated disorders such as coeliac disease and chronic pancreatitis must also be excluded as possible causes of steatorrhoea. In patients with steatorrhoea secondary to the cholestasis a reduction in fat intake is recommended. Deficiencies of fat-soluble vitamins should be sough and supplemented if necessary.

Hyperlipidaemia

Similar to other chronic cholestatic liver disorders, PSC is associated with hypercholesterolaemia and hypertrigliceridaemia. If lipids are raised on a fasting serum sample, dietary changes are advised in the first instance. Statin therapy may be required if dietary modification is ineffective. Concern has arisen over the use of statin therapy in patients with chronic liver disease due to the association of the drug with severe hepatitis. However, this has recently been shown not to be a concern, although close monitoring of the serum liver biochemistry is advised after initiation of therapy.

Portal hypertension

PSC patients may develop complications as a consequence of portal hypertension with the most important being oesophago-gastric varices. Primary prophylaxis with non-selective beta-blockers has been demonstrated to reduce the incidence of variceal development and bleeding. More recently variceal band ligation has shown to be more efficacious at reducing the risk of a primary bleed as opposed to beta-blockade. In patients who have already bled a programme of variceal ligation and beta-blockade is appropriate.

TIPS (transvenous intrahepatic portocaval shunt) may be life saving for variceal bleeding unresponsive to endoscopic therapy. In patients with previous colectomy and ileostomy formation may develop peristomal varices. These are also amenable to local endoscopic therapy but may require, in recalcitrant cases, the use of a TIPS.

Ascites is best managed in the first instance with low salt diet, fluid restriction and diuretics. TIPS may be effective in patients intolerant of, or resistant to, maximal diuretic therapy. Otherwise large volume paracentesis with intravenous albumin replacement may be required. Patients with an episode of spontaneous bacterial peritonitis and low ascitic fluid protein levels should be given long-term antibiotic prophylaxis e.g. norfloxacin 400 mg daily.

Encephalopathy is managed by the regular use of lactulose to ensure a frequency of bowel openings of 2x/day. It should be noted that patients who have complications of portal hypertension should be considered for liver transplantation.

Surgical treatments

Early reports of surgical management of

biliary obstruction in patients with extra-hepatic disease were not favorable with little effect on the progression of the disease and the possible increase in septic complications. Primary surgical intervention is generally now avoided except in the case of a dominant extrahepatic stricture in patients who have been shown to be non-cirrhotic on liver biopsy.

• *Proctocolectomy*

There is no evidence demonstrating any PSC ameliorating effect in patients who have had a colectomy. In patients requiring a colectomy for their CUC, careful assessment including a liver biopsy may be required to assess risk and reduce postoperative mortality. Patients with established cirrhosis are at risk of postoperative hepatic decompensation.

Endoscopic treatment

The main aim of endoscopic treatment is to maintain bile flow. It remains a palliative approach. Therapeutic endoscopic options include balloon dilatation, sphincterotomy and endoscopic stenting and removal of calculi and biliary debris.

Endoscopic intervention improves liver biochemistry in excess of 75% with a complication rate of 7-45%. In a study of 63 patients a survival advantage for endoscopic therapy was noted when outcome was compared to the predicted survival using the Mayo risk score at 83% versus 65%, respectively. This study has been criticized due to the fact that serum bilirubin in these obstructed patients would overestimate the severity of their liver disease and Mayo risk score. A degree of support for this observation was gleaned from a further study which showed that survival with UDCA treatment alone was inferior to UDCA in combination with endoscopic intervention.

• *Cholangiocarcinoma*

The majority of patients who develop CCA have disease that is not amenable to transplantation or surgical resection. Relief of biliary obstruction leads to a reduction in the degree of jaundice and an improvement in the quality of life. A metal stent has advantages over plastic stents, as the latter is more prone to occlusion. Adequate axial imaging is necessary prior to stent insertion to avoid atrophied liver segments and to enable targeting of the most appropriate ducts.

A more novel endoscopic approach is photodynamic therapy. Here the patient is administered an IV nontoxic photosensitizing agent. This agent accumulates in the CCA. Two days later the patient undergoes ERCP and during the procedure the photosensitizing agent is activated by the use of a non-thermal laser inserted in to the bile duct leading to apoptosis of the malignant cells. A recent multi-centre study demonstrated a highly significant improvement in median survival for patients treated with biliary stenting and PDT (median survival 493 days) compared to stenting alone (median survival 98 days) and seemed to be related to an improved amelioration of biliary obstruction in the combination group as opposed to tumor load reduction. Brachytherapy using iridium 192 can be placed across malignant strictures at ERCP or PTC. This approach in theory allows focal and localized delivery of radiation. There is at present no clear consensus on the use of this modality.

Surgical options for CCA in patients with PSC are generally limited due to the extent of the disease at diagnosis, underlying cirrhosis and an inability to tolerate major hepatic resection. However, In patients without a major contraindication surgical resection should be considered. CCA involving the distal CBD require pancreaticoduodenectomy. Patients with hilar CCA deemed surgical candidates are further staged by laproscopy where some 20-30% will be found to be inoperable. The 5-year survival in patients with free resection margins post surgery is in the region of 20-40%. In patients with resectable intrahepatic CCA the 5 year survival is in the region of 30%.

Liver transplantation

Liver transplantation is the only therapeutic option for patients with end stage liver disease. The indications for liver transplantation are outlined in Table 4. Retrospective analysis using prognostic models have demonstrated a clear survival benefit for patients undergoing transplanted compared to their predicted survival. Patient and graft survival in patients with PSC is equivalent to patients transplantion for other autoimmune based liver disorders in the short term (Table 5).

The largest study to date was a retrospective analysis of the UNOS database comparing PSC (3,309 patients) and PBC (3,254 patients) outcomes post transplantation. Overall patient survival for the PSC cohort was 88%, 86%, 83%, 80% and 67%

TABLE 4

INDICATIONS FOR LIVER TRANSPLANTATION

Indications for Liver Transplantation

End stage liver disease
Poor synthetic function
Diuretic resistant ascites
Recurrent encephalopathy
Spontaneous bacterial peritonitis
Persistent hyperbilirubinaemia without a dominant
    stricture amenable to endoscopic stenting
Intractable pruritus
Progressive lethargy/malaise
Severe portal hypertension with recurrent variceal
    bleeding
Hepatocellular carcinoma within established trans-
    plant staging

at 1,2,3,5 and 10 years respectively. Patient and graft survival curves were similar for both the PSC and PBC patients until 7 years post liver transplant when survival curves began to diverge, with PSC patients 20% more likely to dye at 7 years and thereafter. The rate of retransplantation was higher in the PSC group than in the PBC group (12.4% versus 8.8%). PSC was an independent predictor for retransplantation on multivariate analysis. The cause of the higher rates of retransplantation and poorer patient and graft survival is multifactoral and includes higher incidence of biliary complications, PSC recurrence and higher incidence of chronic ductopenic rejection.

A recent single centre report from the Mayo clinic of 150 consecutive PSC patients demonstrated patient survival at 1,2,5, and 10 years of 93.7%, 92.2%, 86.4% and 69.8% respectively. Graft survival in the same time frame was 83.4%, 83.4%, 79% and 60.5%. These results have been substantiated by other centers. The Mayo study demonstrated an increase incidence of chronic ductopenic rejection, anastomotic and non-anastomotic biliary strictures (16.2% and 27.2%, respectively) and a 20% recurrence rate for PSC.

The question of recurrent PSC post transplantation has until recently been controversial. The heart of the controversy lies in the difficulty in excluding alternative potential causes of biliary disease, in particular anastomotic and non-anastomotic biliary strictures. Secondary causes of biliary structuring include preservation injury, ischaemia secondary to hepatic artery thrombosis, chronic rejection, and chronic bacterial infection, particularly in patients with Roux-en-Y biliary anastamosis.. The reported rates of recurrence range up to 41%. In one such study the outcomes of 22 patients transplanted for PSC were compared with those of 185 controls of which 22 patients had a Roux-en-Y biliary

TABLE 5

PATIENT SURVIVAL POST LIVER TRANSPLANTATION FOR PRIMARY SCLEROSING CHOLANGITIS

Auther	Patient Number	% Patient Survival				
		1year	2 year	3year	5year	10year
Narumi	37	97	92		88	
Goss	127	90	86		85	
Grazaidei	150	93.7	92.2		86.4	69.8
Liden	61	82			73	64
Solano	111	84.5		84.5	83.4	68.9
Maheshwari	3309	88	86	83	80	67

anastamosis. Histological examination demonstrated evidence of biliary obstruction in 32% of PSC patients, 10% controls without Roux-en-Y anastomosis and 14% of those with Roux-en-Y anastomosis. The incidence of fibrotic cholangiopathy in the same study was 27%, 2% and 5%, respectively. Numerous studies have now supported the recurrence of PSC post transplantation.

Prior to a diagnosis of recurrent PSC it is mandatory to confirm well-defined cholangiographic and histological findings and to exclude secondary causes. In the short term it appears that recurrence does not influence graft and patient outcomes but would seem to impact on longer-term outcomes. A number of patients have required re-transplantation for recurrent disease and it is anticipated that longer follow up will see the incidence increase. Potential risk factors for recurrence included male sex and an intact colon prior to transplantation. There is no difference between CNI used in disease recurrence but a higher incidence has been noted in patients treated with OKT3. Corticosteroid use did not significantly influence the timing of or incidence of recurrence but there was a trend towards a reduced incidence of recurrence in patients whose steroid therapy was withdrawn early as opposed to those on long-term CS.

Liver transplantation in patients with complicating CCA

Until recently the development of a CCA on a background of PSC was deemed a contraindication to liver transplantation. This nihilistic position was supported by the poor outcome of patients transplanted for PSC with CCA due to a high rate of recurrence and poor survival figures, with overall 5-year survival in the 5-15% range.

Recently the Mayo clinic has reported on an expanding but highly selected group of patients who were transplanted after their CCA was deemed unresectable and having endured an intensive treatment regimen prior to transplantation. For eligibility, extrahepatic and intrahepatic metastasis had to be excluded with axial CT imaging, lymph node biopsies at EUS and isotope bone scan. Eligible patients were treated with a combination of external beam irradiation, chemotherapy with 5-flourouracil, and local brachytherapy with iridium 192. On completion of this neoaduvent chemoradiation stage patients underwent a staging laparotomy. Those with laparotomies demonstrating no progression of their disease were referred for transplantation. In the Mayo study, 29% had staging laparotomies that demonstrated disease progression and were thus not referred for transplantation. Of those transplanted the actuarial survival rates were 88% at 1 year and 82% at 5 years, which is equivalent to patients transplanted for non-oncological indications. These initial encouraging data has more recently been reproduced from another centre using a similar management protocol.

A recent comparison of liver transplant with neoaduvant chemoradiation and surgical resection has demonstrated advantage for the former with 1,3 and 5 year survival for transplantation of 92%, 82% and 82% as compared with 82%, 48% and 21% for resection, respectively. There was also a lower rate of recurrence 13% v 27% in the transplanted patients. In highly selected patients intensive neoaduvent chemoradiation and liver transplantation would seem to offer a viable treatment option.

IBD and colonic carcinoma post liver transplantation

Intuitively remission of CUC in the face of combined inmmunosuppresive regimens would be expected, but the true situation is more varied with some patients improving, others deteriorating and some developing CUC for the first time. Generally flares were controlled with increases in the dose of corticosteroids.

After liver transplantation there remains a significant and indeed an increased risk of colonic carcinoma in those patients with ulcerative colitis with an intact large bowel. A negative colonoscopy by an experienced colonoscopist is mandatory prior to transplantation but it is important to recognize that in one study 3/27 patients (11%) transplanted for PSC developed colonic carcinoma within the first 13 months post transplantation. These cancers probably represent "missed" cancers prior to liver transplantation but consideration to re-

peat colonscopy within the first year post transplant should be considered.

Larger studies have identified cumulative incidences of severe colonic dysplasia of nearly 30% at 8 years post transplant. The increased incidence of colonic carcinoma in the post transplant setting warrants close and long-term colonic screening at yearly intervals, care being taken to ensure that multiple biopsies are taken every 10 cm along the bowel.

REFERENCES

Aadland E, Schrumpf E, Fausa O, Elgjo K, Heilo A, Aakhus T, Gjone E. Primary sclerosing cholangitis: a long-term follow-up study. Scand J Gastroenterol. 1987 Aug;22(6):655-64.

Angulo P, Larson DR, Themeau TM, LaRusso NF, Batts KP, Lindor KD. Time course of historogical progression in primary sclerosing chloangitis. Am J Gastroenterol. 1999 Nov;94(11):3310-3.

Bambha K, Kim WR, Talwalkar J, Torgerson H, Benson J.T., Themeau T.M., Loftus EV Jr, Yawn BP, Dickson ER, Melton LJ 3rd. Incidence, clinical spectrum, and outcomes of primary sclerosing sholangitis in a United States community. Gastroenterology. 2003 Nov;125(5):1364-9.

Bernal W, Moloney M, Underhill J, Donaldson PT. Association of tumor necrosis factor polymorphism with primary sclerosing cholangitis. J. Hepatol. 1999 Feb;30(2):237-41.

Boberg KM, Spurkland A, Rocca G, Egeland T, Saarinen S, Mitchell S, Broome U, Chapman R, Olerup O, Pares A, Rosina F, Schrompf E. The HLA-DR3, DQ2 heterozygous genotype is associated with and accelerated progression of primary sclerosing cholangitis. Scand J Gastroenterol. 2001 Aug;36(8): 886-90.

Boberg K.M., Aadlang E, Jahnsen J, Raknerud N, Stiris M., Bell H. Incidence and prevalence of primary biliary cirrhosis, primary sclerosing cholagitis, and autoimmune hepatitis in a Newegian population. Scand J Gastroenterol. 1998 Jan;33(1):99-103.

Broome U, Olsson R, Loof L, Bodemar G, Hultcrantz

R, Danielsson A, Prytz H, Sandberg-Gertzen H, Wallerstedt S, Lindberg G. Natural history and prognostic factors in 305 Swedish patients with primary sclerosing cholangitis. Gut. 1996 Apr;38(4):610-5.

Chapman RW, Varghese Z, Gaul R, Patel G, Kokinon N, Sherlock S. Association of primary sclerosing cholangitis with HLA-B8. Gut. 1983 Jan;24(1):38-41.

Donaldson PT, Norris S, Constantini PK, Bernal W, Harrison P., Williams R. The interleukin-1 and interleukin-10 gene polymorphisms in primary sclerosing cholangitis: no association with disease susceptibility/resistance. J Hepatol. 2000 Jun;32(6):882-6.

Donaldson PT, Farrant JM, Wilkinson ML, Hayllar K, Portmann BC, Williams R. Dual association of HLA DR2 and DR3 with primary sclerosing cholangitis. Hepatology. 1991 Jan;13 (1): 129-33.

Escorsell A, Pares A. Rodes J, Solis-Herruzo JA, Miras M, de la Morena E. Epidemiology of primary sclerosing cholangitis in Spain. Spanish Association for the Study of the Liver. J. Hepatol. 1994 Novq 21(5):787-91.

Farrant JM, Hayllar KM, Wilkinson ML, Karani J, Portmann BC, Westaby D, Williams R. Natural history and prognostic variables in primary sclerosing cholangitis. Gastroenterology. 1991 Jun;100(6):1710-7.

Farrant JM, Doherty DG, Donaldson PT, Vaughan RW, Hayllar KM, Welsh KI, Eddleston AL, Williams R. Amino acid substitutions of position 38 of the DR beta polypeptide confer susceptibility to and protection from primary sclerosing cholangitis. Hepatology. 1992 Aug; 16(2):390-5

Mehal WZ, Lo YM, Wordsworth BP, Neuberger JM, Hubscher SC, Fleming KA, Chapman RW. HLA DR4 is a marker for rapid disease progression in primary sclerosing cholangitis. Gastroenterology. 1994 Jan;106(1):160-7.

Norris S, Kondeatis E, Colling R, Satsangi J, Clare M, Chapman R, Stephens H, Harisson P, Vaughan R, Donaldson P. Mapping MHC-encoded susceptibility and resistance in primary sclerosing cholangitis: thw role of MICA polymorphism. Gastreenterology. 2001 May;120(6):1475-82.

Olerup O, Olsson R, Hultcrantz R, Broome U. HLA-DR and HLA-DQ are not markers for rapid disease progression in primary sclerosing cholangitis. Gastroenterology. 1995 Mar;108(3):870-8.

Ponsioen CY, Vrouenraet SM, Prawirodirdjo W, Rajaram R, Rauws, EA, Mulder CJ, Reitsma JB, Heisterkamp SH, Tytgat GN. Natural history of primary sclerosing chloangitis and prognostic value of cholangiography in a Dutch population. Gut. 2002 Oct;51(4):562-6.

Shepherd HA, Selby WS, Chapman RW, Nolad D, Barbatis C, McGee JO, Jewell DP. Ulcerative colitis and persistent liver dysfunction. Q J Med. 1983 Autumn;52(208):503-13.

Spurkland A, Saarinen S, Boberg KM, Miitchell S, Broome U, Caballeria L, Ciusani E, Chapman R, Ercilla G, Fausa O, Knutsen I, Pares A, Rosina F, Olerup O, Thorsby E, Schrumpf E HLA class II haplotypes in primary sclerosing cholangitis patients from five European populations. Tissue Antigens. 1999 May;53(5):459-69.

Wiesner RH, Grambsch PM, Dickson ER, Ludwig J, MacCartyh RL, Hunter EB, Fleming TR, Fisher LD, Beaver SJ, LaRusso NF. Primary sclerosing cholangitis: natural history, prognostic factors and survival analysis. Hepatology. 1989 Oct;10(4): 430-6.

Wiesner RH, LaRusso NF. Clinicopathologic features of the syndrome of primary sclerosing cholangitis. Gastroenterolgy. 1980 Aug;79(2):200-6.

Worm infestations causing obstructive jaundice

Misra S.P., Dwivedi Manisha

Worm infestations that results in obstructive jaundice are those due to the nematode *Ascaris lumbricoides,* liver flukes as *Fasciola Hepatica, Opisthorchis viverrini* and *Clonorchis sinenses* and tapeworms as *Echinococcus granulosus* and *multilocularis.*

The pathological changes depend on how well the parasite is adapted to the host organ. Severe injury results if the parasite is poorly adapted to the host organ. The above mentioned worms cause acute inujury as well as chronic irritation to the liver parenchyma and bile ducts.

ASCARIASIS

This is a helminthic infection of man caused by the nematode *Ascaris lumbricoides.* The adult parasite enters and resides in the jejunum after the ingestion of embryonoted eggs. The larvae penetrate the intestinal mucosa to enter the portal circulation, and thus reach the liver, pulmonary artery and lungs. They are regurgitated and swallowed to finally reach the intestine, where the adult worm is found.

Clinical presentation

Depending on the worm burden, the pa-tient may be asymptomatic or have fever, cough, substernal pain, wheezing and hepatomegaly in the first 2 weeks. Chronic infection is characterized by episodic periumbilical pain. With a heavy worm burden, intestinal obstruction, volvulus, perforation or appendicitis may result.

Hepatobiliary and pancreatic ascarasis (HPA) is the result of migration of the worm to the ductal system via the papillary opening. The clinical manifestation of HPA is in the form of biliary colic, acalculus cholecystitis, acute cholangitis or pancreatitis, and hepatic abscess. In the biliary tree, the fragmented worm may act as a nidus for stone formation. HPA is more common in females, with a female-to-male ratio of 3:1 and a mean age of 35 years (range 4-70 years).

Pregnant women and those who have undergone previous surgery on the biliary tree, such as cholecystectomy, choledocholithotomy or sphincteroplasty, are particularly prone to HPA. Recurrent pyogenic cholangitis (RPC) may be the aftermath of recurrent biliary invasion by Ascaris, as ascariasis and RPC have a similar geographic distribution. Nearly 5% of patients with HPA develop RPC over a follow-up period of 2 years. Papillitis and other abnormalities of the sphincter of Oddi may be related to mechanical injury to the papilla by worms invading the ampullary orifice.

Diagnosis

The diagnosis of HPA is made by ultrasonography (USG) or ERCP. The characteristic USG findings are single or multiple echogenic structures, which may contain a central anechoic tube, representing the digestive tract of the worm, without acoustic shadowing seen in the bile duct (Figure 1). USG examination may also show liver abscesses or edematous pancreatitis. A history of regurgitation of the adult worm may be obtained and characteristic Ascaris eggs may be found in stool specimens, sputum or gastric washings. At ERCP, the worm(s) maybe found dangling from the papilla of vater (Figure 2) or the whole worm (s) may be inside the bile ducts and are seen as ling thread-like structures when contrast is injected. Ascarides may also be noted elsewhere in the gut in patients with biliary ascariasis (Figure 3).

Treatment

Cholangitis is treated conservatively, and the worms are paralysed by the oral administration of antithelminthic agents, after which they are expelled by effective peri-

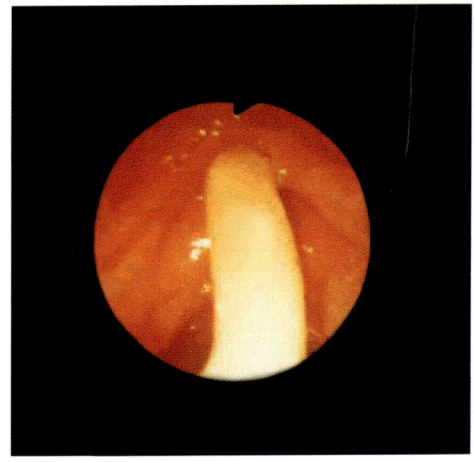

FIGURE 2: *Ascaris lumbricoides* seen entering the common bile duct through the papilla of Vater.

stalsis. Endoscopic intervention from the ampullary orifice is successful in all patients and worms can be removed from the bile or pancreatic duct in nearly 90% of patients, resulting in a rapid amelioration of symptoms; 6% of patients may develop cholangitis and hypotension after the endoscopic procedure.

Roundworm infestation is a common cause of biliary tract disease in countries

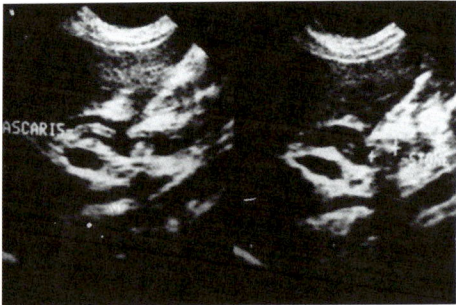

FIGURE 1: Ultrasonography of the abdomen showing ascaris in the bile duct. The frame on the right also shows evidence of choledcholithiasis.

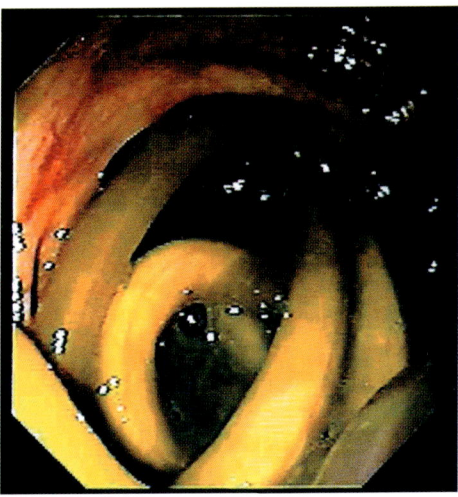

FIGURE 3: Multiple ascarides in the duodenum of a patient with biliary ascariasis.

in which it is endemic and even in nonendemic areas. Endoscopy is the mainstay in treatment for biliary ascariasis Using a Dornia basket, extraction of worm is easy when it is protruding from the ampulla of vater. Extraction of worms using a polypectomy snare should be avoided as it tends to cut the worm and the remnant might be retained. For worms fully migrated in the bile duct EST or endoscopic sphincteroplasty is an alternative to retrieve the parasite and associated calculi. Extraction of worms is usually associated with rapid relief of symptoms. Following endotherpy, patients should receive antihelmithic therapy to eradicate the remaining worms.

FACIOLASIS

Fasciola hepatica (sheep liver fluke) infects humans accidentally in Asia, Africa, Europe and the Americas, where sheep are intensively raised. The mode of infection is by consuming watercress on which the larval stages of *E. hepatica* are present.

Most cases of acute fascioliasis present with fever for up to 3 months, right upper quadrant discomfort and hepatomegaly. In the liver, the tract along which the worm moves in characterized by coagulation necrosis in association with an intense eosinophilic response. At laparoscopy, characteristic yellowish-white, subcapsular serpiginous cords are seen, whereas on CT scan the tracks look like linear array of small 1-3 cm abscess-like lesions. Eosinophilia is a predominant feature in the majority of patients. Due to penetration of the ductal system, haemobilia or abscess formation may occur. Subcutaneous nodules may be present due to eosinophilic infiltration surrounding a dead worm; esinophilic pericarditis or pleuritis may also occur.

The infective metacercariae of *Clonorchis sinensis* occasionally migrate into the ampulla of vater and into the bile ducts from the small intestine and mature into adult flukes. Most of the infected patients are clinically silent or have non-specific symptoms as fever, abdominal pain or diarrhea.

Chronic facioliasis results from the irritation of the bile duct epithelium by proline produced by the adult worm in the bile ducts. Proline is a major nitrogen excretion product and a key precursor of collagen. Chronic irritation results in ductal hyperplasia, fibrosis and episodes of acute cholangitis. USG, CT scan or cholangiography may show dilated ducts in addition to adult flukes.

Diagnosis is made on the basis of the dietary history, clinical presentation, eosinophilia and suggestive findings on imaging. Serology testing by ELISA using cathepsin L1 (purified Fasciola-specific protease) as antigen could detect 20 out of 26 patients with fascioliasis with no false-positive results. A 97% sensitivity and high specificity was seen for the detection of fascioliasis when a crude Fasciola worm antigen was used. Stool examination for eggs may be negative in acute fascioliasis and also at times in chronic disease.

Drug treatment for this condition is with bithionol and triclabendazole. The latter is better tolerated and more effective than the former. Bithionol may result in GI irritation, rash, leucopenia and photosensitivity. The dose is 25 mg/kg for 10 days.

Fasciola hepatica enter the human body through the ingestion of contaminated vegetables. Fasciola usually have an affinity to live in the biliary system where they develop in adults. Clinical presentation can be acute corresponding to migration of young flukes through the liver, latent corresponding to the settling of flukes into the bile ducts and chronic obstructive as a consequence of intrahepatic and extrahepatic bile ductal inflammation and hyperplasia evoked by the presence of adult flukes. Eggs or dead parasites form a nidus for calculus formation, potentially leading to intra or extrahepatic biliary lithiasis.

The worms can be extracted using a balloon catheter or Dormia basket following EST. Dowidar and colleagues treated nine patients with fluke infestation that were resistant to oral therapy by flushing the biliary system with a 2.5% solution of povidone iodine and found it to be highly effective.

OPISTHORCHIASIS, CLONORCHIASIS

Bile duct flukes may be acquired by humans who eat raw fish containing the parasite in the infective metacercaria stage. The life cycle is completed when human hosts excrete eggs that hatch in water, and pass through the snail and fish stages to infect other humans and animals. The major liver flukes that infect human beings are *Clonorchis sinensis, Opisthorchis viverrini* and *O. felineus.* The adult flukes are about 1 cm in size and have a ventral sucker with which they attach themselves to the bile duct epithelium. These flukes have a life span of nearly 10 years. Nearly 25% of Chinese immigrants to the US have been shown to have active infection with *C.sinensis.* while 33% of the population in northeastern Thailand is infected with *O.viverrini. O. felineus* infects cats and humans in some parts of Russia and Eastern Europe.

Pathogenesis

Adult Opisthorchis and *Clonocrhis* flukes inhabit the bile ducts of humans and cause mechanical irritation of the bile ducts. Metabolic products secreted by them cause desquamation of the biliary epithelium, later leading to hyperplasia, dysplasia, and eventual fibrosis and can-

cer, Increased activity of P450 2A6, an enzyme that promotes the activation of carcinogenic nitrosamines, was seen with *O.viverrini* infection. As the adult flukes are long-lived, symptoms can occur even after the host has emigrated from an endemic area. There is strong evidence to link flukes to bilary tract abnormalities and cholangiocarcinoma in areas of endemicity.

Clinical manifestations

Mild liver fluke infections are usually asymptomatic. The worm burden increases with age and symptoms usually manifest in adults more than 30 years of age. Mild symptoms include epigastric pain, anorexia and nausea. With heavy infection, relapsing cholangitis is a common presentation, especially with opisthorchiasis. Cholangitis occurs due to secondary bacterial infection and stone formation in chronically infected, strictured bile ducts. Oriental cholangiohepatitis is a chronic illness characterized by attacks of cholangitis and multiple pigment stones in the bile ducts, which are strictured and irregularly dilated. Cholangitis due to clonorchiasis is a common indication for emergency abdominal surgery in bile ducts that harbor adult liver flukes in Hong Kong Chronic opisthorchiasis can account for a sizeable chunk of hepatobiliary disease in endemic areas, resulting in jaundice, pancreatitis and cholangiocarcinoma. In many patients with severe distortion of the ductal system, recurrent episodes of cholangitis appear to be self-perpetuating in the absence of active parasitic infection.

Chronic manifestations correlate with fluke burden and are dominated by hepatobiliary features. With a heavy worm burden in the bile ducts, chronic or intermittent biliary obstruction, can ensure, with frequent development of cholelithiasis, cholecystitis, jaundice, and ultimately, recurrent pyogenic cholangitis. Cholangiocarcinoma originating from clonorchiasis tend to be multicentric and arises in the secondary biliary ducts of the hilum of liver.

The diagnosis is made by demonstrating typical eggs in the stool, duodenal fluid or bile. On USG, fluke aggregates can be seen as non-shadowing echogenic foci in the bile ducts.

Treatment

Residents from areas with a high prevalence of infection and cholangiocarcinoma should modify their dietary habits and eliminate existing infection with praziquantel at a dose of 25 mg/kg every 8 hours for a total of three doses.

Emergency biliary drainage following EST is the treatment of choice for patients presenting with acute cholangitis. PTCSL is a promising method for treating patients with predominant hepatolithiasis as an alternative to surgical therapy.

ECHINOCOCCOSIS

The metacestodes of all four species of the genus *Echinococcus* cause various forms of echinococcosis in man. However, the two important clinical forms are cystic echinococcosis (CE) caused by *Echinococcous granulosus* and alveolar echinococcosis (AE) caused by *E.multilocularis*. Progress in the management of these conditions has been possible due to the availability of better imaging modalities and better immunodiagnostic tests.

Life cycle

The adult tapeworm inhabits the small intestine of a definitive host; dogs or other canines in the case of *E. granulosus*, and foxes and rarely cats in the case of *E. multilocularis*. Dogs get infected by eating the infected viscera of sheep, cattle or oth-

er livestock. Humans get infected by eating vegetables contaminated by dog faeces containing embryonated eggs. On hatching in the small intestine, the eggs liberate oncospheres that penetrate the mucosa and migrate via the blood vessels or lymphatics to distant sites. The liver is the commonest visceral site involved (70%). The lungs are involved in 20% of cases and other sites of involvement, including the kidney, spleen, brain and bone, constitute the remaining 10%.

In these visceral sites, the parasities develop into metacestodes. The life cycle is completed when the intermediate host containing fertile metacestodes with protoscolices is eaten by a definitive host. Direct human -to -human transmission of *Echinococcus* is impossible, as it requires two mammalian hosts to complete its life cycle.

Organ localization and cyst characteristics

Primary echinococcosis results due to the metacestode cysts inhabiting nearly all anatomical sites after oral ingestion of the eggs of *E. granulosus*. Secondary echinococcosis results due to rupture of the cysts into the peritoneum, pleural space, bile duct or bronchial tree, or release of viable parasitic material during invasive procedures, Rupture of the cyst into the hepatic vein or inferior vena cava may result in pulmonary emboli. In most series of hydatid cyst due to *E. granulosus,* single organ involvement, usually with a solitary cyst, was found. Simultaneous involvement of more than one organ was seen in only 13% of cases.

The liver cysts range in size from 1 to 15 cm, and commonly involve the right lobe of the liver. The usual rate of growth of hydatid cysts as documented by serial USG was shown to be 1-5 mm per year. The triple-layered hydatid cyst consists of a pericyst, which is derived from the host tissue; an endocyst of metacestode origin, which forms daughter cysts; and an acellular middle layer. Protoscolices or daughter cysts usually take 0-12 months or longer to form after infections.

Clinical features

The initial phase of infection is always asymptomatic. Cysts of *E. granulosus* grow in the liver resulting in low-grade fever and tender hepatomegaly. Rupture of the cyst into the lungs presents as acute asthma or haemoptysis, rupture into the peritoneal cavity may result in anaphylactic shock and rupture into the biliary tree results in biliary colic, cholangitis. Liver abscess, pancreatitis or obstructive jaudice. Uncommonly, anaphylactic reactions such as asthma or anaphylactic shock, which can be life threatening, may be the first clinical manifestation.

E. multilocularis forms solid granulomatous lesions in the liver, which may mimic cirrhosis or carcinoma with a fatality rate of nearly 90%. *E. vogeli* infection presents as multiple fluid-filled cysts with protoscolices, and may show some local invasion.

Diagnosis

Diagnosis is based on X-ray and serology. ELISA and IHA, which may be used for diagnosis, have a sensitivity of 90%. The Casoni skin test is no longer recommended due to its lack of specificity. On plain X-ray of the abdomen, ring-like calcification is visible in nearly 25% of hepatic cysts. Both CT scan and USG have high sensitivity and specificity in confirming the diagnosis. Structures of mixed echogenicity are seen in the cysts, with folded membranes seen in 7%-8% of cysts. Internal septations in the cysts may produce a 'cartwheel' appearance. This is typical of multiple daughter cysts within a large mother cyst. Contrast-enhanced CT may show vascular cysts with ring enhancement.

Though not routinely recommended, the cysts may be aspirated under controlled conditions using a thin needle after giving the patient antihelminthic therapy. The presence of protoscolices and acid-fast hooklets in the cyst fluid will confirm the diagnosis.

In *E. multilocularis* infection, scattered areas of calcified necrotic tissue are seen on CT, whereas in *E. vogeli* infection, polycystic lesions are seen in the liver. Plain X-ray of the abdomen may show a ring like calcification in nearly 25% of cases.

Treatment

The treatment of *Echinococcus* cysts is by surgical means, endoscopic methods medical therapy or the PAIR procedure, which involves percutaneous puncture of the cyst, aspiration of fluid, injection of the scolicidal agent and reaspiration.

Surgical treatment

Surgical therapy consists of resection of the cyst after aspiration of the cyst fluid and injection of a scolicidal agent, such as hypertonic saline or liver nitrate, if the cyst fluid is clear. If there is a suspicion that the cyst is in communication with the biliary tree, as evidenced by a turbid fluid in the cyst, sclerosants are avoided. The surrounding pericyst is usually left untouched while the cyst and its membrane are removed. Other surgical approaches are cystectomy, omentoplasty or marsupialization. Hemihepatectomy or hepatic lobectomy may be needed in complicated cases. However, long-term recurrences occur in 2%-25% of cases.

ENDOSCOPIC THERAPY

Diagostic and therapeutic ERCP has been used successfully in the management of hepatic hydatid disease. ERCP is mainly used to resolve acute complications, such as cholangitis and obstruction caused by the cyst material in the preoperative period. The cysts and daughter cysts that have ruptured in the bile duct can be removed using either a Dormia basket (Figure 4) or a balloon extraction catheter (Figure 5). In the postoperative cases, ERCP has additional value for management of external biliary fistula and secondary biliary strictures.

Medical treatment

Albendazole is rapidly metabolized in the liver after intestinal absorption to its main metabolite albendazole sulphoxide, which has potent antihelminthic activity. The dose is 10-15 mg/kg/day. According to WHO recommendations, chemotherapy should be recommended for patients with inoperable disease and to prevent secondary echinococcosis after spontaneous or traumatic rupture of the cysts. After chemotherapy with albendazole, 30% of cysts disappear, 30%-35% show considerable reduction in size and 20%-40% remain unchanged. In nearly 25% of patien-

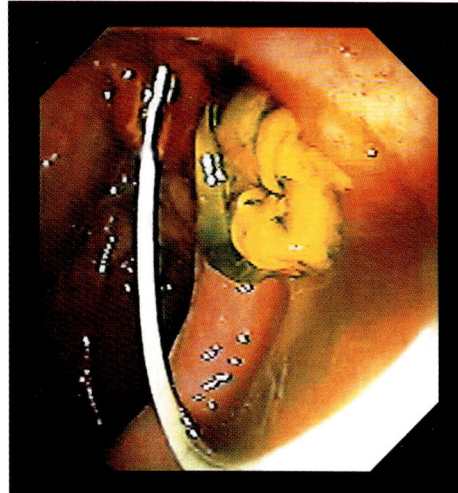

FIGURE 5: Daughter cysts being extracted from the common bile duct using a balloon extraction catheter.

ts, cysts may recur after regression or resolution. Due to the risk of teratogenicity, albendazole should not be given to pregnant females. Alopecia, insomnia and leucopenia may occur, but these are usually mild and transient. If aminotransferase levels increase more than 4 times the normal value or marked leucopenia develops, the drug should be discontinued

The PAIR technique

This procedure is safe and useful for the long-term control of echinococcal cysts.[53-56] One or more days of percutaneous catheter drainage may be needed for large cysts. The usual practice is to start oral albendazole several days before the PAIR procedure. Antihistamines and steroids are administered immediately pre-procedure to prevent anaphylaxis in the event of cyst leakage at puncture. Albendazole is continued for 2 months after the PAIR procedure. The advantages of the procedure are early return to activity and a low recurrence rate as compared to 25% for cysts treated only by medical

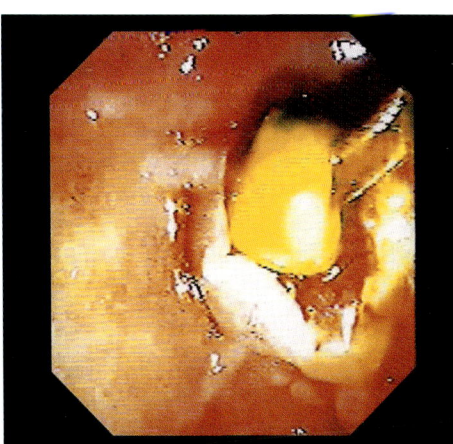

FIGURE 4: Daughter cysts being extracted from the common bile duct using a Dormia basket following endoscopic sphincterotomy.

means. The PAIR procedure and laparoscopic cyst evacuation have shown good results in experienced centers, Anaphylaxis and the potential for haemorrhage should always be considered when treating hepatic hydatid disease.

Echinococcosis is caused by parasitic infestation with the helminth *Echinococcus granulosus* or less frequently Echinococcus multilocularis. The liver is most frequently involved organ (60-74%) with 60-86% of the cysts located in the right lobe. The disease usually does not cause symptoms. Cyst rupture into the biliary tree is a common complication (5-25%) that can lead to obstructive jaundice, cholangitis or both when daughter cyst and fragments obstruct the biliary three. The treatment of this condition may be by surgical means, endoscopically, by drugs or by the PAIR procedure and concomitant albendazole therapy.

REFERENCE

Akinoglu A, Demiyurek H, Guzel C. Alveolar hydatid disease of the liver: A report on thirty-nine surgical cases in eastern Anatolia, Turkey. Am J Trop Med Hyg 1991:45:182-9.

Alonso Casado O, Moreno Gonzalez E, Loinaz Segurola C, et al. Results of 22 years of experience in radical surgical treatment of hepatic hydatid cysts Hepatogastroenterology 2001:48: 235-43

Ammann RW, Eckert J. Clinical diagnosis and treatment of echinococcosis in humans. In Thompson RCA, Lymbery AJ (eds). Echinococcus and hydatid disease. Wallingford, Oxon/UK: CAB International; 1995:411-15.

Ammann RW, Iltsch N, Marincek B, et al, Swiss Echinococcosis Study Group. Effect of chemotherapy on the long-term course of alveolar echinococcosis. Hepatology 1994;19:735-42.

Arjona R, Riancho JA, Aguado JM, el al. Fascioliasis in developed countries: A review of classic and aberrant forms of the disease. Medicine 1995,74:13-23.

Baba H, Messedi H, Masmoudi S, et al. Diagnosis of human hydatidosis: Comparison between imagery and six serological techniques, Am J Trop Med Hyg 1994:50:64-8

Bacq Y, Besnier J-M, Duong T-H. el al. Successful treatment of acute fascioliasis with bithionol. Hepatology 1991:14:1066-9.

Bastani B, Dehdeshti F. Hepatic hydatid disease in Iran, with review of the literature. Mt Sinai J Med 1995:62:62-9.

Dowidar N, El Sayad M, Osman M, Salem A. Endoscopic therapy of fascioliasis resistant to oral therapy. Gastrointest Endosc 1999;50:345-51.

Fenton-Lee D, Morris DL The management of hydatid disease of the liver: Part 1 Trop Doctor 1996:26:173-6.

Franchi C, di Vico B, Tegi A. Long-term evaluation of patients with hydatidosis treated with benzimidazole carbamates. Clin Infect Dis 1999;29:304-9.

Gil-Grande LA, Rodriguez Caabeiro F, Prieto JG. et al. Abdominal hydatid disease. Lancet 1993; 342:1269-72

Gottstein B. Molecular and immunological diagnosis of echinococcosis. Clin Microbiol Rev 1992:5:248-61

Grove DI, Warren KS, Mahmoud AAF. Algorithm in the diagnosis and management of exotic diseases: Echinococcosis. J infect Dis 1976:133: 354-8

Hlaing T. A profile of ascariasis morbidity in Rangoon Children's Hospital, Burma..J Med Hyg 1987:90:165-7.

Halis Simsek, Ersan Ozaslan, Iskender Sayek, et al. Diagnostic and therapeutic ERCP in hepatic hydatid disease. Gastrointest Endosc 2003;58:?

Han JK, Chol BI, Cho JM, et at. Radiological findings of human fascioliasis Abdom Imaging 1993; 18:261-4

Hira PR, Lindberg LG, Francis I, et al. Diagnosis of cystic hydatid disease: Role of aspiration cytology. Lancet 1988:1:655-7.

Kalovidouris A, Pissiotis C, Pontifex C, et al. CT characterization of multivesicular hydatid cysts. J Comput Assist Tomogr 1986:10:428-31

Khuroo MS, Dar MY, Yattoo GN, et al. Percutaneous drainage versus albendazole therapy in hepatic hydatidosis: A prospective, randomized study. Gastroenterology 1993 ;104:1452-9.

Khuroo MS, Zargar SA, Mahajan R. Hepatobiliary and pancreatic ascariasis in India Lancet 1990, 335: 1503-6.

Khuroo MS, Zargar SA, Yattoo GN, el al. Sonographic findings in gallbladder ascariasis J Clin Ultrasound 1992:20:587-91.

Khuroo MS, Mahajan R, Zarqar SA, et al. Biliary and pancreatic ascariasis: A long- term follow-up. Natl Med J India 1989:2:4-6.

Khuroo MS, Zarqar SA, Yattoo GN, et al. Oddi's sphincter motor activity in patients recurrent pyogenic cholangitis. Hepatology 1993:17:53-8.

Khuroo MS, Zarjar SA, Mahajan R, et al. Sonographic appearances in biliary ascariasis Gastroenterology 1987:93:267-72.

Khuroo MS, Zargar SA, Yatoo GN, et al. Worm extraction and biliary drainage in hepatobiliary and pancreatic ascariasis. Gastrointest Endosc 1993;39:680-5.

Kim JB, Kim DJ, Huh S, et al. A human case of invasive fascioliasis associated with liver abscess. Korean J Parasitol 1995,33:395-8

Leung JWC, Sung Y, Banez VP, et al. Endoscopic cholangiopancreatography in hepatic clonorchiasis-a follow-up study. Gastrointest Endosc 1990:36:360-3.

Meeusen E, Rickard MD, Brandon MR. Cellular responses during liver fluke infection in sheep and its evasion by the parasite. Parasite Immunol 1995;17:37-45

Maher K, El Redi R, Elhoda AN, et al. Parasite-specific antibody profile in human fascioliasis: Application for imnnunodiagnosis of infection. Am J Trop Med Hyg 1999;61:738-42.

Misra SP, Dwivedi M. Removal of *Ascaris lumbricoides* from the bile duct using balloon sphincteroplasty. Endoscopy 1998;30-S6-7.

Misra SP, Dwivedi M, Clinical features and management of biliary ascariasis in a non-endemic area. Postgrad Med J 2000;76:29-32.

Moreto M, Barron J. The laparoscopic diagnosis of the liver fascioliasis. Gastrointest Endosc 1980;26:147-9

Odev K, Paksoy Y, Arslan A, et al. Sonographically guided percutaneous treatment of hepatic hydatid cysts: Long term results. J Clin Ultrasound 2000;28:469-78.

Olga Giouleme, ikolaos Nikoliadis, Petros Zezos, et al. Treatment of complications of hydatid disease by ERCP. Gastrointest Endosc 2001;54: 508-10.

Price TA, Tuazon CD, Simon GL. Fascioliasis: Case reports and review. Clin Infect Dis; 1993, 17:426-30

Puspeiro JR, Armesto V, Varela J, et al. Fascioliasis: Findings in 15 patients. Br J Radiol 2001:64:798-801

Salama HM, Ahmed NH, el Deeb N, et al. Hepatic hydatid cysts: Sonographic follow-up after percutaneous sonographically guided aspiration. J Clin Ultraound 1998;26:455-60.

Sandouk F, Haffar S, Zada MM, et al. Pancreatic biliary ascariasis: experience of 300 cases, Am J Gastroenterol 1997;92:2264-7

Satarug S, Lang MA, Yongvanit P, et al. Induction of cytochrome P450 2A6 expression in humans by the carcinogenic parasite infection Opisthorchiasis viverrini. Cancer Epidemiol Biomarkers Prev 1996;5:795-800.

Schaefer JW, Khan MY. Echinococcosis (hydatid disease): Lessons from experience with 59 patients. Rev Infect dis 1991:13:243-7

Schantz PM, Brandt FH, Dickinson CM, et al. Effects of albendazole on Echinococcus multilocularis infection in the Mongolian jird. J Infect Dis 1990;162:1403-7

Schantz PM, Okelo GBA. Echinococcosis (hydatidosis). In: Warren KS, Mahmoud AAF (eds). Tropical and geographical medicine. New York: McGraw-Hill: 1990:505-18.

Schulman A. Non-western patterns of biliary stones and the role of ascariasis. Radiology 1987: 162:425-30.

Schulman A. Intrahepatic biliary stones: Imaging features and a possible relationship with *Ascaris lumbricoides*. Clin Radiol 1993:47:325-32.

Schwartz DA. Cholangiocarcinoma associated with liver fluke infection: A preventable source of morbidity in Asian immigrants. Am J Gastroenterol 1986:81:76-9.

Sithithaworn P, Haswell-Elkins M, Mairiang P, et al. Parasite-associated morbidity: Liver fluke infection and bile duct cancer in northeast Thailand. Int J Parasitol 1994:24:833- 43

Stark ME. Herrington DA, Hillyer GV. et al. An international traveler with fever, abdominal pain, eosinophilia and a liver lesion. Gastroenterology 1993;105:1900-8.

Steiqer U, Corting J, Reichen J. Albendazole treatment of echinococcosis in humans: Effects on microsomal metabolism and drug tolerance. Clin Pharmacol Ther 1990:47:347-53.

Stock FE, Fung JHY. Oriental cholangiohepatitis. Arch Surg 1962,84:409-12.

Uflacker R, Duarte D, Silva P. Association of congenital cystic dilatation of the common bile duct and congenital diverticulum of the hepatic duct with concomitant ascariasis Gastrointest Radiol 1978,3:407-9.

Ustunsoz B, Akhan O, Kamiloglu MA, et al. Percutaneous treatment of hydatid cysts of the liver: Long -term results. Am J Roentgenol 1999;172: 91-6.

Van Beers B, Pringot J, Guebel A, et al. Hepatobiliary fascioliasis: Noninvasive findings. Radiology 1990:174:809-10

Van Steenbergen W, Fevery J, Broechaert L, et al.

Hepatic echinococcosis ruptured into the biliary tract: Clinical, radiological and therapeutic features during five episodes of spontaneous biliary rupture in three patients with hepatic hydatidosis. J Hepatol 1987;4: 133-9

Waianapa P. Cholangiocarcinoma in patients with opisthorchiasis. Br J Surg 1996,83:1062-4

Werczberger A, Golhman J, Wertheim G, et al. Disseminated echinococcosis with repeated anaphylactic shock treated with mebendazole. Chest 1979,76:482-4

Yilmaz bilsel, Turker ulut, Sumer Yamaner, et al. ERCP in the diagnosis and management of complications after surgery for hepatic echonococcosis. Gastrointest Endosc 2003; 57:210-3.

Diagnosis and surgical treatment of hepatocellural carcinoma with obstructive jaundice

Lun-Xiu Qin

INTRODUCTION

Jaundice presents in 19% to 40% of patients with hepatocellular carcinoma (HCC) at the time of diagnosis and usually occurs in later stages. In most situations, it is due to diffuse tumor infiltration of liver parenchyma, hilar invasion, or progressive terminal liver failure (advanced underlying cirrhosis). Obstructive jaundice as the main presenting clinical feature is uncommon. Only 1%-12% of HCC patients manifest obstructive jaundice as the initial complaint. Identification of this group of patients is clinically important, because surgical treatment may be beneficial.

Mallory *et al.* described the first such case in 1947, in which HCC invaded the cystic duct and gave rise to obstructive jaundice caused by hemobilia from the tumor thrombi. Thereafter, there have been few and scattered reports of such presentations of HCC in English literatures. In 1975, Lin et al. clinically classified such cases as "icteric type hepatoma", which manifested as obstructive jaundice in the early stage before the tumor became discernible or palpable. Okuda classified these patients as "cholestatic type of HCC".

Thrombus in bile duct (BDT) is one of the main reasons of obstructive jaundice. The incidence was 1.2-9% in previous reports. Huang et al. collected the cases from the newly diagnosed HCC patients of the admission registration database, and found the incidence of this type HCC was only 0.53%.

Variation in the biological behavior of HCC may partly account for the difference in incidence. It is reported that the incidence is increasing in patients with HCC, and transcatheter arterial chemoembolization (TACE) therapy could increase the possibility of common bile duct obstruction of tumor thrombi.

PATHOLOGICAL FEATURES

HCC may involve the biliary tract in several different ways: tumor thrombi, hemobila, tumor compression, and diffuse tumor infiltration. (Figure 1) Infrequently, jaundice may also result from the external compression on the major bile ducts by direct tumor encasement or by the metastatic lymphoadenopathy at the porta hepatis.

BDT might be benign, malignant, or a combination of both. Benign thrombi

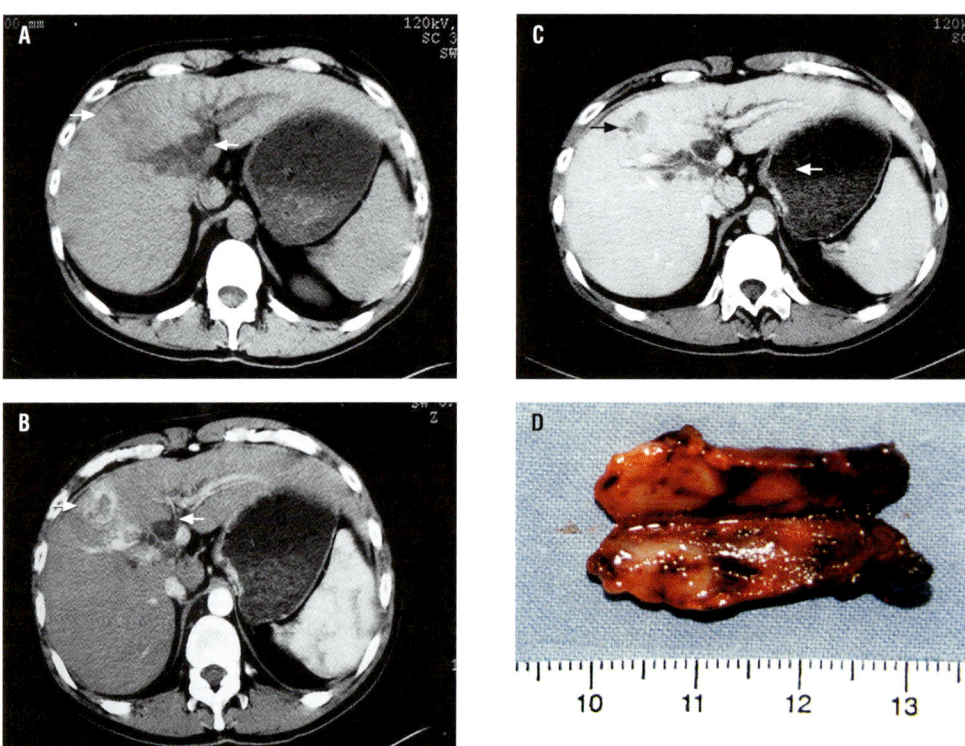

FIGURE 1: The hepatocellular carcinoma (HCC) with tumor thrombosis in common bile duct. **(A-C):** The three phases of CT scan. One small HCC with rich arterial blood flow is shown in the left medial lobe of liver (arrow), with the intrahepatic bile duct of both sides and common hepatic duct dilated obviously (arrow). **(D):** The tumor thrombosis removed from the common bile duct of this HCC patient.

could be blood clots, pus, or sludge. Malignant thrombi could be primary intrabiliary malignant tumors, HCC with invasion to bile ducts, or metastatic cancer with bile duct invasion. HCC invasion into bile duct may be due to one of the three mechanisms: (1) a distal tumor may grow continuously until it fills the entire extrahepatic biliary system; (2) a fragment of necrotic tumor may separate from the proximal intraductal growth, migrate to the distal common bile duct and cause an obstruction; (3) hemorrhage from the tumor may partially or completely fill the biliary tract with tumor-containing blood clots. In this type of HCC, blood clots are inevitably mixed with fresh tumor debris. However, Shimoji et al. reported one case

suspected recurrent HCC during the c-holedochotomy after left hepatectomy for HCC, no HCC was detected by either macroscopic or intra-operative ultrasonographic examination. The course of hemobilia thus remained unclear until the autopsy was performed. Hemorrhage from a ruptured branch of the portal vein into the intrahepatic bile duct, filling the entire common bile duct with solid casts of blood, is uncommon. The hemorrhage into intrahepatic bile duct may be secondary to a portal vein rupture from: (1) a rupture of the engorged or variceal proximal portal vein leading directly into the intrahepatic duct; (2) necrosis of a cirrhotic liver nodule adjacent to both the intrahepatic bile duct and the vein; or (3) either

ical detectable jaundice, and is much better than those with jaundice due to hepatic insufficiency.

There are numerous techniques that can be employed for biliary decompression and drainage. The decision to perform what kind of operations or interventions should be based on the nature and location of the main tumor mass, severity of the symptoms, associated neoplastic strictures, the patient's overall status, and the experience of the surgeon. Wang et al. reported 10 cases with gross evidence of tumor thrombi in the bile duct were treated with different resection methods and interventions. Eight out of the 10 patients underwent exploratory laparotomy (right lobectomy with extrahep-

atic bile duct resection in 2 cases, right lobectomy with tumor thrombectomy in 2 cases, left lobectomy and caudate lobectomy with extra-hepatic bile duct resection in 2 cases including T-tube drainage in 1 case and biopsy only with post-operative internal biliary stent in 1 case). Survival time of these patients was 39 months (still alive); 38 months (still alive); 8 months (died); 8 months (died); 8 months (still alive); 1 month (still alive); 14 months (died); 8 months (died), respectively. Of the 2 non-surgical cases, 1 underwent P-TBD only and the other had endoscopic removal of the thrombi. Their survival time was 18 days (died) and 24 months (still alive with recurrence), respectively. The 4 cases, with right lobectomy or left lobec-

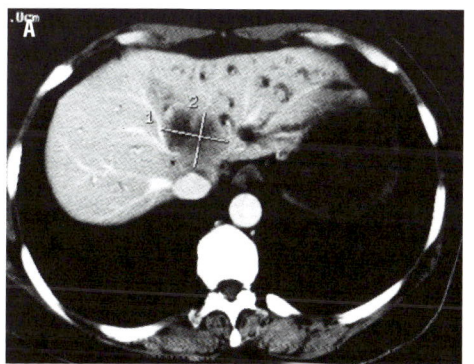

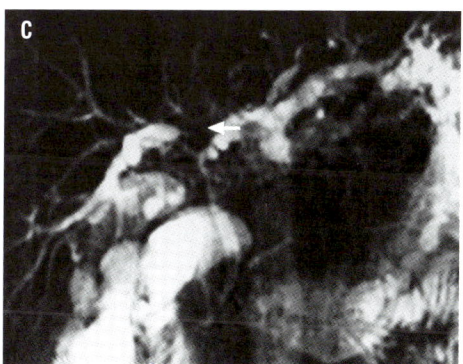

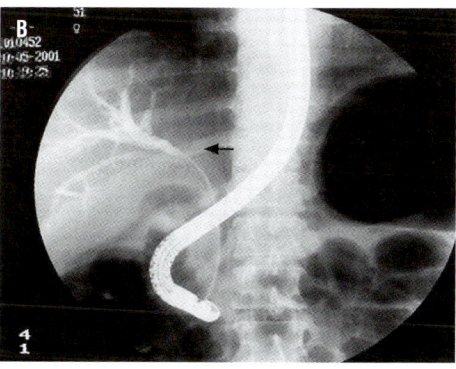

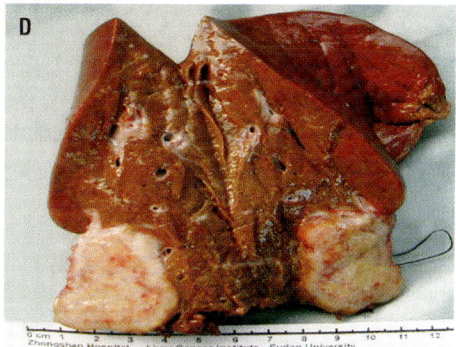

FIGURE 4: Intrahepatic cholangiocarcinoma with invasion of extrahepatic bile duct. **(A).** CT scan showed one tumor in the left middle lobe of the liver, with dilated intrahepatic bile duct. **(B).** ERCP showed obstruction of common and left hepatic duct. **(C).** MRCP showed obstruction of common hepatic duct, with obvious dilated intrahepatic bile duct. **(D).** Surgical specimen of the liver.

tomy including extrahepatic bile duct resection, had relatively long-term disease-free survival (39 months, 38 months, 8 months and 1 month after operation, respectively). However, there were no differences in survival between the partial hepatectomy procedure with removal of tumor thrombi and the simple drainage procedure without tumor resection. So, they suggested that, for the improvement of survival, it was necessary to perform major hepatic resection with removal of the extrahepatic bile duct. If hepatic resection could not be accomplished with bile duct resection due to limited liver function, non-surgical modalities should be considered instead of surgery because there was no difference in prognosis between the 2 groups. Hu et al. reviewed 18 patients with obstructive jaundice by tumor emboli from HCC during a 15-year period of time. Types of surgical procedures were choledochotomy with T-tube drainage alone in 9 patients, choledochotomy with T-tube drainage followed by hepatectomy in six, and T-tube drainage followed by TACE in the remaining three patients. The mean survival time for 9 patients with external drainage alone was 4.5 months. For the 3 patients with T-tube drainage and TACE, the mean survival time was 11 months. Six patients who had undergone hepatectomy had a better postoperative survival time, with 1 surviving for more than 3 years and another alive for 70 months, without evidence of recurrence at the moment. Tantawi et al. reported 5 patients underwent liver resection associated with biliary exploration, clearance and T-tube drainage, 4 of them received major hepatectomy. All of the patients survived more than 1 year with a median survival of 29 months. There were 2 long-term survivors without recurrence at 29 and 80 months.

Intraoperative identification of the nature and location of intraluminal biliary obstruction is crucial for the initial assessment and planning of operative strategy.

In this respect, IOC, cholangiography, and intraoperative US are important adjuncts to formal common bile duct exploration. Direct endoscopic visualization of bile ducts will facilitate differentiation of neoplastic stricture from filling defects demonstrated in cholangiograms. Removal of gross tumor debris as much as possible from the luminal of the bile duct through manual extraction and irrigation is one of the key procedures to the prognosis. This can often be verified at the end of the procedure either by repeated cholangioscopy or cholangiography. Using intra-operative US on the surface of the liver, small or deeply seated tumor and intrahepatic metastasis can be found and an adequate tumor resection margin can be marked out accurately. IOC reveals the characteristic finding of an intraluminal yellowish nodular mass in patients with malignant obstruction of the bile duct due to HCC. Liver resection with a free margin of the involved hepatic duct can be achieved by a choledochoscopically guided operation.

It is not difficult to remove such tumor casts at operation in most cases. The ideal way to remove BDT is *en bloc* resection with the primary tumor. It is also relatively easy to remove BDT either with the exploration of CBD or from the cut-end of bile duct after hepatectomy. However, active hemorrhage occurred during operation in some cases, possibly because of the continuity of the intraductal tumor debris with the main intrahepatic tumor. Suturing, electrocauterization, compression, Pringle's maneuver, or hepatic arterial ligation usually can achieve hemostasis. When noncalculous material is found to be obstructing the extrahepatic ducts, even no obvious primary hepatic tumor was found, tumor embolus must be considered and the material sent routinely for pathological evaluation.

The role of preoperative biliary drainage (PBD) before liver resection in the presence of obstructive jaundice remains controversial. Cherqui et al. found major liver resections without PBD were safe in most patients with obstructive jaundice. Recovery of hepatic synthetic function was identical to that of no jaundiced patients. Transfusion requirements and incidence of postoperative complications, especially bile leaks and subphrenic collections are higher in jaundiced patients. Whether PBD could improve these results remains to be determined. Teda et al. thought a combination of biliary drainage and subsequent TAE is a recommended pre-operative strategy for the successful surgical treatment of IHCC. Nine of the 10 patients achieved sufficient reduction of the jaundice preoperatively. After the evaluation of liver function, 8 patients underwent hepatectomy without any appreciable morbidity or mortality. The median survival time of the resected cases was 18 months.

Non-surgical treatments

Although successfully resected cases of I-HCC have been reported, most of this type of patients are inoperable. The alternative treatment strategy is palliative in intent, including palliative treatment for the tumor and thrombi, and alleviating the jaundice. Palliative treatment strategies, including TACE and/or radiotherapy (R/T) show a beneficial effect in improving the survival.

Biliary drainage is usually used as the initial treatment because of overt cholangitis. Early and effective biliary drainage (percutaneous transhepatic biliary drainage, PTCD) might be necessary in this group of patients with limited hepatic function to prove the prognosis.

To some extent, for icteric type HCC patients with poor and complicated conditions, the palliative strategies are chosen based on experience. In icteric type HCC patients with sufficient reserved liver function, TACE is effective and should be tried as a first choice of therapy. The median survival time among those eight patients who received palliative treatment was 13.4 months (a range of 8-26 months), which was significantly longer than for the other two patients without treatment (2 and 4 months).

External beam radiation therapy may be beneficial in some patients with unresectable icteric-type HCC. Also, US-guided localized radiotherapy, particularly on the critically located CBD and CHD thrombi, could be effective. Huang et al. demonstrated that radiotherapy could be an effective adjuvant strategy in those who showed limited response to TACE or those who had poor liver reserve function. The median survival time of those 8 patients receiving palliative treatment (TACE alone, or radiotherapy alone, or in combination) was longer than that the other two patients without treatment (13.4 months vs. 3 months). When combined with other conventional therapies (such as TACE), radiation therapy may play an important role in the treatment of HCC.

Endoscopic biliary drainage (EBD) for unresectable HCC associated with obstructive jaundice remains controversial because of the short survival of these patients. Some reports suggest EBD is one of the most effective treatments for patients with unresectable malignant biliary stenosis, and even for patients with obstructive jaundice caused by liver metastasis. However, EBD is often difficult in HCC patients with obstructive jaundice and may fail because of proximal biliary obstructive at the hilum, underlying liver cirrhosis, and a poor hepatic functional reserve. Consequently, it is not a commonly used procedure in patients with advanced inoperable HCC and obstructive jaundice, and the indications for EBD in these patients are also controversial because of their short survival.

ERCP can be both diagnostic and therapeutic. Biliary stenting can relieve jaundice and allow further chemotherapy, but at additional expense and potential morbidity. Martin et al. retrospectively analyzed 26 patients with HCC and jaundice undergoing ERCP after CT or US, and found in selected patients, stenting could safely relieve jaundice and allow subsequent chemotherapy. CT or US accurately predicted lesions that responded to stenting. ERCP and stenting provided no benefit in the absence of biliary dilation on CT or US. Placement of metallic stents is the procedure of choice for palliation of malignant biliary obstruction. Stents show a favorable patency rate with regard to patient survival. In patients with hilar obstruction, the clinical efficacy of metallic stents is superior to that in patients with CBD obstruction. In the palliative treatment of HCC patients, a large stent may be necessary, as used in reports of HCC successfully treated by metal stents, if the hepatic functional reserve is not too poor.

EBD is more effective for palliation in the patients with obstructive jaundice caused by tumor fragments and/or blood clots or with tumor protruding into the CBD lumen than in the patients who mainly have tumor invasion. So it is important to understand the causes of obstruction on cholangiograms before performing EBD. And it is difficult in most patients with direct tumor invasion involving both hepatic ducts, and multiple tumors in both lobes. It is important to determine the site, extent, and nature of the obstruction, as well as liver function and the presence of portal thrombus, before performing EBD. In patients with tumor involvement of both the right and left intrahepatic ducts, EBD should be avoided because of the low successful drainage rate and short survival. In HCC patients with obstructive jaundice, considering the progression of hepatic insuf-

ficiency, it is important to achieve complete drainage at the first stenting procedure. In patients with CBD bifurcation tumors, drainage of both lobes should be achieved, if possible. However, attempted drainage of all obstructed liver segments may cause cholangitis or sepsis if it is unsuccessful.

The combination of palliative methods may relieve jaundice, ensure a good quality of life and possibly prolong survival of this type of HCC patients. Lauffer et al. reported 1 case received combination treatment with surgical segment III drainage, TACE and radioembolization with Yttrium-90 resin particles and endoscopic stenting was performed. With these combined procedures, relief of jaundice and a survival time of 32 months could be achieved.

PROGNOSIS

The prognosis of icteric type of HCC patients is generally dismal, but is better than those HCC patients who have jaundice caused by hepatic insufficiency. Cholangitis secondary to tumor obstruction is found to be the major cause of death in these patients.

The prognosis of this type of HCC patients is closely related to the stage of disease, the location and extension of tumor thrombi in bile duct. In 1994, Ueda et al. classified HCC with BDT into 4 types. Type I: BDT located in the secondary branch of the biliary tree. Type II: BDT extending to the first branch of the biliary tree. Type III: BDT extending to CHD (IIIa); an implanted tumor growing in the CHD (IIIb). Type IV: floating tumor debris from the ruptured tumor in the CBD. They also found that the patients with type I, IIIb and IV of BDT had a relative better prognosis than other types.

Different therapies also influence the prognosis of this type of patients. Lau et al. reported that patients who received curative liver resection had a much better survival rate than those without resection (with a median survival of 25.3 vs. 2.1 months, respectively). Huang et al. studied 9 patients who had a patent portal vein and reported that the mean survival of 4 patients with curative resection was 35.8 months, but that of the 5 patients with palliative treatment was only 4.5 months. Thus, the ideal treatment for HCC associated with obstructive jaundice is to reduce the jaundice with preoperatively and perform hepatic resection, but the prognosis of patients who are inoperable is extremely poor. Kojiro et al. reported that 2 of their patients died 40-60 days after the development of obstructive jaundice. In a study of 49 HCC patients with obstructive jaundice, Lau et al. reported that 9 patients received curative resection, 35 had biliary stents, and 5 had supportive treatment, and the overall survival of these patients was similar to that of HCC patients without jaundice. They concluded that good palliation and occasional cure were possible with proper treatment. For biliary drainage in patients with unresectable HCC, the mean survival time or patients with only EBD was 3.9 months, and the patients with external drainage alone was 4.5 months.

AUTHOR'S EXPERIENCE

From July 1987 to January 2003, totally 4324 patients suffering from HCC received surgical treatment in Liver Cancer Institute and Zhongshan Hospital, Fudan University, and 34 cases (0.79%) were found having tumor thrombosis in bile duct. Among of them, 28 cases were male, and 6 cases were female. The mean age of patients was 48.5 years (32–76 years). The history of HBV infection or HBsAg positive was found in all

of the patients, and liver cirrhosis in 94.1% (32/34) of patients. Thirty of them (30/34, 88.2%) were positive for AFP (>20 µg/L), and the highest was over 2000 µg/L. Preoperative obstructive jaundice was found in 12 patients (12/34, 35.3%), and 2 of them had the history of "transient cholangitis" with the manifestation of transient jaundice. The history of "hemorrhage of upper digestive system" was found in 2 patients. Four patients had the history of preoperative TACE (Table 1).

Imaging diagnostic features

Ultrasonography (US) and CT scan were performed in all of the patients. Magnetic resonance cholangiography (MRCP) was also done in 12 patients in recent 3 years. (Figures 1, 2). Eighteen cases were suspected of "obstruction of bile duct" because of the occurrence of preoperative jaundice (12 cases), and/or dilation of intrahepatic bile duct shown in imaging diagnosis (in 6 cases without obstructive jaundice). Only 9 cases of them were obviously shown tumor thrombosis in the bile duct by US, CT scan or MRI preoperatively. One case with neoplasm in the bile duct, while no obvious intrahepatic lesion, was misdiagnosed as cholangiocarcinoma, in spite of the positive AFP.

Characteristics of the primary tumors and BDT

The size of primary tumors was 6.4±2.5 cm in diameter (2-15 cm). All of the primary tumors had no capsule, with unclear tumor margin, and invasive pattern of growth. The primary tumors were located at the segment IV in 13 cases, right anterior section (segments V and VIII) in 14 cases, segment I (caudate lobe) in 1 case, segment II-III in 4 cases, and segment VI in 2 cases. The tumor thrombus located at left hepatic duct (LHD) in 5 cases, LHD to

CHD/CBD in 9 cases, right hepatic bile duct (RHD) in 5 cases, RHD to CHD/CBD in 8 cases, and CBD in 7 cases. According to Ueda classification, 2 cases belonged to type I, 8 cases type II, 16 cases type IIIa, 1 case type IIIb, and 7 cases type IV. In 2 cases, the BDT was as long as 6 cm, and 9 cm, respectively (Table 1, Figure 1).

Treatment strategies

All of the patients received surgical treatment. Thirty-one patients received liver resection and removal of the tumor thrombosis (or thrombectomy). Among them, 12 patients received left hemihepatectomy, 2 cases received left lateral sectionectomy, 11 cases received limited par-

TABLE 1

THE CLINICAL INFORMATION OF THE 34 HCC PATIENTS WITH TUMOR THROMBOSIS IN THE DUCT

Items		Cases (%)
Sex		
	Male	28 (82.4%)
	Female	6
HBV infection		
	HBsAg+	34 (100%)
	Liver cirrhosis	32 (94.1%)
AFP		
	>20 µg/L	30 (88.2%)
	≤20 µg/L	4
Obstructive jaundice		
	+	12 (12, 35.3%)
	–	
Ueda classification		
	Type I	2
	Type II	8
	Type IIIa	16
	Type IIIb	1
	Type IV	7
Treatment		
	Surgical resection	31 (91.2%)
	Removal of BDT +HAL+HAI	2
	Only removal of BDT	1
Survival		
	>1 year	20 (20/28, 71.4%)
	>3 years	3
	>15 years	1
HCC recurrence		
	Within 1 year	14 (14/28, 50.0%)
	Within 3 months	9 (9/31, 29.0%)

tial resection of the liver, 5 cases received right hemihepatectomy, and 1 case received resection of the left lobe and caudate lobe of liver, and CHD, and RHD-jejunum anastomosis. Two patients received removal of CBD thrombosis combined with hepatic artery ligation and cannulation (HAL+HAI), and 1 patient received removal of BDT only because their liver function reservation and general condition could not tolerate the primary tumor resection.

The tumor thrombi were removed by the exploration of CBD in 14 cases, from the cut end of the bile duct after liver resection in 15 cases, and *en bloc* removal with the primary tumor in 5 patients. Intraoperative active bleeding from the CHD after removal of the thrombosis happened in 1 patient, and hemostasis was achieved finally by infusing noradrenalin in normal saline into the bile duct and oppressing locally.

The operations were well tolerated. After operation, the obstructive jaundice due to BDT was successfully relieved in all but two patients. One patient with severe liver cirrhosis and preoperative obstructive jaundice (the total serum bilirubin was 182 µmol/L) received partial resection of the right liver lobe, and died of liver failure at the 35th day after the operation. Another patient with severe preoperative obstructive jaundice (total serum bilirubin was 320 µmol/L, and the direct bilirubin was 210 µmol/L) received right hemihepatectomy and removal of thrombosis in CBD, the total serum bilirubin did not decrease although the general condition of the patient was good, the patient himself chose to give up the treatment and left the hospital at the 40th day after the operation. A third patient with obstructive jaundice (preoperative total serum bilirubin was 156 µmol/L) due to BDT in the CBD received left hemihepatectomy and removal of B-DT. His total serum bilirubin rose to over 700 µmol/L in two weeks after operation, and finally returned to normal in 3 months. By now, this patient has survived for 11 months.

Survivals

The follow-up was up to February of 2003. Twenty-eight patients were followed-up over 1 year. Twenty patients survived over 1 year. One-year survival rate was 71.4% (20/28). The longest disease-free survival time was over 15 years. It occurred in one female patient who received left hemihepatectomy and removal of the tumor thrombosis in CBD (Ueda type IV) in July of 1987. She was still alive without recurrence of cancer up to the last follow-up. Another female patient who received partial resection of right lobe and removal of BDT from the RHD (Ueda type II) in August of 1993 had survived over 9 years without recurrence. The third female patient received right hemihepatectomy and removal of CHD thrombosis (Ueda type IIIa) in May of 1995, and received the second operation due to HCC recurrence 3.5 years later. One male patient who received right hemihepatectomy in September of 1999 (Type II) had also survived over 2 years without recurrence. Fourteen patients (14/28, 50.0%) were found intrahepatic HCC recurrence within 1 year after operation. Nine of them (9/31, 29.0%) were found intrahepatic recurrence within 3 months after operations. The survival times of the 3 patients received biliary decompression were only 2, 3, and 3.5 months, respectively (Table 1).

CONCLUSION

Obstructive jaundice as the main presenting clinical feature of HCC is uncommon. The prognosis of this type of HCC is generally dismal, but is better than those HCC patients who have jaundice caused by hepatic insufficiency. Jaundice is not necessarily a harbinger of advanced disease and a contraindication for surgery. Patients with primary liver cancer and obstructive jaundice due to migrated tumor fragments in the bile duct may benefit from surgical resection. Most patients will have satisfactory palliation and occasional cure if appropriate procedures are selected and carried out safely, which can result in long-term resolution of symptoms and occasional long-term survival.

REFERENCES

Afroudakis A, Bhuta SM, Ranganath KA, Kaplowitz N. Obstructive jaundice caused by hepatocellular carcinoma. *Dig Dis* 1978;23:609-17

Barish MA, Yucel EK, Soto JA, Chuttani R, Ferrucci JT. MR cholangiopancreatography: efficacy of three-dimensional turbo spin-echo technique. *AJR Am J Roentgenol* 1995;165:295-300

Becker FF. Hepatoma--nature's model tumor. A review. *Am J Pathol* 1974;74:179-210

Buckmaster MJ, Schwartz RW, Carnahan GE, Strodel WE. Hepatocellular carcinoma embolus to the common hepatic duct with no detectable primary hepatic tumor. *Am Surg* 1994;60:699-702

Cajot O, Descamps C, Navez B, Lacremans D, Druez P. Hemobilia disclosing very small hepatocellular carcinoma ruptured into the biliary ducts. *Gastroenterol Clin Biol* 1997;21:426-9

Chen CL, Huang SM, Chien CH, Chang TT, Yu CY, Lee JC. Successful resection of a minute icteric hepatocellular carcinoma-case report. *Hepatogastroenterology* 1994;41:503-5

Chen MF, Jan YY, Wang CS, Jeng LB, Hwang TL. Intraoperative fiberoptic choledochoscopy for malignant biliary tract obstruction. *Gastrointest Endosc* 1989;35:545-7

Chen MF, Jan YY, Jeng LB, Hwang TL, Wang CS, Chen SC. Obstructive jaundice secondary to ruptured hepatocellular carcinoma into the common bile duct. *Cancer* 1994;73:1336-40

Chen SC, Lian SL, Chuang WL, Hsieh MY, Wang LY,

Chang WY, Ho YH. Radiotherapy in the treatment of hepatocellular carcinoma and its metastases. *Cancer Chemother Pharmacol* 1992; 31:S103-5

Chen SC, Lian SL, Chang WY. The effect of external radiotherapy in treatment of portal vein invasion in hepatocellular carcinoma. *Cancer Chem Pharm* 1994;33:S124-7

Cherqui D, Benoist S, Malassagne B, Humeres R, Rodriguez V, Fagniez PL. Major liver resection for carcinoma in jaundiced patients without preoperative biliary drainage. *Arch Surg* 2000;135:302-8

Cho HG, Chung JP, Lee KS, Chon CY, Kang JK, Park IS, Kim KW, Chi HS, Kim H. Extrahepatic bile duct hepatocellular carcinoma without primary hepatic parenchymal lesions--a case report. *Korean J Intern Med* 1996;11:169-74

Dodd GD III, Mernel DS, Baron RL, Eichner L, Santiguida LA. Portal vein thrombosis in patients with cirrhosis: does sonographic detection of intrathrombus flow allow differentiation of benign and malignant thrombus? AJR *Am J Roentgenol* 1995;165:573-7

Ducreux M, Liguory CI, Lefebvre JF, Ink O, Choury A, Fritsch J, Bonnel D, Derhy S, Etienne JP. Management of malignant hilar biliary obstrucion by endoscopy: results and prognostic factors. *Dig Dis Sci* 1992;37:778-83

Dusenbery D. Biliary stricture due to hepatocellular carcinoma: diagnosis by bile duct brushing cytology. *Diagn Cytopathol* 1997;16:55-6

Edmondson HA, Steiner PE. Primary carcinoma of he liver, study of case among 43900 necropsies. *Cancer* 1954;7:462-502

Fulcher AS, Turner MA, Capps GW, Zfass AM, Baker KM. Half-Fourier RARE MR cholangiopancreatography: experience in 300 subjects. *Radiology* 1998;207:21-32

Harbin WP, Mueller PR, Ferrucci JT. Transhepatic cholangiography: complications and use pattern of the fine needle technique. *Radiology* 1980; 135:15-22

Huang GT, Sheu JC, Lee HS, Lai MY, Wang TH, Chen DS. Icteric type hepatocellular carcinoma: revisited 20 years later. *J Gastroenterol* 1998; 33:53-6

Huang JF, Wang LY, Lin ZY, Chen SC, Hsieh MY, Chuang WL, Yu MY, Lu SN, Wang JH, Yeung KW, Chang WY. Incidence and clinical outcome of icteric type hepatocellular carcinoma. *J Gastroenterol Hepatol* 2002;17:190-5

Hu J, Pi Z, Yu MY, Li Y, Xiong S. Obstructive jaundice caused by tumor emboli from hepatocellular carcinoma. *Am Surg* 1999;65:406-10

Ihde DC, Sherlock P, Winawer SJ, Fortner JG. Clinical manifestation of hepatoma. A review of 6 years' experience at a cancer hospital. *Am J Med* 1974;56:83-91

Ishikawa I, Kobayashi K, Odajima S, Takada A, Takeuchi J. Primary hepatic cancer with recurrent episodes of obstructive jaundice and distended gall bladder. A case report and review of the literature. *Am J Gastroenterol* 1973;60:496-503

Jan YY, Chen MF, Chen TJ. Long term survival after obstruction of the common bile duct by ductal hepatocellular carcinoma. *Eur J Surg* 1995;161:771-4

Jan YY, Chen MF. Obstructive jaundice secondary to hepatocellular carcinoma rupture into the common bile duct: choledochoscopic findings. *Hepatogastroenterology* 1999;46:157-61

Jurco S, Kim H. Extrahepatic biliary obstruction by hepatocellular carcinoma. *Am J Gastroenterol* 1980;74:176-8

Kew MC, Paterson AC. Unusual presentations of hepatocellular carcinoma. *Trop Gastroenterol* 1985;6:10-22

Kojiro M, Kawabata K, Kawano Y, Shirai F, Takemoto N, Nakashima T. Hepatocellular carcinoma presenting as intrabile duct tumor growth. A clinicopathological study of 24 cases. *Cancer* 1982;49:2144-7

Kojiro M, Nakashima T. Pathology of hepatocellular carcinoma. In: Okuda K, Ishak KG, eds. Neoplasms of the Liver. *Tokyo: Springer-Verlag* 1987:81-107

Kuroyanagi Y, Sawada M, Hidemura R, Aoki S, Kato H. Common bile duct obstruction by hepatoma. *Am J Surg* 1977;133:233-5

Lai ST, Lam KT, Lee KC. Biliary tract invasion and obstruction by hepatocellular carcinoma: report of five cases. *Postgrad Me J* 1992;68:961-3

Lau WY, Leung KL, Leung TW, Ho S, Chan M, Liew CK, Leung N, Johnson P, Li AK. Obstructive jaundice secondary to hepatocellular carcinoma. *Surg Oncol* 1995;4:303-8

Lau WY, Leung JW, Li AK. Management of hepatocellular carcinoma presenting as obstructive jaundice. *Am J Surg* 1990;160:280-2

Lau W, Leung K, Leung TW, Liew CT, Chan MS, Yu SC, Li AK. A logical approach to hepatocellular carcinoma presenting with jaundice. *Ann Surg* 1997;225:281-5

Lauffer JM, Mai G, Berchtold D, Curti CG, Triller J, Baer HU. Multidisciplinary approach to palliation of obstructive jaundice caused by a central hepatocellular carcinoma. *Dig Surg* 1999; 16: 531-6

Lee BH, Choe DH, Lee JH, Kim KH, Chin SY. Metallic stents in malignant biliary obstruction: prospective long-term clinical results. AJR Am *J Roentgenol* 1997;168:741-5

Lee JW, Han JK, Kim TK, Choi BI, Park SH, Ko YH, Yoon CJ, Yeon KM. Obstructive jaundice in hepatocellular carcinoma: response after percutaneous transhepatic biliary drainage and prognostic factors. *Cardiovasc Intervent Radiol* 2002;25:176-9

Lee YC, Wang HP, Huang SP, Chang YT, Wu CT, Yang CS, Wu MS, Lin JT. Obstructive jaundice caused by hepatocellular carcinoma: Detection by endoscopic sonography. *J Clin Ultrasound* 2001;29:363-6

Lee NW, Wong KP, Siu KF, Wong J. Cholangiography in hepatocellular carcinoma with obstructive jaundice. *Clin Radiol* 1984;35:119-23

Lin TY, Chen KM, Chen YR, Lin WS, Wang TH, Sung JL. Icteric type hepatoma. *Med Chir Dig* 1975;4:267-70

Mallory TB, Castleman B, Parris EE. Case records of the Massachusetts General Hospital. *N Eng J Med* 1947;237:673-6

Martin JA, Slivka A, Rabinovitz M, Carr BI, Wilson J, Silverman WB. ERCP and stent therapy for progressive jaundice in hepatocellular carcinoma: which patients benefit, which patients don't? *Dig Dis Sci* 1999;44:1298-302

Matsueda K, Yamamoto H, Umeoka F, Ueki T, Matsumura T, Tezen T, Doi I. Effectiveness of endoscopic biliary drainage for unresectable hepatocellular carcinoma assoicated with obstructive jaundice. *J Gastroenterol* 2001;36:173-180

Matzen P, Malchow-Moller A, Brun B, Gronvall S, Haubek A, Henrksen JH. Ultrasonography, computed tomography and cholescintigraphy in suspected obstruction jaundice. A prospective comparative study. *Gastroenterology* 1983;84: 1492-7

Narita R, Oto T, Mimura Y, Ono M, Abe S, Tabaru A, Yoshikawa I, Tanimoto A, Otsuki M. Biliary obstruction caused by intrabiliary transplantation from hepatocellular carcinoma. *J Gastroenterol* 2002;37:55-8

Okazaki M, Mizuta A, Hamada N, Kawamura N, Nakao K, Kikuchi T, Osada T. Hepatocellular carcinoma with obstructive jaundice successfully treated with a self-expandable metallic stent. *J Gastroenterol* 1998;33:886-90

Okuda K. Clinical aspects of hepatocellular carcinoma: analysis of 134 cases. In: Okuda K, Peters RL, eds. Hepatocellular carcinoma. *New York: John Wiley* 1976: 387-436

Okuda K, Kubo Y, Okazaki N, Arishima T, Hashimoto M. Clinical aspects of intrahepatic bile duct carcinoma including hilar carcinoma *Cancer* 1977;39:232-46

Park SJ, Han JK, Kim TK, Choi BI. Three-diamensional spiral CT cholangiography with minimum intensity projection in patients with suspected obstructive biliary disease: comparison with percutaneous transhepatic cholangiography. *Abdom Imaging* 2001;26:281-6

Polydorou AA, Cairns SR, Dowsett JF, Hatfield ARW, Salmon PR, Cotton PB, Russell RC. Palliation of proximal malignant biliary obstruction by endoscopic endoprosthesis insertion. *Gut* 1991; 32:685-9

Qin LX, Ma ZC, Wu ZQ, Fan J, Zhou XD, Sun HC, Ye QH, Wang L, Tang ZY. Diagnosis and surgical treatments of hepatocellular carcinoma with tumor thrombosis in bile duct: experience of 34 patients. *World J Gastroenterol* 2004;10:1397-401.

Roslyn JJ, Kuchenbecker S, Longmire WP Jr, Tompkins RK. Floating tumor debris. *Arch Surg* 1984;119:1312-5

Saito M, Hige S, Takeda H, Tomaru U, Shibata M, Asaka M. Combined hepatocellular carcinoma and cholangiocarcinoma growing into the common bile duct. *J Gastroenterol* 2001;36:842-7

Shimoji H, Shiraishi M, Hiroyasu S, Isa T, Kusano T, Muto Y. Common bile duct blood clot: an unusual cause of ductal filling defects for calculi. *J Gastroenterol* 1999;34:420-3

Soyer P, Laissy JP, Bluemke DA, Sibert A, Menu Y. Bile duct involvement in hepatocellular carcinoma: MR demonstration. *Abdom Imaging* 1995; 20:118-21

Spahr L, Frossard JL, Felley C, Brundler MA, Majno PE, Hadengue A. Biliary migration of hepatocellular carcinoma fragment after transcatheter arterial chemoembolization therapy. *Eur J Gastroenterol Hepatol* 2000;12:243-4

Sung KF, Tsang NM, Tseng JH, Yeh CT. Effective relief of obstructive jaundice in a patient with nonresectable icteric-type hepatocellular carcinoma by external beam radiation therapy: case report. *Chang Gung Med J* 2001;24:114-8

Tada K, Kubota K, Sano K, Noie T, Kosuge T, Takayama T, Makuuchi M. Surgery of icteric-type hepatoma after biliary drainage and transcatheter arterial embolization. *Hepatogastroenterology* 1999;46:843-8

Takagi H, Yamada S, Abe T, Uehara M, Takezawa J, Nagamine T, Ichikawa K, Kobayashi S, Katakai S. A case report of transcatheter arterial embolization of cholestatic type of hepatoma. *Gastroenterol Jpn* 1989;24:315-9

Tantawi B, Cherqui D, Tran van Nhieu J, Kracht M, Fagniez PL. Surgery for biliary obstruction by tumour thrombus in primary liver cancer. *Br J Surg* 1996;83:1522-5

Terada T, Nakanuma Y, Kawai K. Small hepatocellular carcinoma presenting as intrabiliary pedunculated polyp and obstructive jaundice. *J Clin Gastroenterol* 1989;11:578-83

Tseng JH, Hung CF, Ng KK, Wan YL, Yeh TS, Chiu CT. Icteric-type hepatoma: magnetic resonance imaging and magnetic resonance cholangiographic features. *Abdom Imaging* 2001;26: 171-7

Tseng LJ, Jao YT, Mo LR. Acute pancreatitis caused by hemobilia secondary to hepatoma with bile duct invasion. *Gastrointest Endosc* 2002; 55:240-1

Tsuzuki T, Ogata Y, Iida S, Dasajima M, Takahashi S. Hepatoma with obstructive jaundice due to the migration of a tumor mass in the biliary tract: report of a successful resection. *Surgery* 1979;85:593-8

Ueda M, Takeuchi T, Takayasu T, Takahashi K, Okamoto S, Tanaka A, Morimoto T, Mori K, Yamaoka Y. Classification and surgical treatment of hepatocellular carcinoma (HCC) with bile duct thrombi. *Hepatogastroenterology* 1994;41:349-54

VanSonnenberg E, Ferrucci JT. Bile duct obstruction in hepatocellular carcinoma (hepatoma)-clinical and cholangiographic characteristics. Reports of 6 cases and review of the literature. *Radiology* 1979;130:7-13

Wallner BK, Schumacher KA, Weidenmaier W, Friedrich JM. Dilated biliary tract: evaluation with MR cholangiography with a T2-weighted contrast-enhanced fast sequence. *Radiology* 1991;181:805-8

Wang JH, Chen TM, Tung HD, Lee CM, Changchien CS, Lu SN. Color Doppler sonography of bile duct tumor thrombi in hepatocellular carcinoma. *J Ultrasound Med* 2002;21:767-72

Wang HJ, Kim JH, Kim JH, Kim WH, Kim MW. Hepatocellular carcinoma with tumor thrombi in the bile duct. *Hepatogastroenterology* 1999;46:2495-9

Wang JH, Wang LY, Lin ZY, Chen SC, Kang SC, Chuang WL, Lu SN, Hseih MY, Tsai JF, Chang WY. Doppler sonography of common hepatic duct tumor invasion in hepatocellular carcinoma: report of two cases. *J Ultrasound Med* 1995;14:471-4

Wu CS, Wu SS, Chen PC, Chiu CT, Lin SM, Jan YY, Hung CF. Cholangiography of icteric type hepatoma. *Am J Gastroenterol* 1994;89:774-7

Yeh TS, Jan YY, Tseng JH, Chiu CT, Chen TC, Hwang TL, Chen MF. Malignant perihilar biliary obstruction: magnetic resonance cholangiopancreatographic findings. *Am J Gastroenterol* 2000;95:432-40

Yoshioka T, Uchida H, Kitano S, Makutari S, Maeda M, Taoka T, Ohishi H. Long-term palliative treatment of hepatocellular carcinoma extending into the portal vein and bile duct by chmoembolization and metallic stenting. *Cardiovasc Intervent Radiol* 1997;20:390-3

Zimmon DS, Falkenstein DB, Riccobono C, Aaron B. Complications of endoscopic retrograde cholangiopancreatography. Analysis of 300 consecutive cases. *Gastroenterology* 1975;69:303-9

Pancreatic cancer

Rawat Saumitra, McMahon MJ

EPIDEMIOLOGY

The incidence of pancreatic cancer is approximately nine new cases per 100,000 people. 80% of cases occur in the 60-80 year age group, whereas less than a 2% occur in people younger than 40. Survival in patients with untreated pancreatic cancer is poor. For all stages combined, the 1-year survival rate is 19% and the 5-year survival rate is 4%. Surgical resection (margin negative, node negative) offers the best possibility for cure, with 5-year survival approaching 40% when performed at specialized major medical institutions.

RISK FACTORS

Smoking

Tobacco smoking contributes to the development of 20% to 30% of cases of pancreatic cancer. Smoking cessation can reduce this risk. It has been estimated that moderate reduction in smoking in Europe could save almost 68,000 lives that would otherwise be lost to pancreatic cancer by the year 2020.

Demographic and host risk factors

A number of demographic risk factors have been associated with the development of pancreatic cancer. They are older age (80% of pancreatic cancer cases occur between the ages of 60 and 80), African American race, low socioeconomic status, and Ashkenazi Jewish heritage (related to germ line mutations).

Diabetes mellitus

The incidence of diabetes mellitus is increased in patients with pancreatic cancer, but the relationship of diabetes to pancreas cancer is controversial. Some studies have indicated that diabetes is a risk factor for the development of pancreas cancer (relative risk, 2.0; confidence interval, 1.3 to 2.2), whereas others have argued that diabetes may be a manifestation of the cancer.

Obesity and physical activity

High body mass index (B.M.I.), a measure of obesity, and a low level of physical activity all increase the risk of pancreatic cancer

Occupational Factors

Numerous studies have noted an increased risk of pancreatic cancer with certain occupational factors such as exposures to leather tanning, textiles, and various specific chemicals such as exposure to chlorinated hydrocarbon solvents, nickel and nickel compounds, chromium compounds, polycyclic aromatic hydrocarbons, organochlorine insecticides and silica dust.

Chronic pancreatitis

Chronic pancreatitis is associated with an increased risk of cancer of the order of 5-15-fold.

Other Possible Factors

Factors that have repeatedly been studied, with no consistent association with the development of pancreatic cancer include moderate alcohol intake, nonhereditary and acute pancreatitis. **Coffee drinking,** which was once considered a risk factor, is no longer thought to play a role in the development of pancreatic cancer.

Genetic Predispositions

Pancreatic cancer is characterized by inherited and acquired genetic mutations. Genetic predisposition plays a small but significant role in pancreatic cancer risk. Activation of the oncogene K- ras plus inactivation of tumour suppressor genes (p53, DPC4, p16, and BRCA2) are associated with the development of pancreatic cancer. Nearly 90% of all cases of pancreatic cancer have p16 mutations, 75% have p53 mutations, and 55% have DPC4 mutations.

Inherited Syndromes

Several genetic syndromes (caused by germline mutations) associated with an increased risk of PC have been identified.

Familial breast cancer with germline mutations in the BRCA2 gene. Carriers of germline BRCA2 mutations have a 3.5- to 10.0-fold increased risk of developing pancreatic cancer.

The Peutz-Jeghers syndrome characterized by mucocutaneous melanocytic macules and hamartomatous polyps of the gastrointestinal (GI) tract. Patients with this syndrome have a greater than 100-fold increased risk of developing pancreatic cancer.

Hereditary pancreatitis with germline mutations in the PRSS1 (cationic trypsinogen) gene. Patients develop severe pancreatitis at a young age (often children and adolescents) and have a 50-fold excess risk of developing pancreatic cancer.

Ataxia-telangiectasia, a rare autosomal recessive inherited disorder, characterized by cerebellar ataxia, oculocutaneous telangiectasias, and cellular and humoral immune deficiencies. The gene ATM is associated with an increased risk of leukemia, lymphoma and cancers of the breast, ovaries, biliary tract, stomach and occasionally the pancreas.

Pathology

Neoplasms of the pancreas can be broadly grouped into those with predominantly exocrine differentiation and those with endocrine differentiation. Exocrine neoplasms of the pancreas can be further subdivided into cystic and solid tumours. Although a variety of exocrine pancreatic tumours exist, by far the most common is ductal adenocarcinoma which accounts for well over 90% of all tumours. The term pancreatic cancer is therefore often used synonymously with infiltrating ductal adenocarcinoma.

SOLID NEOPLASMS OF THE EXOCRINE PANCRREAS

The most common solid neoplasms of the exocrine pancreas are the infiltrating ductal adenocarcinoma and its variants, acinar cell carcinoma, and pancreatoblastoma.

Infiltrating ductal adenocarcinomas are malignant epithelial neoplasms that show glandular or ductal differentiation. Most arise in patients between the ages of 60 and 80 years. Roughly 70% of ductal cancers arise in the pancreatic head or uncinate process. Grossly, infiltrating ductal adenocarcinomas form firm, poorly defined white-yellow masses. At the time of diagnosis, they are usually larger than 3 cm in diameter and both nodal and distant metastases are also frequently present. These carcinomas often extend beyond the grossly identifiable tumor, and invasion into large vessels and adjacent organs is common

Microscopically, neoplastic cells show evidence of glandular/ductal differentiation. They frequently induce an intense desmoplastic stromal reaction. This desmoplastic stroma contains myofibroblasts, lymphocytes and extracellular collagen. Another feature that characterizes infiltrating ductal adenocarcinoma is infiltrative growth pattern. This is manifested with extension of the carcinoma beyond the pancreas into adjacent structures, including large vessels, the duodenum, the stomach, the adrenals, and the peritoneum. Perineural growth of the tumour is highly characteristic of this cancer and may account for the propensity of pancreatic cancer to extend into neighbouring neural plexus causing both upper abdominal and back pain. Lymphovascular invasion is associated with lymph node and more distant metastases.

The overall 5-year survival rate is less than 4%, but 5-year survival approaches 20% for all patients who undergo surgical resection.

Several variants of infiltrating adenocarcinoma exist. These include signet-ring cell, medullary, adenosquamous, colloid ductal (mucinous noncystic), and anaplastic carcinomas, as well as the undifferentiated carcinoma with osteoclast-like giant cells. Signet-ring cell carcinomas must be distinguished from metastases from a gastric or breast primary.

Acinar cell carcinomas are derived from glandular epithelium and account for about 4% of pancreatic cancer. Most acinar cell carcinomas arise in adults (mean age 58 years), although cases have been reported in children. Most patients present nonspecifically with signs and symptoms related to a large pancreatic mass, but 15% present with the syndrome of metastatic fat necrosis (subcutaneous fat necrosis and polyarthralgias) caused by the release of lipase into the circulation. Grossly, acinar cell carcinomas are usually softer than most ductal adenocarcinomas, and by light microscopy they grow in sheets and, at least focally, form acinar structures. Immunohistochemical labeling is often needed to establish a diagnosis. In most cases the neoplastic cells label with antibodies to trypsin, chymotrypsin and/or lipase. The presence of zymogen granules can be used to confirm acinar differentiation.

Pancreatoblastomas are malignant epithelial neoplasms that show several directions of differentiation. Acinar differentiation and distinctive squamoid nests may be present. In addition, many pancreatoblastomas show endocrine, ductal, and even mesenchymal differentiation. Most pancreatoblastomas arise in children, but up to a third may arise in adults. At the genetic level, pancreatoblastomas frequently show loss of heterozygosity on the short arm of chromosome 11 near the WT-2 locus, a finding that links them with other embryonal neoplasms such as hepatoblastomas. Pancreatoblastomas are malignant neoplasm. A third of the patients have metastases at diagnosis. The outcome for children is slightly better than for adults.

CYSTIC NEOPLASMS OF THE EXOCRINE PANCREAS

Cystic neoplasms of the pancreas are rare, accounting for 1% of pancreatic neoplasms and 10% of pancreatic cysts. They are more common in women and usually occur in the sixth decade.

The most common cystic neoplasms of the pancreas include mucinous cystic neoplasms, intraductal papillary mucinous neoplasms (IPMNs), serous cystic neoplasms and solid pseudopapillary neoplasms

Mucinous cystic neoplasms are much more common in women (90%) than in men. They arise in the tail of the gland more frequently than the head. Grossly, mucinous cystic neoplasms are composed of large cysts containing thick tenacious mucin. Cysts are separated by thick septae and do not communicate with the larger pancreatic ducts. Based on the degree of cytologic and architectural atypia and the presence or absence of an invasive carcinoma, mucinous cystic neoplasms have been categorized into **mucinous cystadenoma** (no atypia, no invasion), **borderline mucinous cystic neoplasm** (moderate atypia, no invasion), **mucinous cystic neoplasm with in situ carcinoma** (marked atypia, no invasion), and **mucinous cystadenocarcinoma** (an associated invasive carcinoma). The critical prognostic factor for patients with a mucinous cystic neoplasm is the presence or absence of an invasive carcinoma. Patients with completely resected mucinous neoplasms without an associated invasive carcinoma are cured. By contrast, the 5-year survival rate for patients with a completely resected invasive mucinous cystadenocarcinoma is approximately 50%.

Intraductal papillary mucinous neoplasm (IPMN) IPMNs also produce mucin, but in contrast to mucinous cystic neoplasms, they involve the larger pancreatic ducts. Hence, mucin can often be seen on endoscopy oozing from a patulous ampulla of Vater. Grossly, IPMNs reveal villous projections into a dilated pancreatic duct that contains thick mucin. By light microscopy they are composed of papillae lined by tall columnar mucin-producing epithelium. IPMNs generally have an excellent prognosis although one-third of them have an associated invasive carcinoma. The 5-year survival rate for patients with resected invasive carcinomas arising in association with IPMNs is approximately 40%.

Serous cystic neoplasms are almost always benign. The average age is 65 years, and the male to female ratio is 3:7. Serous cystic neoplasm's have a characteristic gross appearance. They are well demarcated and on cross section are composed of multiple small cysts.

Solid pseudopapillary neoplasms are distinctive neoplasms of uncertain histogenesis that almost always arise in young women (90% female; average age 26 years). They are well demarcated and grossly are composed of solid areas admixed with cystic areas with haemorrhage and necrosis. Immunohistochemically, the neoplastic cells label for CD 10 and α1-antitrypsin. Surgical resection is the treatment of choice for these neoplasms, and, if completely resected, most patients are cured of their disease.

Nonepithelial cancers of all types, including leiomyosarcomas, liposarcomas, plasmacytomas, and lymphomas, can also develop within the pancreas, but these tumours are quite rare. Metastatic tumours do occur in the pancreas, with breast, colorectal, renal and melanoma being the most common.

CLINICOPATHOLOGIC STAGING

Staging of pancreatic exocrine cancers depends on the size and extent of the primary tumor, as well as the status of regional lymph node involvement and metastasis to distant sites. American Joint Committee on Cancer (AJCC) Cancer Staging Manual was published in 2002, updated and revised (Table 1).

STAGING

Only a minority of patients with pancreatic cancer are able to undergo surgical resection of the pancreas and adjacent structures, and therefore a single TNM (tumour, node, metastasis) classification system is best applied to the clinical and the pathologic staging. The newest edition of the AJCC Cancer Staging Manual has

---

TABLE 1

AMERICAN JOINT COMMITTEE ON CANCER STAGING: EXOCRINE PANCREAS

Primary Tumor (T)

TX	Primary tumor cannot be assessed
T0	No evidence of primary tumor
Tis	Carcinoma *in situ*
T1	Tumor limited to pancreas, 2 cm or less in greatest dimension
T2	Tumor limited to pancreas, more than 2 cm in greatest dimension
T3	Tumor extends beyond the pancreas but without involvement of the celiac axis or the superior mesenteric artery
T4	Tumor involves the celiac axis or the superior mesenteric artery (unresectable primary tumor)

Regional Lymph Nodes (N)

NX	Regional lymph nodes cannot be assessed
N0	No regional lymph node metastasis
N1	Regional lymph node metastasis

Distant Metastasis (M)

MX	Distant metastasis cannot be assessed
M0	No distant metastasis
M1	Distant metastasis

Stage Grouping

Stage 0	Tis	N0	M0
Stage IA	T1	N0	M0
Stage IB	T2	N0	M0
Stage IIA	T3	N0	M0
Stage IIB	T1	N1	M0
	T2	N1	M0
	T3	N1	M0
Stage III	T4	Any N	M0
Stage IV	Any T	Any N	M1

made two changes, altering the key classification to a more clinically relevant system. First, because pancreatic tumours are judged unresectable when they encase or encircle large arterial structures such as branches of the celiac axis or superior mesenteric artery, T1, T2, and T3 lesions all fulfill criteria for local resectability, whereas T4 lesions that involve the branches of the celiac axis or the superior mesenteric artery are considered unresectable.

The second major change involves stage-grouping III. In the current edition, stage III is used to classify patients with unresectable, locally advanced pancreatic cancer, with major visceral arterial involvement. Stage III no longer is used to denote the presence of lymph node metastasis.

Extent of resection

Although the extent of resection is not part of the TNM staging system, the extent of resection is important for pancreatic adenocarcinoma.

R0 disease: Patients with complete resection, including grossly and microscopically negative margins of resection

R1 disease: Patients with grossly negative but positive microscopic margins of resection.

R2 disease: Patients with grossly and microscopically positive margins of resection

CLINICAL PRESENTATION AND EVALUATION

Clinical Presentation

History
Obstructive jaundice is the commonest presentation of pancreatic cancer. This is due to pancreatic head tumour obstructing the intrapancreatic portion of the common bile duct. Fluctuant jaundice suggests incomplete obstruction by gallstones, although ampullary tumours may occasionally undergo partial necrosis, producing a temporary improvement. Seen with the jaundice are accompanying signs and symptoms such as dark urine, light stools, weight loss, pruritus, weakness, and anorexia.

In a minority of patients, pancreatic cancer presents without jaundice. New-onset diabetes may be the first clinical feature in approximately 10% of all patients. Occasionally, acute pancreatitis is the first manifestation of a pancreatic cancer, related to partial obstruction of the pancreatic duct, which causes pancreatic inflammation. It is important to consider the diagnosis of a pancreatic tumour in elderly patients presenting with pancreatitis, particularly when there is no obvious cause for the pancreatitis such as gallstones or alcohol abuse.

Epigastric pain is a common feature of pancreatic malignancy. Back pain suggests that the tumour has invaded tissues outside the pancreas and is unresectable. Significant weight loss (> 10% of body weight) is common even when the pancreatic cancer is resectable.

A presentation with steatorrhea or diarrhoea is usually the result of a tumour in the uncinate process that obstructs the pancreatic duct but not the bile duct. Often, these symptoms are overlooked until the tumour extends and causes jaundice.

Additional symptoms found in a small percentage of patients may include nausea or vomiting, or both, related to mechanical gastro duodenal obstruction. Mechanical obstruction of the proximal duodenum can be related to right-sided tumour or an obstruction at the ligament of Treitz by tumour of the mid body of the pancreas.

Examination
The most common physical finding at ini-

tial presentation is jaundice. Often, patients with deep jaundice may exhibit cutaneous signs of scratching, related to pruritus. The classical Courvoisier syndrome (palpable gallbladder in the presence of painless jaundice) occurs in less than 25% of cases. In patients with disseminated advanced pancreatic cancer, findings may include hepatomegaly (hepatic metastases), left supraclavicular lymphadenopathy (Virchow's node), periumbilical lymphadenopathy (Sister Mary Joseph's nodes) and ascitis. Migratory thrombophlebitis (the Trousseau sign) is uncommon and usually signifies metastatic disease.

Laboratory investigations
The laboratory findings in patients with pancreatic cancer are usually non-specific. A normochromic anaemia and mild hypoalbuminemia may reflect the chronic nature of the neoplastic process and its nutritional sequelae. Patients with pancreatic head lesions frequently have elevated serum bilirubin and alkaline phosphatase levels suggestive of obstrutive jaundice. There may be mild elevations of the hepatic aminotransferases. Hepatitis serologies are typically negative. Although uncommon, patients with ductal adenocarcinoma of the pancreas may have hyperamylasaemia or hyperlipasaemia, findings more commonly seen in patients with IPMN. A prolongation of the prothrombin time may be seen in deeply jaundiced patients due to malabsorption of fat-soluble vitamins.

Carbohydrate antigen 19-9 is the most commonly used marker. Its efficacy in comparison with other tumour markers (carcinoembryonic antigen, carbohydrate antigen 50, cellular adhesion molecule 17.1) in detecting pancreatic carcinoma has been widely studied; most studies have concluded that serum concentrations of the tumour marker CA 19-9 are often elevated in patients with pancreatic

or biliary adenocarcinomas. With a cut off value of 37 U/ml, CA 19-9 has been reported to have a sensitivity of 86% and a specificity of 87%. Unfortunately the circulating level of the tumour marker is often normal in patients with early, potentially curable, tumours. Thus, using these tumour markers to screen patients with vague symptoms or those in high-risk groups has not been shown to be useful in detecting early disease. Extremely high levels of either the CA 19-9 or CEA usually indicate unresectable and/or metastatic disease. Measurement of CA 19-9 concentrations may be employed to detect recurrences in patients who have elevated CA 19-9 levels that return to normal after tumour resection; a second rise in the CA 19-9 level in the follow-up period is indicative of recurrence in most cases.

Technology has been used to profile gene expression in pancreatic cancer, chronic pancreatitis and the normal pancreas. A review of the literature shows that there are more than 1000 genes that are differentially expressed in pancreatic tumours, and about 50 of these have been repeatedly reported by a number of different investigators using slightly different techniques. The proteins encoded by these genes have potential for early detection of pancreatic cancer.

Diagnostic imaging

ULTRASOUND: In patients presenting with jaundice, a reasonable first diagnostic imaging study is abdominal ultrasound. Its sensitivity for determining cholelithiasis is superior to that of computed tomography (CT). If bile duct dilation is not seen, hepatocellular disease is likely. Demonstration of cholelithiasis and bile duct dilation suggests diagnosis of choledocholithiasis. The primary pancreatic lesion is often visible together with liver metastases and ascites, if present. The use of Doppler ultrasonography gives a reasonably reliable measure of vascular patency and can improve accuracy in measuring vascular invasion. Ultrasonography is operator dependent and may be inaccurate as a result of large body habitus, presence of ascites, or overlying bowel gas (in as many as 20% of patient). Use of echo enhanced power Doppler sonography (power doppler sonography after injection of a contrast agent) has increased the sensitivity (to 87%) and specificity (to 94%). In the absence of gallstones, malignant obstruction of the bile duct is likely and CT scan is the next logical step.

CT SCAN: Thin-cut contrast-enhanced multislice (1.25-mm sliced) pancreas protocol helical CT is the radiological investigation of choice. This technology uses multidetector CT acquisition with three-dimensional reconstruction. Multidetector CT incorporates dual-phase imaging in the arterial and the venous phases of enhancement. Non-ionic contrast medium is administered via a peripheral intravenous catheter at a rate of 3 mL/sec, and slices through the pancreas are obtained every 1.25 mm, with all images being acquired during one 20-second breath hold. The acquired slices are reviewed at a three-dimensional work station using a standard software platform, allowing for three-dimensional viewing of the data which improve detection, staging and surgical planning. Using this technology, adenocarcinoma of the pancreas typically appears as a low-density (hypodense) mass within the pancreas, generally best seen on the venous phase of enhancement). It is approximately 90% sensitive for lesions greater than 2 cm, although this drops to approximately 60% for smaller lesions. CT scan assesses local tumour extension with contiguous organ invasion, vascular involvement, hepatic metastases, and lymph node metastases. The advent of the multidetector dual phase computed tomography, along with three dimensional image reconstructions, has helped in improving the preoperative assessment of surgical resectability, particularly in relation to vascular invasion.

MRI: Advances in MRI, including high-resolution fast imaging, volume acquisitions, and MR cholangiopancreatography have led to an improved ability of MRI to diagnose and stage pancreatic cancer. Most tumours appear with low signal intensity on T1-weighted fat-suppressed images as they have significant desmoplasia with sparse vascularity. The main use of T2 images is in MRCP after the intravenous injection of gadolinium-based contrast. Combining T1/T2 weighted images is useful as the primary tumour can be visualised together with its relationship to biliary and pancreatic ducts. Thus, MRCP can provide detailed ductal images and may clarify diagnostic uncertainty (chronic pancreatitis versus cancer) as well as diagnose intraductal tumours. Additionally, contrast enhanced magnetic resonance angiography or venography can show vascular involvement with the tumour and obviate the need for conventional angiography. MRI is rapidly evolving but currently provides essentially the same information as CT scanning.

ERCP: When used appropriately, endoscopic retrograde cholangiopancreatography can provide a definitive diagnosis. Although it allows direct imaging of the pancreatic duct and its sensitivity for the diagnosis of pancreatic cancer remains high, the current technologic advances in CT scanning and MRI make the routine practice of diagnostic ERCP unsupported. ERCP is important in the diagnosis of ampullary tumours by direct visualisation and providing an opportunity to sample for cytology or histology. It is also an important therapeutic modality for biliary stenting to provide relief of jaundice.

EUS: Has gained popularity and is now increasingly available for pancreatic imaging. Endoscopic ultrasound (EUS) is useful in determining lesions that are e-quivocal on CT scan. EUS is highly sensitive in the detection of small tumours and invasion of major vascular structures. EUS is superior to spiral CT, MR, or positron e-mission tomography in the detection of s-mall tumours. EUS is a sensitive test for portal/superior mesenteric vein invasion, although it is somewhat less effective at detecting superior mesenteric artery invasion. EUS has the added advantage of providing the opportunity for transluminal biopsy of pancreatic masses, although a tissue diagnosis prior to pancreaticoduo-denectomy is not required. However, in specific patients a histological diagnosis may be necessary such as for those in a neoadjuvant clinical trial or before chemotherapy in advanced tumours. EUS-guided biopsy is superior to CT-guid-ed transabdominal biopsy. Access to the head of the pancreas is easier and the chance of needle tracking is reduced (because the biopsy is taken through the duodenal wall, which is resected if a Whipple procedure is done).

Angiography

In the past, preoperative angiography was commonly used to predict resectability and to give information on vascular anatomy. Some studies have shown that angiography adds to the reliability of computed tomography, whereas other studies have shown that multidetector computed tomography can predict unresectability better than angiography alone. Conventional angiography is not currently part of the diagnostic protocol in most centres.

Positron emission tomography

Although CT or MRI remains the mainstay of imaging of patients with suspected pancreatic cancer, the newer technique of positron emission tomography (PET) provides additional imaging opportunities. Positron emission tomography is a non-invasive imaging tool that provides metabolic rather than morphological information on tumours. This diagnostic method is based on greater use of glucose by tumour cells than by normal pancreatic parenchyma. A radioactive glucose analogue termed fluorodeoxyglucose is administered intravenously, followed by detection by the scanner of uptake of fluorodeoxyglucose by the tumour. Malignant tissues will show a higher uptake of fluorodeoxyglucose than normal surrounding tissues. Positron emission tomography (PET) may be of value in diagnosing small pancreatic tumours that escape CT or MRI detection, but the sensitivity and specificity of PET scanning remain to be established. It may also be useful in detecting extra pancreatic disease such as peritoneal or omental metastases. At present it is not routinely used in the diagnosis of pancreatic cancer because of the lack of anatomical detail. With the advent of combined positron emission tomography and computed tomography scanning, both anatomical and functional imaging can be obtained simultaneously. Future information about PET will clarify its role in predicting prognosis and tumour dissemination and in distinguishing between benign and malignant tumours

Histopathologic diagnosis

Most surgeons would not recommend routine preoperative biopsy for confirmation of the diagnosis in the management of patients with potentially resectable lesions. However, in such cases patients should be specifically counselled of a 5-10% rate of resection for benign disease. Biopsy to confirm the presence and identify the type of cancer is usually required before chemoradiation therapy of unresectable pancreatic tumors or neoadjuvant treatment of resectable tumours.

Furthermore, biopsy may be considered in patients whose clinical presentation and imaging studies are not suggestive of pancreatic carcinoma but rather of more uncommon entities such as pancreatic lymphoma. In this situation, the diagnosis of lymphoma would preclude surgical exploration and allow treatment with chemotherapy.

In situations in which a pancreatic biopsy is necessary, options include either a percutaneous or an endoscopic approach. Although percutaneous biopsy is generally safe, serious complications, such as hemorrhage, pancreatitis, fistula, abscess, and death, have been reported. Additionally, there have been reports of tumour seeding along the subcutaneous tract of the needle and concerns regarding tumour dissemination by the act of capsular disruption of the neoplasm. In general, when a pancreatic biopsy is needed, EUS combined with FNA is apparently safer technique and would eliminate the concern of tumour dissemination.

Laparoscopy

The rationale for the use of laparoscopy comes from data indicating that between 20% and 40% of patients staged with modalities such as CT, MR, or EUS will have unanticipated peritoneal or liver metastases at laparotomy. Laparoscopy may be performed immediately before conversion to laparotomy or as an interval staging measure. Staging laparoscopy can be performed with minimal morbidity and mortality and any suspicious lesions are biopsed under direct vision with frozen-section analysis. Patients who are found to have unresectable disease recover more rapidly than following a laparotomy and can receive palliative chemotherapy and radiation sooner. The potential immunosuppressive effects of a major surgical procedure are also avoided, as well as the negative psychologic impact of a major painful operation with little benefit. There are varying degrees of expertise in the application of laparoscopy, with some highly experienced groups performing a more extensive laparoscopic evaluation.

Some surgeons use staging laparoscopy on a selected basis in patients with large tumours (>2 cm), tumours located in the body or tail, or other indications of advanced disease such as marked weight loss or markedly elevated CA19-9.

TREATMENT OF PONENTIALLY RESECTABLE DISEASE

Resectional aproaches

Pancreaticoduodenectomy for tumours of the head, neck, or uncinate process
The first successful resection of head of the pancreas for an ampullary tumour was reported in 1912 by Kausch, a German surgeon from Berlin. In 1935, Allen O. Whipple in New York City reported three cases of pancreatico-duodenal resection for ampullary cancer. Since then operation was performed infrequently until the 1980s because of high hospital mortality (approximately 25%). In 1980s specialist centers developed and it allowed institutions and individuals to gain large experiences which resulted in a significant drop in hospital mortality. There is considerable evidence that operative mortality rates can be kept to low figure values when undertaken in specialist centres.

Procedure widely employed is the Whipple pancreaticoduodenectomy. More radical approaches have been adopted, such as total pancreatectomy or portal vein excision, as well as more conservative approaches to include pylorus preservation with the aim to improve the quality of survival.

Controversies

These include
1. Classic pancreaticoduodenectomy versus pylorus-preserving pancreaticoduodenectomy
2. Partial pancreatectomy versus total pancreatectomy,
3. Classical/Standard pancreaticoduodenectomy versus extended (or radical) pancreaticoduodenectomy.

Classic pancreaticoduodenectomy versus pylorus-preserving pancreatico duodenectomy

The advantages of pylorus preservation have not been conclusively established but it maintains the pyloric sphincter mechanism, preserves the entire gastric reservoir and shortens the operative time. There is also a reduction in enterogastric reflux, improved postoperative nutritional status and weight gain compared with the standard Whipple operation. The two most common causes for sacrificing the pylorus and performing a distal gastrectomy include (1) Tumour involvement of the first portion of the duodenum, pylorus, or distal stomach or (2) Ischemia of the duodenal cuff after resection due to devascularization.

Although some have cautioned that pylorus preservation may compromise cancer therapy, this has not been supported by number of data. Pylorus preserving operation does not compromise long term survival figures compared with the standard Whipple's operation for carcinoma for the head of the pancreas.

Total pancreatectomy versus Whipple's (Partial pancreatectomy)

Total pancreatectomy has no advantage in long-term survival compared with Whipple's resection but has its own troublesome nutritional and metabolic sequelae. Current practice favours the performance of partial resection. Total pancreatectomy requires exogenous pancreatic enzyme supplements and development of insulin-dependent DM. There is also increased intraoperative blood loss. Total pancreatectomy is therefore reserved for cases in which there is diffuse involvement of pancreas without evidence of spread or in rare cases in which the pancreatic remnant is too soft, friable, or inflamed to allow a safe pancreatic-enteric anastomosis.

Standard pancreaticoduodenectomy versus extended (or radical) pancreaticoduodenectomy

Extended or radical pancreatectomy modifications include the portal vein and a block of lymphatic tissue around the origins of the coeliac and superior mesenteric arteries. Several trials have suggested that extended (radical) pancreaticoduodenectomy may improve survival in patients with pancreatic adenocarcinoma but postoperative morbidity and mortality were higher than that encountered in the standard Whipple resection. Prospective randomized trial at Johns Hopkins of extended versus standard lymphadenectomy also failed to demonstrate survival benefit.

COMPLICATIONS

The operative mortality after pancreaticoduodenectomy is currently 2% to 3% in major surgical centers with significant experience. The leading causes of postoperative mortality include cardiovascular events, sepsis, and hemorrhage. Postoperative complications are unfortunately still very common and can approach 30-40%. The leading causes of morbidity include pancreatic fistula, early delayed gastric emptying, hemorrhage and intraabdominal abscess. Some of these complications prolong hospitalization and may require interventional radiological techniques or reoperation.

Haemorrhage can occur either intra-operatively or postoperatively. Intraoperative haemorrhage typically occurs during the dissection around portal vein. Sometimes the Portal vein can be repaired with minimal narrowing. Other times, a patch repair or segmental resection and interposition graft may be needed.

Postoperative hemorrhage can occur from inadequate ligature of any one of numerous blood vessels during the procedure.

Delayed gastric emptying is common after pancreaticoduodenectomy and is treated conservatively as long as complete gastric outlet obstruction is ruled out by a contrast study.

Leakage from pancreatic anastomosis resulting in a pancreatic fistula occurs in 15% to 20% of patients. With adequate drainage, these fistulas usually heal within several weeks. It can result in sepsis and serious haemorrhage. The fistula usually presents about 5 days postoperatively. If the output is low and the patient's general condition is satisfactory, it is reasonable to consider conservative treatment with antibiotics, octreotide and parenteral nutrition. In the presence of sepsis the patient should have a CT scan. If a collection is present it should be drained percutaneously. If bleeding has occurred and patient is stable, an arterial reconstruction should be done from the CT and if possible transcatheter embolization considered. If this fails then laparotomy should be carried out.

Biliary fistulas are much less common than pancreatic fistulas after pancreatico-duodenectomy, but they also usually heal if adequate drainage is achieved.

Distal pancreatectomy for tumors of the body and tail

Tumours arising in the left side of the pancreas typically grow to a larger size before diagnosis as they do not present with early jaundice. Left-sided tumours are associated with a much higher incidence of metastatic disease, and with low likelihood of curative resection. In addition to routine imaging studies including either multidetector three-dimensional CT or modern MR, there appears to be an important role for staging laparoscopy in patients with left-sided tumours. The resectability rates for adenocarcinoma of the left side of the pancreas in the era before routine staging laparoscopy were approximately 10%. With the use of staging laparoscopy, in addition to modern CT and MR, resectability rates have improved. Distal Pancreatectomy (with splenectomy) is indicated for localised carcinomas of the body and tail of the pancreas. Involvement of the splenic vein or artery is not in itself a contraindication to such resection as the entirety of these vessels can be resected en bloc with the tumor. While these procedures can be carried out by laparoscopic, as well as by open means there are no data at present to indicate superiority of either approach.

PALLIATIVE SURGERY

Most of the symptoms experienced by patients with unresectable pancreatic cancer can be relieved by non-surgical means. Palliative surgery for pancreatic adenocarcinoma is indicated in patients discovered to have unresectable disease at the time of planned resection or in good-risk patients whose tumour-related symptoms are poorly alleviated by non-surgical means. Palliative surgery is appropriate to relieve biliary obstruction, avoid or treat duodenal obstruction, palliate tumour-associated pain, and improve quality of life.

OBSTRUCTIVE JAUNDICE

A number of prospective randomized studies have been undertaken to compare palliative biliary drainage surgery with stenting. Stenting can be performed either endoscopically or by a transhepatic approach. Morbidity and mortality rates were lower when the endoscopic route was used compared with the transhepatic route.83 Endoscopic stenting has a lower procedure related complication rate and mortality than surgical bypass, although there is higher risk of recurrent jaundice. All surgical procedures for palliation of obstructive jaundice include some form of an internal biliary bypass. The four techniques used include
- hepatico-jejunostomy,
- choledochojejunostomy,
- choledochoduodenostomy
- cholecystojejunostomy.

The preferred technique in patients with a median life expectancy of 6 months or more is hepatico- or choledochojejunostomy. Choledochoduodenostomy is generally avoided in patients with pancreatic cancer due to concerns regarding the proximity of the biliary-enteric anastomosis to the tumor, with the possibility of recurrent jaundice. Cholecystojejunostomy has been advocated by some surgeons (because it can be performed quickly and can be done laparoscopically) and does not require dissection of the extrahepatic biliary tree but there is an increase risk of recurrent jaundice.

GASTRIC/DOEDENAL OBSTRUCTION

One-third of patients have some symptoms of nausea, early satiety and/or vomiting at the time of diagnosis. Prospective randomized trial has evaluated the role of prophylactic gastrojejunostomy in patients found at laparotomy to have unresectable pancreatic head cancer. Approximately 19% of patients treated by biliary bypass alone without gastrojejunostomy developed late gastric outlet obstruction and required subsequent gastroenterostomy. No patient in the prophylactic gastrojejunostomy group required repeat intervention. Gastrojejunostomy is usually performed as an isoperistaltic loop procedure, using the jejunum 20 to 30 cm beyond the ligament of Treitz, and anastomosing to the most dependent portion of greater curvature of stomach.

PAIN

The abdominal and back pain associated with an unresected pancreatic adenocarcinoma can be unremitting and a major debilitating symptom for the patient. Some surgeons routinely perform operative coeliac plexus block by injecting alcohol at the time of surgical palliation. However, many patients with unresectable pancreatic cancer can be successfully managed with minimal or no narcotic analgesics and, when more severe pain occurs, good results can be achieved by coeliac plexus block using percutaneous approach.

ADJUVANT THERAPY

Surgical resection alone has a 5-year survival rate of 10-20% for ductal adenocarcinoma of the pancreas. Several studies have been carried out to determine whether adjuvant radiotherapy or chemotherapy might improve the survival rate.

Gastrointestinal Tumor Study Group (GITSG) reported prospective randomised controlled study of adjuvant chemoradiation (5-fluorouracil (5-FU) for six days and 40 Gy of radiation followed by maintenance chemotherapy with 5-FU after pan-

creaticoduodenectomy. It was suggested that the combination of 5-fluorouracil with radiation therapy could increase the 2-year survival rate for patients with tumour-free resection margins from 18% to 43%. The median survival was significantly longer in the "adjuvant treatment" group than in the surgery group (20 months vs 11 months). However, the total number of patients in this trial was only 43.

EORTC study of pancreatic and ampullary cancers found no benefit on survival for patients treated with radiation and 5-FU in a chemo radiation protocol.8

The European Study Group for Pancreatic Cancer (ESPAC) reported a large trial (ESPAC-1) of 546 patients, which compared adjuvant chemoradiotherapy with or without maintenance chemotherapy (5-FU with folinic acid) against no treatment. The group concluded that there was no survival benefit for adjuvant chemoradiotherapy and that a potential benefit existed for adjuvant chemotherapy alone after surgical resection.

At present, adjuvant therapy is not considered standard therapy. Further studies are planned or in progress, which should provide additional data regarding the potential benefits of adjuvant therapies. ESPAC-3 trial is in progress to compare adjuvant 5-FU with folinic acid, gemcitabine with no adjuvant therapy

ADVANCED OR METASTATIC PANCREATIC CANCER

The standard treatment of patients with advanced metastatic or recurrent pancreatic adenocarcinoma with adequate performance status is systemic chemotherapy. The best response rates were historically achieved with 5-FU and mitomycin C. However, since the introduction of gemcitabine the scene has changed. Gemcitabine is a chemotherapeutic drug that exerts its action by inhibiting DNA synthesis. It is a nucleoside analogue with a wide spectrum of anti-tumour activity against a variety of solid tumours including pancreatic cancer. Single-blind RCT compared gemcitabine to treatment with 5-FU as a first line treatment used on patients with a Karnofsky score of 50 or more. In this trial 126 patients randomised to gemcitabine had better one-year survival (18% vs 2%, p=0.0002), better median survival (5.6 vs 4.4 months, p=0.0025) and improved median progression free survival (2.3 vs 0.9 months, p=0.0002). There was also evidence of improvement in disease related symptoms, including a clinical benefit response based on pain control, performance status, and weight gain in 24% of gemcitabine treated patients, as opposed to 5% with 5-FU.

NICE guidelines concluded that gemcitabine may be used as a first line chemotherapy for the treatment for patients with advanced or metastatic adenocarcinoma of the pancreas if they have Karnofsky performance score of 50 or more. Karnofsky is a measure given by a health professional to a person's ability to perform certain ordinary tasks: 100 = normal, no complaints, 70 = unable to carry on normal activity, 50 = requires considerable assistance, 40 = disabled, 30 =hospitalisation recommended. Gemcitabine should not be used for people with pancreatic cancer who are suitable for surgery that may cure their cancer, or those who have a Karnofsky performance score of less than 50.

Gemcitabine is generally well tolerated but may cause rashes and mild gastrointestinal side effects such as nausea. Bone marrow suppression, influenza-like symptoms, proteinuria/haematuria, peripheral oedema, bronchospasm, and in rare cases, Adult Respiratory Distress Syndrome (ARDS), and potentially irreversible renal failure have been reported.

Combinations of gemcitabine with other agents, such as cisplatin, irinotecan,

oxaliplatin, and fluoropyrimidines, have not resulted in improvement in survival or quality of life in studies available so far. Such combinations should not be considered standard at the present time, although this could change as the results of randomized studies become available. There are now numerous phase II and phase III studies of doublet and triplet regimens that include gemcitabine as one of the active agent are under way.

REFERENCES

Abraham SC, Klimstra DS, Wilentz RE, et al. Solid-pseudopapillary tumors of the pancreas almost always harbor mutations in the beta-catenin gene. Am J Pathol 2002; 160: 1361

Abraham SC, Wu TT, Klimstra DS, Finn L, Hruban RH. Distinctive molecular genetic alterations in s-poradic and familial adenomatous polyposis-associated pancreatoblastomas: frequent alterations in the AIIX/B-catenin pathway and chromosome 11p. Am J Pathol 2001;159:1619

Adsay NV, Longnecker DS, Klimstra DS. Pancreatic tumors wlth cystic dilatation of the ducts: intraductal papillary mucinous neoplasms and intraductal oncocytic papillary neoplasms. Semin Diagn Pathol 2000; 17:16.

Alazraki N. Imaging of pancreatic cancer using fluorine-18 fluorodeoxyglucose positron emission tomography. J Gastrointest Surg 2002:6:136

American Cancer Society. Facts and figures. Atlanta, GA: American Cancer Society, 2002.

Andren-Sandberg A, Ihse I. Factors influencing survival after total pancreatectomy in patients with pancreatic cancer. Ann Surg 1983; 198:605.

Bansal P, Sonnenberg A. Pancreatitis is a risk factor for pancreatic cancer.Gastroenterology 1995; 109:247-57.

Birkmeyer JD, Siewers AE, Finlayson EV, et al. Hospital volume and surgical mortality in the United States. N Engl J Med 2002; 346:1128-37.

Bluemke DA, Fishman EK. CT and MR evaluation of pancreatic cancer. Surg Oncol Clin N Am 1998; 7:103.

Bret PM, Reinhold C. Magnetic resonance cholangiopancreatography. Endoscopy 1997; 29:472-86.

Burris HA, Moore MJ, Andersen J, et al. Improvements in survival and clinical benefit with gemcitabine as first-line therapy for patients with advanced pancreas cancer: A randomised trial. J Clin Oncol 1997; 15:2403-13.

Cameron JL, Pitt HA, Yeo CJ, et al. One hundred and forty-five consecutive pancreaticoduodenectomies without mortality. Ann Surg 1993; 217:430-8.

Chang KJ, Nguyen P, Erickson RA, et al. The clinical utility of endoscopic ultrasound guided fine-needle aspiration in the diagnosis and staging of pancreatic carcinoma. Gastrointest Endosc 1997; 45:387-93.

Chong M, Freeny PC, Schmiedl UP. Pancreatic arterial anatomy. Depiction with dual phase helical CT. Radiology 1998; 208:537-42.

Clarke DL, Thomson SR, Madiba TE, Sanyika C. Preoperative imaging of pancreatic cancer: a management-oriented approach. J Am Coll Surg 2003;196:119-29

Conlon KC, Dougherty E, Klimstra DS, et al. The value of minimal access surgery in the staging of patients with potentially resectable peripancreatic malignancy. Ann Surg 1996; 223:134.

Edis AJ, Kierman PD, Taylor WF. Attempted curative resection of ductal carcinoma of the pancreas. Mayo Clin Proc 1980; 55:531.

Exocrine pancreas. In: AJCC cancer staging manual, 6th Ed. New York: Springer, 2002:157.

Fernandez-del Castillo C, Warshaw AL. Laparoscopic staging and peritoneal cytology. Surg Oncol Clin N Am 1998; 7:135.

Ferrucci JT, Wittenberg J, Margolics MN, et al. Malignant seeding of the tract after thin needle aspiration biopsy. Radiology 1979; 130:345-6.

Fink AS, DeSouza LR, Mayer EA, et al. Long term evaluation of pylorus preservation during pancreaticoduodenectomy. World J Surg 1988; 12:663-70.

Freeny PC, Traverso LW, Ryan JA. Diagnosis and staging of pancreatic adenocarcinoma with dynamic computer tomography. Am J Surg 1993; 165:600-6.

Fuhrman GM, Charnsangavej C, Abbruzzese JL, et al. Thin section contrast enhanced computed tomography accurately predicts the resectability of malignant pancreatic neoplasms. Am J Surg 1994; 167:104-111.

Gambil EF. Pancreatitis associated with pancreatic carcinoma: study of 26 cases. Mayo Clin Proc 1971; 46:174.

Gastrointestinal Tumour Study Group. Further evidence of effective adjuvant combined radiation and chemotherapy following curative resection of pancreatic cancer. Cancer 1987; 59:2006-10.

Giardiello FM, Brensinger JD, Tersmette AC, et al. Very high risk of cancer in familial Peutz-Jeghers syndrome. Gastroenterology 2000; 119:1447-53.

Gordis L, Gold EB. Epidemiology of pancreatic cancer. World J Surg 1984; 8:808-21.

Grace PA, Pitt HA, Longmire WP. Pancreatoduodenectomy with pylorus preservation for adenocarcinoma of the head of the pancreas. Br J Surg 1986; 73:647.

Hahn SA, Greenhalf W, Ellis I, et al. BRCA2 germ line mutations in familial pancreatic carcinoma. J Natl Cancer Inst 2003; 95:214-21.

Haycox A, Lombard M, Neoptolemos JP, et al. Current treatment and optimal patient management in pancreatic cancer. Aliment Pharmacol Ther 1998;12:49-964.

Herter FP, Cooperman AM, Ahlborn TN, et al. Surgical experience with pancreatic and peri-ampullary cancer. Ann Surg 1982; 195:274.

Hosten N, Lemke AJ, Wiedenmann B, Bohmig M, Rosewicz S. Combined imaging techniques for pancreatic cancer. Lancet 2000; 356:909-10.

Howard TJ, Chin AC, Streib EW, et al. Value of helical computed tomography, angiography and endoscopic ultrasound in determining resectability of periampullary carcinoma. Am J Surg 1997;174:237-41

Howes N, Wong T, Greenhalf W, et al. Pancreatic cancer risk in hereditary pancreatitis in Europe. Digestion 2000; 61:300.

Hruban RH, Petersen GM, Ha PK, Kern SE. Genetics of pancreatic cancer: from genes to families. Surg Oncol Clin N Am 1998; 7:1.

Iacobuzio-DonahueCA,Maitra A,Olsen M.et al: Exploration of global gene expression patterns in pancreatic adenocarcinoma using cDNA microarrays. Am J Pathol 162:1151,2003.

Karlson BM, Ekbom A, Lindgren PG, et al. Abdumi-

nal US for diagnosis of pancreatic tumor: prospective cohort analysis. Radiology 1999; 213:107-11.

Kausch W. Das carcinoma der papilla duodeni und seine radikale entfeinung. Beitr Z Clin Chir. 1912; 78:439-486.

Klimstra DS, Heffess CS, Oertel JE, Rosai J. Acinar cell carcinoma of the pancreas. A clinicopathologic study of 28 cases. Am J Surg Pathol 1992; 16:815.

Klimstra DS, Wenig BM, Adair CF, Heffess CS. Pancreatoblastoma. A clinicopathologic study and review of the literature. Am J Surg Pathol 1995; 19:1371.

Klinkenbijl JH, Jeekel J, Sahmoud T, et al. Adjuvant radiotherapy and 5- fluorouracil after curative resection of cancer of the pancreas and periampullary region: phase III trial of the EORTC gastrointestinal tract cancer cooperative group. Ann Surg 1999; 230:776-82.

Lees WR. Imaging diagnosis of pancreatic cancer. Curr Pract Surg 1994; 6:143-6.

Legmann P, Vignaux O, Dousset B, et al. Pancreatic tumors: Comparison of dual phase helical CT and endoscopic sonography. AJR Am J Roentgenol 1998; 170:1315-22.

Lillemoe KD, Cameron JL, Hardacre JM, et al. Is prophylactic gastrojejunostomy indicated for unresectable periampullary cancer? A prospective randomized trial. Ann Surg 1999; 230:322.

Lillemoe KD, Cameron JL, Kaufman HS, et al. Chemical splanchnicectomy in patients with unresectable pancreatic cancer: a prospective randomized trial. Ann Surg 1993; 217:447.

Lowenfels AB, Maisonneuve P, DiMagno EP, et al. Hereditary pancreatitis and the risk of pancreatic cancer. J Natl Cancer Inst 1997; 89:442-6.

Lowenfels AB, Maisonneuve P. Environmental factors and risk of pancreatic cancer. Pancreatology 2003; 3:1.

Lowenfels AB, Maisonneuve P, Cavallini G, et al. Pancreatitis and the risk of pancreatic cancer. N Engl J Med 1993; 328:1433-7.

McCarthy MJ, Evans J, Sagar G, et al. Prediction of resectability of npancreatic malignancy by computed tomography. Br J Surg 1998; 85:320-5.

McLeod RS, Taylor BR, O'Conner BI, et al. Quality of life, nutritional status and gastrointestinal hormonal profile following the Whipple procedure. Am J Surg 1995; 169:179-85.

Mertz HR, Sechopoulos P, Delbeke D, et al. EUS, PET and CT scanning for evaluation of pancreatic adenocarcinoma. Gastrointest Endosc 2000; 52:367-71.

Mertz HR, Sechopoulos P, Delbeke D, Leach SD. EUS, PET, and CT scanning for evaluation of pancreatic adenocarcinoma. Gastrointest Endosc 2000; 52:367-71.

Michaud DS, Giovannucci E, Willett WC, et al. Physical activity, obesity, height, and the risk of pancreatic cancer. JAMA 2001; 286:921.

Midwinter MJ, Beveridge CJ, Wilsdon JB, et al. Correlation between spiral computed tomography, endoscopic ultrasonography and findings at operation in pancreatic and ampullary tumours. Br J Surg 1999;86:189-93.

Mulder I, van Genugten MLL, Hoogenveen R, de Hollander AE, Bueno-de-Mesquita HB. The impact of smoking on future pancreatic cancer: a computer simulation. Ann Oncol 1999; 10:S74.

Neoptolemos JP, Stocken DD, Dunn JA, et al. Influence of resection marginsn on survival for patients with pancreatic cancer treated by adjuvant chemoradiation and/or chemotherapy within the ESPAC-1 randomized controlled trial. Ann Surg 2001; 234:758-68.

Nguyen TC, Sohn TA, Cameron JL, et al. Standard versus radical pancreaticoduodenectomy for periampullary adenocarcinoma: a prospective randomized trial evaluating quality of life in pancreaticoduodenectomy survivors. J Gastrointest Surg 2003; 7:1.

NICE (National Institute for Clinical Excellence). Guidance on the use of gemcitabine for pancreatic cancer May 2001. http://www.nice.org.uk

Ojajarvi I, Partanen T, Ahlbom A, et al. Occupational exposures and pancreatic cancer: a meta-analysis. Occup Environ Med 2000; 57:316.

Ozkan H, Kaya M, Cengiz A. Comparison of tumor marker CA 242 withCA 19-9 and carcinoembryonic antigen (CEA) in pancreatic cancer. Hepatogastroenterology 2003; 50:1669-74.

Rashleigh-Bilcher HJC, Russell RCG, Lees WR. Cutaneous seeding of pancreatic carcinoma by fine needle aspiration biopsy. Br J Radiol 1986; 59:182-3.

Reinhold C. Magnetic resonance imaging of the pancreas in 2001. J Gastrointest Surg 2002;6:133.

Reuther G, Kiefer B, Tuchmann A, et al. Imaging studies of pancreaticobiliary duct diseases with single shot MR cholangiopancreatography. AJR Am J Roentgenol 1997; 168:453-59.

Rickes S, Unkrodt K, Neye H, Ocran KW, Wermke W. Differentiation of pancreatic tumours by conventional ultrasound, unenhanced and echo-enhanced power Doppler sonography. Scand J Gastroenterol 2002; 37:1313-20.

Rosch T, Lightdale CJ, Botet JF, et al. Endosonographic localization of pancreatic endocrine tumours. N Engl J Med 1992; 326:1721-6.

Safi F, Schlosser W, Falkenreck S,et al: Ca 19-9 Serum course and prognosis of pancreatic cancer. Int J Pancreatol 20:155-162, 1996.

Sarfeh IJ, Rypins EB, Jakwatz JG, et al. A prospective randomised clinical investigation of cholecystoenterostomy and choledochoenterostomy. Am J Surg 1988; 155:411-14.

Sarr MG, Cameron JL. Surgical management of unresectable carcinoma of the pancreas. Surgery 1983;91:123.P.984

Satake K, Nishiwaki H, Yokomatsu H, et al. Surgical curability and prognosis for standard versus extended resections for T1 carcinoma of the pancreas. Surg Gynecol Obstet 1992; 175:259.

Shmulewitz A, Teefey SA, Robinson BS. Factors effecting image quality and diagnostic efficacy in abdominal sonography: a prospective study of 140 patients. J Clin Ultrasound 1993; 21:623-30.

Smith CD, Behrns KE, van Heerden JA, et al. Radical pancreaticoduodenectomy for misdiagnosed pancreatic mass. Br J Surg 1994; 81:585-9.

Sohn TA, Yeo CJ, Cameron JL, et al. Pancreaticoduodenectomy: role of interventional radiologists in managing patients and complications. J Gastrointest Surg 2003; 7:209.

Sohn TA, Yeo CJ, Cameron JL, et al. Resected adenocarcinoma of the pancreas-616 patients: results, outcomes and prognostic indicators. J Gastrointest Surg 2000; 4:567.

Sohn TA, Yeo CJ, Cameron JL, et al. Resected adenocarcinoma of the pancreas- 616 patients: results, outcomes, and prognostic indicators. J Gastrointest Surg 2000; 4:567.

Solcia E, Capella C, Kloppel G. Atlas of tumor pathology: tumors of the pancreas, 3rd ed. Washington, DC: Armed Forces Institute of Pathology, 1997.

Sosa JA, Bowman HM, Gordon TA, et al. Importance of hospital volume in the overall management of pancreatic cancer. Ann Surg 1998; 228:429-38.

Speer AG, Cotton PB, Russell RCG, et al. Randomized trial of endoscopicversus percutaneous stent insertion in malignant obstructive jaundice. Lancet1987; ii: 57-62.

Taylor KJW, Buchin PJ, Viscomi GN, et al. Ultrasonographic scanning of the pancreas prospective study of clinical results. Radiology 1981; 138:211-13.

Tio TL, Sie LH, Tytgat GNJ. Endosonography and cytology in diagnosing and staging pancreatic body and tail carcinoma. Dig Dis Sci 1993; 38:59-64.

Tomiyama T, Ueno N, Tano S, et al. Assessment of arterial invasion in pancreatic cancer using color doppler ultrasonography. Am J Gastroenterol 1996; 91:1410-16.

Trede M, Carter DC. Clinical evaluation and pre-operative assessment. In: Trede M, Carter DC, eds. Surgery of the pancreas. Edinburgh: Churchill Livingstone, 1993:423-31.

Vargas R, Nino-Murcia M, Trueblood W, Jeffrey RB Jr. MD. CT in pancreatic adenocarcinoma: prediction of vascular invasion and respectability using a multiphasic technique with curved planar reformations. AJR Am J Roentgenol 2004;182:419-25

Vitellas KM, Keogan MT, Spritzer CE, et al. MR cholangiopancreatography of bile and pancreatic duct abnormalities with emphasis on single-shot fast spin-echo technique. Radiographics 2000; 20:1108-12.

Wade TP, Virgo KS, Johnson FE. Distal pancreatectomy for cancer: results in US Department of Veterans Affairs Hospitals, 1987-1991. Pancreas 1995; 11:341.

Watanapa P, Williamson RCN. Surgical palliation for pancreatic cancer: developments during the past two decades. Br J Surg 1992; 79:8-20.

Whipple A, Parsons WB, Mullins CR. Treatment of carcinoma of the ampulla of Vater. Ann Surg. 1935; 102:763-779.

Wiersema MJ. Endoscopic ultrasonography. J Gastrointest Surg 2002; 6:129.

Wilentz RE, Albores-Saavedra J, Zahurak M, et al. Pathologic examination accurately predicts prognosis in mucinous cystic neoplasms of the pancreas. Am J Surg Pathol 1991; 23:1320.

Williamson RCN, Bliouras N, Cooper MJ, et al. Gastric emptying and enterogastric reflux after conservative and conventional pancreatoduodenectomy. Surgery 1993; 114:82-6.

Yeo CJ, Cameron JL, Lillemoe KD, et al. Pancreaticoduodenectomy with or without distal gastrectomy and extended retroperitoneal lymphadenectomy for periampullary adenocarcinoma: randomized controlled trial evaluating survival, morbidity and mortality. Ann Surg 2002; 236:355.

Yeo CJ, Cameron JL, Sohn TA, et al. Six hundred fifty consecutive pancreaticoduodenectomies in the 1990s; pathology, complications, outcomes. Ann Surg 1997; 226:248.

Yeo CJ. Management of complications following pancreaticoduodenectomy. Surg Clin North Am 1995; 75:913.

Yeo TP, Hruban RH, Leach SD, et al. Pancreatic cancer. Curr Probl Cancer 2002; 26:176

Gallbladder cancer: Diagnosis and treatment

Jonathan Koea

INTRODUCTION

Primary carcinoma of the gallbladder is not infrequently encountered by both general and oncology surgeons. It is generally regarded as an obscure tumour that is difficult to manage. However carcinoma of the gallbladder is the most common malignancy affecting the human biliary tract and the fifth most common cancer of the digestive tract following colorectal carcinoma, gastroesophageal cancer, hepatocellular carcinoma and pancreatic carcinoma. Gallbladder carcinoma was first described in 1777 by Maximilian Stoll and, since this original description, many clinical reports have established the characteristic pattern of late diagnosis, advanced disease and limited treatment options. In 1924 Alfred Blalock stated that an operation should be avoided at all costs if the diagnosis of gallbladder carcinoma was made preoperatively. This nihilistic attitude toward gallbladder cancer has dominated surgical thinking for several decades. However a number of recent advances in the diagnosis of gallbladder cancer and the improved understanding of the role of radical surgical resection in managing the disease as well as an emerging role for chemotherapy and radiotherapy means that a true multimodality approach to its management can now be developed.

This chapter briefly reviews the etiology, epidemiology and clinical features of gallbladder cancer. Recent advances in diagnostic modalities and in multimodality management of potentially curable disease and palliation of advanced tumours will be discussed.

EPIDEMIOLOGY

The incidence of gallbladder cancer varies with geography and race. The incidence in the United States is 2.5 cases/100,000 while it rise to 8 cases/100,000 in parts of South America. However in Boliva the incidence of gallbladder cancer in whites is 1 case/100,000 but affects 7.2/100,000 native Bolivian Indians. Similar ethnic variations are seen in the Pacific and in Asia. Piehler and Crichlow reviewed cases of gallbladder carcinoma published between 1960 and 1978 and found 303 cases in 55,543 autopsies giving an overall incidence of 0.55%. Earlier reviews published between 1949 and 1960 reported an incidence of between

0.43% and 1.41%, while in the 15 years between 1960 and 1975 Piehler and Crichlow documented an incidence of 1.91% with 1091 cases found in 57,170 biliary tract procedures. It is unclear whether this apparent increase represents a true increase in incidence or is a reflection of more accurate diagnosis and reporting. More recently there is evidence that the incidence of gallbladder cancer is decreasing in parallel with a rising rate of cholecystectomy. In the United Kingdom and North America there was a decline in mortality from gallbladder cancer from 1977 to 1987 while in Sweden there was a 33% rise in mortality. These changes are inversely related to the rates of cholecystectomy in these countries.

A high incidence of gallbladder carcinoma is also seen in a number of at risk population groups. The incidence of gallbladder cancer in Native Americans is six times that of the non Native American population and, particularly in the Southwest of America, carcinoma of the gallbladder has been found in 4.5 to 6% of all patients undergoing biliary tract procedures. A similar incidence has also been recorded in Americans of Mexican origin. The incidence of gallbladder carcinoma is also increased in the New Zealand Maori population as well as in the native populations of Bolivia and Peru. However the tumour is rare amongst Polynesians and Melanesians.

Carcinoma of the gallbladder is predominantly a disease of elderly females. Of 2998 patients in 51 series reviewed by Piehler and Crichlow 76% were female with a female to male ratio of 3.2:1. When stratified by age at diagnosis, the incidence of gallbladder cancer in patients at New York Hospital was 0.3% in those less than 50 years of age, and 3.8% in patients greater than 50 years of age. This incidence increased to 8.8% in those over 65 years.

ETIOLOGY

Genetic factors

Gallbladder cancer can occur in family clusters and various oncogenes have been implicated in this process. Kamel found that mutations in p53 and c-erbB-2 play a major role in the neoplastic transformation of gallbladder epithelial cells. The p53 oncogene is also expressed in epithelial dysplasia suggesting that this is an early event in the development of carcinoma. More recently, microarray studies have demonstrated an increased number of candidate genes involved in gallbladder carcinogenesis.

Congenital abnormalities

Cystic dilatation of the biliary tree is known to predispose to extrahepatic cholangiocarcinoma. The pathogenesis of choledochal cysts is poorly understood but is associated with an anomalous high junction of the pancreatic and common bileducts. Anomalous pancreatic/biliary duct union without the presence of choledochal cyst has also been reported in association with gallbladder carcinoma. It has been suggested that longstanding pancreaticobiliary reflux causes inflammation in the extrahepatic bile ducts and gallbladder and induces epithelial metaplasia.

Sex hormones

Both the incidence and prevalence of gallbladder cancer is higher in females than in males. This suggests that female sex hormones may play a role in the development of this condition. The estrogen receptor (ER) is present in gallbladder cancers and poorly differentiated tumours have higher levels of ER positivity than well differentiated tumours. However there is no evidence that exogenous estrogens are associated with an increased risk of gallbladder cancer, although a history of gallstones is a strong risk factor.

Cholelithiasis

Carcinoma of the gallbladder and c-holelithiasis are frequently associated. In 2352 patients with gallbladder cancer reported between 1960 and 1978, gallstones were present in 74%. Other clinical reviews reported similar findings. This association is strengthened by the finding of a greater incidence of gallstones in patients with carcinoma than in the general population at all age levels, a similar frequency of gallstones in both males and females with carcinoma despite a higher frequency of gallstones in females in the general population, and the long history of abdominal symptoms attributed to gallstones in many patients with gallbladder cancer. Warren and Balch also demonstrated that only 16% of metastatic carcinomas of the gallbladder are associated with cholelithiasis, making the formation of gallstones secondary to mucosal irregularity or stasis unlikely. The relative risk of carcinoma is also increased when symptoms and signs of c-holecystitis have previously occurred indicating that chronic inflammation in association with cholelithiasis is an important element in carcinogenesis. A higher incidence of gallbladder carcinoma has also been found in patients with Mirizzi syndrome emphasizing the close association of cholelithiasis, and chronic cholecystitis in the development of gallbladder carcinoma.

Diehl has also shown a strong relationship between gallstone size and gallbladder carcinoma. For stones of 2.0 to 2.9 cm in diameter, the odds ratio (versus stone size of <1 cm) was 2.4, while for stones of 3 cm or larger the ratio was 10.1. Lowenfels et al have also reported similar results and estimated that 30% of all carcinomas are associated with large gallstones (>3 cm diameter). However the relationship of gallstone size with the risk of developing carcinoma has not been a universal finding.

ABO blood groups

The increased incidence of cancers of the stomach, colon, pancreas, bladder and female reproductive tract in patients with group A blood has been recognized for several decades. Pandey et al determined the distribution of ABO and Rh blood groups in 69 patients with gallbladder cancer and 152 patients with cholelithiasis and found an increased frequency of both gallstones and gallbladder cancer in patients with group A blood. The mechanism and reasons for this association are unclear.

Diffuse calcification of the gallbladder (porcelain gallbladder)

Diffuse calcification of the gallbladder is found in less than 0.1% of cholecystectomies and over 95% are associated with gallstones. Porcelain gallbladder is five times more frequent in females than males, and between 10% and 25% are associated with gallbladder carcinoma.

Typhoid carrier state

The chronic typhoid carrier state has been found to be associated with an increased risk of gallbladder and bile duct cancers. It has been suggested that a combination of bile stasis and alteration in bile salts by organisms surviving in the gallbladder may be responsible.

Occupation

Specific substances within industry have been shown to be associated with the development of carcinoma of the liver, bile ducts and gallbladder. Most frequently implicated is 3,3 dichlorobenzidine and chemicals used in the rubber industry.

Chronic inflammatory bowel disease

Inflammatory bowel disease is associated with an increased risk of carcinoma within the biliary tree and up to 13% of these tumours will originate in the gallbladder. The risk is highest in those patients with a long history of colitis, particularly those with a pancolitis. The causation of these carcinomas is not understood but they frequently occur without pre-existing hepatobiliary disease including cholelithiasis and, in general, these patients present 10 to 15 years before the peak incidence in the general population.

Previous biliary surgery

In two uncontrolled studies, patients who have undergone previous gallbladder surgery, particularly cholecystostomy, appear to have a higher incidence of gallbladder carcinoma. This finding must be viewed with caution as tumors were found between 1.3 and 50 years following the procedure suggesting that carcinomas were misdiagnosed at the time of the original procedure or developed later for reasons unrelated to the original procedure.

Benign neoplasms

Benign tumours of the gallbladder have been found in between 0.15 to 8.5% of cholecystectomy specimens. Inflammatory lesions and cholesterol polyps are not associated with any risk of malignant degeneration. Similarly, adenomatous and adenomyomatous hyperplasia do not appear to carry any risk of later malignant change. Carcinoma has been reported in the presence of adenomyomatous hyperplasia but this association is probably coincidental. However reports from Japan and France describe several patients in whom gallbladder carcinoma developed in areas of adenomyomatosis. Currently the pre-malignant potential of this lesion is unsettled.

Papillary and non-papillary adenomas have been shown to be associated with malignant change and to be precursor lesions for gallbladder carcinomas. In a review of the benign tumours of the gallbladder from the Armed Forces Institute of Pathology, 3 of 29 non-papillary adenomas were found to contain carcinoma *in situ* while 22 papillary adenomas had no evidence of carcinoma. Further evidence for the adenoma-carcinoma sequence comes from the study of Kozuka *et al* who reviewed the histology of 1605 gallbladders and found 11 benign adenomas, 7 adenomas with malignant change and 79 invasive carcinomas. The transformation from benign adenoma to invasive carcinoma can be traced histologically and there was a significant correlation between the presence of malignancy and adenoma size. All adenomas less than 12 mm in diameter were benign, while all adenomas showing dysplasia or in situ carcinoma were greater than 12 mm in diameter. Most invasive carcinomas were over 30 mm in diameter.

PATHOLOGY

Ninety-eight percent of malignant tumours of the gallbladder are carcinomas and they are generally classified according to their histological differentiation into adenocarcinoma, squamous cell carcinoma, adenosquamous carcinoma and oat cell carcinoma. The clinical behaviour and principles of management of these different tumours is similar although papillary carcinomas may have a more favourable prognosis. Macroscopically carcinomas produce diffuse thickening of the gallbladder with infiltration of surrounding structures. Papillary projections into the gallbladder lumen can occur.

The mode of spread of gallbladder cancer has been studied by Fahim *et al.* Gallbladder carcinoma spreads primarily by local invasion of hepatic segments IV and V and other adjacent structures, usually duodenum, colon and abdominal wall. The common hepatic duct can be involved by direct distension and gallbladder carcinoma is an important differential in patients presenting with a hilar stricture (Figure 1). Hematogenous spread can occur by invasion of the veins draining the gallbladder into the liver, and also along the cystic veins into segment IV. Lymphatic spread follows lymphatics to the cystic and portal lymph nodes with more distant drainage to retropancreatic and celiac basins. Hematogenous spread and transperitoneal spread usually occurs when the tumour is locally advanced. In the series of Piehler and Crichlow which included 984 patients with gallbladder carcinomas, 679 (69%) demonstrated hepatic invasion and 443 (45%) had regional lymph node metastases at presentation.

Other histological tumours can rarely affect the gallbladder. These include primary carcinoid tumor, adenoendocrine carcinoma, primary melanoma, lymphoma, rhabdomyosarcoma and spindle cell tumours.

CLINICAL FEATURES

The early stages of gallbladder carcinoma are often clinically silent and therefore prevent the early detection of this tumor at an easily resectable stage. Clinical signs commonly mimic benign gallbladder disease and, because of its rarity, often the diagnosis of carcinoma is not made until following simple cholecystectomy.

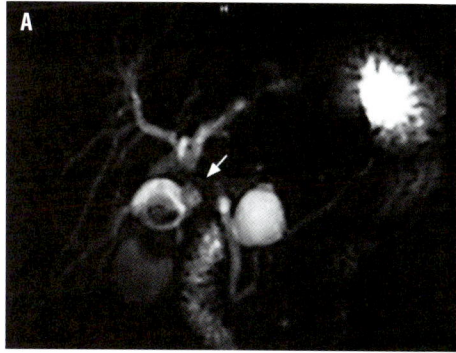

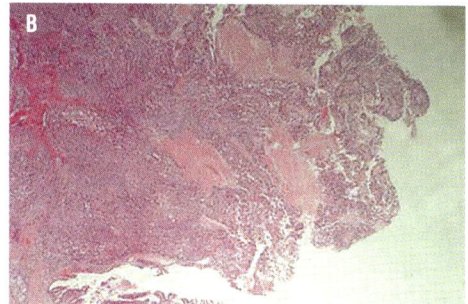

FIGURE 1: **(A)**. MR cholangiogram demonstrating obstruction of the common hepatic duct with a small impacted calculus (arrow). **(B)**. Final pathology showing a well differentiated carcinoma of the gallbladder arising in mucosa adjacent to the obstructing calculus.

Piehler and Crichlow reviewed the common presentation characteristics in over 2000 patients with gallbladder carcinoma reported in the literature. These investigators found that 16% of patients present with acute cholecystitis (right upper quadrant pain, nausea, vomiting and localized tenderness on examination) caused by cystic duct obstruction with tumour or calculus. Thorbjarnarson found that 1% of all cholecystectomy specimens for acute cholecystitis will contain an unsuspected carcinoma. At least 40% of patients with gallbladder cancer present with histories consistent with chronic cholecystitis and patients with longer histories were more likely to have carcinomas found in the resected gallbladder.

Thirty percent of patients presented with symptoms suggesting malignant biliary disease. These symptoms included jaundice, malaise, weight loss, generalised weakness, and persistent upper abdominal and back pain. Fourteen percent of patients with gallbladder cancer presented with symptoms of metastatic disease or advanced unresectable disease. This included symptomatic invasion and fistularisation of the tumour into adjacent colon or duodenum. Physical findings in gallbladder carcinoma are often non-specific and are difficult to differentiate from benign biliary disease. A right upper quadrant mass was present in 42% of patients and right upper quadrant tenderness was found in 38% of patients in the series of Piehler and Crichlow.

Gallbladder carcinoma is unique in that it will normally present to the surgeon either as an incidental finding following laparoscopic or open cholecystectomy for assumed benign disease, or as a suspected or confirmed gallbladder carcinoma. Approximately 1% of patients undergoing cholecystectomy will be found to have an unsuspected carcinoma in the surgical specimen. This incidental group accounts for one third of cases surgically explored with curative intent for gallbladder cancer. Patients presenting with suspected gallbladder cancers *de novo* form two thirds of the cases surgically explored for cure. Previous authors have maintained that the treatment of gallbladder carcinoma is dictated by the mode of presentation, with patients who are re-explored following cholecystectomy often having a more aggressive disease and one which is less able to be managed surgically. However more recent evidence suggests that this is not the case and patients in whom carcinoma of the gallbladder is diagnosed following laparoscopic cholecystectomy should be managed in a manner similar to those presenting with *de novo* disease.

INVESTIGATIONS

Laboratory and simple radiological investigations are usually not useful in establishing either the diagnosis or stage of carcinoma of the gallbladder. Many patients present with a mild anemia, a mild leucocytosis and abnormal liver function tests usually with an obstructive picture. Nearly two thirds of patients presenting with gallbladder carcinoma have an isolated elevation of serum alkaline phosphatase due to early invasion of segments IV and V, unilateral hepatic duct occlusion or liver metastases. Vaittinen has emphasized that an isolated rise in serum alkaline phosphatase is an important finding that warrants further investigation in all patients.

TUMOUR MARKERS

There is evidence that both carcinoembryonic antigen (CEA) and CA19-9 may have a role in the diagnosis of and screening for carcinoma of the gallbladder. Strom et al measured plasma CEA and CA19-9 concentrations in 20 patients with invasive carcinoma and compared these results to CEA and CA19-9 levels in patients with both high grade and low grade dysplasia of the gallbladder mucosa, 12 patients with mucosal hyperplasia and 10 patients with acute or chronic cholecystitis. These investigators found that levels of CEA and CA19-9 were increased in patients with invasive cancer but not in those with dysplasia or benign hyperplasia. Subsequent investigations have confirmed that CA19-9 and CEA are elevated in many patients with invasive carcinoma of the gallbladder, although the exact role of these markers has yet to be clarified. Stefanovic et al have demonstrated that CA19-9 is elevated in carcinoma *in situ* as well as invasive tumor suggesting a role for this marker in screening in a defined high risk population. De Arctxabala et al measured CEA and CA19-9 levels in 54 patients with gallbladder cancer both before and after surgical resection and found that CEA and CA19-9 had similar sensitivities (approximately 70%), but that CA19-9 was more specific than CEA (90% versus 71% respectively) at detecting both primary and recurrent disease. Ritts et al have also measured marker levels in icteric and non-icteric patients with gallbladder and biliary cancer. In non-icteric patients, in whom gallbladder carcinoma may be more difficult to diagnose, CA19-9 had a sensitivity of 55% but a specificity of >99% leading these investigators to suggest that CA19-9 determination is a "useful adjunct to imaging in non-jaundiced patients". Consequently measurement of CEA and CA19-9 levels in patients with suspected gallbladder cancer is useful both in obtaining a diagnosis and in detecting recurrence after resection. However this cannot be undertaken in isolation from appropriate radiological and clinical investigations.

RADIOLOGICAL INVESTIGATIONS

Radiological diagnosis of gallbladder carcinoma is difficult. Plain radiology may show evidence of a tumour mass, gallbladder calcification, or gas within the biliary tree if biliary-enteric fistula has developed. Similarly oral cholecystography will fail to opacify the gallbladder in over 90% of cases due to cystic duct obstruction. Percutaneous cholangiography now has a limited place in the diagnosis of hepatobiliary cancers. However it can be undertaken in the jaundiced patient and Collier et al have emphasised that the pruning or distortion of segment V ducts is highly suggestive of gallbladder carcinoma. Endoscopic retrograde cholangiopancreatography is a useful investigation in the nonjaundiced patient in whom malignancy is suspected. The most common finding is obstruction or distortion of the common hepatic duct with non-filling of the gallbladder (Figure 2) and ERCP will detect 60 to 80% of gallbladder carcinomas using these criteria.

The first reported preoperative diagno-

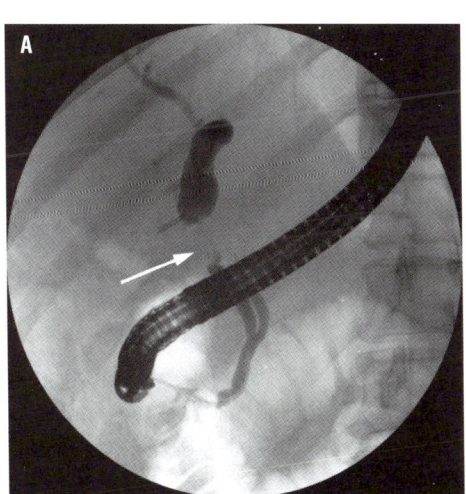
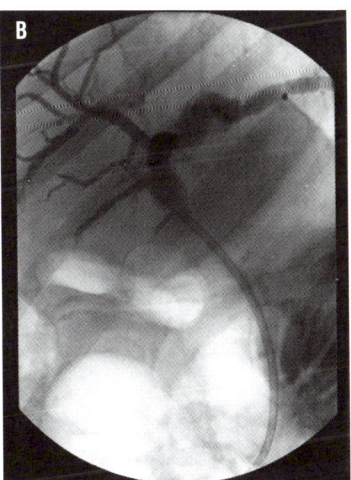

FIGURE 2: (A). Endoscopic retrograde cholangiogram demonstrating a malignant stricture in the common bile duct (arrow). Twelve months previously the patient had undergone a laparoscopic cholecystectomy for a T_2 carcinoma of the gallbladder. No sudsequent reexcision had been undertaken. **(B).** An endoscopic stent was placed traversing the stricture.

sis of gallbladder carcinoma using transabdominal ultrasound was by Olken et al. Transabdominal ultrasound has become the primary investigation for patients with suspected biliary disease and it remains an important investigation in patients with suspected gallbladder carcinoma. The ultrasonographic features of gallbladder cancer are irregular thickening of the gallbladder wall, an intraluminal mass and evidence of direct invasion of the hepatic parenchyma with a poorly defined boundary between gallbladder and liver bed. In addition the presence of cholelithiasis, hepatic metastases, retroperitoneal lymphadenopathy and biliary dilatation at the hilus also suggest the diagnosis. Early series defining the role of ultrasound in detecting gallbladder cancers showed that this modality accurately diagnosed 50% of tumours preoperatively. Contemporary series suggest that careful ultrasound examination of the gallbladder will diagnose nearly 70% of all carcinomas on the basis of an intraluminal mass, gallbladder wall thickening, or hepatic invasion although many of these cancers are locally advanced T_3 or T_4 tumours.

In an attempt to better define the ability of ultrasound to detect early (T_1 and T_2) tumours Onoyama et al retrospectively analysed 53 cases of early gallbladder cancer. Preoperative diagnosis with ultrasound was suspected in only 34% of early cancers and all of the visualised tumours were polypoid lesions. No infiltrating lesions were defined. Thus ultrasound should be performed in all cases when carcinoma is suspected. A high rate of accuracy is possible for advanced lesions but the more subtle changes of early tumors, particularly the infiltrating type are less easily defined.

Computed tomography (CT) also accurately demonstrates gall bladder cancers. Itai et al reported 27 patients with gallbladder carcinoma in whom CT demonstrated a gallbladder mass in 70%, abnormal thickening of the gallbladder wall in 22%, 15% had intraluminal masses and 78% had a low density area of liver adjacent to the gallbladder suggesting invasion. Overall CT scan correctly diagnosed 20 of 27 gallbladder cancers. However a false positive diagnosis was made in 5 patients with chronic inflammatory disease of the gallbladder emphasising the difficulty defining early tumours radiologically. In a more detailed study of 80 gallbladder cancers Oikarinen et al. found that CT was able to define the primary tumour within the gallbladder in 59% of cases. However CT scan defined direct hepatic invasion and intrahepatic metastases in 67% and 75% of cases respectively suggesting that this modality is most useful in advanced tumours.

Magnetic resonance cholangiopancreatography (MRCP) has almost replaced endoscopic or percutaneous cholangiography in the investigation of biliary tract disease. A number of investigations have demonstrated its accuracy in the investigation of perihilar biliary obstruction and differentiating benign lesions of the gallbladder from malignant lesions. MRCP is more accurate than ERCP in differentiating obstructing hilar cholangiocarcinomas from primary gallbladder cancers. Axial magnetic resonance scanning also accurately detects hepatic invasion, discontiguous hepatic and lymph node metastases, and is a useful investigation in the preoperative staging of the disease. MR imaging also provides information regarding the presence of either portal venous or hepatic arterial involvement and MR angiography has replaced transfemoral visceral arteriography. Unlike other modalities MRCP does not require biliary intubation which may contribute to bacterbilia and increase postoperative morbidity. Most importantly magnetic resonance imaging provides the opportunity to undertake definitive radiological staging with arteriography, cholangiography, sagittal and axial scans obtainable during a single examination.

Dynamic scans with fluorodeoxyglucose positron emission tomography (FDG-PET) have been used as a tool for differentiating between inflammation and malignant infiltration of the gallbladder. In a small series of 16 patients with thick walled gallbladders, FDG-PET was found to have a sensitivity of 80% and a specificity of 82%. There was one false positive reading in a patient with benign inflammation and one false negative reading in a patient with a mucinous adenocarcinoma. Other investigators have shown that FDG-PET is more effective at detecting nodular tumours of the gallbladder rather than the more diffuse infiltrating subtype. Currently the role of FDG-PET in the assessment of gallbladder carcinoma is restricted to the detection of metastatic disease.

In summary a variety of radiological imaging techniques have been applied to the diagnosis of gallbladder carcinoma. Advanced tumours can be diagnosed with CT and MRI scans. However early lesions remain a diagnostic challenge and will probably continue to be diagnosed following cholecystectomy for suspected benign disease. A high index of suspicion is required and careful interpretation of preoperative radiology by both surgeon and radiologist is necessary in patients who are being considered for cholecystectomy. In a series of patients referred with carcinoma of the gallbladder to the Hammersmith Hospital following simple cholecystectomy, careful review of their preoperative radiology demonstrated unequivocal findings of gallbladder carcinoma in over 50%.

CLINICOPATHOLOGICAL STAGING

Three clinicopathological staging systems for gallbladder cancer are currently in clinical use. These are the modified Nevin system, the Japanese Biliary Surgical Society, and the AJCC/UICC TNM staging system (Table 1). All three staging systems consider the extent of invasion of the gallbladder wall, the adjacent liver, the presence of lymph node metastases and distant metastases. The major difference between both the TNM, modified Nevin stage and the Japanese system is the importance of lymph node metastases. In both the TNM and modified Nevin systems patients with lymph node metastases in N_1 or N_2 basins are staged as stage III or IV reflecting the poor survival of node positive patients in Western series. In contrast patients with metastases in the cystic node or portal nodes (N_1) are classified as stage II in the Japanese classification, reflecting the better survival reported in Japanese series for patients with nodal metastases. The reasons for this relatively improved outcome in Japanese patients is unclear. All three systems are based on pathological analysis following surgical resection. The TNM system is the most useful preoperative staging since the depth of primary tumour invasion (T stage) can be determined from a simple cholecystectomy specimen or inferred from radiological imaging and, clinically, therapy for gallbladder cancer is currently dictated by T stage.

MANAGEMENT

Aims of treatment

In their review of over 6000 cases of gallbladder carcinoma reported in the English language literature until 1978 Piehler and Crichlow documented a 16.5% five year survival in resected tumours. This poor survival had been attributed to late diagnosis and stage at presentation. However

TABLE 1

STAGING OF GALLBLADDER CARCINOMA

Stage	TNM	Modified Nevin	Japanese Biliary Surgical Society
I	Mucosal/muscular invasion ($T_1N_0M_0$)	In situ carcinoma	No capsular invasion
II	Transmural invasion ($T_2N_0M_0$)	Mucosal/muscular invasion	Suspected capsular invasion Lymph node metastasis (N_1) Suspected hepatic/bile duct invasion
III	Hepatic invasion <2 cm; Nodal metastasis ($T_3N_1M_0$)	Transmural liver invasion	Marked capsular invasion Lymph node metastasis (N_2/N_3) Marked hepatic/bile duct invasion
IV	(A) Liver invasion >2 cm ($T_4N_0M_0$, $T_xN_1M_0$) (B) Distant metastasis ($T_xN_2M_0$, $T_xN_xM_1$)	Lymph node metastasis	Invasion adjacent viscera Lymph node metastasis (N_4) Liver metastasis Extensive hepatic/bile duct invasion
V		Distant metastasis	

of all patients managed surgically with this disease, only 5% were treated with a surgical procedure other than simple cholecystectomy. Consequently the implication in this data is that the majority of 5 year survivors were patients with early stage disease restricted to the mucosa who were treated with simple cholecyctectomy. The majority of deaths in this series were due to obstructive liver failure from local recurrence and not from distant metastases emphasising the inadequacy of simple cholecystectomy alone to control local disease and the importance of complete resection of all tumour. Since gallbladder cancer spreads to the adjacent liver and regional lymph nodes it has been suggested that rational surgical therapy for this condition should include resection of the gallbladder with *en bloc* removal of the gallbladder bed (segments IV and V) and regional lymphadenectomy of the hepatoduodenal ligament. In patients with tumours that involve the cystic duct, extended right hepatectomy with excision of the extrahepatic bile ducts may be required to obtain tumour clearance. Piehler and Crichlow reported in 1978 that radical surgical approaches had not been used frequently enough to permit statistical analysis, and of the small series published at that time no clear survival benefit was observed. However longterm survivors were documented in patients following radical resections for advanced cancers and this provided sufficient encouragement for a number of centres to undertake an aggressive surgical approach to resection for this disease.

Preoperative assessment

All patients presenting with a diagnosis of gallbladder cancer should be critically reviewed with a view to surgical resection. The patient's radiological investigations should be reviewed in detail with attention focussed on defining the extent of hepatic resection required and any criteria for unresectability (Table 2). In addition note should be made of any atypical features to suggest an alternative diagnosis. Consent should be taken by the operating surgeon following discussion of the planned procedure, possible benefits and alternatives. Patients should be carefully assessed preoperatively from both a cardiological and pulmonary perspective and cardiopulmonary function should be optimised.

Virtually all patients presenting with gallbladder carcinoma and jaundice have advanced disease with infiltration of the hilar plate and segment IV or nodal metastases causing ductal obstruction. The presence of jaundice can be considered a relative contraindication to surgical exploration and these patients should be considered for palliative biliary drainage and stent placement.

Since up to one third of patients with carcinoma of the gallbladder will have occult peritoneal metastases a staging laparoscopy should be undertaken prior to formal open surgical exploration. Staging laparoscopy permits the assessment of the parietal peritoneum, portal and celiac nodal basins as well as direct and ultrasound guided assessment of the liver for metastases.

Careful preoperative review of any pathology will provide valuable information on the extent of resection required to obtain clear margins. The depth of tumour in any resected specimen is particularly important. Patients with T_1 lesions can be safely observed following simple cholecystectomy provided the cystic duct margin is not positive. For thicker tumours (T_2 or greater) reexcision is indicated. If the tumour is sited distally in the gallbladder and the cystic duct margin is negative then reexcision of the gallbladder bed (segments IV and V) is

TABLE 2	CRITERIA FOR UNRESECTABILITY IN PATIENTS WITH GALLBLADDER CANCER

Patient Factors
  Medically unfit for operation.
  Cirrhosis/portal hypertension
  Jaundice

Local Factors
  Bilateral hepatic duct involvement up to
    secondary biliary radicals contralaterally
  Encasement or occlusion of the main portal vein
  Encasement of the common hepatic artery or
    left hepatic artery

Metastatic Disease
  Histologically proven metastases to N_2 lymph
    nodes (retroduodenal, retropancreatic, celiac,
    paraaortic)
  Liver, lung, peritoneal metastases

indicated. If the tumour lies proximally within the gallbladder and the cystic duct margin is positive then right hepatic lobectomy or extended right hepatic lobectomy, with resection of the extrahepatic bile ducts, is indicated with Roux-en-Y hepaticojejunostomy. All patients who are re-explored should undergo portal lymphadenectomy taking all lymphatic tissue superior to the upper border of the duodenum including tissue along the common hepatic artery. Reports from Japan have described more extensive lymphadenectomy removing paraaortic tissue and retropancreatic lymph nodes. However the results achieved with this approach in Japan have not been obtained in the West.

Wound site management and tumour recurrence

A clinical feature of gallbladder carcinoma is its ability to grow in surgical wounds. This was first described in 1955 following open cholecystectomy and this phenomenon has received renewed attention following the recognition of port site metastases following laparoscopic cholecystectomy. It is unclear whether port site recurrence following laparoscopic cholecystectomy is more common than following open cholecystectomy. A recent survey of wound recurrence following open cholecystectomy for cancer found a 6.5% rate of recurrence. In comparison 3.5% of patients treated with laparoscopic cholecystectomy were found to have port site recurrence in a series of patients treated at Memorial Sloan-Kettering Cancer Center. All patients presenting for further treatment should have either the original surgical wound or port sites excised. However this is probably only a staging procedure as wound site recurrence is generally a marker of diffuse intraabdominal disease and patients with recurrent disease have a median survival of less than 12 months.

RESULTS OF SURGICAL RESECTION

The nature and results of surgical resection are dependant on tumour stage. Patients with T_1 tumors are adequately treated by simple cholecystectomy alone as this provides adequate tumour clearance and 5 year survival rates of over 90% are the norm. Unfortunately tumours of this stage are rare. Simple cholecystectomy was also thought to be adequate treatment for T_2 tumours as these tumors are subserosal but have invaded the muscularis. However the plane of dissection in simple cholecystectomy is usually subserosal between gallbladder and liver bed. Consequently the tumour may be violated and a microscopically positive margin left. In a recent review of 25 patients with T_2 tumours, 11 patients had a positive margin after simple cholecystectomy. Similarly between 33% and 43% of patients with T_2 tumours have lymph node metastases at

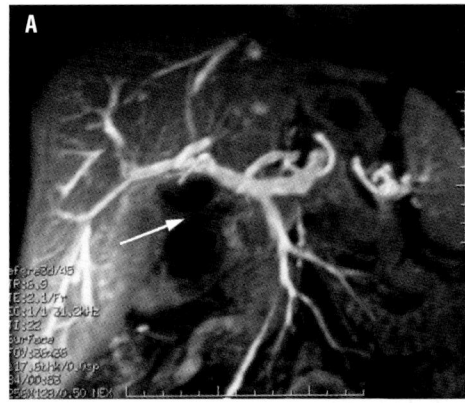

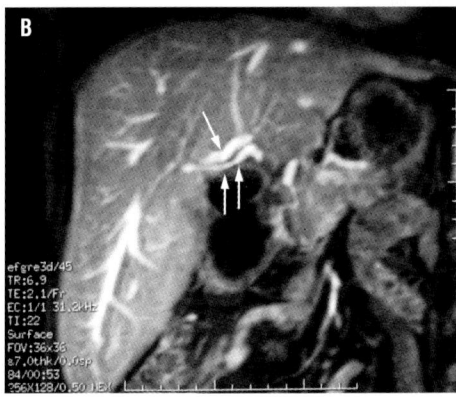

FIGURE 3: **(A).** MR venogram demonstrating approximation but no narrowing of the right portal vein from a large gallbladder cancer (arrow). **(B).** MR angiogram from the same patient showing narrowing of the right hepatic artery from carcinoma of the gallbladder (double arrow). The right portal vein is spared (single arrow).

presentation. Consequently T_2 tumours should also be managed with a radical resection encompassing gallbladder, segments IV and V as well as a portal lymphadenectomy. If the tumor lies proximally and involves the cystic duct then the extrahepatic bile ducts will need to be resected. Radical resections of T_2 tumors are associated with a 5 year survival of between 60 and 80%. In comparison, treating T_2 tumours with simple cholecystectomy alone is associated with a 5 year survival of approximately 20%.

The role of radical resections in advanced carcinoma of the gallbladder remains more controversial. Many series report no long term survivors even following surgical resections. However a number of institutions now report a 25% to 50% 5 year survival in patients with aggressively resected stage III and stage IV disease. Fong et al have recently reported similar 5 year survival rates (21% and 28%) after radical resection in T_3 and T_4 tumours. This included five actual 5 year survivors in the T_4 stage grouping. This emphasises the importance of complete surgical resection and the benefits of an aggressive surgical philosophy in treating patients who were, until recently, felt to be incurable.

RADIATION AND CHEMOTHERAPY

Several studies have investigated the benefit of adjuvant or palliative radiation therapy in advanced carcinoma of the gallbladder. In a review of the role of radiation therapy in carcinoma of the gallbladder Houry et al concluded that gallbladder carcinoma is not radioresistant and that radiotherapy can be administered with minimal morbidity. While some investigators have shown no survival benefit from radiation therapy in gallbladder cancer, Todoroki et al suggested that radiation may improve survival in patients with advanced gallbladder cancer with histologically positive margins, and both Lindell and Czito also noted a tendency to improved survival in patients undergoing surgical resection and adjuvant radiotherapy. However in neither study did the improved survival reach statistical significance and Jarnagin et al have demonstrated that only a minority of patients recur locally with gallbladder cancer with most occurring at distant sites making systemic therapy more attractive than local radiation therapy alone.

However the role of chemotherapy in the management of carcinoma of the gallbladder remains undefined, 5-fluorouracil (5FU) being the best studied agent in the systemic treatment of gallbladder carcinoma. Gebbia et al reported a multicentre trial of systemic 5FU combined with oral hydroxyurea in the treatment of advanced gallbladder cancer and found a 30% partial response rate with minimal toxicity. This agent has also been used as a neoadjuvant agent in conjunction with radiation therapy. This therapy was associated with significant hematological toxicity (leukopenia or thrombocytopenia in 83%). However 83% of patients were able to undergo resection with residual tumor present in 23%. Other investigators have also utilised hepatic arterial infusion of 5FU with some success. It must be emphasised none of these studies involving chemotherapy or radiation therapy were randomised and most consist of relatively small clinical series of selected patients. There is currently no data to support the routine use of chemotherapy or radiation therapy in the pre or postoperative management of gallbladder carcinoma. However these investigators do emphasise the urgent need for an effective adjuvant therapy for this disease and should stimulate the performance of randomized clinical trials.

PALLIATION

Up to two thirds of patients presenting with gallbladder cancer are unsuitable for resection. In these patients the aims of management include supportive care, relief of jaundice and gastric outlet obstruction. In patients who present with advanced disease and significant comorbidities, supportive care is indicated. Jaundice is usually a sign of advanced disease and these patients are rarely resectable. The indications for biliary decompression in these patients are intractable pruitis, cholangitis, and the need to improve hepatic function in the patient contemplating chemotherapy. The therapeutic option to achieve biliary decompression in these patients will be determined by their presentation. In patients who are not subjected to surgical exploration percutaneous biliary drainage with a self-expandable metallic wallstent will provide adequate biliary drainage for several months. In patients who are found to be unresectable at operation, intrahepatic biliary-enteric bypass can be considered. Segment III bypass appears to give the best results with patency rates of greater than 60% at 1 year, and is less prone to occlusion by tumour than are wallstents.

SUMMARY

The surgical management of gallbladder carcinoma is evolving. The safer performance of major hepatic resections has encouraged a more radical approach to its resection and discouraged a nihilistic approach to its management. New developments in preoperative radiological investigations have improved the surgeon's ability to accurately stage and select patients for appropriately radical operations. However an aggressive surgical approach remains the only therapy available that is potentially curative and this must be undertaken with the aim of complete tumour resection. Partial hepatic resection will usually be necessary to achieve this. Unfortunately there are no effective non operative therapies available for patients who are at high risk of recurrent disease following resection (for example those with node positive tumors) or those who have advanced and unresectable tumours. However combined radiation and systemic chemotherapy with 5 fluorouracil shows some

promise and should be formally assessed in a clinical trial.

REFERENCES

Adson MA. Carcinoma of the gallbladder. Surg Clin North Am 1973;53:1203-10.

Albores-Saave I; Henson DE. Tumors of the gallbladder and extrahepatic bile ducts. Armed Forces Institute of Pathology. Atlas of tumor pathology. Fasc 22. 1986;17-123.

Aldridge MC; Bismuth H. Gallbladder cancer: the polyp-cancer sequence. Brit J Surg 1990;77:363-364.

American Cancer Society. Cancer facts and figures 2000; 4-5.

American Joint Committee on Cancer. AJCC Cancer Staging Handbook. 1998:98-99.

Anderson CD; Rice MH; Pinson CW; Chapman WC; Chari RS; Delbeke D. Fluorodeoxyglucose PET imaging in the evaluation of gallbladder carcinoma and cholangiocarcinoma. J Gastrointestinal Surg 2004;8:90-97. 2004.

Anderson JB; Hughes RG; Williamson RCN. Malignant melanoma of the gallbladder. Postgraduate Med J 1983;59:390-391.

Arminski TC. Primary carcinoma of the gallbladder; a collective review with the addition of twenty-five cases from Grace Hospital, Detroit, Michigan. Cancer 1949;2:379-85.

Barbosa E; Rate RG. Primary cholecystic carcinoma; a vanishing entity. J Int Coll Surg 1963;40: 429-35.

Bartlett D; Fong Y; Fortner J; Brennan MF; Blumgart LH. Long-term results after resection for gallbladder cancer. Implications for staging and management. Ann Surg 1996;224:639-646.

Beran G. Acalculous adenomyomatosis of the gallbladder. Gut 1979;11:1029-36. 1979.

Berk RN; Armbuster TG; Saltzstein SL. Carcinoma in the porcelain gallbladder. Radiology 1973;106: 29-31.

Blalock AA. A statistical study of 888 cases of biliary tract disease. Johns Hopkins Hosp Bull 1924; 35:391-409.

Borgerson RJ; DelBeccaro EJ; Callaghan PJ. Polypoid lesions of the gallbladder. Arch Surg 1962;85: 234-9.

Broden G; Bengtsson L. Carcinoma of the gallbladder, its relation to cholelithiasis and the concept of prophylactic cholecystectomy. Acta Chirurgica Scandinavica Supplementum 1980; 500:15-18.

Burdette WJ. Carcinoma of the gallbladder. Ann Surg 1957;145:832-40.

Chatila R; Fiedler PN; Vender RJ. Primary lymphoma of the gallbladder. Am J Gastroenterol 1996;91:2242-2244.

Christensen AH; Ishak KG. Benign tumors and pseudotumors of the gallbladder; report of 180 cases. Arch Pathol 1970;90:423-32. Collier N; Carr D; Hemingway A; Blumgart LH. Preoperative diagnosis and its effect on the treatment of carcinoma of the gallbladder. Surg Gynecol Obstet 1984;159: 465-470.

Collier N; Blumgart LH. Tumors of the gallbladder. Blumgart LH. Surgery of the Liver and Biliary TracT. [Vol 2], 960. 1994. Churchill Livingstone.

Collier N; Carr D; Hemingway A; Blumgart LH. Preoperative diagnosis and its effect on the treatment of carcinoma of the gallbladder. Surg Gynecol Obstet 1984;159:465-470.

Czito BG; Hurwitz HI; Clough RW; Tyler DS; Morse MA; Clary BM; Pappas TN; Fernando NH; Willett CG. Adjuvant external-beam radiotherapy with concurrent chemotherapy after resection of primary gallbladder carcinoma: a 23 year experience. Int J Radiation Oncol, Biology, Physics 2005;62:1030-1034.

de Arctxabala X; Riedeman JP; Roa I; Wenzel C; Inostrosa J; Burgos L; Carlos Araya J; Siegel S; Millaqueo L; Espinoza R. CA19-9 and carcinoembryonic antigen in gallbladder cancer. Revista Medica de Chile 1996;124:11-20. 1996.

de Arctxabala X; Roa IS; Mora JP; Orellana JJ; Riedeman JP; Burgos LA; Silva VP; Cuadra AJ; Wanebo HJ. Laparoscopic cholecystectomy: its effect on the prognosis of patients with gallbladder cancer. World J Surg 2004;28: 544-547.

de Arctxabala X; Roa I; Burgos L; Cartes R; Silva J; Yanez E; Araya JC; Villaseca M; Quijada I; Vittini C. Preoperative chemoradiotherapy in the treatment of gallbladder cancer. American Surgeon 1999;65:241-246.

Diehl AK; Beral V. Cholecystectomy and changing mortality from gallbladder cancer. Lancet 1981;ii: 187-189.

Diehl AK. Epidemiology of gallbladder cancer: a synthesis of recent data. J Natl Cancer Inst 1980; 65:1209-1214.

Diehl AK. Gallstone size and the risk of gallbladder cancer. JAMA 1983;250: 2323-2326.

Dixon E; Vollmer CM Jr; Sahajpal A; Cattral M; Grant D; Doig C; Hemming A; Taylor B; Langer B; Grieg P; Gallinger S. An aggressive surgical approach leads to improved survival in patients with gallbladder cancer: a 12-year study at a North American Center. Ann Surg 2005;241:385-394.

Donohue JH; Nagorney DM; Grant CS; Tsushima K; Ilstrup DM; Adson MA. Carcinoma of the gallbladder. Does radical resection improve outcome. Arch Surg 990;125:237-241.

Fahim RB; McDonald JR; Richards JC; Ferris DO. Carcinoma of the gallbladder; a study of its modes of spread. Ann Surg 1962;156:114-124.

Flanagan DP. Biliary cysts. Ann Surg 1975;82:635-643.

Fong Y; Heffernan N; Blumgart LH. Gallbladder carcinoma discovered during laparoscopic cholecystectomy. Aggressive resection is beneficial. Cancer 1998;83:423-427.

Fong Y; Jarnagin W; Blumgart LH. Gallbladder cancer: comparison of patients presenting initially for definitive operation with those presenting after prior noncurative intervention. Ann Surg 2000; 232:557-569.

Gall FP; Kockerling F; Scheele J; and et al. Radical operations for carcinoma of the gallbladder: present status in Germany. World J Surg 1991; 15:328-336.

Gebbia V; Majello E; Testa A; Pezzella G; Giuseppe S; Giotta F; Riccardi F; Fortunato S; Colucci G; Gebbia N. Treatment of advanced adenocarcinomas of the exocrine pancreas and gallbladder with 5-fluorouracil, high dose levofolinic acid and oral hydroxyurea on a weekly schedule. Results of a multicenter study of the Southern Italy Oncology Group. Cancer 1996;78:1300-1307.

Glattli A; Stain S; Baer HU; Schweizer W; Triller J; Blumgart LH. Unresectable malignant biliary obstruction: treatment by self-expandable biliary endoprosthesis. Hepatobiliary Surgery 1993;6: 175-184.

Glenn F; Hays DM. The scope of radical surgery in the treatment of malignant tumors of the extrahepatic biliary tract. Surg Gynecol Obstet 1954; 99:529.

Hansel DE;, Rahman A; Hildago M; Thuluvath PJ; Lillemoe KD; Shulick R; Ku JL; Park JG; Miyazaki K; Asfaq R; Wistuba II; Varma R; Hawthorne L; Geradts J, Argani P; Maitra A. Identification of novel cellular targets in biliary tract cancers using global gene expression technology. Am J Pathol 2003;163, 217-229.

Hara H; Nomura E; Watanabe I; Sako S; Otani M; Tanigawa N. Advanced gallbladder carcinoma with liver metastasis showing a favourable response after intra-arterial infusion chemotherapy: report of a case. Surgery Today 1999;29: 1102-1105.

Hart J; Modan B; Shani M. Cholelithiasis in the aetiology of gallbladder neoplasms. Lancet1971; i:1151-3.

Hawkins WG; DeMatteo RP; Jarnagin WR; Ben-Porat L; Blumgart LH; Fong Y. Jaundice predicts advanced disease and early mortality in patients with gallbladder cancer. Ann Surg Oncol 2004; 11:310-315.

Hemminki K; Li X. Familial liver and gallbladder cancer: a nationwide epidemiological study from Sweden. Gut 2003;52:592-596.

Heslin M; Brooks AD; Hochwald SN; Harrison LE; Blumgart LH; Brennan MF. A preoperative biliary stent is associated with increased complications after pancreaticoduodenectomy. Arch Surg 1998;133:149-154.

Hochwald SN; Burke EC; Jarnagin WR; Fong Y; Blumgart LH. Preoperative biliary stenting is associated with increased postoperative infectious complications in proximal cholangiocarcinoma. Arch Surg 1999;134:261-266.

Houry S; Haccart V; Huguier M; Schlienger M. Gallbladder cancer: role of radiation therapy. Hepato-Gastroenterology 1999;46:1578-1584.

Itai Y; Araki T; Yoshikawa K; Furui S; Yashiro N; Tasaka A. Computed tomography of gallbladder carcinoma. Radiology 1980;137:713-718.

Jarnagin WR; Browne W; Klimstra DS; Ben-Porat L; Roggin K; Cymes K; Fong Y; DeMatteo RP; D'Angelica M; Koea J; Blumgart LH. Papillary phenotype confers improved survival after resection of hilar cholangiocarcinoma. Ann Surg 2005;241:703-714.

Jarnagin W; Burke EC; Power C; Fong Y; Blumgart LH. Intrahepatic biliary enteric bypass provides effective palliation in selected patients with malignant obstruction at the hepatic duct confluence. Am J Surg 1998;175:453-460.

Jarnagin W; Ruo L; Little SA; Klimstra DS; D'Angelica M; DeMAtteo RP; Wagman R; Blumgart LH; Fong Y. Patterns of initial disease recurrence after resection of gallbladder carcinoma and hilar cholangiocarcinoma: implications for adjuvant therapeutic strategies. Cancer 2003;98:1689-1700. 2003.

Kamel D; Paakko P; Nuorva K; Vahakangas K. p53 and c-erb-2 protein expression in adenocarcinomas and epithelial dysplasia of the gallbladder. J Pathol 1992;170: 67-72.

Katoh T; Nakai T; Hayashi S; Satake T. Noninvasive carcinoma of the gallbladder arising in localized type adenmyomatosis. Am J Gastroenterol 1988;83:670-674.

Kawarada Y; Sanda M; Mizumoto R; Yatani R. Early carcinoma of the gallbladder, noninvasive carcinoma originating in a Rokitansky-Aschoff sinus. Am J Gastroenterol 1986;81:61-66.

Koea J; Findlay M; Ramsdorp R; MacCormack M. Adeno-endocrine cancer of the gallbladder. ANZ J Surg 2004;74:808-809.

Koea JB; Phillips A; Lawes C; Rodgers M; Windsor J; McCall J. Gallbladder cancer, extrahepatic bile duct cancer and ampullary carcinoma in New Zealand: Demographics, pathology and survival. ANZ J Surg 2002;72:857-861.

Kozuda S; Tsubone M; Yasui A; Hachisuka K. Relation of adenoma to carcinoma in the gallbladder. Cancer 1982;50:2226-2234.

Lindell G; Holmin T; Ewers SB; Tranberg KG; Stenram U; Ihse I. Extended operation with or without intraoperative (IORT) and external beam (EBRT) radiotherapy for gallbladder carcinoma. Hepato-Gastroenterology 2003;50: 310-314.

Lowenfels AB; Walker AM; Althaus DP; Townsend G; and Domellof L. Gallstone growth, size and risk of gallbladder cancer; an interracial study. Int J Epidemiol, 1980;1:50-54.

Lundberg O; Kristoffersson A. Wound recurrence from gallbladder cancer after open cholecystectomy. Surgery 2000;127:296-300.

Mahe M; Stampfli C; Romestaing P; Salerno N; Gerer, US cannot reliably depict the full extent of disease and is insensitive in detecting early cases of CaGB (sensitivity 26%).

Computed tomography

CT defines the tumor extent and spread better than US and is the most commonly performed imaging modality for staging. Although CT is very sensitive in detecting advanced cases of CaGB (sensitivity 55-100%), detection rate for early cases is far from satisfactory. The tumor may be seen as a heterogenously enhancing mass replacing the gall bladder, as mural thickening (Figure 2), or as a polypoidal lesion. The mass is generally hypovascular, typically hypodense with areas of necrosis. However, it may show heterogenous enhancement in the arterial phase. Preoperative CT staging has an overall accuracy ranging from 83 to 86%, and is valuable in determining resectability of CaGB.

Magnetic resonance imaging

CaGB is usually hypointense on T1 and hyperintense relative to liver parenchyma

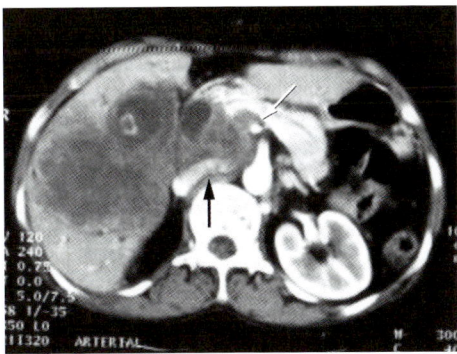

FIGURE 2: Carcinoma gallbladder showing diffuse thickening of gall bladder wall with extensive liver involvement and infiltration into the adjacent duodenum and pancreatic head. There is also encasement of the retroperitoneal vessels (inferior vena cava [black arrow], aorta - right anterolateral aspect, proximal superior mesenteric artery [white arrow]). - Unresectable.

on T2 weighted images (Figure 3, 4). Recent reports suggest that like CT, MRI is a sensitive modality for the detection and preoperative evaluation of CaGB. Kim et al performed gadolinium enhanced MRI along with MR angiography and magnetic resonance cholangiography in patients with CaGB and compared MRI features with surgical findings. They reported a diagnostic accuracy of 77%, 94% and 89% for hepatic invasion, bile duct invasion and hepatic vascular invasion respectively. But the sensitivity of MRI for lymphadenopathy and peritoneal dissemination was less in this study.

Cholangiography

Biliary obstruction is seen in around 30-40% of the cases with CaGB. The correct diagnosis and level of biliary obstruction is crucial in the appropriate management of these patients, because involvement of the bile duct is an important factor governing resectability. Most of these cases are inoperable and need palliation in the form of percutaneous or transhepatic biliary drainage. The global map of the dilated biliary system as seen with cholangiography also helps in planning the biliary drainage procedure.

Endoscopic or percutaneous cholangiography (PTC), alone or in combination, are accurate in diagnosing the extent of biliary tree involvement. These are nevertheless invasive procedures with a high rate of complications ranging from 0.5 to 5% and do not depict isolated portions of the biliary tree. Noninvasive cholangiography techniques using CT or MRI have overcome these drawbacks. The signs of biliary tree involvement on any of these modalities are focal or eccentric narrowing, or abrupt cut off of the bile ducts with proximal dilatation.

MRCP is obtained using heavily T2 weighted sequences like HASTE (Figure 3c, 4c) and RARE, and is reported to be

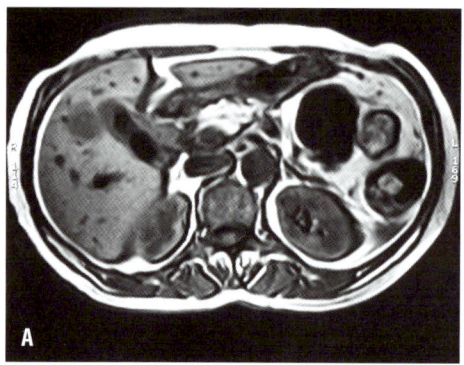

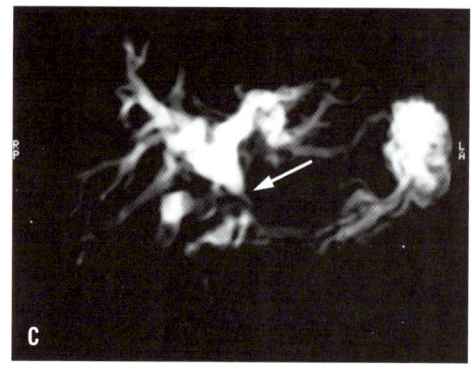

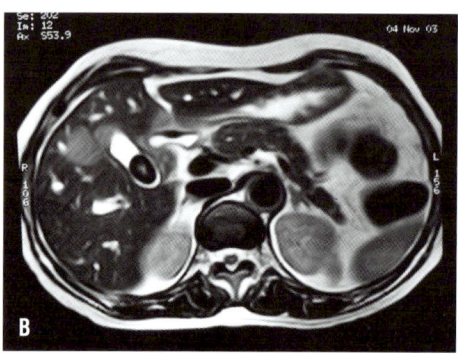

FIGURE 3: Breathhold axial MRI **(A,B)** showing irregular thickening of the gall bladder wall with contiguous invasion of adjacent liver segment 4b. Mass is hypointense on TI weighted **(A)** and hyperintense on T2 weighted images **(B)** relative to the liver parenchyma. Thick-slab coronal MRCP **(C)** showing malignant stricture of the proximal common duct (arrow) and dilatation of intrahepatic biliary radicals.

100% sensitive for bile duct invasion with a diagnostic accuracy of 94%.

CT cholangiography (CTC) used to be performed following oral or intravenous administration of cholangiographic contrast agents. However use of such contrast agents has fallen out of favor because of the high rate of associated contrast reactions and the inability to opacify the biliary tree in patients with impaired liver function. The technique of minimum intensity projection has revived interest in CT cholangiography (CTC). In this method, the hypodense dilated biliary radicals are depicted in the coronal plane without interference from other high-density structures like the enhancing vessels and liver parenchyma (Figure 5). Three Dimensional CTC (3D CTC) using minimum intensity projection (minIP) was found to

be comparable to MRCP and PTC in the evaluation of CaGB patients in a study published from our center by the authors. In this study, 25 consecutive patients with proven CaGB, presenting with clinical and biochemical features of obstructive jaundice, were included. Dual phase helical CT data was obtained in the arterial and venous phases respectively, after intravenous contrast injection was made using a pressure injector. Axial CT data (both arterial and venous phase) was studied for staging and resectability of tumor. 3D CTC using minIP obtained from the venous phase data set, was used to assess the level of biliary obstruction and isolation of hepatic segmental ducts. 3D CTC findings were compared with MRC and percutaneous transhepatic cholangiography (PTC) (gold standard). In all

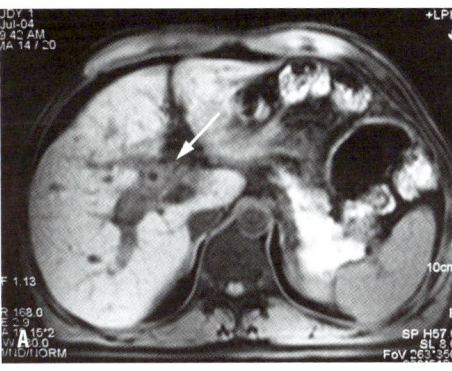

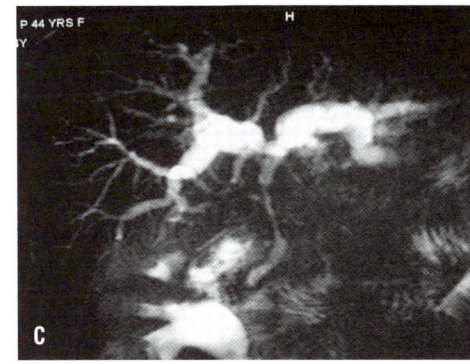

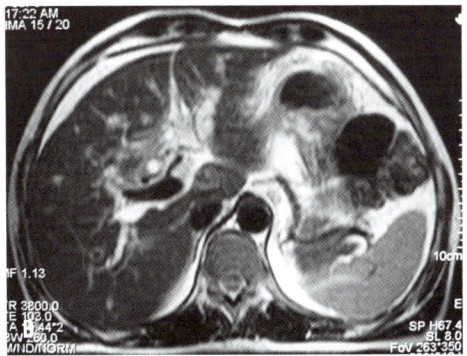

FIGURE 4: Breath hold axial MRI **(A,B)** showing an ill defined mass arising from the neck of the gall bladder (arrow). Mass is hypointense on T1 weighted image **(A)** and hyperintense to liver parenchyma on T2 weighted image **(B)**. Mass is encasing the common hepatic artery and fat plane with the main portal vein is lost. Thick slab coronal MRCP **(C)** showing dilated right and left hepatic ducts with blocked primary confluence. All of the above mentioned features make the tumour unresectable.

patients, 3D CTC demonstrated dilated intrahepatic ducts up to tertiary branch level. 3D CTC correctly diagnosed the level of biliary obstruction and demonstrated isolated segmental ducts in all patients and correlated well in all cases with MRC and PTC findings in this regard. It was concluded that 3D CTC with minIP can correctly determine the level of biliary obstruction in patients with CaGB and may be a strong competitor with MRC, because it gives equivalent information with regard to the level of ductal obstruction even while being a part of an overall comprehensive CT staging study.

Radiological differential diagnosis

Mural thickening is the most non-specific imaging appearance of CaGB and has a wide differential diagnosis. These include inflammatory conditions like cholecystitis, tuberculous involvement of GB, xanthogranulomatous cholecystitis, pancreatitis, and some systemic and noninflammatory conditions like heart failure, cirrhosis, renal failure, hypoalbuminemia and adenomyomatosis. Wall thickening due to CaGB tends to be thicker and more irregular, often with ancillary findings such as biliary tree dilatation, lymphadenopathy or hepatic metastases. On the other hand a layered appearance of the thickened GB wall on US, CT, MRI or endoscopic US favors a benign etiology.

Xanthogranulomatous cholecystitis is an inflammatory condition of the gall bladder that may mimic chronic cholecystitis or CaGB. Imaging features include

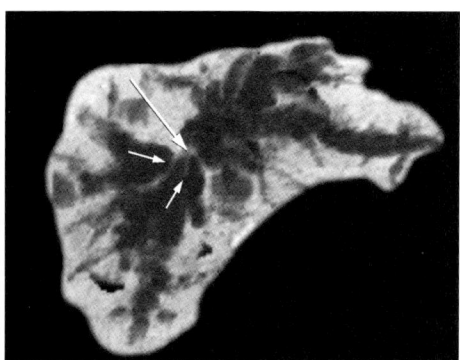

FIGURE 5: Malignant hilar biliary obstruction secondary to carcinoma gall bladder. CT cholangiogram axial minimum intensity projection (as seen from below) shows blocked primary confluence (large arrow) and right secondary confluence (small arrows). Reproduced with permission from Tropical Gastroenterology.

of gall bladder wall thickening. This is best accomplished with T2 weighed MRI which depicts them as hyperintense structures.

The differential diagnosis of a small polypoidal CaGB includes cholesterol, hyperplastic or adenomatous polyps. Benign polyps are typically less than 1 cm in size, while polypoidal cancers are usually larger. Presence of intratumoral vascularity and an irregular contour are suggestive of CaGB. Recently FDG-PET was shown to be useful in differentiating CaGB from other protuberant lesions of the gall bladder like cholesterol polyp and adenomyomatosis with an accuracy of 81.3%. FDG-PET may aid conventional imaging in differentiating benign from malignant conditions of the gall bladder.

Resectability criteria

The imaging based resectability criteria for CaGB were recently described on dual phase helical CT from our center. The authors reported that helical CT was very accurate in determining both resectable and unresectable cases with an overall accuracy of 93%. The factors governing resectability of CaGB include not only the presence of lymph nodal or distant metastases but also contiguous organ invasion and involvement of the crucial hepatic hilar structures (hepatic artery, portal vein and bile ducts).

The following **Criteria for Unresectability** were described: The presence of any of these features makes the tumor unresectable, and surgery with curative intent should be undertaken only in the absence of these findings:
– Peritoneal metastasis (Figure 6).
– Hepatic metastasis (Figure 6).
– Lymph nodes greater than 1.5 cm in size and heterogenous in appearance
– Contiguous involvement of greater than 2 segments each in both lobes of the liver
– Contiguous extensive involvement of

a distended gall bladder with irregularly thickened nodular wall and frequent association with gallstones. In some cases intramural nodules representing abscesses or xanthogranulomas are seen. These appear as nodular hypodense (on CT) or hypoechoic (on US) lesions, and are considered characteristic of this condition. An aggressive variant of this condition is also described in which there is a prominent inflammatory mass involving contiguous structures. This appearance is indistinguishable from that of advanced CaGB on imaging and often times even at surgery.

Adenomyomatosis is characterized by hypertrophy of the gall bladder wall and mucosal –submucosal diverticula (termed Rokitansky Aschoff sinuses). On US, CT or MRI it appears as segmental or diffuse wall thickening, or as focal nodule which may mimic CaGB. Anechoic areas and echogenic foci with ring down artifacts can be seen in the thickened wall. Visualization of the Rokitansky Aschoff sinuses is essential to differentiate adenomyomatosis from other causes

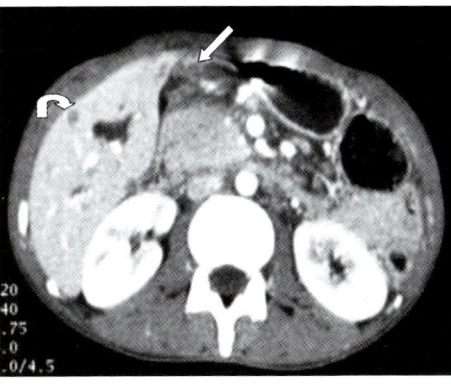

FIGURE 6: Ca GB with multiple hepatic metastases (arrow), peritoneal thickening around the liver anteriorly and in the subhepatic space (arrow), and mesenteric nodules (around mesenteric vessels).

colon, duodenum and/or pancreas (Figure 2).
– Involvement of secondary confluence (confluence of segmental ducts to form right or left bile ducts) of both lobes of liver
– Involvement of main portal vein or proper hepatic artery (Figure 7).

– Simultaneous involvement of either both hepatic arteries or both portal veins supplying both lobes of liver
– Simultaneous involvement of ipsilateral hepatic artery and contralateral portal vein
– Simultaneous involvement of ipsilateral hepatic artery and/or portal vein along with contralateral secondary confluence of bile ducts.

The signs of vascular invasion on CT are: direct contact of the mass with the artery or vein with loss of intervening fat plane, presence of mass on both sides of the vessel and vascular narrowing or irregularity. The advent of multidetector CT scanners and latest MRI technology like parallel imaging and high field magnets should further improve the ability to accurately select the resectable cases while avoiding laprotomy in patients with inoperable disease.

To conclude, CaGB is a morbid disease with a high proportion of unresectable tumours at presentation. US is the best initial modality for diagnosis and has the potential for giving most of the infor-

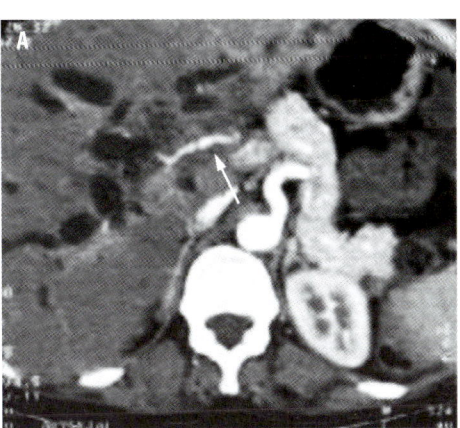
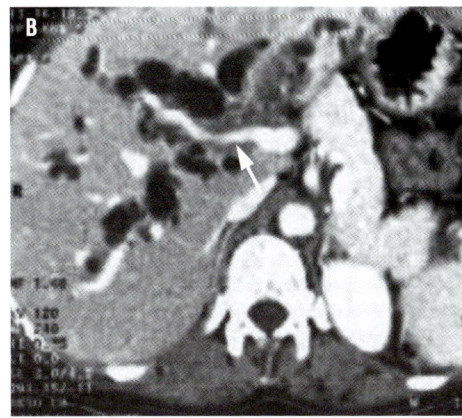

FIGURE 7: Arterial **(A)** and venous phase **(B)** helical CT shows carcinoma gallbladder encasing both the proper hepatic artery (arrow) and main portal vein (arrow), and the corresponding right branches of both vessels. The mass is seen on both sides of the vessels and is causing irregularity of the lumen. The primary confluence of bile ducts is also blocked. The tumour was suggested to be and found unresectable. Reproduced with permission from European Radiology.

mation. This technique is however, heavily dependant on the skill of the operator. It is further limited by lack of information on peritoneal disease. It is useful for providing guided biopsy for diagnosis. MRI has shown some promise in recent reports in providing good information in this setting. Overall, dual phase CT remains the mainstay at present for comprehensively defining the true extent of the disease including vascular invasion. In combination with value-added features such as 3D CTC, it may be possible to overcome limitations in elegantly displaying biliary anatomy for the benefit of the treating surgeons.

ACKNOWLEDGEMENT

The authors wish to thank Dr. A.L.Baert (Editor, European Radiology) and Dr. S.K.Acharya (Editor, Tropical Gastroenterology) for kindly granting permission to reproduce part of the text and figures from the articles published in these journals by the authors.

REFERENCES

Belbao MK, Dotter CT, Lee TG et al. Complications of endoscopic retrograde cholangiopancreatography (ERCP): A study of 10,000 cases. Gastroenterology 1976;70:314-20.

Casas D, Andres RP, Jimenez JA et al. Xanthogranulomatous cholecystitis: a radiological study of 12 cases and a review of literature. Abdom Imaging 1996;21:456-60.

Chijuwa K, Tanaka M. Carcinoma of the gallbladder: An appraisal of surgical resection. Surgery 1994;115:751-57.

Das DK, Tripathi RP, Bhambhani S et al. US guided fine needle aspiration cytology of gallbladder lesions: A study of 82 cases. Diagn Cytopathol 1998;18:258-64.

De Aretxabala X, Rao I, Burgos L et al. Gallbladder cancer in Chile. A report on 54 potentially respectable tumors. Cancer 1992;69:60-65.

Donabu JH, Nagorney DM, Grant CS et al. Carcinoma of the gall bladder. Arch Surg 1990;125:237-41.

Engles JT, Balfe Dm, Lee JK. Biliary carcinoma: CT evaluation of extrahepatic spread. Radiology 1989;172:35-40.

Enomoto T, Todoroti T, Koike N et al. Xanthogranulomatous cholecystitis mimicking stage IV gall bladder cancer. Hepatogastroenterology 2003; 50:1255-58.

Franquet T, Montes M, deAzua YR et al. Primary gall bladder carcinoma: Imaging findings in 50 patients with pathologic correlation. Gastrointest Radiol 1991;16:143-48.

Gore RM, Yaghmai V, Newmark GM et al. Imaging benign and malignant diseases of the gall bladder. Radiol Clin N Am 2002;40:1307-23.

Grenlee RT, Murray T, Bolden S et al. Cancer Statistics 2000. Cancer Clin 2000;50:7-33.

Gulati MS, Srinivasan A, Agarwal PP, Paul SB, Garg P, Rao NDLV. Percutaneous management of malignant biliary obstruction: the Indian perspective. Trop Gastroenterol 2003;24:47-58.

Henson DE, Albores-Saavedra J, Corle D. Carcinoma of the gall bladder: Histologic types, stage of disease, grade and survival rates. Cancer 1992;70:1493-97.

Kim JH, Kim TK, Eun HW et al. Preoperative evaluation of gall bladder carcinoma: Efficacy of combined use of MR imaging, MR choangiography and contrast enhanced dual phase three dimensional MR angiography. J of Mag Res Imaging 2002;16: 676-84.

Kim PN, Lee SH, Gong GY et al. Xanthogranulomatous cholecystitis: Radiologic findings with histologic correlation that focuses on intramural nodules. AJR 1999;172:949-53.

Koh T, Taniguchi H, Yamaguchi A et al. Differential diagnosis of gall bladder cancer using positron emersion tomography with fluonne-18-labelled Fluorodeoxyglucose (FDG-PET). J of Surg Oncol 2003;84:74-81.

Kumaran V, Gulati MS, Paul SB et al. The role of dual phase helical CT in assessing resectability of carcinoma of the gall bladder. Eur Radiol 2002; 12:1993-99.

Levy DA, Murkata AL, Rohrmam CA. Gall bladder carcinoma: Radiologic-pathologic correlation. Radiographics 2001;21:295-314.

Miyazaki M, Ioh H, Ambiru S et al. Radical surgery for advanced gall bladder carcinoma. Br J Surg 1996;83:478-81.

Mizuguchi M, Kudo S, Fukahon T et al. Endoscopic ultrasonography for demonstrating loss of multiple layer pattern of the thickened gall bladder wall in the preoperative diagnosis of gall bladder cancer. Eur Radiol 1997;7:1323-27.

Mueller PR, Harbin WP, Ferrucce JT Jr et al. Fine needle transhepatic cholangiography: reflection over 450 cases. Am J Roenterogenol 1981;136: 85-90.

Nakamura S, Sagaguchi S, Suzuki S et al. Aggressive surgery for carcinoma of the gallbladder. Surgery 1989;106:467-73.

Nimura Y, Hayakawa N, Kamuga J et al. Combined portal vein and liver resection for carcinoma of the biliary tract. Br J Surg 1991;78:727-31.

Ohtani T, Shirai Y, Tsukada K et al. Spread of gall bladder carcinoma: CT evaluation with pathologic correlation. Abdom Imaging 1996;21:195-201.

Onoyama H, Yamamoto M, Takada M et al. Diagnostic imaging of early gall bladder cancer: Retrospective study of 53 cases. World J Surg 1999; 23:708-12.

Rao ND, Gulati MS, Paul SB et al. Three dimensional helical computed tomography cholangiography with minimum intensity projection in gall bladder carcinoma patients with obstructive jaundice: comparison with magnetic resonance cholangiography and percutaneous transhepatic cholangiography. J of Gastroenterol and Hepatol 2005 Feb;20(2):304-8.

Soyer P, Gouhiri MH, Spelle IB et al. Carcinoma of the gall bladder: Imaging features with surgical correlation. Am J Roentgenol 1997;169:781-85.

Shirai Y, Yoshida K, Tsukada K et al. Early carcinoma of the gall bladder. Eur J Surg 1992;158: 545.

Sons HU, Borchard F, Joel BS. Carcinoma of the gall bladder: Autopsy findings in 287 cases and review of the literature. J Surg Oncol 1985;28: 199-206.

Todoraki T, Kawamoto T, Takahashi H et al. Treatment of gall bladder cancer by radical resection. Br J Surg 1999;86:622-27.

Tsukada K, Kurosaki I, Uchid K et al. Lymphnode spread from carcinoma of the gall bladder. Cancer 1997;80:661-67.

Wanebo HJ, Vezeridis MP. Carcinoma of the gall bladder. J Surg Oncol. Suppl. 1993;3:134-39.

Yoshimitsu K, Honda H, Shinozaki et al. Helical CT of the local spread of carcinoma of the gall bladder: Evaluation according to the TNM system in patients who underwent surgical resection. AJR 2002;179:423-28.

Zandrino F, Benzi L, Ferretti ML et al. Multislice CT cholangiography without biliary contrast agent: technique and initial clinical results in the assessment of patients with biliary obstruction. Eur Radiol 2002;12:1155-61.

Causes and treatment of obstructive jaundice due to malignant non-pancreatic periampullary tumours

Al-Bahrani Ahmed, Ammori Basil

SUMMARY

This chapter discusses the management of non-pancreatic periampullary cancers (*non*P-PAC), which arise from the ampulla, distal bile duct or duodenum. These tumours constitute approximately one-quarter of all PAC. Some of these tumours arise from premalignant conditions, such as familial polyposis coli, sclerosing cholangitis, choledochal cysts, and adenomatous polyps. Almost all *non*P-PAC are adenocarcinomas, and lymph node involvement is present in up to one-third of resected tumours. There is no reliable tumour marker for the diagnosis and monitoring of PAC. Computed tomography, magnetic resonance cholangiography and ERCP with biopsies or brush cytology are the main diagnostic tools. Positron emission tomography is useful in differentiating malignant from benign distal biliary strictures. Endoscopic ultrasound-guided fine needle aspiration for cytology may assist diagnosis. Staging laparoscopy is not routinely necessary in patients with ampullary or duodenal cancer. A selective approach to preoperative biliary drainage in jaundiced patients is advised. Surgical resection of PAC is the only curative option. Pancreaticoduodenectomy, either conventional or pylorus-preserving, is the standard procedure for radical resection. Randomised trials failed to demonstrate a survival benefit from extended lymphadenectomy. Transduodenal or endoscopic ampullectomy may be considered in elderly and high risk surgical patients with ampullary cancer. Adjuvant chemotherapy, radiotherapy or chemo-radiation offer limited survival benefits. Pancreas-sparing duodenectomy is applicable to patients with premalignant duodenal polyps. Palliative therapy is the only option for the majority of patients, and minimally invasive endoscopic and surgical palliation modalities include insertion of expandable biliary and duodenal stents, laparoscopic gastric and biliary bypass and thoracoscopic splanchnicectomy for pain relief.

INTRODUCTION

Periampullary tumours may be defined as those tumours that originate within 2 cm of the major papilla of Vater. They include four subgroups according to their anatomical origin: pancreatic (arising from the head of the pancreas), ampullary, duodenal and distal common bile duct (CBD).

When the pancreatic group of periampullary cancers (P-PAC) is excluded, the remainder will be referred to in this chapter as non-pancreatic periampullary cancers (nonP-PAC).

Most periampullary tumours are malignant while some are pre-malignant such as periampullary and duodenal adenomas. The nonP-PAC carry better prognosis than its equivalent P-PAC. However, the complexity of the anatomy of the periampullary region makes it very difficult at times to determine the origin of some tumours. Although periampullary cancers (PAC) often share similar clinical presentation, anatomical location and imaging and therapeutic approaches, their long-term outcome may vary according to tumour origin with a decline in survival in the following order: duodenal and ampullary, then bile duct and lastly tumours of pancreatic origin. PAC remains the fourth leading cause of cancer death in adults in the United States as it contributes to 30,000 deaths annually.

In this chapter we have endeavoured to focus our discussion on nonP-PAC and to highlight differences from P-PAC whenever possible, although some overlap is inevitable. Indeed most publications in the literature present these tumours as one group and very few discuss the nonP-PAC separately.

INCIDENCE

PAC constitutes 5% of all the gastrointestinal cancers, amongst which 20-27% are of the nonP-PAC. Some 15-25% of PAC originate from the ampulla of Vater, 10% from the bile duct, 10% from the duodenum and the remainder are of pancreatic origin. PAC affects male subjects slightly more frequently than female and often presents in the seventh decade with patients of White origin constituting some four-fifths of patients. While these ob-

servations also apply to patients presenting with ampullary carcinoma others report a female predominance of 1:2 in this subgroup.

Duodenal adenocarcinoma constitutes one-third of all the small bowel cancers and some three-quarters of all duodenal cancers, while cholangiocarcinoma of the distal CBD constitutes 20-25% of all cholangiocarcinomas. The incidence of distal CBD carcinoma has risen dramatically in recent years.

PREMALIGNANT CONDITIONS

An increase in the incidence of distal CBD cancer has been reported in patients with ulcerative colitis, primary sclerosing cholangitis (PSC) and disorders leading to biliary stasis such as pancreatobiliary maljunction (PBM) and choledochal cyst. Reflux of pancreatic juice into the biliary tract caused by PBM is considered important in the development of carcinogenesis in choledochal cysts. In patients with choledochal cysts, the risk of cancer is less than 1% in the first decade, but increases with age to over 10% in the third decade. Biliary adenomas could also give rise to bile duct cancer.

Villous adenomas of the duodenal mucosa, particularly in patients with familial adenomatous polyposis (FAP) may progress to adenocarcinoma. In one study, the relative risk of duodenal adenocarcinoma in patients with FAP was 331 (95% confidence limits, 133 and 681; p <0.001). Duodenal adenocarcinoma is the second commonest malignancy in FAP patients. In addition, colorectal carcinoma, hereditary non-polyposis colorectal cancer (HNPCC), Peutz-Jeghers Syndrome, celiac disease and sprue are recognized risk factors for development of duodenal carcinoma.

FAP also increases the incidence of ampullary carcinoma and so does neurofibromatosis. In one study, the relative risk of ampullary adenocarcinoma in FAP patients was 124 (95% confidence limits, 3334 and 317; p <0.001). Patients with ampullary carcinoma tend to have twice the incidence of colon cancer compared with the general population and *vice versa*.

CANCER PATHOLOGY

Virtually all *non*-PAC are adenocarcinomas of moderate to well differentiation except for those of duodenal origin, which often follow the line of P-PAC of poor tumour differentiation.

Some 90% of ampullary tumours are adenocarcinomas of low grade malignancy and tend to be polypoidal and soft.[13] The papillary variant of bile duct or ampullary carcinoma is associated with the most favourable outcome, whereas the mucinous type has a poor prognosis. A very small minority of duodenal cancers are of the carcinoid type or sarcomas, and in these, surgical excision is often curative. Rarely, what is presumed to be a *non*P-PAC proves histologically to be a metastatic adenocarcinoma.

Resectable tumours of the *non*P-PAC origin tend to be considerably smaller than those of the P-PAC origin with 50% measuring less than 2 cm compared with 33% respectively. Ampullary tumours tend to be the smallest among all *non*P-PAC and some 75% of those measures less than 4 cm.

Lymph node (LN) involvement, an important staging and prognostic factor, is present in up to one-third of resected *non*P-PAC compared to more than two-thirds of P-PAC. Some reports however revealed nodal involvement in 50% of patients with resected cholangiocarcinoma. The incidence of nodal involvement increases with the stage of the tumour with 5-10% LN involvement in T_1 ampul-

lary cancer that increases by three-folds in T_2 tumours.

The resection margins of the *non*P-PAC may be expected to be involved in less than 10% of cases compared with 50% of patients with resectable P-PAC.

Local infiltration of the tumour to the surrounding tissue may be seen in one-third of patients with resected PAC. There is more than a five-fold increase in the frequency of perineural and vascular infiltration in patients with P-PAC compared with *non*P-PAC (49% vs. 9% in one report)·

Metastases that preclude tumour resectability occur in more than two-thirds of patients presenting with PAC (pancreatic and *non*-pancreatic), and more frequently involve the liver than the peritoneum (42% vs. 25% in one report.

The ability of malignant epithelial cells to produce matrix metalloproteinases (MMP) to degrade extracellular matrix and basement membrane is an important step in the process of metastatic invasion and tumour spread. The ratio of expression of matrix metalloproteinases (MMP)-2 to tissue inhibitor of matrix metalloproteinase (TIMP)-2 in the resected LN and primary tumour is significantly higher in resected patients with eventually fatal disease compared to those with prolonged disease-free survivals.

TNM AND STAGE GROUPINGS

The tumour, node, metastases (TNM) classification and stage grouping of cancers were based on the Union Internacional Contra la Cancrum (UICC) system, established in 1977, with separate classifications for pancreatic and non-pancreatic periampullary carcinomas. The staging is important to communicate a uniform definition of extent of disease, to plan treatment and to predict prognosis. The latest TNM classification systems and stage groupings for ampullary, extrahepatic bile ducts and duodenal carcinomas produced in 2002 uniformly by the UICC and the American Joint Committee on Cancer (AJCC) and published in their 6th edition are shown in Tables 1, 2 and 3 respectively. Compared with the 5th edition, the 6th edition introduced important changes for carcinomas of the pancreas, extrahepatic biliary system, and ampulla. The changes were made based on new prognostic information and analysis of available data sets.

CLINICAL FEATURES

Although the clinical presentation in patients with nonP-PAC often mimics that of P-PAC, some clinical features might give a clue to the anatomical origin of the PAC and to its potential resectability or otherwise.

Symptoms

The duration of symptoms before diagnosis is largely determined by the rapidity

TABLE 1a

TNM CLASSIFICATION SYSTEM FOR CARCINOMAS OF THE AMPULLA OF VATER

TNM		Description
T	Tx	Primary tumour cannot be assessed
	T0	No evidence of primary tumour
	Tis	Carcinoma in situ
	T1	Tumour limited to ampulla of Vater or sphincter of Oddi
	T2	Tumour invades duodenal wall
	T3	Tumour invades 2 cm or less into pancreas
	T4	Tumour invades more than 2 cm into pancreas and/or into other adjacent organs
N	Nx	Regional lymph nodes cannot be assessed
	N0	No regional lymph node metastasis
	N1	Regional lymph node metastasis
M	Mx	Distant metastasis cannot be assessed
	M0	No distant metastasis
	M1	Distant metastasis

T: tumour, N: lymph node, M: metastasis

TABLE 1b

TNM STAGE GROUPING OF CARCINOMAS OF THE AMPULLA OF VATER

Stage	Tumour (T)	Lymph Node (N)	Metastasis (M)
0	Tis	N0	M0
I	T1	N0	M0
II	T2, T3	N0	M0
III	T1-3	N1	M0
IVA	T4	Any N	M0
IVB	Any T	Any N	M1

TABLE 2a TNM CLASSIFICATION SYSTEM FOR CARCINOMAS OF THE EXTRAHEPATIC BILE DUCTS (INCLUDING THOSE OF CHOLEDOCHAL CYSTS)

TNM		Description
T	Tx	Primary tumour cannot be assessed
	T0	No evidence of primary tumour
	Tis	Carcinoma in situ
	T1a	Tumour invades subepithelial connective tissue
	T1b	Tumour invades fibromuscular layer
	T2	Tumour invades perifibromuscular connective tissue
	T3	Tumour invades adjacent structures: liver, pancreas, duodenum, gallbladder, colon, stomach
N	Nx	Regional lymph nodes cannot be assessed
	N0	No regional lymph node metastasis
	N1	Metastasis to cystic duct, pericholedochal, and/or hilar lymph nodes (i.e. in the hepatoduodenal ligament)
	N2	Metastasis to peripancreatic (head only), periduodenal, periportal, coeliac, superior mesenteric, posterior peripancraetico-duodenal lymph nodes
M	Mx	Distant metastasis cannot be assessed
	M0	No distant metastasis
	M1	Distant metastasis

T: tumour, N: lymph node, M: metastasis

TABLE 2b TNM STAGE GROUPING OF CARCINOMAS OF THE EXTRAHEPATIC BILE DUCTS

Stage	Tumour (T)	Lymph Node (N)	Metastasis (M)
0	Tis	N0	M0
I	T1	N0	M0
II	T2	N0	M0
III	T1-2	N1-2	M0
IVA	T	Any N	M0
IVB	Any T	Any N	M1

with which the PAC obstructs the flow of bile and varies with the origin of the tumour; Shao *et al* reported 18 weeks for duodenal cancer, 11 weeks for P-PAC, and approximately 6 weeks for both ampullary and distal CBD cancers. Some 25-50% of patients with PAC tumours e-

lude the diagnosis until the time of surgery.

Jaundice is the commonest presenting symptom of PAC and is seen in 73-100% of patients with resectable P-PAC, ampullary and distal common bile duct tumours, but in only half of the patients with unresec-

TABLE 3a

TNM CLASSIFICATION SYSTEM FOR CARCINOMAS OF THE DUODENUM (AND SMALL BOWEL)

TNM		Description
T	Tx	Primary tumour can not be assessed
	T0	No evidence of primary tumour
	Tis	Carcinoma in situ
	T1	Tumour invades lamina propria or submucosa
	T2	Tumour invades muscularis propria
	T3	Tumour invades through muscularis propria into subserosa or into non-peritoneal-ized perimuscular tissue (mesentery or retroperitoneum) with extension of less than 2 cm
	T4	Tumour perforates visceral peritoneum or directly invades other organs or structures (includes other loops of small intestine, mesentery, or retroperitoneum for more than 2 cm and invasion of pancreas)
N	Nx	Regional lymph nodes (LN) can not be assessed
	N0	No regional LN metastasis
	N1	Regional LN metastasis
M	Mx	Distant metastasis can not be assessed
	M0	No distant metastasis
	M1	Distant metastasis

T: tumour, N: lymph node, M: metastasis

TABLE 3b

TNM STAGE GROUPING OF CARCINOMAS OF THE DUODENUM (AND SMALL BOWEL)

Stage	Tumour (T)	Lymph Node (N)	Metastasis (M)
0	Tis	N0	M0
I	T1, T2	N0	M0
II	T3, T4	N0	M0
III	Any T	N1	M0
IV	Any T	Any N	M1

table PAC. While jaundice is progressive in most of patients with PAC, it fluctuates in 5-29% of ampullary tumours. Occult gastrointestinal bleeding from duodenal cancer could present itself with iron deficiency anaemia, while frank bleeding is usually a sign of ampullary or duodenal cancer. Silver stools, which are the result of combi-nation of biliary obstruction and melaena, are a characteristic feature of ampullary cancers. Gastric outlet obstruction is more likely to present in patients with duodenal cancer. Acute pancreatitis either as single or recurrent attacks is a rare presentation of PAC and is more likely to feature in patients with ampullary cancers.

Signs

A palpable tumour mass, splenomegaly as a result of splenic vein involvement by the tumour and thrombosis, and enlarged left supraclavicular lymph glands (Trousier's sign) are rare features that usually indicates an advanced P-PAC (usually of the body of the pancreas) rather than a nonP-PAC.

DIAGNOSIS AND STAGING

Tumour markers

There is no reliable tumour marker for the diagnosis and monitoring of PAC that has a high accuracy rate for clinical use. In one study the sensitivity of carbohydrate antigen (CA) 19-9 in the diagnosis of nonP-PAC was 49% in comparison with 73% for P-PAC. On the other hand, CA 19-9 appears useful for the detection of cholangiocarcinoma in patients with PSC with a reported sensitivity and specificity (cut-off, 100 U/L) of 75% and 80% respectively. However, CA 19-9 is of poor diagnostic value for cholangiocarcinoma in non-PSC patients.

Radiology

• *Ultrasonography (US)*
An abnormal pulsed Doppler signal obtained from the portal venous system due to severe narrowing or occlusion is highly suspicious for major involvement and irresectability of the tumour. However, a normal pulsed Doppler signal does not exclude involvement, if the tumour has continuity with the vessel with interruption of the hyperechoic tumour vessel interface.

Endoscopic ultrasound (EUS) is highly operator dependent and is not widely available. EUS is useful in assessing local tumour infiltration, regional LN involvement, vascular invasion and possibly peritoneal seedlings but its accuracy is reduced in the presence of endobiliary stents. Some studies reported higher accuracy for EUS than computed tomography (CT) in detecting pancreatic tumours, especially if less than 2 cm in size and in predicting vascular invasion. Therefore, EUS is beneficial in patients with unidentifiable tumour on CT and when vascular invasion is suspected on CT. EUS however is not superior to endoscopic retrograde cholangiopancreatography (ERCP) in detecting ampullary tumours. The use of three-dimensional linear EUS enhanced the evaluation of vascular involvement compared with linear echoendoscopy alone. EUS may also facilitate fine needle aspiration (FNA) of PAC or regional LN to assist in preoperative staging. EUS-guided FNA appears safe, and in one report there were no false-positive results and a 13% false-negative results due to inadequate sampling.

More recently, an intraluminal or intraductal mini-probe US has become available and was shown to have a greater diagnostic sensitivity than ERCP +/- endoscopic transpapillary biopsy in clarifying the nature of bile duct strictures, 75-90% vs. 52-67% though its diagnostic sensitivity for lesions of the distal CBD is lower due to the high resemblance of benign processes.

Three dimensional intra-ductal US is more useful for the precise diagnosis of cancer extension in cholangiocarcinoma, especially invasion into the portal vein and pancreas, than CT scan and angiography. In a study of 33 patients with obstructive jaundice secondary to bile duct strictures, the addition of intra-ductal US to ERCP significantly increased the accuracy of differentiation of malignant from benign lesions from 76% to 88%.

• *Computed tomography (CT)*
Imaging studies such as US and CT could

differentiate distal CBD strictures (dilated proximal biliary tree and normal pancreatic duct) from pancreatic head cancer; the latter may be associated with dilatation of both ducts or of the pancreatic duct only. It is advisable to obtain a CT in patients suspected to have PAC on abdominal US prior to biliary stent insertion as stenting considerably reduces the accuracy of CT diagnosis of malignancy (from 88% to 73% in one report).

The radiographic assessment of extent of tumour burden and local vascular invasion appears to be enhanced with three-dimensional CT. House *et al* compared three-dimensional CT scan findings with intraoperative findings in a prospective study and reported CT accuracy in predicting disease resectability and negative resection margins in 115 patients with proven PAC of 98% and 86%, respectively.

• *Magnetic resonance imaging (MRI)*

Although MRI is usually used as a second line of imaging after CT, it is probably the best imaging modality for the detection of CBD lesions. Magnetic resonance cholangiopancreatography (MRCP) has an accuracy of 85-100% in the detection of CBD obstruction and 90-100% accuracy in the detection of level of obstruction. Cholangiocarcinoma of the distal CBD manifests as luminal obliteration and wall thickening or as an intra-ductal polypoid mass. A dilated proximal bile duct, a non-dilated distal CBD, and a dilated or non-dilated pancreatic duct may form the three-segment sign characteristic of distal cholangiocarcinoma. Ampullary carcinoma manifests on MRI as a small mass, peri-ductal thickening, or bulging of the duodenal papilla. Dilatation of the side branches of the pancreatic duct is frequently seen in P-PAC but not in *non*P-PAC. Abdominal MRI may be combined with MRCP and magnetic resonance angiography to provide an 'all-

in-one' examination in the evaluation of suspected cholangiocarcinoma.

Endoscopic MRI involves the insertion into the second part of the duodenum of a magnetic resonance endoscope with a small radiofrequency coil attached to its tip. The patient is then placed in a MRI scanner and the acquisition of fast spoiled pulse sequences. Endoscopic MRI (virtual endoscopy) facilitates the reconstruction of an intraluminal vision of the biliary and pancreatic ducts. Virtual endoscopy for pancreatic cancer has potential clinical utility particularly that it is associated with minimal discomfort compared to real endoscopic examination, and it can access cystic lesions as well as the pancreatic duct behind the stricture. Virtual endoscopy is also useful for surgical planning of minimally invasive resection of the pancreas.

• *Positron emission tomography (PET)*

PET is useful in differentiating malignant from benign distal biliary strictures with an accuracy of up to 92%. PET however is less accurate than CT and EUS in the diagnosis of other types of PAC. In one study, PET missed more than 10% of PAC and was not able to identify the anatomical details needed to decide their resectability. PET on the other hand is more accurate than CT in the detection of LN and distant metastases and is beneficial when the diagnosis of PAC remains equivocal.

• *Endoscopic retrograde cholangiopancreatography (ERCP)*

ERCP is as accurate as EUS in detecting ampullary tumours and has its role in obtaining biopsies and brush cytology from biliary strictures and in performing endoscopic interventions *(see below)*. It is advisable however to defer ERCP and stent insertion till after completing all the imaging procedures needed for localizing and staging PAC in order to avoid the confounding effects of the stent.

- *Preoperative cytological confirmation*

There is no place for routine preoperative cytological confirmation of malignancy with percutaneous fine needle aspiration (FNA) in patients with potentially resectable PAC, particularly if the surgical team has low perioperative mortality. The sensitivity of percutaneous FNA cytology in assessing a 'pancreatic mass' is quite variable (57-96%) and sampling errors are frequent. Complications such as pancreatitis, pancreatic fistula and stomach or colon injury may occur, albeit rare. In a review of more than 38,000 patients, percutaneous FNA had an overall mortality and morbidity rates of 0.006-0.008% and 0.005-0.16% respectively. The risk of tumour seedling along the needle track is not negligible with an incidence of up to 1.4% in patients with P-PAC as a recent report from Japan revealed. Therefore, percutaneous FNA of PAC should continue to be reserved to patients unfit for resection and those with unresectable disease if histological confirmation is required.

In patients with nonP-PAC however, histological confirmation may be obtained safely through endoscopic biopsies of ampullary or duodenal cancers, and from brush cytology in patients with distal cholangiocarcinoma. It is advisable however to avoid endoscopic biopsies of suspected ampullary lesions for 7-10 days after endoscopic sphincterotomy as high artefact changes occur and preclude the reliability of histological analysis.

Endoscopic brush cytology at time of ERCP in 86 patients with biliary strictures of unknown status was uncomplicated and had a sensitivity of 80% for confirming cholangiocarcinoma (compared with 35% for P-PAC) and a specificity of 90% due to misinterpretation of dysplastic cells in patients with chronic pancreatitis and inflammatory strictures. In another study of 58 patients with obstructive jaundice due to biliary strictures and external biliary drains, percutaneous transhepatic endobiliary brush cytology had a high sensitivity (75%) and specificity (100%) but a low negative predictive value (12.5%). On the other hand, brush cytology in patients with PSC and biliary stricture has a rather poor sensitivity and positive predictive value but a reasonably good specificity and negative predictive value.

There appears to be no additional value from p53 immunocytochemistry and K-ras mutation analysis to brush cytology in patients with PSC and biliary strictures. EUS-guided FNA cytology, of diagnostic value in potentially operable patients with hilar cholangiocarcinoma, has not been clearly evaluated in patients with suspected distal cholangiocarcinoma.

- *Laparoscopy and laparoscopic ultrasound:*

There is no longer a place for staging laparotomy in patients with PAC. A recent study of staging laparotomy and proceed to either resection of PAC or bypass in 186 patients showed limited value for laparotomy in disease staging with 35% unresectability rate due to distant metastasis and loco-regional tumour spread. Staging laparoscopy on the other hand is of benefit in patients with P-PAC but is not routinely necessary in patients with ampullary or duodenal cancer. In a study that investigated whether staging laparoscopy and laparoscopic ultrasound in patients with PAC could change the imaging-based clinical decisions, found no benefit for laparoscopy in patients with ampullary or duodenal tumours while it detected metastatic disease and vascular invasion in one-third of patients with P-PAC. In another study in 121 patients with suspected nonP-PAC, a selective use of staging laparoscopy was advocated as the addition of diagnostic laparoscopy to dynamic CT scan identified an additional 10% of patients with unresectable disease. Staging laparoscopy however may underestimate portal vein and regional LN involvement. On the other hand, laparoscopic ultrasound in experienced hands is of some benefit in detecting vascular involvement in patients with P-PAC but is of little value in those with nonP-PAC.

TREATMENT

Surgical resection of periampullary tumours is the only curative option, but resectability rates vary with the type of the tumour with the lowest rates reported for P-PAC (20-44%) and the highest rates for ampullary tumours (90-94%).

Preoperative preparations

The role of *preoperative nutrition* and *biliary drainage* is briefly discussed.

• *Nutrition*
Patients with cancer tend to suffer from malnutrition due to anorexia and increased metabolic rate by the tumour, and this is particularly true for patients with P-PAC. The perioperative enteral administration of immune-enhancing nutrition (IEN) appears beneficial with enhancement of cell-mediated immunity in patients with gastric or colorectal cancer undergoing surgery when compared to conventional enteral nutrition. These favourable results however could not be reproduced in severely malnourished patients with head and neck cancer that were fed preoperatively. In a randomised trial that involved 100 patients with pancreatic cancer undergoing pancreaticoduodenectomy (PD), the postoperative administration of IEN reduced the incidence and severity of postoperative complications when compared with intravenous nutrition. The observed difference however might have been related to the increased risk of infections with intravenous nutrition. The role of a com-

bined approach of preoperative and postoperative IEN in patients with PAC has not been evaluated.

• *Preoperative biliary drainage*
The role of preoperative biliary drainage in jaundiced patients undergoing PD remains controversial. Some investigations suggested that preoperative biliary stenting increased operative time, intraoperative blood loss and incidence of wound infection and other infectious complications as well as operative mortality while others showed no increase in major morbidity or mortality. Others reported that preoperative endoscopic biliary drainage significantly reduced operative morbidity and postoperative hospital stay. However, a meta-analysis of eight retrospective and two prospective randomised controlled clinical trials found no evidence of either a positive or adverse effect of preoperative endoscopic biliary stent placement on the outcome of PD in patients with PAC and obstructive jaundice. A selective approach to preoperative biliary stenting is therefore advised, such as in patients with infective cholangitis, long-standing and deep jaundice, those with impaired renal function and when definitive surgery is expected to be delayed (e.g. for more than 10-14 days).

Surgical resection

Surgical resection of localised PAC offers the only option for cure. The standard procedure for radical resection of nonP-PAC is pancreaticoduodenectomy (PD), either conventional or pylorus-preserving, while localised resection of ampullary tumours is of some proposed applicability in the occasional patient.

Unlike P-PAC, which continues to have a rather low resectability rate, there is no doubt that the resectability rates for nonP-PAC have improved in recent years. In a report that compared two periods;

1988-1998 (147 patients) and 1999-2003 (130 patients), the resectability rates for ampullary, duodenal and distal bile duct cancers increased from 75% to 100%, 66.7% to 83.3% and 50% to 75% respectively while those for pancreatic cancer remained unchanged (20.2% to 20.4%). In another report, the resectability rates for ampullary, duodenal and distal CBD cancers have considerably increased to 94%, 83% and 83% respectively with the lowest rate (44%) remaining for pancreatic cancer.

• *Pancreaticoduodenectomy*

The advancements in preoperative preparation and optimization of patients for surgery as well as the improvement in surgical and anaesthetic techniques and the concentration of surgery for PAC in high-volume specialist centres has resulted in marked reductions in operative morbidity (from 40-60% to 30%) and mortality (from 20-40% to 5%).

Randomised controlled trails have demonstrated that both the pylorus preserving PD and the classical PD (Whipple procedure) were equally effective in treating P-PAC and nonP-PAC with comparable morbidity, mortality, hospital stay, and overall long-term and disease-free survival. Whilst there is some evidence to suggest that the pylorus preserving PD offers some early postoperative nutritional advantages over the classical PD, these differences are not maintained in the long term. Neither technique appears superior with regard to the incidence of postoperative delayed gastric emptying. The pylorus preserving PD is particularly oncologically sufficient for *non*P-PAC, but is contraindicated for carcinomas of the anterior-superior part of the head of the pancreas.

The proposal of an improved survival for patients with pancreatic and other periampullary adenocarcinomas when subjected to an extended lymphadenectomy at the time of PD remains unsupported by randomised trials. In an American randomised trial that involved 299 patients with resectable PAC, radical PD (extended to include distal gastrectomy and retroperitoneal lymphadenectomy) increased operative morbidity compared to standard pylorus preserving PD and incurred no survival benefit at 1, 3 and 5 years. However, no differences in operative mortality and long-term quality of life between the two procedures were observed. In an Italian randomised trial of 81 patients undergoing PD for P-PAC, the addition of an extended lymphadenectomy to PD did not significantly increase morbidity and mortality rates but failed to offer a survival advantage.

Two studies from Japan had suggested a disease-free survival benefit to a 'non-touch' approach to PD for PAC in which the feeding and draining vessels of the pancreatic carcinoma are ligated and divided prior to pancreatectomy in order to reduce the potential risk of postoperative liver metastases. Mimura et al reported a 6 and 12 months survival advantage for the 'non-touch' technique with extensive retroperitoneal lymphadenectomy compared with conventional resection (0% vs. 22.9% and 16.7% vs. 31.3% respectively), while Kobayashi et al reported neither operative mortality nor liver metastasis during the follow up after 'non-touch' PD.

Some 20%-40% of the patients with an adenoma of the ampulla of Vater will have a co-existent malignant transformation. PD is therefore recommended in patients with ampullary adenomas that have high-grade dysplasia.

The recurrence rate after potentially curative resection of duodenal, ampullary and distal bile duct adenocarcinoma has been reported to be 37%, 50% and 74% respectively, compared to 81% for P-PAC.

Localised resection

Transduodenal ampullectomy may be safely applied to patients with an endoscopic pathologic diagnosis of ampullary adenoma with or without mild to moderate dysplasia or with ampullary polypoidal tumours of less than 2 cm in size. Endoscopic snare excision of presumed benign ampullary adenomas is a relatively new approach that has been shown to resolve symptoms of obstruction, but long-term follow up is necessary to detect early malignant transformation. Snare ampullectomy carries lower morbidity (12-15%) and mortality (0%-1%) compared with transduodenal local excision, but is highly dependent on local availability of experienced operators and endoscopic modalities of haemostasis, requires multiple procedures (mean, 2.0 procedures) to effect complete excision, and requires continued endoscopic surveillance.

Ampullectomy however is best avoided in fit patients with high-grade dysplasia and in those with carcinoma in favour of PD. In a retrospective pathological analysis of 201 resected specimens of PD for ampullary cancer Yoon *et al* demonstrated that some one-third of patients had at least one risk factor for failure after ampullectomy, such as LN metastasis, perineural invasion, or mucosal tumour infiltration along the CBD or pancreatic duct. With a background of a 5-year survival of approximately 84% with PD for ampullary cancer, Yoon *et al* concluded that ampullectomy with re-implantation of the pancreatic and distal CBD into the duodenal wall should be reserved for patients who have *p*Tis or *p*T1 cancer sized 1.0 cm or less with high operative risk. Although local excision (transduodenal or endoscopic) in patients with ampullary malignancy may be associated with lower morbidity and quicker recovery compared with PD, its has its drawbacks such as high recurrence rate (5-30%), worse prognosis and

need for long term endoscopic surveillance. Local resection of ampullary cancer may therefore be reserved to elderly high risk patients who cannot withstand PD.

In Japan, the screening programme for gastric cancer tends to detect some duodenal cancers at their very early stages where the tumour is confined to mucosa (the extent of duodenal wall invasion may be assessed with EUS). Some of these patients have been successfully and effectively treated with endoscopic mucosal resection with very low morbidity (6%) and no disease recurrence after a mean follow-up of more than 4 years.

PANCREAS-SPARING DUODENECTOMY:

Pancreas-sparing duodenectomy (PSD) is a safe and effective procedure for patients with premalignant duodenal polyps such as those with FAP. Although technically demanding, PSD is associated with good quality of life and may reduce the risk of subsequent malignancy. However, PSD is contraindicated in the setting of malignancy. PSD is yet to be performed laparoscopically.

Adjuvant therapy

Recent studies of adjuvant chemotherapy, radiotherapy or chemo-radiation have, by and large, failed to demonstrate clear survival benefits in patients with PAC with few exceptions. Studies at the John Hopkins Hospital, USA, have shown some limited value for the combination of adjuvant chemo-radiation for periampullary adenocarcinoma with improvement of short-term disease-free survival, especially for *non*P-PAC. In another study however, adjuvant chemo-radiation had no effect on local recurrence of resected duodenal cancer. A more recent study of intraoperative radiotherapy for PAC has shown significant improvement in the incidence of isolated lo-co-regional recurrence and systemic recurrence pattern, but disease-free survival and overall survival remained unchanged.

Adjuvant photodynamic therapy (PDT) appears safe with improved survival in patients with bile duct cancer undergoing surgical resection. In patients with advanced biliary tract malignancies however, chemotherapy with gemcitabine demonstrated notable activity with an overall response rate of 12.5% and a tolerable toxicity profile.

Palliative therapy

The majority of patients presenting with PAC have unresectable disease, and the focus of treatment is on palliation. The three main symptoms to palliate include obstructive jaundice, duodenal obstruction and pain, and these could be managed operatively or non-operatively.

NON-OPERATIVE PALLIATION

Obstructive jaundice may be palliated by insertion of biliary plastic or metal **biliary stents** through endoscopic, percutaneous, or combined approaches. Although metal stents remain patent longer than plastic stents, the optimal palliation of inoperable malignant biliary strictures remains controversial because of the high cost of metal stents and short patient survival. The stent choice however is largely dependent on the extent of disease and predicted patient survival. In a randomised controlled trial of metal versus plastic stents in the palliation of obstructive jaundice in 118 patients with inoperable malignant strictures of the distal CBD, metal stent placement were more effective with significantly longer time to first stent obstruction (median not reached vs. 5 months, $p=0.007$). The number of additional days of hospitalization, days of antibiotic therapy, and the numbers of

ERCPs and transabdominal US procedures was significantly higher in the plastic stent group. Placement of a metal stent was cost effective in patients without hepatic metastases who had significantly longer survival, whereas placement of plastic stent was recommended in patients with liver metastases. A similar randomised trial that involved 101 jaundiced patients with inoperable PAC found the use of metal stents more cost effective in patients surviving more than 6 months, whereas plastic stents were more cost effective in patients surviving 6 months or less. In another randomised trial, the overall cost of treatment of obstructive jaundice was higher in the plastic stent than the metal stent group due to the added cost of re-stenting and treatment of stent-related complications.

Endoscopic sphincterotomy does not seem to be necessary for placement of 10-Fr plastic stents in patients with malignant CBD obstruction. In a randomised trial of 172 consecutive patients with inoperable malignant CBD strictures endoscopic sphincterotomy before stent insertion did not increase the success rate of stenting but was associated with a slight (but statistically not significant) increase in morbidity.

Photodynamic therapy (PDT) involves the endoscopic delivery of red light (630 nm) to ampullary tumours pre-sensitized with intravenous haematoporphyrin. or Photofrin. This method includes subjecting the tumour to 3-4 light applications for up to five sessions over 3-6 months period. In a randomised multi-centre trial of PDT versus stenting in patients with unresectable cholangiocarcinoma, PDT was associated with significant prolongation of survival that resulted in premature termination of the trial. Photodynamic therapy has been shown to improve survival compared with plastic stent for unresectable cholangiocarcinoma (intrahepatic or extrahepatic).

Endoscopic palliation of malignant

duodenal stenosis or obstruction with insertion of large calibre self-expandable metallic *duodenal stents* is safe and effective in the majority of patients with an overall success rate in clinical relief of obstruction of approximately 85%. Complications occur in 6-8% of patients including, bleeding, jaundice, stent migration and mucosal hyperplasia. However, there is a considerable re-obstruction rate of 12-30% due to tumour ingrowth, overgrowth or stent migration.

The role of neurolytic pain relief through *coeliac plexus block* (CPB) delivered percutaneously, endoscopically with EUS guidance or intraoperatively is largely applicable to patients with pancreatic rather than *non*P-PAC and has been discussed in the previous chapter.

External *radiotherapy* could be utilized as a second alternative for pancreatic pain control after recurrence of pain following percutaneous nerve block. In a recent non-randomised study that investigated pain management in 98 patients who underwent palliative bypass surgery for unresectable PAC, the pain medication-free survival in patients who received radiotherapy was significantly longer than in patients who had bypass surgery alone or who received CPB, and the hospital-free survival and overall survival were significantly longer in the radiotherapy group than in the CPB group. However, there are no randomised trials to confirm these findings in patient with *non*P-PAC.

OPERATIVE PALLIATION

Obstructive jaundice may be palliated through the construction of a *biliary bypass* at conventional laparotomy or laparoscopically. The minimal invasive approach has been promoted as a safe and effective alternative to traditional surgical biliary bypass. Although it is well recognised that hepatico-jejunostomy produces superior long-term patency rates compared with cholecysto-jejunostomy, it is worth noting that the difference in patency rates at 1-year is less than 5% and that only a small proportion of patients with inoperable PAC remain alive after 1 year. When biliary imaging shows a cystic duct insertion at 1 cm or more above a distal CBD stricture, it is preferable to laparoscopically construct a cholecysto-jejunostomy as this is technically less demanding and time consuming than hepatico-jejunostomy and is associated with a more rapid recovery and shorter hospital stay.

Whilst the indication for *gastric bypass* for palliation of duodenal obstruction is evident, it is also of value as a prophylactic procedure in patients with locally advanced disease. In a randomised controlled trial that addressed this issue in 87 patients with PAC who were found to have unresectable disease at exploratory laparotomy, Lillemoe *et al* reported that the construction of a prophylactic gastric bypass significantly reduced the incidence of late gastric outlet obstruction (19% vs. 0%) without increasing the incidence of postoperative complications (33% vs. 32%) or extending the length of hospital stay (mean 8.5 vs. 8.0 days). These findings have conclusively favoured the addition of a prophylactic gastric bypass at the time of a palliative biliary bypass. In another randomised multi-centre trial, the addition of a prophylactic gastric bypass at the time of an open biliary bypass significantly decreased the incidence of gastric outlet obstruction without increasing complication rates.

The operative mortality of palliative procedures for unresectable PAC is generally greater than that of resectable disease (3.1% vs. 1.9% in one report).

Palliative gastric bypass may be safely accomplished laparoscopically with advantages over open surgery. In a comparative study, laparoscopic gastric bypass for gastric outlet obstruction was associated with significantly lower morbidity, more rapid recovery, and shorter hospital stay compared with open surgery. The addition of a prophylactic laparoscopic gastric bypass at the time of a palliative laparoscopic biliary bypass in patients with locally advanced but non-metastatic PAC who have better prognosis may be accomplished safely without an increase in morbidity or hospital stay.

Thoracoscopic division of the splanchnic nerves *(thoracoscopic splanchnicectomy)* is an effective minimally invasive approach for the palliation of intractable pancreatic pain and provides an alternative solution to percutaneous nerve block. Bilateral thoracoscopic splanchnicectomy eliminates the need for progressive doses of analgesics, with their side effects, and allows recovery of daily activity. The efficacy of this procedure in palliation of intractable abdominal pain in cancer patients with very short life expectancy is currently the subject of a multi-centre randomised trial in the UK that compares medical therapy alone and in combination with either coeliac plexus block or thoracoscopic splanchnicectomy.

The role of *palliative pancreaticoduodenectomy* remains controversial and to date there are no prospective randomized data to support its role in palliation of locally advanced PAC.

Conventional chemotherapy and radiotherapy have not been shown to be effective in prolonging long-term survival in patients with cholangiocarcinoma.

PREVENTION

Patients with *FAP* have a cumulative lifetime risk of over 90% for developing duodenal adenomas, and a 5% to 10% lifetime risk of periampullary or duodenal adenocarcinoma, making this the leading cause of cancer death in FAP patients who have had prophylactic colectomy. Almost all cases of adenocarcinoma occur in patients with advanced polyposis (Spigelman stage IV disease) (Table 4), and approximately 33% of this group will go on to develop adenocarcinoma if left untreated. The cumulative risk of stage IV duodenal polyposis has been evaluated at 20% and 30% at ages 60 and 65 years, respectively, in two recent series and reaches 40% at age 60 and 50% at age 70 in a third study. *Endoscopic duodenal surveillance* is therefore generally adopted in patients with FAP, particularly that the prognosis of duodenal cancer is rather poor. A high initial Spigelman's score (>7 points) is considered a risk factor for development of high-grade dysplasia and subsequent malignancy. These patients may therefore be offered prophylactic PD or PSD. Endoscopic snare excision of adenomas and ampullectomy offers an alternative to surgery in selected patients, though its role in the prevention of duodenal cancer requires further evaluation.

Nonsteroidal anti-inflammatory drug therapy with sulindac, a nonselective cy-

TABLE 4 SPIGELMAN STAGING SYSTEM OF DUODENAL POLYPS IN FAP PATIENTS

Endoscopic & histological findings	No. of points scored		
	1	2	3
No. of polyps	1-4	5-20	>20
Polyp size (mm)	1-4	5-20	>20
Histology	tubulous	tubulovillous	villous
Dysplasia	mild	moderate	severe

Spigelman's stage	No. of points
0	0
I	1-4
II	5-6
III	7-8
IV	9-12

clooxygenase (COX) inhibitor, or cele-coxib, a COX-2 selective inhibitor, may be of benefit after the development of duodenal polyposis by inducing the regression or stabilization of the polyposis, although there is limited evidence from randomized controlled trials to support its routine use.

Early excision of the extrahepatic biliary tree and Roux-en-Y hepatico-jejunostomy is recommended in patients with PBM and extrahepatic *choledochal cysts* to prevent the development of cholangiocarcinoma. However, the relative risk of cholangiocarcinoma after excision of the extrahepatic bile ducts seems to remain high compared with that of the general population despite a slight reduction by surgery. Careful long-term follow-up is therefore necessary in these patients, especially after operations that leave dilated bile ducts, such as in patients with Todani type IV-A (Figure 1 & Table 5). Laparoscopic resection of choledochal cysts in experienced hands appears safe.

PROGNOSIS

Resection of PAC is associated with significantly longer survival compared with non-resectable disease. As an example, Sohn *et al* reported 1, 2 and 4 year survival for

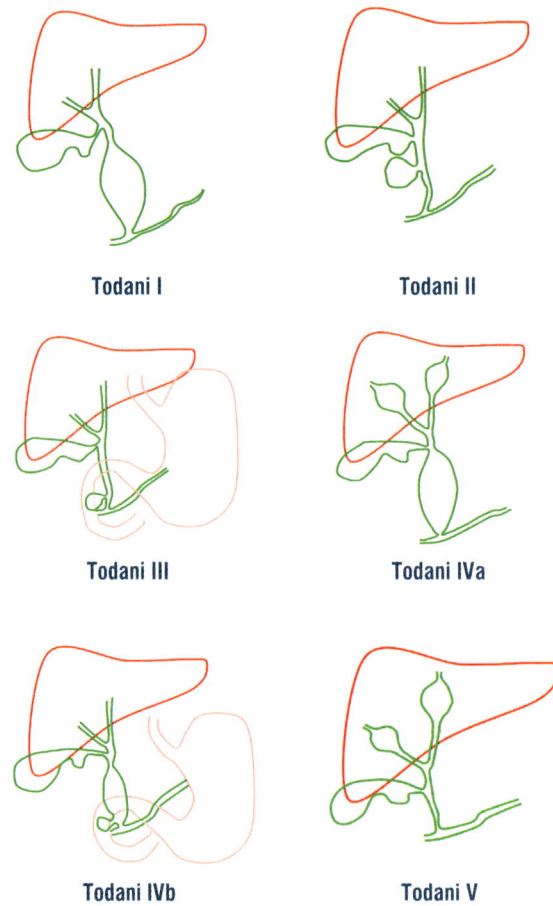

Todani I   Todani II

Todani III   Todani IVa

Todani IVb   Todani V

FIGURE 1: Todani's classification of choledochal cysts.

TABLE 5	TODANI'S CLASSIFICATION OF CHOLEDOCHAL CYSTS

Todani's type	Description
I	Solitary, fusiform
II	Extrahepatic supraduodenal diverticulum of the choledochus
III	Intraduodenal diverticulum (choledochocele proper)
IVA	Fusiform intra- and extrahepatic cysts
IVB	Multiple extrahepatic cysts
V	Multiple intrahepatic cysts (Caroli's syndrome)

resectable and palliative PAC to be 75% and 25%, 47% and 9%, and 24% and 6% respectively, with a median survival of 21 and 6.5 months respectively.

Although the complication rate and 30-day mortality for resectable P-PAC may not vary from that of resection for nonP-PAC, survival after the latter is significantly longer. In a recent report, the actuarial 5-year survival for PAC was 30%; being 11% for P-PAC and 46% for nonP-PAC. Survival also differs between different histological subtypes of PAC, with some reports showing a median survival of 13-16 months for pancreatic cancer, 16-25 months for distal bile duct cancer, and 24-36 months for ampullary cancer.

Similar to resected P-PAC, multivariable analysis of prognostic factors in 51 patients with ampullary cancer who underwent PD showed that node-negative disease was of an independent prognostic significance with a 5-year survival of 78% in patients with node-negative disease. Similar findings were reported by Su et al in a multivariate analysis of factors influencing survival after PD in 132 patients with ampullary cancer. In another report of 47 radical PD for ampullary cancer, multivariate analysis showed that the TNM stage and tumour differentiation were independently correlated with the survival. In a multivariate analysis, Ryder et al examined factors influencing survival in 49 patients with resected and unresectable duodenal adenocarcinoma and reported large tumour size, advanced histological grade, and transmural invasion to be associated with decreased survival.

REFERENCES

Abrams RA, Yeo CJ. Combined modality adjuvant therapy for resected periampullary pancreatic and nonpancreatic adenocarcinoma: a review of studies and experience at The Johns Hopkins Hospital, 1991-2003. Surg Oncol Clin N Am 2004; 13:621-38.

Abulafi AM, Allardice JT, Williams NS, van Someren N, Swain CP, Ainley C. Photodynamic therapy for malignant tumours of the ampulla of Vater. Gut 1995; 36:853-6.

Al-Rashedy M, Issa ME, Ballester P, Ammori BJ. Laparoscopic surgery for the management of obstruction of the gastric outlet and small bowel following previous laparotomy for major upper gastrointestinal resection or cancer palliation: a new concept. J Laparoendosc Adv Surg Tech A 2005;15:153-9.

Albores-Saavedra J, Henson DE, Klimstra D. Atlas of Tumor Pathology: Tumors of the Gallbladder, Extrahepatic Bile Ducts, and Ampulla of Vater, 3rd series, fascicle 27. Washington, DC: Armed Forces Institute of Pathology; 2000.

Asbun HJ, Rossi RL, Munson JL. Local resection for ampullary tumors. Is there a place for it? Arch Surg 1993; 128:515-20.

Bakaeen FG, Murr MM, Sarr MG, Thompson GB, Farnell MB, Nagorney DM, Farley DR, van Heerden JA, Wiersema LM, Schleck CD, Donohue JH. What prognostic factors are important in duodenal adenocarcinoma? Arch Surg 2000; 135:635-41.

Beger HG, Treitschke F, Gansauge F, Harada N, Hiki N, Mattfeldt T. Tumor of the ampulla of Vater: experience with local or radical resection in 171 consecutively treated patients. Arch Surg 1999; 134:526-32.

Benjamin IS. Biliary cystic disease: the risk of cancer. *J Hepatobiliary Pancreat Surg* 2003; 10:335-9.

Bjork J, Akerbrant H, Iselius L, Bergman A, Engwall Y, Wahlstrom J, Martinsson T, Nordling M, Hultcrantz R. riampullary adenomas and adenocarcinomas in familial adenomatous polyposis: cumulative risks and APC gene mutations. *Gastroenterology* 2001; 121:1127-35.

Bottger T, Hassdenteufel A, Boddin J, Kuchle R, Junginger T, Prellwitz W. Value of the CA 19-9 tumor marker in differential diagnosis of space-occupying lesions in the head of the pancreas. *Chirurg* 1996; 67:1007-11. [German]

Brooks AD, Mallis MJ, Brennan MF, Conlon KC. The value of laparoscopy in the management of ampullary, duodenal, and distal bile duct tumors. *J Gastrointest Surg* 2002; 6:139-45.

Brown KM, Tompkins AJ, Yong S, Aranha GV, Shoup M. Pancreaticoduodenectomy is curative in the majority of patients with node-negative ampullary cancer. *Arch Surg* 2005; 140:529-32.

Carriaga MT, Henson DE. Liver, gallbladder, extrahepatic bile ducts, and pancreas. *Cancer* 1995; 75:171-90.

Chakravarthy A, Abrams RA, Yeo CJ, Korman LT, Donehower RC, Hruban RH, Zahurek ML, Grochow LB, O'Reilly S, Hurwitz H, Jaffee EM, Lillemoe KD, Cameron JL. Intensified adjuvant combined modality therapy for resected periampullary adenocarcinoma: acceptable toxicity and suggestion of improved 1-year disease-free survival. *Int J Radiat Oncol Biol Phys* 2000;48: 1089-96.

Chalasani N, Baluyut A, Ismail A, Zaman A, Sood G, Ghalib R, McCashland TM, Reddy KR, Zervos X, Anbari MA, Hoen H. Cholangiocarcinoma in patients with primary sclerosing cholangitis: a multicenter case-control study. *Hepatology* 2000; 31:7-11.

Chan C, Herrera MF, de la Garza L, Quintanilla-Martinez L, Vargas-Vorackova F, Richaud-Patin Y, Llorente L, Uscanga L, Robles-Diaz G, Leon E, et al. Clinical behavior and prognostic factors of periampullary adenocarcinoma. *Ann Surg* 1995;222: 632-7.

Chen CH, Tseng LJ, Yang CC, Yeh YH. Preoperative evaluation of periampullary tumors by endoscopic sonography, transabdominal sonography, and computed tomography. *J Clin Ultrasound* 2001;29:313-21.

Cheng CL, Sherman S, Fogel EL, McHenry L, Watkins JL, Fukushima T, Howard TJ, Lazzell-Pannell L, Lehman GA. Endoscopic snare papillectomy for tumors of the duodenal papillae. *Gastrointest Endosc* 2004; 60:757-64.

Das A, Neugut AI, Cooper GS, Chak A. Association of ampullary and colorectal malignancies. *Cancer* 2004; 100:524-30.

de Castro SM, Kuhlmann KF, van Heek NT, Busch OR, Offerhaus GJ, van Gulik TM, Obertop H, Gouma DJ. Recurrent disease after microscopically radical (R0) resection of periampullary adenocarcinoma in patients without adjuvant therapy. *J Gastrointest Surg* 2004; 8:775-84

Di Carlo V, Gianotti L, Balzano G, Zerbi A, Braga M. Complications of pancreatic surgery and the role of perioperative nutrition. *Dig Surg* 1999; 16:320-6.

Di Giorgio A, Alfieri S, Rotondi F, Prete F, Di Miceli D, Ridolfini MP, Rosa F, Covino M, Doglietto GB. Pancreatoduodenectomy for tumors of Vater's ampulla: report on 94 consecutive patients. *World J Surg* 2005; 29:513-8.

Domagk D, Poremba C, Dietl KH, Senninger N, Heinecke A, Domschke W, Menzel J. Endoscopic transpapillary biopsies and intraductal ultrasonography in the diagnostics of bile duct strictures: a prospective study. *Gut* 2002;51: 240-4.

Domagk D, Wessling J, Reimer P, Hertel L, Poremba C, Senninger N, Heinecke A, Domschke W, Menzel J. Endoscopic retrograde cholangiopancreatography, intraductal ultrasonography, and magnetic resonance cholangiopancreatography in bile duct strictures: a prospective comparison of imaging diagnostics with histopathological correlation. *Am J Gastroenterol* 2004;99: 1684-9.

Eloubeidi MA, Chen VK, Eltoum IA, Jhala D, Chhieng DC, Jhala N, Vickers SM, Wilcox CM. Endoscopic ultrasound-guided fine needle aspiration biopsy of patients with suspected pancreatic cancer: diagnostic accuracy and acute and 30-day complications. *Am J Gastroenterol* 2003; 98:2663-8.

Eloubeidi MA, Gress FG, Savides TJ, Wiersema MJ, Kochman ML, Ahmad NA, Ginsberg GG, Erickson RA, Dewitt J, Van Dam J, Nickl NJ, Levy MJ, Clain JE, Chak A, Sivak MV Jr, Wong R, Isenberg G,

Scheiman JM, Bounds B, Kimmey MB, Saunders MD, Chang KJ, Sharma A, Nguyen P, Lee JG, Edmundowicz SA, Early D, Azar R, Etemad B, Chen YK, Waxman I, Shami V, Catalano MF, Wilcox CM. Acute pancreatitis after EUS-guided FNA of solid pancreatic masses: a pooled analysis from EUS centers in the United States. *Gastrointest Endosc* 2004; 60:385-9.

Farnell MB, Sakorafas GH, Sarr MG, Rowland CM, Tsiotos GG, Farley DR, Nagorney DM. Villous tumors of the duodenum: reappraisal of local vs. extended resection. *J Gastrointest Surg* 2000; 4:13-21.

Pisters PW, Hudec WA, Hess KR, Lee JE, Vauthey JN, Lahoti S, Raijman I, Evans DB. Effect of preoperative biliary decompression on pancreaticoduodenectomy-associated morbidity in 300 consecutive patients. *Ann Surg* 2001; 234:47-55.

Fletcher DR, Jones RM. Laparoscopic cholecystjejunostomy as palliation for obstructive jaundice in inoperable carcinoma of pancreas. *Surg Endosc* 1992; 6:147-9.

Freeman JS, Jr. *Cancer: principles and practice of oncology,* 6th ed. Philadelphia, Pa: Lippincott Williams & Wilkins, 2001; 1126-217.

Fritscher-Ravens A, Broering DC, Knoefel WT, Rogiers X, Swain P, Thonke F, Bobrowski C, Topalidis T, Soehendra N. EUS guided fine-needle aspiration of suspected hilar cholangiocarcinoma in potentially operable patients with negative brush cytology. *Am J Gastroenterol* 2004; 99:45-51.

Fritscher-Ravens A, Knoefel WT, Krause C, Swain CP, Brandt L, Patel K. Three-dimensional linear endoscopic ultrasound-feasibility of a novel technique applied for the detection of vessel involvement of pancreatic masses. *Am J Gastroenterol* 2005;100:1296-302.

Fong Y, Blumgart LH, Lin E, Fortner JG, Brennan MF. Outcome of treatment for distal bile duct cancer. *Br J Surg* 1996; 83:1712-5.

Gianotti L, Braga M, Fortis C, Soldini L, Vignali A, Colombo S, Radaelli G, Di Carlo V. A prospective, randomized clinical trial on perioperative feeding with an arginine-, omega-3 fatty acid-, and RNA-enriched enteral diet: effect on host response and nutritional status. *J Parenter Enteral Nutr* 1999; 23:314-20.

Giorgio PD, Luca LD. Comparison of treatment outcomes between biliary plastic stent placements with and without endoscopic sphincterotomy for inoperable malignant common bile duct obstruction. *World J Gastroenterol* 2004; 10:1212-4.

Glasbrenner B, Ardan M, Boeck W, Preclik G, Moller P, Adler G. Prospective evaluation of brush cytology of biliary strictures during endoscopic retrograde cholangiopancreatography. *Endoscopy* 1999; 31:712-7.

Greene F, Page D, Fleming I, Fritz A, Balch C, Haller D, Morrow M. AJCC *Cancer Staging Manual,* 6th ed. New York: Springer-Verlag, 2002.

Greene FL. TNM staging for malignancies of the digestive tract: 2003 changes and beyond. *Semin Surg Oncol* 2003; 21:23-9.

Groves CJ, Saunders BP, Spigelman AD, Phillips RK. Duodenal cancer in patients with familial adenomatous polyposis (FAP): results of a 10 year prospective study. *Gut* 2002; 50:636-41.

Haarmann W, Busing M, Reith HB, Wysocki P, Kozuschek W. The oncological approach to pylorus preserving pancreatoduodenectomy (PP-PD) in pancreas malignancies. *Wiad Lek* 1997;50:140-4.

Hamade AM, Al-Bahrani AZ, Owera AM, Hamoodi AA, Abid GH, Hani OI, O'shea S, Lee SH, Ammori BJ. Therapeutic, prophylactic, and preresection applications of laparoscopic gastric and biliary bypass for patients with periampullary malignancy. *Surg Endosc* 2005; [Epub ahead of print].

Hodul P, Creech S, Pickleman J, Aranha GV. The effect of preoperative biliary stenling on postoperative complications after pancreaticoduodenectomy. *Am J Surg* 2003; 186:420-5.

Holt AP, Patel M, Ahmed MM. Palliation of patients with malignant gastroduodenal obstruction with self-expanding metallic stents: the treatment of choice? *Gastrointest Endosc* 2004; 60:1010-7.

Horstmann O, Markus PM, Ghadimi MB, Becker H. Pylorus preservation has no impact on delayed gastric emptying after pancreatic head resection. *Pancreas* 2004; 28:69-74.

House MG, Yeo CJ, Cameron JL, Campbell KA, Schulick RD, Leach SD, Hruban RH, Horton KM, Fishman EK, Lillemoe KD. Predicting resectability of periampullary cancer with three-dimensional computed tomography. *J Gastrointest Surg* 2004; 8:280-8.

Howe JR, Klimstra DS, Moccia RD, Conlon KC, Brennan MF. Factors predictive of survival in ampullary carcinoma. *Ann Surg* 1998; 228:87-94.

Ihse I, Axelson J, Dawiskiba S, Hansson L. Pancreatic biopsy: why? When? How? *World J Surg* 1999; 23:896-900.

Inui K, Miyoshi H. Cholangiocarcinoma and intraductal sonography. *Gastrointest Endosc Clin N Am* 2005; 15:143-55.

Inui K, Nakazawa S, Yoshino J, Ukai H. Endoscopic MRI. *Pancreas* 1998; 16:413-7.

Jarnagin WR, Shoup M. Surgical management of cholangiocarcinoma. *Semin Liver Dis* 2004;24: 189-99.

Jarnagin WR, Shoup M. Surgical management of cholangiocarcinoma. *Semin Liver Dis* 2004; 24:189-99.

Jarufe NP, Coldham C, Mayer AD, Mirza DF, Buckels JA, Bramhall SR. Favourable prognostic factors in a large UK experience of adenocarcinoma of the head of the pancreas and periampullary region. *Dig Surg* 2004;21:202-9.

Jemal A, Thomas A, Murray T, Thun M. Cancer statistics, 2002. *CA Cancer J Clin* 2002; 52:23-47.

Johnson JC, DiSario JA, Grady WM. Surveillance and Treatment of Periampullary and Duodenal Adenomas in Familial Adenomatous Polyposis. Curr Treat Options *Gastroenterol* 2004; 7:79-89.

Kaassis M, Boyer J, Dumas R, Ponchon T, Coumaros D, Delcenserie R, Canard JM, Fritsch J, Rey JF, Burtin P. Plastic or metal stents for malignant stricture of the common bile duct? Results of a randomized prospective study. *Gastrointest Endosc* 2003; 57:178-82.

Kadmon M, Tandara A, Herfarth C. Duodenal adenomatosis in familial adenomatous polyposis coli. A review of the literature and results from the Heidelberg Polyposis Register. *Int J Colorectal Dis* 2001;16:63-75.

Kalady MF, Clary BM, Clark LA, Gottfried M, Rohren EM, Coleman RE, Pappas TN, Tyler DS. Clinical utility of positron emission tomography in the diagnosis and management of periampullary neoplasms. *Ann Surg Oncol* 2002; 9:799-806.

Katz MH, Bouvet M, Al-Refaie W, Gilpin EA, Moossa AR. Non-pancreatic periampullary adenocarcinomas: an explanation for favorable prognosis. *Hepatogastroenterology* 2004; 51:842-6.

Kaw M, Singh S, Gagneja H, Azad P. Role of self-expandable metal stents in the palliation of malignant duodenal obstruction. *Surg Endosc* 2003; 17:646-50.

Khan AW, Dhillon AP, Hutchins R, Abraham A, Shah SR, Snooks S, Davidson BR. Prognostic significance of intratumoural microvessel density (IMD) in resected pancreatic and ampullary cancers to standard histopathological variables and survival. *Eur J Surg Oncol* 2002; 28:637-44.

Kim JH, Kim MJ, Park SI, Chung JJ, Lee WJ, Yoo HS, Lee JT. Differential diagnosis of periampullary carcinomas at MR imaging. *Radiographics* 2002; 22:1335-52.

Klapman JB, Chang KJ. Endoscopic ultrasound-guided fine-needle injection. *Gastrointest Endosc Clin N Am* 2005; 15:169-77.

Klempnauer J, Ridder GJ, Pichlmayr R. Prognostic factors after resection of ampullary carcinoma: multivariate survival analysis in comparison with ductal cancer of the pancreatic head. *Br J Surg* 1995; 82:1686-91.

Klempnauer J, Ridder GJ, Pichlmayr R. Prognostic factors after resection of ampullary carcinoma: multivariate survival analysis in comparison with ductal cancer of the pancreatic head. *Br J Surg* 1995; 82:1686-91.

Klinkenbijl JH, Jeekel J, Schmitz PI, Rombout PA, Nix GA, Bruining HA, van Blankenstein M. Carcinoma of the pancreas and periampullary region: palliation versus cure. *Br J Surg* 1993; 80:1575-8.

Kitoh H, Ryozawa S, Harada T, Kondoh S, Furuya T, Kawauchi S, Oga A, Okita K, Sasaki K. Comparative genomic hybridization analysis for pancreatic cancer specimens obtained by endoscopic ultrasonography-guided fine-needle aspiration. *J Gastroenterol* 2005; 40:511-7.

Kluge R, Schmidt F, Caca K, Barthel H, Hesse S, Georgi P, Seese A, Huster D, Berr F. Positron emission tomography with [(18)F]fluoro-2-deoxy-D-glucose for diagnosis and staging of bile duct cancer. *Hepatology* 2001; 33:1029-35.

Knyrim K, Wagner HJ, Pausch J, Vakil N. A prospective, randomized, controlled trial of metal stents for malignant obstruction of the common bile duct. *Endoscopy* 1993; 25:207-12.

Kobayashi S, Asano T, Yamasaki M, Kenmochi T, Nakagohri T, Ochiai T. Risk of bile duct carcinogenesis after excision of extrahepatic bile ducts in pancreaticobiliary maljunction. *Surgery* 1999;126:939-44.

Kobayashi S, Asano T, Ochiai T. A proposal of no-touch isolation technique in pancreatoduodenectomy for periampullary carcinomas. *Hepatogastroenterology* 2001; 48:372-4.

Kosugi C, Furuse J, Ishii H, Maru Y, Yoshino M, Kinoshita T, Konishi M, Nakagohri T, Inoue K, Oda T. Needle tract implantation of hepatocellular carcinoma and pancreatic carcinoma after ultrasound-guided percutaneous puncture: clinical and pathologic characteristics and the treatment of needle tract implantation. *World J Surg* 2004; 28:29-32.

Kuriansky J, Saenz A, Astudillo E, Cardona V, Fernandez-Cruz L. Simultaneous laparoscopic biliary and retrocolic gastric bypass in patients with unresectable carcinoma of the pancreas. *Surg Endosc* 2000;14:179-81.

Lee H, Hirose S, Bratton B, Farmer D. Initial experience with complex laparoscopic biliary surgery in children: biliary atresia and choledochal cyst. *J Pediatr Surg* 2004; 39:804-7.

Lillemoe KD, Cameron JL, Hardacre JM, Sohn TA, Sauter PK, Coleman J, Pitt HA, Yeo CJ. Is prophylactic gastrojejunostomy indicated for unresectable periampullary cancer? A prospective randomized trial. *Ann Surg* 1999; 230:322-8.

Lln MH, Chcn JS, Chen HH, Su WC. A phase II trial of gemcitabine in the treatment of advanced bile duct and periampullary carcinomas. *Chemotherapy* 2003; 49:154-8.

Lin PW, Lin YJ. Prospective randomized comparison between pylorus-preserving and standard pancreaticoduodenectomy. *Br J Surg* 1999;86:603-7.

Lindell G, Borch K, Tingstedt B, Enell EL, Ihse I. Management of cancer of the ampulla of Vater: does local resection play a role? *Dig Surg* 2003; 20:511-5.

Liu JF, Li A, Liu Q, Zhou JS, Sun JB, Li D. Surgical treatment of 475 patients with periampullary carcinoma. *Zhonghua Zhong Liu Za Zhi* 2005; 27:251-3. [Article in Chinese].

Madjov R, Chervenkov P. Carcinoma of the papilla of Vater. Diagnostic and surgical problems. *Hepatogastroenterology* 2003; 50:621-4.

Madjov R, Chervenkov P. Carcinoma of the papilla of Vater. Diagnostic and surgical problems. *Hepatogastroenterology* 2003; 50:621-4.

Marcus SG, Dobryansky M, Shamamian P, Cohen H, Gouge TH, Pachter HL, Eng K. Endoscopic biliary drainage before pancreaticoduodenectomy for periampullary malignancies. *J Clin Gastroenterol* 1998;26:125-9.

Martignoni ME, Wagner M, Krahenbuhl L, Redaelli CA, Friess H, Buchler MW. Effect of preoperative biliary drainage on surgical outcome after pancreatoduodenectomy. *Am J Surg* 2001; 181:52-9.

Martin JA, Haber GB. Ampullary adenoma: clinical manifestations, diagnosis, and treatment. *Gastrointest Endosc Clin N Am* 2003; 13:649-69.

McKenna GJ, Meneghetti A, Chen YL, Mui AL, Ong C, Scudamore CH, McMaster WR, Owen DA, Chung SW. Predictive value of lymph node and tumor matrix metalloproteinase expression in the analysis of metastatic periampullary tumors. *J Surg Oncol* 2005; 90:239-46.

Menack MJ, Spitz JD, Arregui ME. Staging of pancreatic and ampullary cancers for resectability using laparoscopy with laparoscopic ultrasound. *Surg Endosc* 2001; 15:1129-34.

Menzel J, Poremba C, Dietl KH, Bocker W, Domschke W. Tumors of the papilla of Vater--inadequate diagnostic impact of endoscopic forceps biopsies taken prior to and following sphincterotomy. *Ann Oncol* 1999; 10:1227-31.

Michelassl F, Erroi F, Dawson PJ, Pietrabissa A, Noda S, Handcock M, Block GE. Experience with 647 consecutive tumors of the duodenum, ampulla, head of the pancreas, and distal common bile duct. *Ann Surg* 1989; 210:544-54.

Mimura H, Mori M, Hamazaki K, Tsuge H. Isolated pancreatectomy for ductal carcinoma of the head of the pancreas. *Hepatogastroenterology* 1994; 41:483-8.

Minnard EA, Conlon KC, Hoos A, Dougherty EC, Hann LE, Brennan MF. Laparoscopic ultrasound enhances standard laparoscopy in the staging of pancreatic cancer. *Ann Surg* 1998; 228:182-7.

Moossa AR, Gamagami RA. Diagnosis and staging of pancreatic neoplasms. *Surg Clin North Am* 1995; 75:871-90.

Naef M, Buhlmann M, Metzger D, Baer HU. Periampullary carcinomas: a special entity of duodenal tumors. *Swiss Surg* 1999; 5:11-3.

Nakagohri T, Jolesz FA, Okuda S, Asano T, Kenmochi T, Kainuma O, Tokoro Y, Aoyama H, Lorensen WE, Kikinis R. Virtual pancreatoscopy of mucin-producing pancreatic tumors. *Comput Aided Surg* 1998; 3:264-8.

Nakaizumi A, Uehara H, Iishi H, Tatsuta M, Kitamura T, Kuroda C, Ohigashi H, Ishikawa O, Okuda S. Endoscopic ultrasonography in diagnosis and staging of pancreatic cancer. *Dig Dis Sci* 1995; 40:696-700.

Nakazawa S, Inui K. Endosonography and endoscopic magnetic resonance imaging. *Baillieres Best Pract Res Clin Gastroenterol* 1999; 13:21-31.

Nanashima A, Yamaguchi H, Shibasaki S, Ide N, Sawai T, Tsuji T, Hidaka S, Sumida Y, Nakagoe T, Nagayasu T. Adjuvant photodynamic therapy for bile duct carcinoma after surgery: a preliminary study. *J Gastroenterol* 2004; 39:1095-101.

Nathanson LK. Laparoscopic cholecyst-jejunostomy and gastroenterostomy for malignant disease. *Surg Oncol* 1993; 2:19-24.

Nguyen TC, Sohn TA, Cameron JL, Lillemoe KD, Campbell KA, Coleman J, Sauter PK, Abrams RA, Hruban RH, Yeo CJ. Standard vs. radical pancreaticoduodenectomy for periampullary adenocarcinoma: a prospective, randomized trial evaluating quality of life in pancreaticoduodenectomy survivors. *J Gastrointest Surg* 2003; 7:1-9.

Nikfarjam M, Muralidharan V, McLean C, Christophi C. Local resection of ampullary adenocarcinomas of the duodenum. *ANZ J Surg* 2001; 71:529-33.

Offerhaus GJ, Giardiello FM, Krush AJ, Booker SV, Tersmette AC, Kelley NC, Hamilton SR. The risk of upper gastrointestinal cancer in familial adenomatous polyposis. *Gastroenterology* 1992; 102:1980-2.

Ogilvie H. Thomas's sign, or the silver stool in cancer of the ampulla of Vater. *Br Med J* 1955; 4907:208.

Oka S, Tanaka S, Nagata S, Hiyama T, Ito M, Kitadai Y, Yoshihara M, Haruma K, Chayama K. Clinicopathologic features and endoscopic resection of early primary nonampullary duodenal carcinoma. *J Clin Gastroenterol* 2003; 37:381-6.

Okorie MI, Hussain SA, Riley PL, McCafferty IJ. The use of self-expandable metal stents in the palliation of malignant bowel obstruction. *Oncol Rep* 2004; 12:67-71.

Ortner ME, Caca K, Berr F, Liebetruth J, Mansmann U, Huster D, Voderholzer W, Schachschal G, Mossner J, Lochs H. Successful photodynamic therapy for nonresectable cholangiocarcinoma: a randomized prospective study. *Gastroenterology* 2003; 125:1355-63.

Paksoy N, Lilleng R, Hagmar B, Wetteland J. Diagnostic accuracy of fine needle aspiration cytology in pancreatic lesions. A review of 77 cases. *Acta Cytol* 1993; 37:889-93.

Parsons L Jr, Palmer CH. How accurate is fine-needle biopsy in malignant neoplasia of the pancreas? *Arch Surg* 1989; 124:681-3.

Pavone P, Laghi A, Panebianco V, Catalano C, Lobina L, Passariello R. MR cholangiography: techniques and clinical applications. *Eur Radiol* 1998;8:901-10.

Pedrazzoli S, Beger HG, Obertop H, Andren-Sandberg A, Fernandez-Cruz L, Henne-Bruns D, Luttges J, Neoptolemos JP. A surgical and pathological based classification of resective treatment of pancreatic cancer. Summary of an international workshop on surgical procedures in pancreatic cancer. *Dig Surg* 1999; 16:337-45.

Pedrazzoli S, DiCarlo V, Dionigi R, Mosca F, Pederzoli P, Pasquali C, Kloppel G, Dhaene K, Michelassi F. Standard versus extended lymphadenectomy associated with pancreatoduodenectomy in the surgical treatment of adenocarcinoma of the head of the pancreas: a multicenter, prospective, randomized study. Lymphadenectomy Study Group. *Ann Surg* 1998; 228:508-17.

Pietrabissa A, Vistoli F, Carobbi A, Boggi U, Bisa M, Mosca F. Thoracoscopic splanchnicectomy for pain relief in unresectable pancreatic cancer. *Arch Surg* 2000; 135:332-5.

Ponsioen CY, Vrouenraets SM, van Milligen de Wit AW, Sturm P, Tascilar M, Offerhaus GJ, Prins M, Huibregtse K, Tytgat GN. Value of brush cytology for dominant strictures in primary sclerosing cholangitis. *Endoscopy* 1999; 31:305-9.

Popovici A, Popescu I, Ionescu MI, Vasilescu C, Ciurea S, Tonea A, David L. The periampullary carcinoma. Clinical and therapeutic alternatives. *Chirurgia (Bucur)* 2000; 95:407-24. [Romanian]

Posner S, Colletti L, Knol J, Mulholland M, Eckhauser F. Safety and long-term efficacy of transduodenal excision for tumors of the ampulla of Vater. *Surgery* 2000; 128:694-701.

Povoski SP, Karpeh MS Jr, Conlon KC, Blumgart LH, Brennan MF. Preoperative biliary drainage: impact on intraoperative bile cultures and infectious morbidity and mortality after pancreaticoduodenectomy. *J Gastrointest Surg* 1999; 3:496-505.

Prat F, Chapat O, Ducot B, Ponchon T, Pelletier G, Fritsch J, Choury AD, Buffet C. A randomized trial of endoscopic drainage methods for inoperable malignant strictures of the common bile duct. *Gastrointest Endosc* 1998; 47:1-7.

Pungpapong S, Noh KW, Wallace MB. Endoscopic ultrasonography in the diagnosis and management of cancer. *Expert Rev Mol Diagn* 2005; 5:585-97.

Rashleigh-Belcher HJ, Russell RC, Lees WR. Cutaneous seeding of pancreatic carcinoma by fine-needle aspiration biopsy. *Br J Radiol* 1986; 59:182-3.

Razzaq R, Laasch HU, England R, Marriott A, Martin D. Expandable metal stents for the palliation of malignant gastroduodenal obstruction. *Cardiovasc Intervent Radiol* 2001; 24:313-8.

Rhodes M, Nathanson L, Fielding G. Laparoscopic biliary and gastric bypass: a useful adjunct in the treatment of carcinoma of the pancreas. *Gut* 1995; 36:778-80.

Riddell RH, Petras RE, Williams GT, Sobin LH: *Atlas of tumour pathology: Tumours of the intestines.* Washington DC: Armed forces institute of Pathology; 2003.

Ridder GJ, Klemprauer J. Clinical symptoms in cancer of the exocrine pancreas in peri-ampullary region. Old and new knowledge from the analysis of a surgical patient sample. *Zentralbl Chir* 1996; 121:557-64. [German]

Ross WA, Bismar MM. Evaluation and management of periampullary tumors. *Curr Gastroenterol Rep* 2004; 6:362-70.

Ryder NM, Ko CY, Hines OJ, Gloor B, Reber HA. Primary duodenal adenocarcinoma: a 40-year experience. *Arch Surg* 2000; 135:1070-4.

Saenz A, Kuriansky J, Salvador L, Astudillo E, Cardona V, Shabtai M, Fernandez-Cruz L. Thoracoscopic splanchnicectomy for pain control in patients with unresectable carcinoma of the pancreas. *Surg Endosc* 2000; 14:717-20.

Saleh MM, Norregaard P, Jorgensen HL, Andersen PK, Matzen P. Preoperative endoscopic stent placement before pancreaticoduodenectomy: a meta-analysis of the effect on morbidity and mortality. *Gastrointest Endosc* 2002; 56:529-34.

Sarmiento JM, Nagomey DM, Sarr MG, Farnell MB. Periampullary cancers: are there differences? *Surg Clin North Am* 2001; 81:543-55.

Sarmiento JM, Thompson GB, Nagorney DM, Donohue JH, Farnell MB. Pancreas-sparing duodenectomy for duodenal polyposis. *Arch Surg* 2002; 137:557-62.

Saurin JC, Gutknecht C, Napoleon B, Chavaillon A, Ecochard R, Scoazec JY, Ponchon T, Chayvialle JA. Surveillance of duodenal adenomas in familial adenomatous polyposis reveals high cumulative risk of advanced disease. *J Clin Oncol* 2004;22:493-8.

Schiefke I, Zabel-Langhennig A, Wiedmann M, Huster D, Witzigmann H, Mossner J, Berr F, Caca K. Self-expandable metallic stents for malignant duodenal obstruction caused by biliary tract cancer. *Gastrointest Endosc* 2003; 58:213-9.

Schlippert W, Lucke D, Anuras S, Christensen J. Carcinoma of the papilla of Vater. A review of fifty-seven cases. *Am J Surg* 1978; 135:763-70.

Schwarz A, Beger HG. Biliary and gastric bypass or stenting in nonresectable periampullary cancer: analysis on the basis of controlled trials. *Int J Pancreatol* 2000; 27:51-8.

Schwarz M, Pauls S, Sokiranski R, Brambs HJ, Glasbrenner B, Adler G, Diederichs CG, Reske SN, Moller P, Beger HG. Is a preoperative multidiagnostic approach to predict surgical resectability of periampullary tumors still effective? *Am J Surg* 2001;182:243-9.

Schwarz RE, Smith DD, Keny H, Ikle DN, Shibata SI, Chu DZ, Pezner RD. Impact of intraoperative radiation on postoperative and disease-specific outcome after pancreatoduodenectomy for adenocarcinoma: a propensity score analysis. *Am J Clin Oncol* 2003; 26:16-21.

Scott-Coombes DM, Williamson RC. Surgical treatment of primary duodenal carcinoma: a personal series. *Br J Surg* 1994; 81:1472-4.

Seiler CA, Wagner M, Bachmann T, Redaelli CA, Schmied B, Uhl W, Friess H, Buchler MW. Randomized clinical trial of pylorus-preserving duodenopancreatectomy versus classical Whipple resection-long term results. *Br J Surg* 2005; 92:547-56.

Sewnath ME, Birjmohun RS, Rauws EA, Huibregtse K, Obertop H, Gouma DJ. The effect of preoperative biliary drainage on postoperative complications after pancreaticoduodenectomy. *J Am Coll Surg* 2001; 192:726-34.

Shao YF, Wu TC, Shan Y, Wu JX, Wang X, Zhao P. Clinico-pathological characteristics of surgical effect on periampullary cancers: report of 631 cases. *Zhonghua Yi Xue Za Zhi* 2005; 85:510-3. [Chinese]

Sherlock S, Dooley J. Diseases of the ampulla of Vater and pancreas. In: Sherlock S, Dooley J, eds. *Diseases of the liver and biliary system,* 10th ed. London: Blackwell Science; 2000 p. 633-640.

Shim CS. Photodynamic therapy in gastroenterology. *Korean J Gastroenterol* 2005; 45:153-61. [Korean]

Shin HJ, Lahoti S, Sneige N. Endoscopic ultrasound-guided fine-needle aspiration in 179 cases: the M. D. Anderson Cancer Center experience: *Cancer* 2002; 96:174-80.

Shoup M, Hodul P, Aranha GV, Choe D, Olson M, Leya J, Losurdo J. Defining a role for endoscopic ultrasound in staging periampullary tumors. *Am J Surg* 2000; 179:453-6.

Shyr YM, Su CH, Lo SS, Wang HC, Lui WY. Is pancreatoduodenectomy justified for periampullary cancers with regional lymph node involvement? *Am Surg* 1995; 61:288-93.

Smits NJ, Reeders JW. Imaging and staging of biliopancreatic malignancy: role of ultrasound. *Ann Oncol* 1999; 10:20-4.

Sobin LH, Wittekind C. UICC TNM *Classification of Malignant Tumours.* 6th ed. New York: Wiley-Liss; 2002.

Sohn TA, Lillemoe KD, Cameron JL, Huang JJ, Pitt HA, Yeo CJ. Surgical palliation of unresectable periampullary adenocarcinoma in the 1990s. *J Am Coll Surg* 1999;188:658-66.

Song HY, Shin JH, Yoon CJ, Lee GH, Kim TW, Lee SK, Yook JH, Kim BS. A dual expandable nitinol stent: experience in 102 patients with malignant gastroduodenal strictures. *J Vasc Interv Radiol* 2004; 15:1443-9.

Spigelman AD, Williams CB, Talbot IC, Domizio P, Phillips RK. Upper gastrointestinal cancer in patients with familial adenomatous polyposis. *Lancet* 1989; 2:783-5.

Staats PS, Hekmat H, Sauter P, Lillemoe K. The effects of alcohol celiac plexus block, pain, and mood on longevity in patients with unresectable pancreatic cancer: a double-blind, randomized, placebo-controlled study. *Pain Med* 2001; 2:28-34.

Stefaniak T, Basinski A, Vingerhoets A, Makarewicz W, Connor S, Kaska L, Stanek A, Kwiecinska B, Lachinski AJ, Sledzinski Z. A comparison of two invasive techniques in the management of intractable pain due to inoperable pancreatic cancer: neurolytic celiac plexus block and videothoracoscopic splanchnicectomy. *Eur J Surg Oncol* 2005; [Epub ahead of print]

Stojadinovic A, Brooks A, Hoos A, Jaques DP, Conlon KC, Brennan MF. An evidence-based approach to the surgical management of resectable pancreatic adenocarcinoma. *J Am Coll Surg* 2003;196:954-64.

Su CH, Shyr YM, Lui WY, P'eng FK. Factors affecting morbidity, mortality and survival after pancreaticoduodenectomy for carcinoma of the ampulla of Vater. *Hepatogastroenterology* 1999; 46:1973-9.

Tamada K, Tomiyama T, Wada S, Ohashi A, Satoh Y, Ido K, Sugano K. Endoscopic transpapillary bile duct biopsy with the combination of intraductal ultrasonography in the diagnosis of biliary strictures. *Gut* 2002; 50:326-31.

Tan HL, Shankar KR, Ford WD. Laparoscopic resection of type I choledochal cyst. *Surg Endosc* 2003;17:1495.

Tanasijtchouk T, Vaisbein E, Lachter J, Nassar F. Carcinoma of Papilla Vateri presenting as recurrent acute pancreatitis. *Acta Gastroenterol Belg* 2004; 67:309-10.

Tanizawa Y, Nakagohri T, Konishi M, Inoue K, Oda T, Takahashi S, Kawahira H, Nakamura T, Nishimori T, Nagase M, Ueda T, Kinoshita T. Virtual pancreatoscopy of pancreatic cancer. *Hepatogastroenterology* 2003; 50:559-62.

Telford JJ, Carr-Locke DL, Baron TH, Tringali A, Parsons WG, Gabbrielli A, Costamagna G. Palliation of patients with malignant gastric outlet obstruction with the enteral Wallstent: outcomes from a multicenter study. *Gastrointest Endosc* 2004; 60:916-20.

Tilleman EH, Kuiken BW, Phoa SS, de Castro SM, Busch OR, Obertop H, Gouma DJ. Limitation of diagnostic laparoscopy for patients with a peri-ampullary carcinoma. *Eur J Surg Oncol* 2004;30: 658-62.

Todani T, Watanabe Y, Narusue M, Tabuchi K, Okajima K. Congenital bile duct cysts: Classification, operative procedures, and review of thirty-seven cases including cancer arising from choledochal cyst. Am J Surg 1977; 134:263-9.

Tomazic A, Pegan V, Ferlan-Marolt K, Pleskovic A, Luzar B. Cyclin D1 and bax influence the prognosis after pancreatoduodenectomy for periampullary adenocarcinoma. *Hepatogastroenterology* 2004;51:1832-7.

Tran KT, Smeenk HG, van Eijck CH, Kazemier G, Hop WC, Greve JW, Terpstra OT, Zijlstra JA, Klinkert P, Jeekel H. Pylorus preserving pancreaticoduodenectomy versus standard Whipple procedure: a prospective, randomized, multicenter analysis of 170 patients with pancreatic and periampullary tumors. *Ann Surg* 2004; 240:738-45.

Tran TC, Vitale GC. Ampullary tumors: endoscopic versus operative management. *Surg Innov* 2004; 11:255-63.

Tsiotos GG, Farnell MB, Sarr MG. Are the results of pancreatectomy for pancreatic cancer improving? *World J Surg* 1999; 23:913-9.

Urbach DR, Bell CM, Austin PC. Differences in operative mortality between high- and low-volume hospitals in Ontario for 5 major surgical procedures: estimating the number of lives potentially saved through regionalization. *CMAJ* 2003; 168:1409-14.

Urbach DR, Bell CM, Swanstrom LL, Hansen PD. Cohort study of surgical bypass to the gallbladder or bile duct for the palliation of jaundice due to pancreatic cancer. *Ann Surg* 2003; 237:86-93.

van Bokhorst-De Van Der Schueren MA, Quak JJ, von Blomberg-van der Flier BM, Kuik DJ, Langendoen SI, Snow GB, Green CJ, van Leeuwen PA. Effect of perioperative nutrition, with and without arginine supplementation, on nutritional status, immune function, postoperative morbidity, and survival in severely malnourished head and neck cancer patients. *Am J Clin Nutr* 2001; 73:323-32.

van Geenen RC, Keyzer-Dekker CM, van Tienhoven G, Obertop H, Gouma DJ. Pain management of patients with unresectable peripancreatic carcinoma. *World J Surg* 2002; 26:715-20.

van Geenen RC, van Gulik TM, Offerhaus GJ, de Wit LT, Busch OR, Obertop H, Gouma DJ. Survival after pancreaticoduodenectomy for periampullary adenocarcinoma: an update. *Eur J Surg Oncol* 2001;27:549-57.

Van Heek NT, De Castro SM, van Eijck CH, van Geenen RC, Hesselink EJ, Breslau PJ, Tran TC, Kazemier G, Visser MR, Busch OR, Obertop H, Gouma DJ. The need for a prophylactic gastrojejunostomy for unresectable periampullary cancer: a prospective randomized multicenter trial with special focus on assessment of quality of life. *Ann Surg* 2003;238:894-902.

Vazquez-Sequeiros E, Baron TH, Clain JE, Gostout CJ, Norton ID, Petersen BT, Levy MJ, Jondal ML, Wiersema MJ. Evaluation of indeterminate bile duct strictures by intraductal US. *Gastrointest Endosc* 2002; 56:372-9.

Vogt M, Jakobs R, Riemann JF. Rationale for endoscopic management of adenoma of the papilla of Vater: options and limitations. *Langenbecks Arch Surg* 2001; 386:176-82.

Vollmer CM, Drebin JA, Middleton WD, Teefey SA, Linehan DC, Soper NJ, Eagon CJ, Strasberg SM. Utility of staging laparoscopy in subsets of peripancreatic and biliary malignancies. *Ann Surg* 2002;235:1-7.

Wade TP, Coplin MA, Virgo KS, Johnson FE. Periampullary cancer treatment in U.S. Department of Veterans Affairs hospitals: 1987-1991. *Surgery* 1994; 116:819-25.

Wade TP, Prasad CN, Virgo KS, Johnson FE. Experience with distal bile duct cancers in U.S. Veterans Affairs hospitals: 1987-1991. *J Surg Oncol* 1997; 64:242-5.

Wang CH, Mo LR, Lin RC, Kuo JJ, Chang KK, Lin YW, Yang DM, Yau MP, Cho CY. A survival predictive model in patients undergoing radical resection of ampullary adenocarcinoma. *Hepatogastroenterology* 2004; 51:1495-9.

Warshaw AL, Fernandez-del Castillo C. Pancreatic carcinoma. *N Engl J Med* 1992; 326:455-65.

Warshaw AL. Implications of peritoneal cytology for staging of early pancreatic cancer. *Am J Surg* 1991; 161:26-9.

Watanapa P, Williamson RC. Surgical palliation for

pancreatic cancer: developments during the past two decades. *Br J Surg* 1992; 79:8-20.

Wray CJ, Ahmad SA, Matthews JB, Lowy AM. Surgery for pancreatic cancer: recent controversies and current practice. *Gastroenterology* 2005;128:1626-41.

Xing GS, Geng JC, Han XW, Dai JH, Wu CY. Endobiliary brush cytology during percutaneous transhepatic cholangiodrainage in patients with obstructive jaundice. *Hepatobiliary Pancreat Dis Int* 2005; 4:98-103.

Yeo CJ, Cameron JL, Lillemoe KD, Sohn TA, Campbell KA, Sauter PK, Coleman J, Abrams RA, Hruban RH. Pancreaticoduodenectomy with or without distal gastrectomy and extended retroperitoneal lymphadenectomy for periampullary adenocarcinoma, part 2: randomized controlled trial evaluating survival, morbidity, and mortality. *Ann Surg* 2002; 236:355-66.

Yeo CJ, Sohn TA, Cameron JL, Hruban RH, Lillemoe KD, Pitt HA. Periampullary adenocarcinoma: analysis of 5-year survivors. *Ann Surg* 1998;227: 821-31.

Yim HB, Yap WM, Chong PY. Clinical usefulness of endoscopic ultrasonography with or without fine needle aspiration in the diagnosis and staging of pancreatic carcinoma. *Ann Acad Med Singapore* 2005; 34:124-9.

Yoon YS, Kim SW, Park SJ, Lee HS, Jang JY, Choi MG, Kim WH, Lee KU, Park YH. Clinicopathologic analysis of early ampullary cancers with a focus on the feasibility of ampullectomy. *Ann Surg* 2005; 242:92-100.

ABBREVIATIONS

AJCC	American Joint Committee on Cancer
CA	Carbohydrate antigen
CBD	Common bile duct
COX	Cyclooxygenase
CPB	Coeliac plexus block
CT	Computed tomography
ERCP	Endoscopic retrograde cholangiopancreatography
EUS	Endoscopic ultrasound
FAP	Familial adenomatous polyposis
FNA	Fine needle aspirate
HNPCC	Hereditary non-polyposis colorectal cancer
IEN	Immune-enhancing nutrition
LN	Lymph node
MMP	Matrix metalloproteinases
MRCP	Magnetic resonance cholangiopancreatography
MRI	Magnetic resonance imaging
*non*P-PAC	Non-pancreatic periampullary cancer
PAC	Periampullary cancer
PBM	Pancreatobiliary maljunction
PD	Pancreaticoduodenectomy
PDT	Photodynamic therapy
PET	Positron emission tomography
P-PAC	Pancreatic periampullary cancer
PSC	Primary sclerosing cholangitis
PSD	Pancreas-sparing duodenectomy
TIMP	Tissue inhibitor of matrix metalloproteinase
US	Ultrasonography

Current advances in the diagnosis and treatment of cholangiocarcinoma

Mairiang P., Mairiang E.

ABSTRACT

Cholangiocarcinoma (CCA) is malignant tumor of the bile duct. In western countries, CCA is associated with primary sclerosing cholangitis. In Asia, CCA is associated with liver fluke infestation (Opisthorchiasis, Clonorchiasis) and hepatolithiasis. The pathogenesis of CCA is related to inflammation induced malignancy. CCA can be classified into Intrahepatic, perihilar and extrahepatic types.

The most common presentation of intrahepatic CCA is liver mass. The most common presentation of extrahepatic and perihilar CCA is obstructive jaundice. The diagnosis is based on imagings, tumor markers, histology and cytology. The treatment of choice is hepatic resection. Most are diagnosed at an advanced stage. Many palliative treatment modalities are introduced to improve quality of life of the patients. Liver transplantation in selective patients with pretransplantation treatment with neoadjuvant radiotherapy, and chemosensitization is the potential treatment to improve the survival. To control of liver fluke infestation may reduce the incidence of CCA in the endemic area.

DEFINITION OF CHOLANGIOCARCINOMA (CCA)

Cholangiocarcinoma is the primary malignant tumor of the bile duct epithelium. The carcinoma of the gall bladder and the ampulla of Vater are excluded. The tumor can be originated from intrahepatic bile duct (intrahepatic or peripheral type) perihilar (Klatskin type) and distal extrahepatic bile ducts.

Intrahepatic bile duct is defined as the portion that is proximal to the hepatic confluence. The tumor can occur in any sites of intrahepatic biliary tree from bile ductules to segmental bile ducts and the right or the left hepatic ducts.

The perihilar bile duct is defined as the bile duct at hepatic confluence including the right main and left main bile ducts and the common hepatic duct.

The extrahepatic bile ducts include the cystic duct and common bile duct (excluding ampulla of Vater). Uttaravichein T et al has a different definition. The intrahepatic CCA includes peripheral type and perihilar type. This classification is similar to Nakamura et al.

RISK FACTORS

Primary sclerosing cholangitis (PSC)

The most common risk factor of CCA in western countries is primary sclerosing cholangitis. The incidence of CCA in PSC ranges from 8-40%. The CCA is commonly multifocal and leads to progression of the clinical course of the disease.

Parasitic infestation

Opisthorchis viverrini and *Clonorchis* sinensis are the most common causes of CCA in Eastern countries. More than 9 million people in Thailand, Laos and Cambodia are infected by *Opisthorchis viverrini* and more than 7 million people in Korea, Taiwan, China, Hong Kong and Vietnam are infected by *Clonorchis sinensis*. The incidence of CCA in endemic areas of the liver flukes is 25-40 times higher than non-endemic areas.

Intrahepatic duct stone

The condition is common among Japanese and Chinese. The prevalence of CCA in patient with intrahepatic duct stone is 2-10%.

Thorotrast exposure

Thorotrast was a radionuclide used in the past for lymphangiography. After 30-35 years of exposure to thorotrast, CCA developed.

Congenital cystic disease of biliary tract

Choledochal cyst and Calori's disease are congenital cystic abnormalities of biliary tract that increased risk of CCA. The incidence of CCA in this condition is approximately 15-20%.

Genetic disorders

Multiple biliary papillomatosis, Gardner's syndrome and Lynch syndrome are reported to increase the risk of CCA.

PATHOGENESIS OF CHOLANGIOCARCINOMA

Biliary tract carcinogenesis has been studied extensively only in PSC associated CCA and Opisthorchis associated CCA.

Pathogenesis of PSC associated with CCA

PSC is a cholestatic liver disease associated with chronic inflammation of the biliary tree. It is slowly progressive disease, resulting in terminal biliary cirrhosis. CCA is the consequence of chronic inflammatory process generating proinflammatory cytokines that induce cholangiocytes to express the inducible form of nitric oxide syntase (iNOS). INOS generates nitric oxide (NO). NO may modified or alter DNA bases, leading to DNA damages and eventually mutation. Interleukin 6 (IL-6) is the important proinflammatory cytokines that alternates the growth of cholangiocytes.

Proliferation of cholangiocytes under mutagenic environment is the key process of carcinogenesis. Bile stasis is the characteristic of PSC. Bile acids in static bile under chronic inflammatory environment are changed to toxic bile acids. Toxic bile acids activate the epidermal growth factor receptor in cholangiocytes and induce cyclooxygenase -2-expression (COX-2). COX-2 enzyme inhibits apoptosis, promotes angiogenesis and enhances growth of malignancies. Mutation at p14, p16 and p53 are commonly found in PSC associated CCA. Exceptionally, p16 inactivation is potentially used as molecular diagnostic test for the cancer.

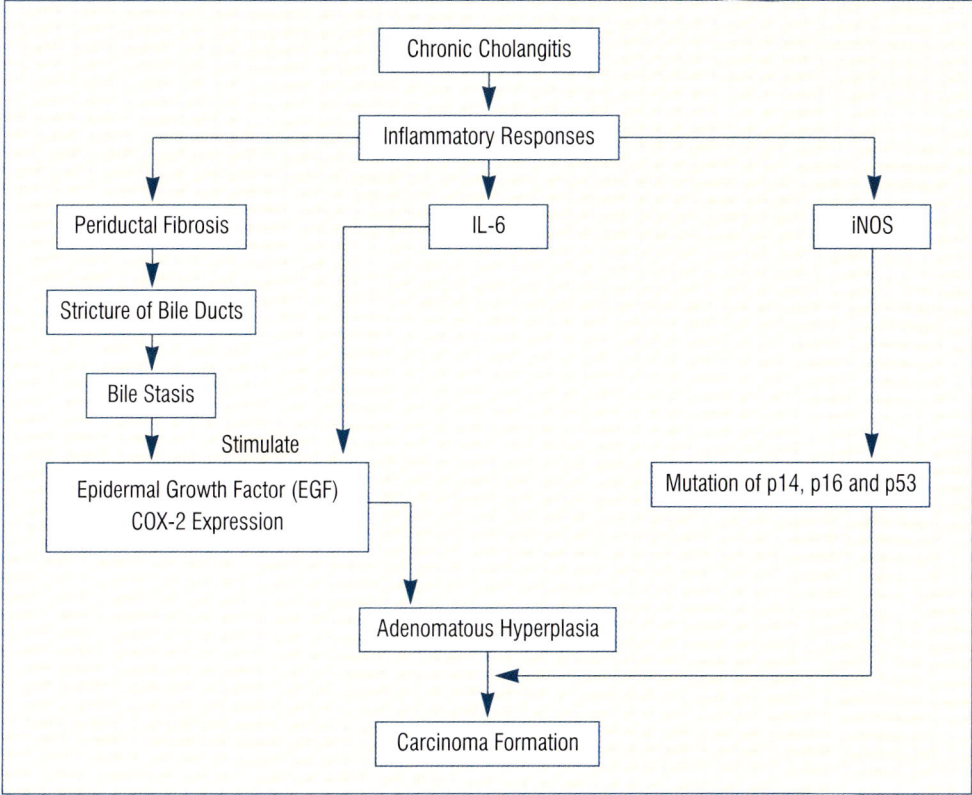

FIGURE 1: Diagram show pathogenesis of PSC associated CCA.

Pathogenesis of *O. viverini* associated CCA

Thammawit et al was able to induce CCA in Syrian hamsters by feeding *O. viverini* metacercariae and adding dimethylni-trosamine (DMN) in drinking water. The effects were dose-dependent. When giving an animal 50 metacercariae with DMN, 20% of animals developed CCA while giving 100 metacercariae with DMN all animals developed CCA. They suggested that *O. viverini* infection was the promoter and DMN was an initiator of CCA formation in the animal model. They also postulated that chronic *O. viverrini* infection and eating of nitrosamine-rich diet might be pathogenesis of human CCA.

The nitrosamine rich diets are commonly found in daily diet intake of people in the northeast of Thailand such as fermented fish (Pla-ra). Many scientists believed in this hypothesis of exogenous nitrosamine as a carcinogen. Recent reports suggested that liver fluke infection can produce endogenous nitrosation by inducing nitric oxide synthase production in macrophages, mast cells and eosinophils around the inflamed area surrounding the bile ducts. Endogenous nitrosation in *O. viverini* infected subjects is abolished by anti parasitic (Praziquantel) treatment and by co-administration of ascorbic acid. Both endogenous and exogenous nitrosamine formation lead to DNA damage of inflamed tissue and exert direct toxicity and mutation of biliary epithelium. Eventually the bilianct epithelium is transformed to CCA.

O. viverrini infection enhances host susceptibility to CCA by activation of drug metabolizing enzymes, particularly cytochrome P450 isoenzymes. The enzyme family is known to involve in activation and metabolism of various hepatic carcinogens including N-nitroso compounds and aflatoxins. Satarug et al observed that humans infected by liver flukes increased in CYP 2A6-related enzyme activity. This enzyme induction might play an important role in the activation of nitrosamine generated within inflamed tissue of the biliary tract.

K-ras proto-oncogene activation by point mutations is the most common genetic mutation of CCA. Most K-ras mutation at codon 12 are G to A (GGT to GAT).The model of nitrosamine induced *K-ras* mutation had been reported in pancreatic cancer and CCA induced in hamster. However, *K-ras* mutation among Thai CCA occurred only 16.7%. Other genetic mechanisms to stimulate bile duct epithelial hyperplasia such as over expression of COX-2, c-erB-2 (an epidermal growth factor receptor) and c-met (a hepatocyte growth factor receptor) have been reported in carcinoma of gall bladder and primary sclerosing cholangitis associated CCA.These mechanisms has not yet been explored in *O. viverrini* associated CCA. Mutation of *p53* is the most common tumor suppressor gene that had been reported in various cancers, this mutation occurred in 35% in Thai patients. Mutation of another tumor suppressor gene, *p15,* had also been reported in bile duct cancers.

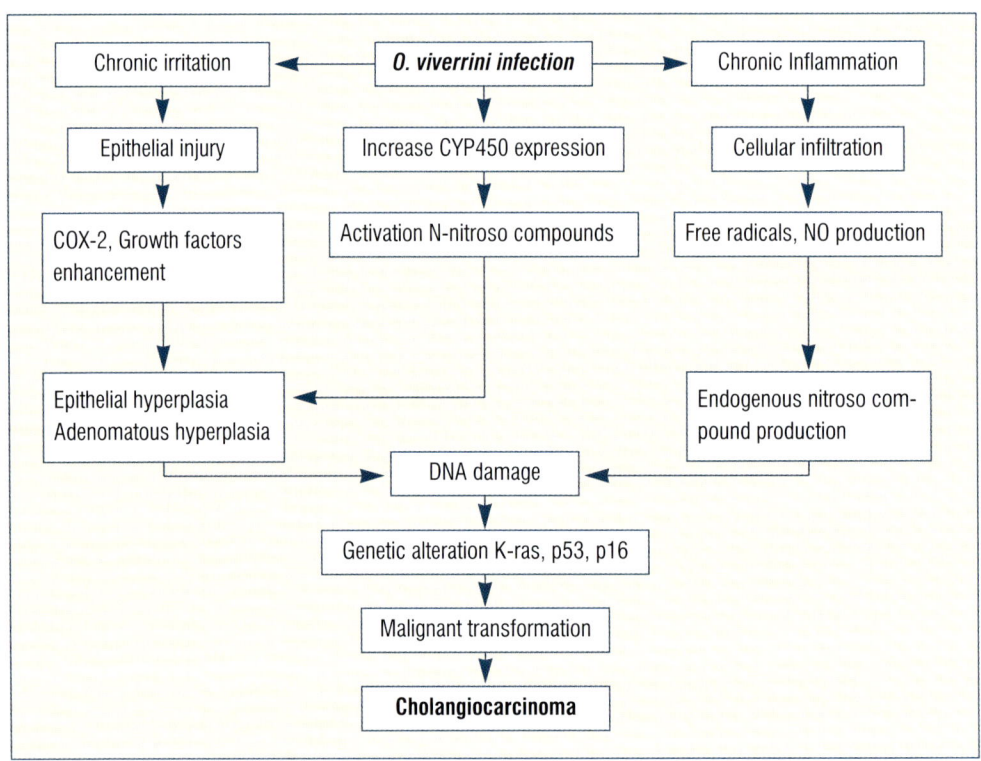

FIGURE 2: Diagram show pathogenesis of *O.viverini* associated CCA.

Pathology of CCA

Pathologic findings in patients with CCA are the combination of preexisting pathology (opisthorchiasis, clonorchiasis, primary sclerosing cholangitis, choledochal cyst etc) and pathology of Cholangiocarcinoma per se. In this chapter, we described only the pathology of Cholangiocarcinoma.

Many classifications of CCA have been reported. The liver cancer study group of Japan has introduced a classification based on growth characteristics as: a) mass forming, b) periductal infiltrating and c) intraductal growth type. This classification can be used in intrahepatic, perihilar and extrahepatic CCA.

a) Mass forming type
The tumor originates from the bile duct epithelium and grows to form mass around the bile duct. In the intrahepatic CCA, the tumor presents as a non capsulated liver mass. The peritumoral bile duct dilatation occurs occasionally. The tumor occurs commonly in segments VI, VII, and VIII. Cystic necrosis of a large mass is reported and misdiagnosed as a liver abscess. In the perihilar mass forming CCA, the tumor presents with mass at bile duct confluence leading to obstruction of the right and/or the left hepatic ducts. The gross specimens of the tumors are firm and whitish gray on cut-surface. The histology is adenocarcinoma with large amount of fibrous stroma. The tumor tends to invade branch of portal vein.

b) Periductal infiltrating type
The tumor originates from the bile duct epithelium and grows or spreads along the bile duct wall. The tumor of this type causes narrowing of bile duct lumen leading to dilatation of bile ducts proximal to the tumor. In the intrahepatic CCA, tumor presents as localized bile duct dilatation with irregular and thickening of bile duct at the lesions.

The tumor is not obviously detected as a tumor mass. Most perihilar CCAs, are of this type. The bile ducts proximal to the tumor are dilated. The involved bile ducts are diffusely narrow or obliterated. Nonunion of the right and left hepatic ducts with or without a thickened wall is a common finding. The tumor can spread both intra and extrahepatic duct in the same patient, leading to the skipped lesions.

c) Intraductal growth type
The tumor originates from bile duct epithelium and grows slowly as polypoid mass in the bile duct lumen. The tumor p-resents with localized bile duct obstruction either intrahepatic or extrahepatic ducts. The tumor tends to grow slowly. It has much better prognosis than type a) and b). It is commonly misdiagnosed as an intrahepatic or a common bile duct stone. Occasionally, the tumor produces large amount of mucus, resulting in mucoid discharge form the papilla.

Histological findings of CCA

The most common histology of CCA is adenocarcinoma with glandular or papillary pattern. The adenocarcinoma can be sub-classified into papillary, well- differentiated, moderately differentiated, or poorly differentiated types. Papillary adenocarcinoma is a well- differentiated type with papillary growth pattern. Well- differentiated adenocarcinoma has a uniform glandular structure with cuboidal malignant cell. Moderately differentiated tumor has moderately distorted gland. Poorly differentiated adenocarcinoma has very distorted glandular structure with cellular pleomorphism.

Mucin production is commonly found in the lesion. Mucus core proteins (MUC) are detected in the lesion as well as in the serum. Some type of CCA produce large amount of mucin called mucinous carcinoma. It produces both intra and extra

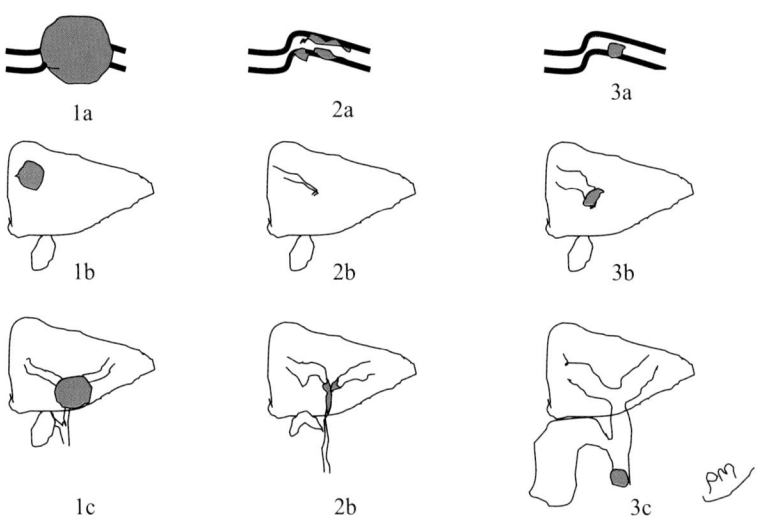

FIGURE 3: The morphologic classification of CCA 1) Mass forming type (1a growth pattern, 1b intrahepatic mass forming, 1c perihilar mass forming type) 2) periductal infiltrative type (2a growth pattern, 2b intrahepatic periductal infiltrative type, 2c perihilar periductal infiltrative type) 3) intraductal growth or papillary type (3a growth pattern,3b intrahepatic intraductal growth type, 3c extrahepatic intraductal growth type)

cellular mucin. The intra cellular mucin produces the so call "signet- ring cell".

Mucinous cystadenocarcinoma is the tumor arises from cell lining of the cystic lesions. The cyst fills with abundant mucin. Rare types of CCA are adenosquamous and squamous cell carcinoma with or without keratinization.

Tumor spreading and metastasis

Intrahepatic mass forming CCA tends to spread out of the bile duct wall and spread between hepatic plates and sinusoid. The tumor tends to invade and spread via small portal venous branches to form daughter tumor nodules. The direct invasion to the right diaphragm,the right 12th rib, the gall bladder and hepatic flexure of colon can be found at the operation. Extrahepatic mass-forming CCA tends to invade the bile duct wall and spread out of the duct. The tumor commonly causes obstructive jaundice.

Intrahepatic periductal infiltrating CCA tends to invade the wall and penetrates to the serosa. The tumor cells those are outside the bile duct tend to spread along the bile duct wall via the perineural tissue toward the porta hepatis. Extrahepatic periductal infiltrating CCA invades the bile duct and spreads longitudinally along the bile duct and cause concentric thickening of bile duct wall.

Intraductal growth CCA can spread intraluminally by implanting the detached tumor cells at the lumen of the adjacent bile duct. This results in multiple intraductal papillary tumors.

Intrahepatic metastasis occurs in almost all cases at the diagnosis. The regional lymph nodes metastasis is more common as compare to hepatocellular carcinoma. Blood-borne spreading occurs in advanced cases.The common sites of metastasis are the lungs, bone, adrenal glands, kidneys and brain. Direct spreading into peritoneal cavity is commonly seen in advanced cases.

CLINICAL PRESENTATION

The clinical manifestation of CCA is depended on the underlying conditions. In western countries, CCA is associated with primary sclerosing cholangitis (PSC) whereas in Asian countries CCA is associated with Opisthorchiasis and Clonorchiasis.

PSC associated cholangiocarcinoma

The most common symptoms in patients with PSC are fatigue, jaundice, pruritus and abdominal pain. The mean age at diagnosis of PSC is 32-42 years. The patients progress slowly with intermittent fever with abdominal pain. These symptoms can subside spontaneously. If the clinical and biochemical profiles deteriorate rapidly, the concomitant CCA is suspected.[62] The ERCP is recommended to detect the dominant stricture cause by CCA. Brushing cytology, therefore, should be done at the strictures. Although the false negative for brush cytology is high but it has high specificity. Serum tumor markers (CA19-9, CEA) have been used for evaluation of PSC with suspected CCA. The incidence rate of CCA is 1.5% per year in PSC patients.

Clonorchiasis associated CCA

Clinical manifestation of Clonorchiasis is not similar to Opisthorchiasis. Clonorchis sinensis causes more periductal fibrosis, more mucin production and more biliary stricture than Opisthorchis viverrini. The mucin- rich bile incorporate with the eggs can initiate nidus of the intrahepatic duct stones. Therefore, intrahepatic duct stones are commonly occur in Clonorchis sinensis. Biliary obstruction, ascending cholangitis and liver abscess are common complications in Clonorchiasis without CCA. The diagnosis of the concomitant CCA in Clonorchiasis is difficult. Rapid

clinical deterioration such as progressive weight loss and persistent obstructive jaundice are the clues for the diagnosis of Clonorchiasis associated CCA. Recently, using intrahepatic cholangioscopy makes the direct visualization of bile duct epithelium possible. The suspected lesions can be brushed and biopsy for histology.

O.viverrini associated CCA

The prevalence of CCA is high in the patient's age between 45-55 years old. The male/female ratio is 2.4/1. The main clinical manifestations are obstructive jaundice with or without cholangitis, acute abdomen, right upper abdominal pain, abdominal mass and distant metastasis.

Obstructive jaundice is the most common presentation of the pontural CCA. The jaundice progresses slowly and may become very severe at the late stage. Majority of these patients develop fever due to ascending cholangitis. The common associated symptoms are pruritus, pale stool, anorexia and weight loss. The pruritus is usually severe enough to disturb the patient's sleep. The common physical findings are hepatomegaly, moderate to severe jaundice, fever and palpable gall bladder. The right upper abdominal tenderness is common in the patient with cholangitis and acalculous cholecystitis. Secondary biliary cirrhosis is a late complication. This can lead to developing of ascites and esophageal variceal bleeding. The patients who have severe jaundice and sepsis may die of septicemic shock and acute renal failure.

Abdominal mass and *hepatomegaly* are the common findings in the intrahepatic CCA. The tumor tends to involve the intrahepatic vessels. This may cause atrophic change in the unilateral lobe and compensate hypertrophy of the contralateral lobe of the liver. Obstruction of the cystic duct by the tumor or the lymph node can cause the hydrop of the gall bladder. 31 of 187 CCA cases seen at Khon Kaen presented with palpable gall bladder with or without jaundice.

Acute abdomen can be a presenting symptom when it is complicated by acalculous cholecystitis, liver abscess and bile peritonitis.

Intra peritoneal metastasis present with ascites and rectal shelf occur in 10% of the cases. Left supraclavicular node and bone metastasis are also the common distant metastases in the advanced CCA.

Trousseau's syndrome as a recognized manifestation of CCA, is occasionally seen in our cases. It presents as a DVT and pulmonary embolism.

DIAGNOSIS

The diagnosis of CCA depends on the stage of disease (asymptomatic to advanced disease).The early CCA can be diagnosed by screening program among the high risk population. The advance CCA can be diagnosed, mainly, by imaging, tumor markers and histopathology.

CCA screening

Population-based ultrasound screening

The Khon Kaen cohort study took place in an endemic area of Opisthorchiasis in Thailand. 25,000 subjects enrolled in the study and 4154 subjects received ultrasound screening to identify the linkage between liver fluke infestation and CCA. Only 0.51% was suspected to have CCA by ultrasound criteria. The ultrasound screening is not cost effective and need many support facilities. It also needs other radiological investigation for the confirmation of the diagnosis.Other study in Northeast Thailand enrolled 15,000 subjects. Subject who had Opisthorchis egg more than 6,000 eggs per gram (epg) of feces underwent ultrasound examination. There were 15 sub-

jects who were confirmed to have CCA by ERCP. The odd ratio of subjects who were OV positive and having CCA was 4.1 as compared to the OV negative group. The odd ratio of subjects who had stool OV egg count over 6,000 epg to have CCA was 16.1. In conclusion: screening of early fluke associated CCA by ultrasound should be performed in only the patients who have heavy OV infestation and have hepatobiliary symptoms.

Liver function test

The serum alkaline phosphatase bilirubin and gamma glutamyl transpeptidase have low sensitivity and low specificity to be used for screening.

Serum tumor markers

Tumor markers that have been used in Cholangiocarcinoma screening are CEA, CA19-9, Ca125, CA 195 CA 242, IL 6, trypsinogen 2. Elevation of CA19-9 over 100 u/ml has sensitivity 75% and specificity 80% in PSC. But the level of CA19-9 could be very high in benign obstructive jaundice. Serum CEA is elevated in 30% of CCA, but it can be found in other tumors such as carcinoma of the colon, stomach and pancreas. Other tumor markers rise in advanced CCA. So, using them in screening is limited.

Tumor marker in bile

These markers are CEA, Mac-2-binding protein, CA19-9 and K-ras mutation in bile. They are sensitive but needs endoscopy to obtained bile. Therefore they are not appropriate for the screening.

Tumor markers in feces

This type of markers is being investigated and has the potential use in the future.

Diagnostic guidelines for CCA

Most patients with CCA present with advanced disease as mentioned.CCA is suspected in any patients with the risk conditions (primary sclerosing cholangitis, chronic liver fluke infestation, chronic intrahepatic duct stone, choledochol cyst, Calori's disease, multiple biliary papillomatosis and thorotrast exposure) whom present as an obstructive jaundice or a liver mass/masses. The liver function test shows elevation of alkaline phosphatase with or without hyperbilirubinemia. The low serum albumin is seen in late cases. The serum tumor markers such as CEA and CA 19-9 are elevated in CCA as common as 80-90%.Alpha fetoprotein, the tumor marker specific for hepatocellular carcinoma, is rarely observed in CCA.The imaging is the important tool for making diagnosis.

Imaging of CCA

Intrahepatic type

Most patients with intrahepatic CCA present with palpable liver mass. The mass may be single or multiple and may involve one or both lobes of the liver. Majority of the tumor mass is located in segment 8 of the liver adjacent to the diaphragm. Ultrasonography (US) is used initially to localize the tumor. Small tumors are hypoechoic or isoechoic, but large tumors may exhibit a hyperechoic

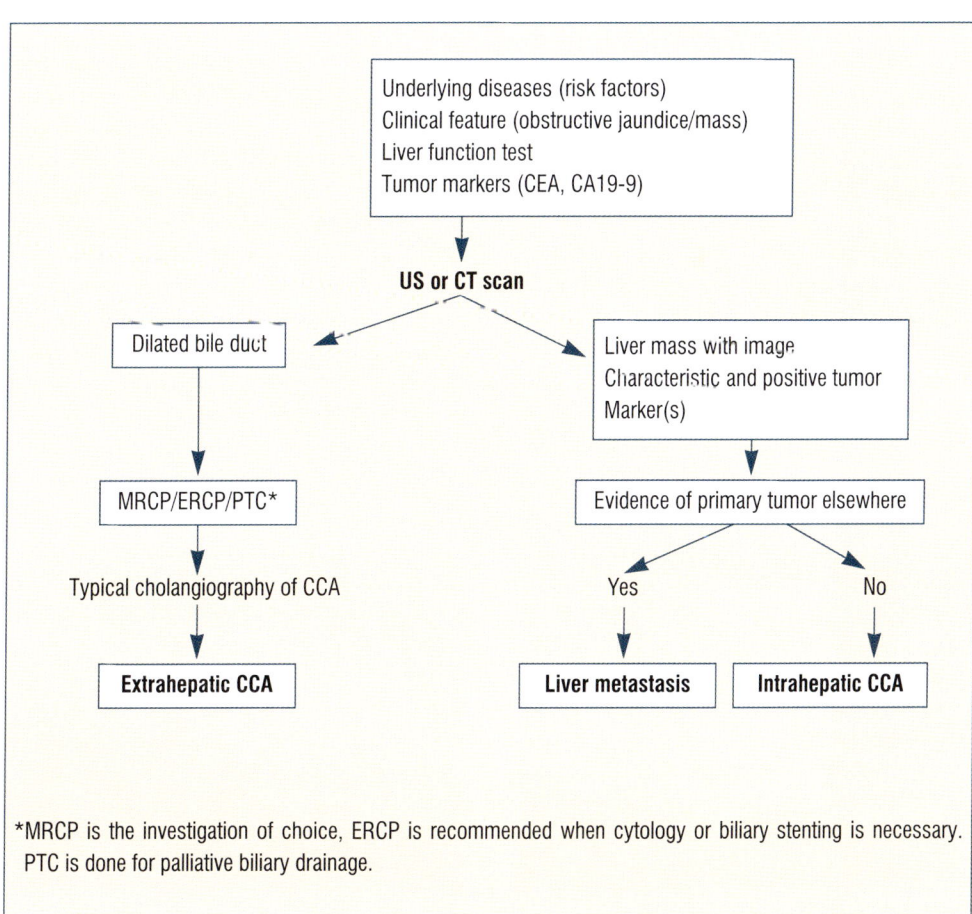

FIGURE 4: Diagnostic flow chart for CCA.

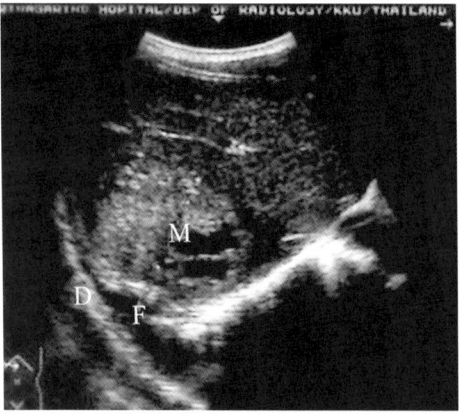

FIGURE 5: US demonstrates a non capsulated hyperechoic mass with necrosis in segment 8 of the liver, adjacent to diaphragm. (M = mass, F = pleural effusion, D = diaphragm).

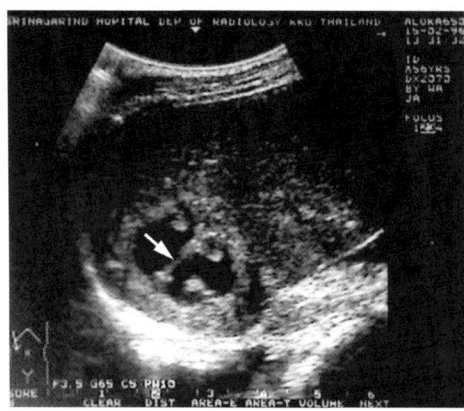

FIGURE 7: US demonstrates cystic cholangiocarcinoma. Papillary projection is shown along the wall (arrow).

or a mixed echoic pattern. Peritumoral bile duct dilatation is occasionally found. Pre-enhanced computed tomography (CT) shows an inhomogeneous hypodense mass with an ill-defined border. On enhanced dynamic CT, a mild to moderate peripheral enhancement with progressive central filling is observed. Calcification may be present. The tumor mass as detected by angiography is relatively hypovascular with late arterial phase neovascularity with no arteriovenous shunting. Lesions are usually hypointense on T1-weighted MRI. They may be slightly to strong hyperintense on T2-wighted MRI. The hyperintense foci contain prominent mucous secretion and/or necrosis. Gadolinium enhanced image shows initial rim enhancement with progressive central filling. Delayed contrast enhanced T1-weighted MRI shows incomplete and hertergeneous contral fill-in. There are other findings that may suggest the diagnosis of CCA, such as capsular retraction, segmental or lobar atrophy.

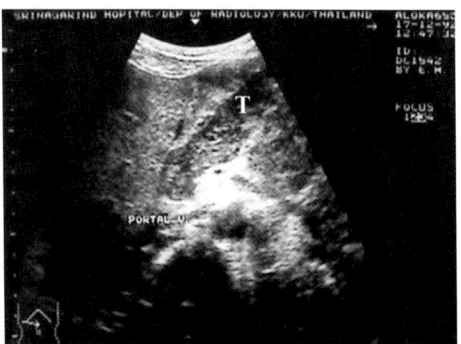

FIGURE 6: US demonstrates tumor invasion of portal vein (T = tumor).

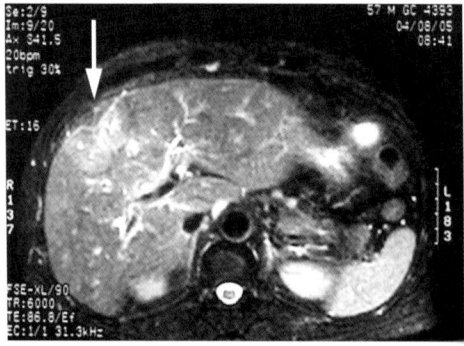

FIGURE 8: T2W MRI shows a heterogeneous hyperintense mass with retraction of liver capsule (arrow).

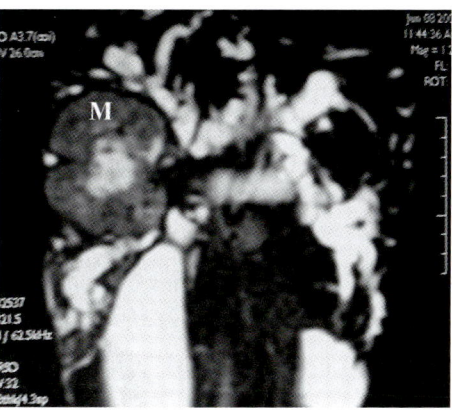

FIGURE 9: MRCP shows a heterogeneous hyperintense mass compressing hepatic duct confluence (M=mass).

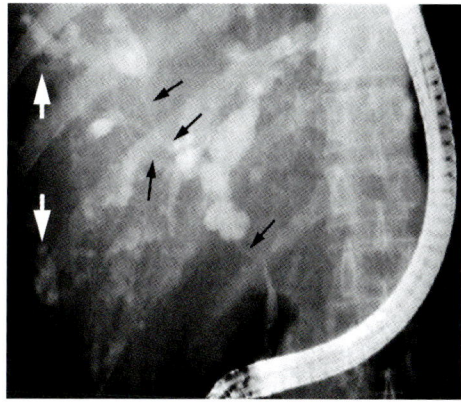

FIGURE 11: ERCP shows circumferential masses along segment 8 duct and at common hepatic duct. Sacular dilatation(white arrows) and strictures of intrahepatic ducts are shown (black arrows).

Extrahepatic type

US is very useful in the diagnosis of this type of CCA. Endoscopic retrograde cholangiopancreatography (ERCP) gives the details of the level and degree of bile duct obstruction. It is also useful in differentiating papillary growth of CCA in the common bile duct from common bile duct stone. The information obtained from through ERCP is very important if endo-scopic retrograde biliary drainage is being considered for palliative treatment. ERCP has the risk of post ERCP pancreatitis and cholangitis. Cytologic examination of aspiration bile gives low diagnostic sensitivity of 34-50%. Brushing cytologic performed at ERCP has a sensitivity of 40-60%. Endoscopic needle aspiration has a sensitivity of 83%. Biliary imaging can also be obtained with magnetic resonance cholan-

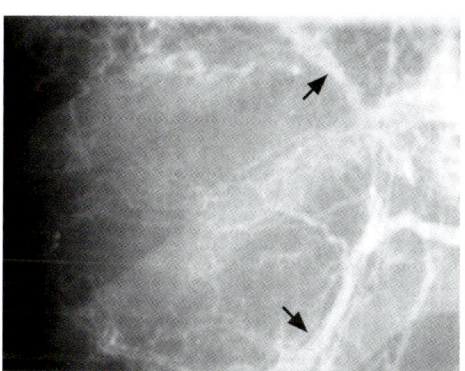

FIGURE 10: Angiography shows a hypovascular mass with stretching branches of right hepatic artery (arrows)

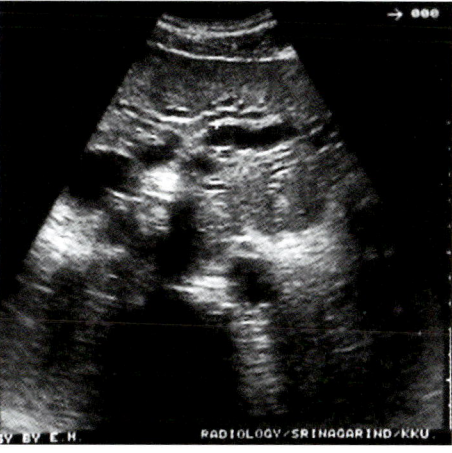

FIGURE12: US demonstrates dilated intrahepatic ducts in both lobes of the liver.

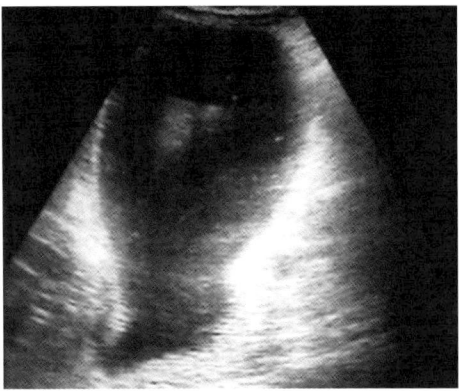

FIGURE13: US demonstrates markedly distended gall bladder, commonly seen in CCA involves common hepatic duct and cystic duct.

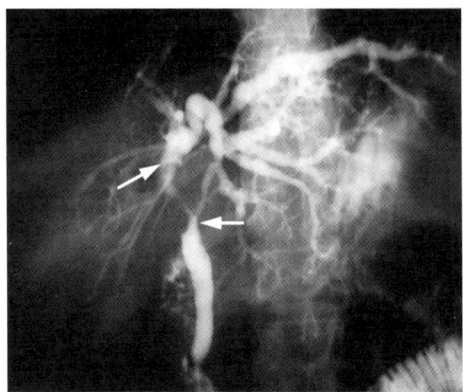

FIGURE 15: ERCP demonstrates a circumferential mass at common hepatic duct(arrow).

giopancreatography (MRCP). MRCP is a non-invasive for imaging of biliary tree and required no ionizing radiation or iodinated contrast material. MRCP can detect both hepatic mass or biliary obstruction.

Endoscopic ultrasonography (EUS)

EUS is very useful in preoperative assessment of nodal metastasis by EUS-guided fine needle aspiration of the lymph node. The accuracy, sensitivity and specificity are 91, 89, 100% respectively.

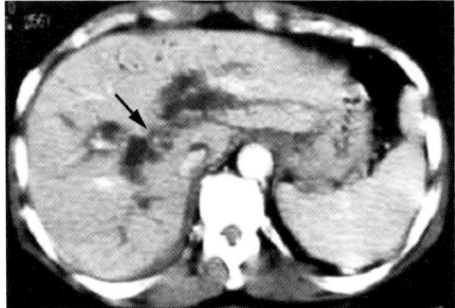

FIGURE 14: Contrast enhanced CT demonstrates dilated intrahepatic ducts around isodense mass at the confluence (arrow).

Positron emission tomography (PET) with (18F)-2-deoxy-D-glucose

Cholangiocarcinoma cells can uptake glucose but cannot metabolize (^{18}F)-2-deoxy-D-glucose, therefore, leads to accumulation of the substrate. This causes hot spot in PET scan. PET scan has not been reported in Opisthorchiasis associated Cholangiocarcinoma.

Clinical staging

Intrahepatic cholangiocarcinoma can be staged in TMN classification as table 1. The **T** is not classified by size of tumor but by using the invasion of tumor through the bile duct wall. The tumors which only confined to stage I and II are consider suitable for the curable resection. Most tumors are detected at stage III and IV. Therefore surgical outcome in this type of tumor is poor.

Hilar Cholangiocarcinoma can also be staged in TMN classification as table 2. Hilar CCA tends to involved vascular and tends to early metastasize to regional lymph node, therefore, the curative resection is occasionally possible. Most common palliative treatments are surgical by-

TABLE 1 INTRAHEPATIC CHOLANGIOCARCINOMA STAGING

Stage I	T1	N0	M0
Stage II	T2	N0	M0
Stage III	T1,T2	N1	M0
Stage IVA	T3	any N	M0
Stage IVB	any T	any N	M1

TI: Infiltrate mucosa, muscular

T2: Limited to Perimuscular connective tissue

T3: Infiltrate adjacent structure (Liver, GB, Duodenum, Pancreas, Stomach etc)

N0: Negative node, N1 positive node

M1: Distant metastasis

pass, endoscopic biliary drainage and percutaneous biliary drainage (PTBD). Recently extensive resection with removal of the caudate lobe, the invaded vascular and affected nodes has been recommended.

The tumor staging for respectability should be done by multi modality investigations to obtain the most accurate preoperative condition. CT scan gives 60-80%, MRI+MRCP 80%, EUS 91% accuracy in detection of tumor respectability.

TREATMENT

Surgical treatment is the mainstay treat-

TABLE 2 HILAR CHOLANGIOCARCINOMA STAGING

Stage 0	Carcinoma in situ
Stage I	Carcinoma limited to mucosa
Stage II	Carcinoma with local invasion
Stage III	Hepatoduodenal ligament invasion and Invasion of adjacent tissue
Stage IV	Peripancreatic, celiac, superior mesenteric Lymph nodes involvement and Distant metastasis

ment of CCA. As mentioned before, most CCA patients present at advanced stage, the curative resection is occasionally possible. The National Comprehensive Cancer Network proposed the clinical practice guidelines for CCA as Figure 16a and Figure 16b.

Surgical treatment is the best option for patient with intrahepatic cholangiocarcinoma. The surgical approach is the same as the other mass lesion of the liver. Bhudhisawasdi studed preoperative condition of 125 cholangiocarcinoma by using multivariate analysis of prognostic factors. The factor that correlate with perioperative mortality were haematocrit less than 30%, neutrophil count >80%, serum albumin <2.7 mg%, prothrombin activity <85%, serum creatinine >3.0 mg/dl, serum BUN >30 mg%, serum SGOT >150 U. The perioperative mortality in his case series is 17.6%. Most of the patients in this series had >3 risk factors; these can explain the high perioperative mortality.

The biliary bypass surgery for 125 non selected extrahepatic CCA, also reported. The mean survival was 3.5 months and 1 year survival is 20%. 4 types of biliary bypass had been performed; a) peripheral bilateral bypass b) peripheral unilateral bypass c) central high bilateral bypass d) central high unilateral bypass. The best result was in the patients who had central high bilateral bypass as shown in the figure 17.

To improve the surgical outcome, many techniques had been reported. The preoperative biliary drainage to improve the function of the liver had been reported from Barcelona group. The study showed no significant differences in postoperative mortality between drained and undrained groups. Launois B et al reported French experience on 552 cases of primary carcinoma of the extrahepatic bile ducts (gallbladder and periampullary tumors were excluded) from 55 surgical centers. Three

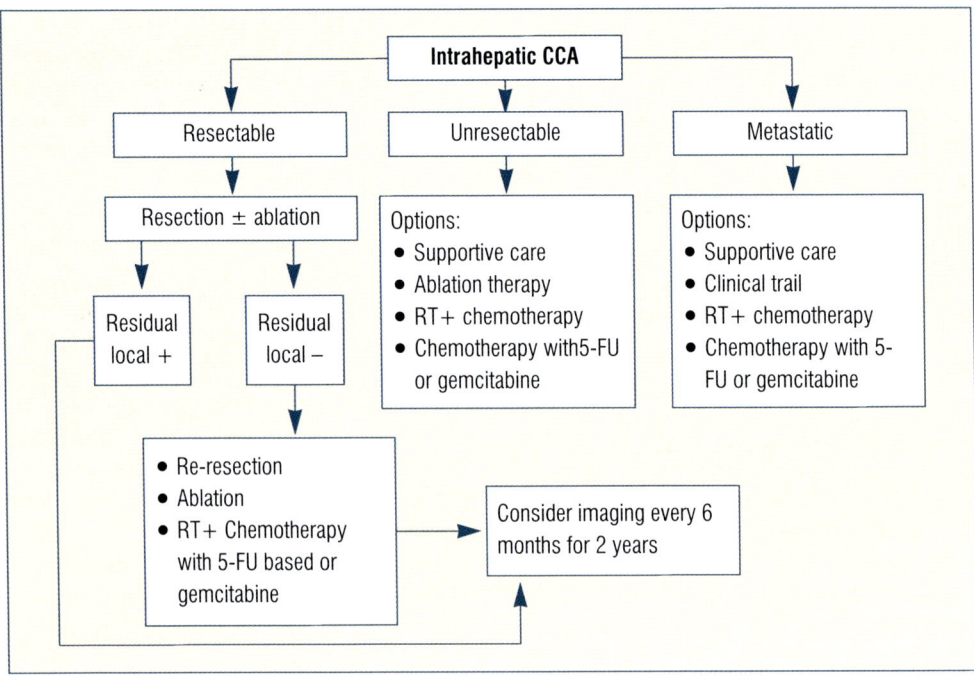

FIGURE 16a: Clinical practice guidelines for intrahepatic CCA.

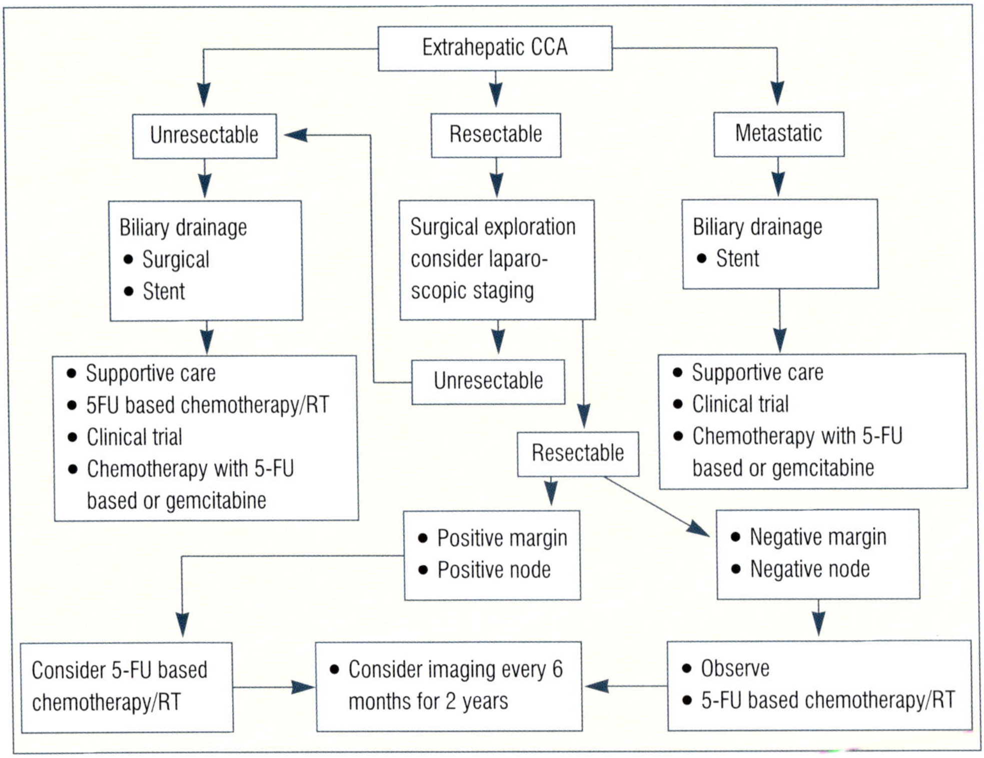

```
                          Intrahepatic CCA

        Resectable            Unresectable            Metastatic

    Resection ± ablation    Options:                Options:
                            • Supportive care       • Supportive care
                            • Ablation therapy      • Clinical trail
    Residual    Residual    • RT+ chemotherapy      • RT+ chemotherapy
    local +     local −     • Chemotherapy with5-FU • Chemotherapy with 5-
                              or gemcitabine          FU or gemcitabine

                • Re-resection
                • Ablation              Consider imaging every 6
                • RT+ Chemotherapy      months for 2 years
                  with 5-FU based or
                  gemcitabine
```

FIGURE 16b: Clinical practice guidelines for extrahepatic CCA.

```
                          Extrahepatic CCA

        Unresectable          Resectable              Metastatic

    Biliary drainage      Surgical exploration    Biliary drainage
    • Surgical            consider laparo-         • Stent
    • Stent               scopic staging

    • Supportive care        Unresectable         • Supportive care
    • 5FU based chemotherapy/RT                    • Clinical trial
    • Clinical trial           Resectable          • Chemotherapy with 5-FU
    • Chemotherapy with 5-FU                         based or gemcitabine
      based or gemcitabine
                          • Positive margin        • Negative margin
                          • Positive node          • Negative node

    Consider 5-FU based   • Consider imaging every 6   • Observe
    chemotherapy/RT         months for 2 years          • 5-FU based chemotherapy/RT
```

hundred and seven patients (56%) had upper-third carcinoma, whereas 71 (13%) had middle-third and 101 (18%) had lower-third bile duct carcinoma. The remaining patients had diffuse lesions. Resectability rates were 32% for upper-third lesion compared with 47% and 51% for middle-third and lower-third lesion, respectively. The operative mortality rate for proximal carcinoma was significantly lower with resection (16%) compared with palliative surgery (31%) (P <0.05). Overall 1 year survival (operative deaths were excluded) was 68% after tumor resection compared to 31% after palliative surgery (P <0.001). The results suggested that resection of extrahepatic bile duct carcinomas had better prognosis than palliative bypass surgery. Kawarada Y et al used percutaneous transhepatic portal vein embolization before doing extended right hepatectomy (S4a +S5 +S1) for the hilar CCA instead of conventional resection. They improved the rate of curative resection from 54.8% to 88% and the 3-year survival rate improved from 27.1% to

59.9%. Ebata T et al reported that the hilar CCA patients with macroscopic portal invasion had poorer survival rate than without portal vein resection (5-year survival, 9.9% vs. 36.8%; P <0.0001). They suggested that hepatectomy with portal vein resection should be attempted in every hilar CCA with portal vein invasion. Yi, B et al conducted a retrospective cohort study in 198 patients with hilar CCA.They used Cox's regression model analysis to determine the significant prognostic factors for long-term survival. The result suggested that operative procedure was the most important prognostic factor affecting the operative results of the hilar CCA. Radical resection is still the primary treatment for a cure and long-term survival of the patients. For patients with irresectable hilar CCA, no evidence had shown that treatment with endoscopic retrograde biliary drainage was inferior to palliatve bypass surgery.

Hepatic resection is the treatment of choice of intrahepatic CCA. Uttaravichien T, et al reported of 16.6% of 2 years

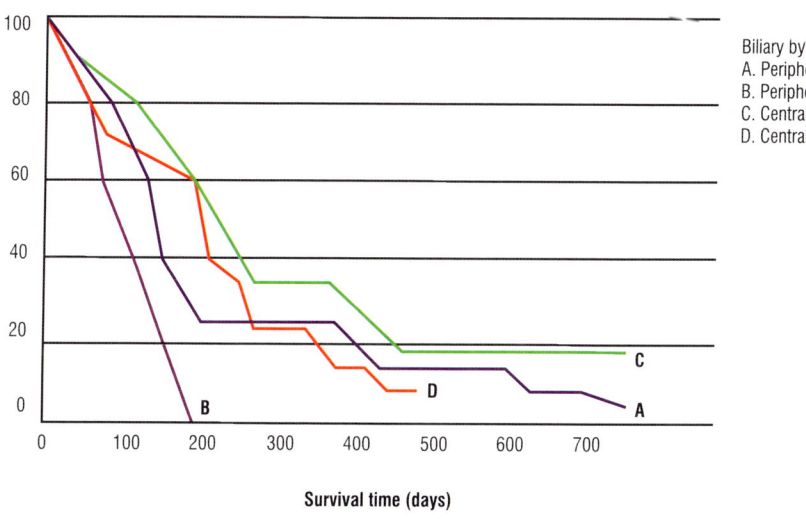

FIGURE 17: Survival analysis of 125 cases of extrahepatic CCA with different bypass procedures.

survival after hepatic resection with mean survival of 48 weeks in the non selected intrahepatic CCA. Weber S M et al reported 53 patients with intrahepatic CCA underwent exploration; the overall resectability rate was 62% (33 of 53). Median survival for patients submitted to resection was 37.4 months versus 11.6 months for patients undergoing biopsy only (p = 0.006) and the 3-year survival was 55% versus 21%, respectively. Factors predicting of poor survival after resection included: vascular invasion (p = 0.0007), histological positive margin (p = 0.009) and multiple tumors (p = 0.003). Suzuki S et al found that the intrahepatic CCA with periductal infiltration, perineural invasion, portal vein invasion, presence of intrahepatic metastasis, and two or more lymph node metastases had poor prognosis. Kawarada Y et al used the multivariate analysis to evaluate the factors that affected the outcome of 37 intrahepatic CCA treated by hepatic resection. The actuarial 1-, 3-, and 5-year survival rates in the 37 resected cases were 54.1%, 34.0%, and 23.9%, respectively. The stage of the intrahepatic CCA influenced their overall survival rate. Multivariate analysis revealed that non-curative resection, lymph node metastasis, and less differentiated histological type were significant risk factors for poor outcome. They also suggested that extensive resection was not indicated if lymph node metastasis was identified pre-operatively or intraoperatively. However, Akatsu T et al recently reported a very rare 6-year disease-free survivor of a 76-year-old female with intrahepatic CCA who also had hilar lymph node metastasis and portal vein involvement. They performed hepatectomy, reconstruction of the portal vein and extensive lymph node resection. They suggested that aggressive surgery may be a potential approach to provide a hope of long-term survival for patients with intrahepatic CCA despite the presence of regional lymph node metastasis and vascular invasion. Their result has to be confirmed before making further recommendation.

Endoscopic treatment: The hilar CCA in Khon Kaen can classified as 16.8% Bismuth I, 24.1% Bismuth II, 19.5 Bismuth IIa, 17.2% Bismuth IIIb and 32.2% Bismuth IV. Endoscopic biliary plastic stenting has been successfully placed in 80% of cases but adequate drainage occurs in less than 50%. Therefore, post ERCP cholangitis is a common complication. Many palliative endoscopic biliary drainage techniques had been reported to improve the outcomes in unresectable hilar CCA.

The pre-ERCP anatomic evaluation of the biliary tree by MRCP is essential for planning of stent insertion: plastic or metallic, unilateral or bilateral. De Palma G D et al conducted an randomized controlled trial on 157 patients with CCA, gallbladder cancer, or periportal lymph node metastases to has unilateral stenting (group A) or bilateral stenting (group B). The patients in group A had a significantly higher rate of successful endoscopic stent insertion than group B (88.6% vs. 76.9%, p = 0.041). Group B had a significantly higher rate of complications than group A (26.9% vs. 18.9%, p = 0.026). The rate of successful drainage, complications, and mortality did not differ between the two groups. They concluded that the bilateral stenting would not appear justified as a routine procedure in patients with biliary bifurcation tumors. Rerknimitr R et al compared the incidence of post endoscopic plastic stenting cholangitis among different Bismuth groups. They found that incidence of cholangitis in Bismuth I was 4%, in Bismuth II was 10% and in Bismuth III/IV was 57.7%. They also found that the mean duration of stent patency was only 41.3 days in Bismuth III/IV. They concluded that the plastic stenting might not give an adequate biliary drainage in advanced hilar CCA. Therefore, the metallic stenting might be the first option in the advanced unresectable hilar CCA. De Palma, G. D et al treated 61 patients with malignant hilar obstruction by insertion unilateral metallic stent across the stricture into the duct that technically was easiest to access. The success rate of stent insertion was 59 of 61 (96.7%) patients. The median stent patency was 169 days. They concluded that the unilateral metallic stent insertion was safe, feasible, and achieved adequate drainage in the majority of patients with nonresectable hilar CCA. Shah R et al conducted a randomized controlled trail comparison between insertion of 10-mm diameter Wallstent or a 10-mm diameter Z-stent in the patients with unresectable malignant biliary obstruction distal to the bile duct bifurcation. Sixty-four patients received a Z-stent and 68 patients had a Wallstent. The metallic stents were successfully placed in all patients. Median time of patency was 162 days in Z-stents and 150 days in Wallstents (p = 0.22). The study showed that the Z-stent was comparable with the Wallstent in terms of sucessful placement, and overall patency. The patients whom received biliary stent insertion not only became less jaundice,they also had better quality of life in term of improvement in emotional, anorexia, diarrhoea, sleep pattern, cognitive and global health scores (P <0.01). The cost of surgical bypass and endoscopic biliary drainage,for unresectable CCA, were compared. The median total lifetime cost for surgical therapy was $60,986 vs $24,251 for endoscopic therapy. Endoscopic therapy is an effective palliative therapy for unresectable CCA and costs less than surgical treatment.

Percutaneous transhepatic biliary drainage (PTBD) is an alternative option for palliative biliary drainage by inserting the catheter from skin into liver parenchyma and placeing into a intrahepatic duct. Nowadays, this method is not commonly practiced and is replaced by endoscopic biliary stent insertion.However, PTBD is a common palliative treatment in advanced unresectable extrahepatic CCA at Khon Kaen, Thailand. The mean survival of 137 hilar CCA was 163.9 days after PTBD. 14.28% of the patients survived more than one year. The irrigation with normal saline and periodic exchange of the catheter whenever clogging occurred were the key factors for long survival rate.

Radiotherapy is used to 1) reduce the pain from tumor metastasis, 2) delay tumor recurrence after surgery, 3) relief biliary obstruction from tumor by using intraluminal brachytherapy. Sagawa N et al reported that radiation therapy after surgery did not show any clinical benefits for patients with hilar CCA. However, it may be effective as adjuvant therapy after curative resection in a small subgroup of patients with stage III or IV disease. Shinchi H et al retrospectively reviewed 51 patients with unresectable hilar CCA. 30 patients received external beam radiotherapy combined with endoscopic metallic stenting (EMS + RT group), 10 patients were treated with EMS alone, and the remaining 11 patients underwent PTBD alone. The mean survival of 6.4 months in the EMS group was significantly longer than that of 4.4 months in the PTBD group (P <0.05). The EMS+RT group with a mean survival of 10.6 months had a significantly longer survival than the EMS group (P <0.05). EMS+RT group had a longer stent patency than the EMS group (mean: 9.8 vs. 3.7 months; P <0.001).Ede R et al reported pilot study of 14 patients with inoperable CCA using endoscopic intraluminal radiotherapy with iridium-192 wire. The wire was inserted down via a nasobiliary catheter placed within a previously inserted endoscopic biliary prosthesis. A total radiation dose of 6000 cGy at 0.5 cm from the source was administered over a median of 85 hr (range 77-116 hr).The radiation reduced the tumor size and temporary relieved the obstruction. Chen Y et al conducted a controlled trail comparison between intraluminal brachytherapy with HDR-192 Ir wire (n = 14) and control group (n = 12 Mean stent patency of H-DR-192 Ir group was significantly longer than that of control group (12.6 months vs 8.3 months; P <0.05). The brachytherapy combined with external beam radiotherapy increased survival from a median of 3.9 months (non-brachytherapy group) to 9.1 months in the brachytherapy group. The common adverse effects of brachytherapy are portal vein thrombosis and radiation injury to adjacent organs.

Chemotherapy are aimed for prolong survival and improvement of quality of life in unresectable CCA. 5-Fluorouracil (5-FU), used as a single agent for treatment of CCA, gave the response rate 0-10%. 5-FU combined with Leucovorin increased response rate to 32%. 5-FU combined with cisplatin gave the response rate only 24%. However adding epirubicin as the third agent increased the response rate to 40% and median survival of 11 months. Paclitaxel is commonly used as a single agent for treatment of many adenocarcinoma such as colorectal carcinoma,had been reported as a single agent in treatment of CCA. Papakostas P et al used paclitaxel as the first-line chemotherapy for 21 unresectable CCA. They reported that only one patient had complete response and three patients had partial response (overall response rate was 14.3%). Gemcitabine is the most effective agent in treatment of CCA. Using gemcitabine alone gave the response rate 8-60% and median survival of 6.3-16 months. Gemcitabine combined with cisplatin gave the response rate of 27.5-50% and median survival of 5-15.3 months. Gemcitabine combined with oxaliplatin had the response rate of 36% and median survival of 15.4 months. Gemcitabine combined with capecitabine gave no better outcome than gemcitabine alone. In conclusion: chemotherapy in CCA is recommended as a palliative treatment in only unresectable cases. The chemotherapy regimens with gemcitabine give better outcome.

Tumor ablation

Radiofrequency (RFA) is a common technique for treatment hepatocellular carcinoma. Slakey D P presented the first case of a recurrent intrahepatic CCA successfully treated with RFA and the patient remained free of detectable disease 10 months after the ablation. Livraghi, T et al conducted a large multi center study of 2320 liver cancer treated with RFA. Most of the cases were hepatocellular carcinoma, only 17 cases were CCA. There were only 0.3% procedure related deaths and complications occurred in 2.2% of the cases (peritoneal hemorrhage, tumor seeding, liver abscess and intestinal perforation). They concluded that RFA was safe and could be used in any kinds of liver cancers (hepatocellular carcinoma, CCA, metastasis etc). Chiou Y et al reported of 10 intrahepatic CCA patients who were treated by US-guided percutaneous RFA. Complete necrosis in all five tumors (100%) with diameters of 3.0 cm or less, two of three tumors (67%) with diameters of 3.1-5.0 cm, and one of two tumors (50%) with diameters of more than 5.0 cm. They suggested that RFA was effective and successful in the treatment of intrahepatic CCA of 3 cm or less. RFA can not only be done via percutaneous but also via laparoscopy. Therefore, laparoscopic radiofrequency ablation is an option when other treatment methods have failed. Ablation of intraductal CCA can be done by using photodynamic therapy. Ortner M used photodynamic therapy (PDT) combined with biliary stenting to evaluate the additional therapeutic effect. He intravenously infused hematoporphyrin derivative (Photofrin) into 21 perihilar unresectable CCA patients. The substance was taken up by Cholangiocarcinoma cells. By using intraluminal photo activation (wavelength 630 nm) via ERCP, the cells were sensitized and sloughed off. The results showed decreasing serum bilirubin from a mean level of 201.26 +/- 189.25 micromol/l after stenting alone to 68.87 +/- 78.27 micromol/l (P = 0.0051).To confirm the positive result, Ortner M conducted another prospective, open-label, randomized, multicenter study to compare PDT in addition to stenting (n = 20) with stenting alone (n = 19) in patients with nonresectable CCA. PDT resulted in prolongation of survival as comparison to stenting alone (median survival 493 vs 98 days; P <0.0001). Wiedmann M et al conducted a five-year follow-up study of 23 nonresectable CCA patients treated with PDT. Median survival after treatment was 11.2 months for patients without distant metastases (M0) and 9.3 months for all patients (M0+M1). The 1-year, 2-year, 3-year, and 4-year survival rates were estimated to be 47%, 21%, 11% and 5%, respectively, for patients with stage M0 CCA, and 39%, 17%, 9%, and 4%, respectively, for patients with stages M0 and M1. Of the patients who died, 73.9% (n = 17) were because of tumor progression. This 5-year follow-up study confirmed that photodynamic therapy was effective for nonresectable hilar CCA, although it does not prevent progression of the disease.

Liver transplantation

Primary sclerosing cholangitis (PSC) is the most common predisposing condition of CCA in the western countries whereas liver flukes are the most common predisposing of CCA in Asia. Median survival of patients condition with primary PSC has been estimated to be 12 years. Cholangiocarcinoma are found 10% of the cases. Approximately 8% of PSC has undergone liver transplantation for progressive liver failure. Long-term survival after liver transplantation for

PSC related CCA has been disappointing. One year survival was 53%, and disease-free survival at 3 years was only 13%. Recently, the Mayo study of transplantation of CCA under special protocol gave a very good result. They developed a protocol combining external beam irradiation, brachytherapy, chemotherapy, PDT, and orthotopic liver transplantation for patients with operatively confirmed stage I and II hilar CCA. One-, 3-, and 5-year survival were 92%, 82%, and 82% after transplantation. The study of transplantation in liver fluke-related CCA has no enough data to make any suggestion. We conclude that the transplantation for CCA has a potential to improve survival if the disease is early diagnosed (stage I, II) and pre transplantation treatment with neoadjuvant radiotherapy, chemosensitization has been done.

Gene therapy and future trends of treatment

By using adenovirus as a vector to carry a desirable gene to cholangiocarcinoma cells cause apoptosis. p27kip1, one of the cyclin-dependent kinase inhibitors, is known to limit proliferation of the cells. Over expression of p27kip1 by a recombinant adenoviral vector expressing p27kip1 (Adp27) induces apoptosis. The role of COX-2 inhibitors as chemo-prevention of adenoma of colon, perhaps can be beneficial in prevention of bile duct cancer.

Prevention

To decrease incidence of liver fluke related CCA is to control liver fluke infection. The national opisthorchiasis control program had been initiated in 1987 with collaboration between the department of communicable disease control of the Ministry of Public Health of Thailand and the Federal Republic of Germany government. 1,839,813 cases received stool examination and 531,175 positive cases were treated. The crucial activity designated for the control strategies include the following elements: 1) the organizing of mobile stool examination teams 2) community preparation through mobilization of individuals, family and community participation 3) continuing effective health education. The result of this program leaded to decrease prevalence of opisthorchiasis in Thailand from 15.2% (1991) to 9.6% (2001) for all regions and for high prevalence of opisthorchiasis in Northeast, the prevalence dropped from 34.6% (1981) to 15.7% (2001). By effective control program of the fluke may reduce the prevalence of opisthorchiasis associated CCA in the future.

REFERENCES

Ahrendt SA, Eisenberger CF, Yip L et al. Chromosome gb21 less and p16 inactivation in primary sclerosing cholangitis-associated cholangiocarcinoma. J Surg Res 1999;84:88-93.

Akatsu T, Shimazu M, Kawachi S et al. Long-term survival of intrahepatic cholangiocarcinoma with hilar lymph node metastasis and portal vein involvement Hepatogastroenterology 2005; 52:603-5.

Andre T, Tournigand C, Rosmorduc O et al Gemcitabine and oxaliplatin (GEMOX) inadvanced biliary tract carcinoma: a GERCOR study Ann Oncol 2004; 15:1339-43.

Arroyo G, Gallardo J, Rubio B gemcitabine in advanced biliary tract cancer: Experience from Chile and Argentina in phase II trails. Proc Am Soc Clin Oncol2001; 157a.

Berber E, Ari E, Herceg N Siperstein A. Laparoscopic radiofrequency thermal ablation for unusual hepatic tumors: operative indications and outcomes Surg Endosc 2005;19:1613-7.

Bergquist A, Ekborn A, Olsson R, et al. Hepatic and extrahepatic malignancies in primary sclerosing cholangitis. J Hepatol 2002;36;321-7.

Bhargava AK, Petrelli NJ, Karna A, et al. Serum levels of cancer-associated antigen CA-195 in gastrointestinal cancers and its comparison with CA19-9. J Clin Lab Anal 1989;3:370-7.

Bhudhisawasdi V. Survival analysis of hilar cholangiocarcinoma after different surgical bypass procedures. Asian J Surg 1996;19:269-70.

Bhudhisawasdi V. Place of surgery in opisthorchiasis associated cholangio-carcinoma Southeast Asian J Trop Med Public Health 1998; 28(supl. 1):85-90.

Boonla C, Sripa B, Thuwajit P, et al. MUC1 and MUC5AC mucin expression in liver fluke-associated intrahepatic cholangiocarcinoma. World J Gastroenterol 2005;11(32):4939-46.

Broome U, Olsson R, Loof L et al. Natural history and prognostic factors in 305 Swedish patients with primary sclerosing cholangitis. Gut 1996;38: 610-5.

Carraro S, Servienti PJ, Bruno MF Gemcitabine and cisplatin in locally advanced or metastatic gallbladder and bile duct adenocarcinomas Pro Am Soc Cli Oncol 2001;20: 146B(A2333).

Chen Y, Wang X,/Yan Z.et al HDR-192Ir intraluminal brachytherapy in treatment of malignant obstructive jaundice World J Gastroenterol 2004;10:3506-10 117) Schleicher M, Staatz G, Alzen G, Andreopoulos D. Combined external beam and intraluminal radiotherapy for irresectable Klatskin tumors Strahlenther Onkol 2002;178:682-7.

Chijiwa H, Yamashita H, Yashider J et al. Current management of long term prognosis of hepatolithiasis. Arch Surg 1995;130:194-7.

Chiou Y, Hwang I, Chou, Y et al Percutaneous ultrasound-guided radiofrequency ablation of intrahepatic cholangiocarcinoma. Kaohsiung J Med Sci2005; 21:304-9.

Choi BI, Han JK, Hong ST and Lee KH. Clonorchiasis and Cholangiocarcinoma: Etiologic relationship and imaging diagnosis. Clinical Microbiology Reviews 2004;17(3):540-52.

Clinical practice guidelines in oncology volume1.2005 National Comprehensive Cancer Network. http://www.nccn.org/.

Cong WM, Bakker A, Swalsky PA et al. Multiple genetic alteration in involved in the tumorigenesis of human cholangiocarcinoma: a molecular genetic and clinicopathological study. J Cancer Res Clin Oncol 2001:127:187-92.

Daytan MT, Longmire WP, Tomkin H. Calori's disease: a premalignant condition. Am J Surg 1983; 145:41-8.

De Palma G D, Galloro G, Siciliano S et al. Unilateral versus bilateral endoscopic hepatic duct drainage in patients with malignant hilar biliary obstruction: results of a prospective, randomized, and controlled study Gastrointest Endosc 2001; 53:547-53.

De Palma G D Pezzullo A Rega M et al. Unilateral placement of metallic stents for malignant hilar obstruction: a prospective study Gastrointest Endosc 2003;58:50-3.

Dobrila-Dintinjana R, Kovac D, Depolo A et al Gemcitabine in patients with nonresectable cancer of the biliary system or advanced gallbladder Am J Gastroent 2000; 95:2476.

Doval DC, Sekhon JS, Gupta SK et al.A phase II study of gemcitabine and cisplatin in chemotherapy naive, unresectable gallbladder cancer. Br J Cancer 2004;90:1516-1520.

Ducreux M,Rougier P,Fandi A et al Effective treatment in advanced biliary tract carcinoma using 5-FU continuous infusion with cisplatin, Ann Oncol 1998;9:653-6.

Ebata T, Nagino M, Kamiya J, et al Hepatectomy with portal vein resection for hilar cholangiocarcinoma: audit of 52 consecutive cases Ann Surg 2003; 7(2):128-34.

Ede R,Williams S, Hatfield A, McIntyre S, Mair G. Enduscopic management of inoperable cholangiocarcinoma using iridium-192 Br J Surg 1989;76:867-9.

Ellis PA, Norman A, Hill A et al Epirubicin, cisplatin and infusion 5-FU in Hepatobiliary tumours Eur J Cancer 1995;31A(10):1594-8.

Falkson G, McIntyne J M, Moertel CG Eastern cooperative Oncology Group experience with chemotherapy for inoperable gallbladder and bile duct cancer Cancer 1984;54:965-9.

Figueras J, Llado L,Valls C, et al. Changing strategies in diagnosis and management of hilar Cholangiocarcinoma. Liver Transpl 2000;6(6): 786-94

Fritscher-Ravens A, Broering DC, Knoefel WT et al EUS-guided fine-needle aspiration of suspected hilar cholangiocarcinoma in potentially operable patients with negative brush cytology. Am J Gastroenterol. 2004;99(1):45-51.

Gebbia V, Giuliani F, Maiello E et al Treatment of inoperable and/or metastasis biliary tract carcinomas with single agent gemcitabine or in combination with levofolinic acid and infusional fluorouracil: result of a multicentre phase II study. J of Clin oncol 2001;19:4089-91.

Georgopoulos SK, Schwartz LH, Jarnagin WR, et al. Comparison of magnetic resonance and endoscopic retrograde cholangiopancreatography in malignant pancreaticobiliary obstruction. Arch Surg. 1999;134(9):1002-7.

Gores GJ. Early detection and treatment of Cholangiocarcinoma. Liver Traspl 2000;6:530-4.

Goydos JS, Brumfield AM, Frezza E, et al. Marked elevation of serum interleukin-6 in patients with Cholangiocarcinoma: validation of utility as a clinical marker. Ann Surg 1998;227: 398-404.

Green A, Uttaravichien T, Bhudhisawasdi V, et al Incidence and presentation of Cholangiocarcinoma in Northeast Thailand: A hospital-based study. Trop Geo Med 1992; 43:193-8.

Hann LE,Getrajdman GI,Brown KT,et al Hepatic atrophy:association with ipsilateral portal vien obstruction.Am J Roentgenol 1996;167:1017-21.

Haswell-Elkins MR, Mairiang E, Mairiang P, Chaiyakum J, Chamadol N, Loapaiboon V, Sithithaworn P, Elkins DB. Cross sectional study of Opisthorchis viverrini infection and cholangiocarcinoma in communities within a high-risk area in northeast Thailand. Int J Cancer 1994;59(4): 505-9.

Haswell-Elkins M.R., Satarug S., Tsuda M., et al. Liver Fluke Infection and CCA:Model of Endogenous Nitric Oxide and Extragastric Nitrosation in Human Carcinogenesis. Mut Res 1994; 305: 241-52.

Hedstorm J, Haglund C, Haapiainen R, et al. Serum trypsinogen-2 and trypsin-2-Alpha(1)-antitrypsin complex in malignant and benign digestive tract disease: preferential elevation in patients with cholangiocarcinoma. Int J Cancer 1996;66:326-31.

Hernander J, Riancho J, Gonzcellez, Macias J. Cholangiocarcinoma present as Trousseau's syndrome. Am J Gastroenterol 1998; 93:847-8.

Hou PC. The relationship between primary carcinoma of the liver and infestation with Clonorchis sinensis. J pathol Bacteriol 1956;72:239-46.

Howell DA, Beviridge RP,Bosco J Jones M Endoscopic needle aspiration at ERCP in the diagnosis of biliary strictures Gastrointest Endosc.1992;38: 531-5.

Ito y, Kojiro M, Nakashima T, Mori T. Patho-morpho-logic characteristics of the 120 cases of Thorotrast-related hepatocellular carcinoma, cholangiocarcinoma and hepatic angiosarcoma. Cancer 1988;62:1153-62.

Jaiwal M, La Russo NF, Burgart LJ, Gores GJ. Inflammatory cytokines induced ANA damage and inhibit DNA repair in Cholangiocarcinoma cells by a nitric oxide -dependent mechanism. Cancer Res 2000;60:184-90.

Jeyarajah D R, Klintmalm G B. Is liver transplantation indicated for cholangiocarcinoma? J Hepatobiliary Pancreat Surg 1998;5:48-51.

Jongsuksuntikul P. Evaluation of helminthiasis control program in Thailand at the end of the eighth health development plan. J Trop Med Parasitol Assoc Thai 2003; 26:38-45.

Kawarada Y, Das B C, Naganuma T, Tabata M, Taoka H, Surgical Treatment of Hilar Bile Duct Carcinoma.J of Gastrointestinal Surgery 2002;6 (4):617-24

Kawarada Y, Yamagiwa K, Das B. Analysis of the relationships between clinicopathologic factors and survival time in intrahepatic Cholangiocarcinoma Am J Surg 2002;183:679-85.

Khan SA, Davidson BR, Goldin R, et al. Guidelines for the diagnosis and treatment of cholangiocarcinoma: consensus document. Gut 2002; 5 (Suppl6): V11-V19.

Kiba T, Tsuda H, Pairojkul C, Inoue S, Sugimura T, Hirohashi S. Mutation of the P53 Tumor Suppressor Gene and the Ras Gene Famaly in Intrahepatic Cholangio-carcinoma in Japan and Thailand. Molecular Carcinogenesis 1993;8: 312-8.

Kim MH, Sekijima J, Lee SP. Primary intrahepatic stones. Ann J Gastroenterol 1995;90:540-8.

Kim TK, Choi BI, Han JK, Jang HJ, Cho SG, Han MC. Peripheral cholangiocarcinoma of the liver: two phase spiral CT findings. Radiology 1997;204:539-43.

Kluge R, Schmidt F, Caca K et al. Positron emission tomography with (^{18}F)-2- deoxy-D-glucose for diagnosis and staging of bile duct cancer. Hepatology 2001;33(5):1029-35.

Koopmann J, Thuluvath PJ, Zahurak ML, et al. Mac-2-binding protein in a diagnostic marker for biliary tract carcinoma. Cancer 2004;101(7): 1609-15.

Kristiansen TZ, Bunkenborg J, Gronborg M, et al. A proteomic analysis of human bile. Mol Cell Proteomics 2004;3(7):715-28.

Kubicka S, Rudolf KL, Tietze MK, et al Phase II study of systemic gemcitabine chemotherapy for advanced unresectable hepatobiliary carcnomas Hepatogastroenterology 2001;22:498-501.

Kurathong S, Lerdverasinkul P, Wongpaiboon V et al. Opisthorchiasis infection and Cholangiocarcinoma. A prospective case control study. Gastroenterol 1985;89:151-6.

Kuusela P, Haglund C, Robert PJ. Comparison of a new tumor marker CA 242 withCA 19-9, CA 50 and carcinoembryonic antigen (CEA) in digestive tract disease. Br J Cancer 1991;63:636-40.

Launois B, Reding R, Lebeau G, Buard J. L, Surgery for hilar cholangiocarcinoma: French experience in a collective survey of 552 extrahepatic bile duct cancers. J Hepatobiliary Pancreat Surg 2000;7(2):128-34.

Lee SS, Kim MH, Lee SH et al. Clinicopathological review of 58 patients with biliary papillomatosis. Cancer 2004; 100(4):783-93.

Levi S., Urbano-Ispizua A., Gill R., et al Multiple K-ras Mutations in CCA Demonstrated with a Sensitive Polymerase Chain Reaction Technique. Cancer Res 1991; 51: 3497-502.

Liver Cancer Study Group of Japan. The general rules for the clinical and pathological study of primary liver cancer,4 th ed, Tokyo, Kanehara 2000.

LivraghiT, Solbiati L, Meloni M F, et al Treatment of focal liver tumors with percutaneous radio-frequency ablation: complications encountered in a multicenter study Radiology 2003;226:441-5.

Luman W,Cull A, Palmer K R. Quality of life in patients stented for malignant biliary obstructions Eur J Gastroenterol Hepatol 1997;9: 481-4.

Maeda I, Ku Y, Iwasaki T, et al. A case of advanced cholangiocarcinoma treated successfully by percuatneous isolated liver perfusion with cisplatin. Gan To Kagaku Ryoho 1996;23:1607-9. (In Japanese)

Maeda T,Takenaka K,Taguchi K, et al Adenosquamous carcinoma of the liver: clinicopathologic characteristics and cytokeratin profiles Cancer 1997;80:34-71.

Mairang P, Bhudhisawasdi V, Borirakchanyavat V, Sitprija V. Acute renal failure in obstructive jaun-

Biological tests for cholestasis

Tantau Marcel

Cholestasis occurs in case of a mechanical blockage of the biliary ducts or in liver diseases.

ALKALINE PHOSPHATASE

Alkaline phosphatase (AP) comprises a group of enzymes with a generally unclear physiological role. These enzymes are most active at alkaline pH - hence the name, and are present in a variety of tissues, including liver, bone, intestine, placenta, leukocytes, kidney.

Each tissue produces a slightly different AP called isoenzymes. In the laboratory, AP is measured as the total amount or the amount of each of the four isoenzymes. The isoenzymes react differently to heat, certain chemicals, and other processes in the laboratory. Gel electrophoresis enables qualitative differentiation of this isoenzymes, their precise identification is made with monoclonal antibodies.

The AP from blood originate mainly from liver and bones. AP serum activity is higher in adolescence because of rapid bone growth and during late pregnancy because of placental growth and metabolism. Persons with group O and B may have elevated levels of AP derived from small bowel.

The AP of the liver is located in the cells lining the small bile ducts (ductoles) and on the apical (i.e., canalicular) domain of the hepatocyte plasma membrane.

Abnormal rises of AP appear predominantly in liver diseases but also in bone diseases. Elevation of AP in the setting of cholestatic liver disease results from increased synthesis and release of the enzyme into serum rather than from impaired biliary secretion. Bile acids retained in cholestase will solubilize the cell membrane and so will release the AP into blood. Because half time of AP is approximately 7 days, the level in serum may remain elevated for several days after resolution of biliary obstruction, and normalisation of serum bilirubin.

Important elevations of AP are seen in metastatic tumor infiltration of the liver or biliary obstruction, either in the liver as in primary biliary cirrhosis or in extrahepatic biliary tree, but the level of AP cannot be used to distinguish reliably between these diseases. For example, identical levels can be seen with hepatic metastases, obstructing choledocholithiasis, cholangiocarcinoma and primary biliary cirrhosis. In some cases of Hodgkin's disease and renal cell carcinoma, elevations of AP can occur without obvious direct liver involvement, maybe because of a nonspecific hepatitis.

Mild elevations of AP are seen in hepatic granulomatosis, abscesses, or amyloidosis.

Lower levels of AP are encountered in conditions such as: hypothyroidism, pernicious anaemia, conditions that lead to malnutrition (such as celiac disease) or are caused by a lack of necessary nutrients in the diet (such as scurvy).

Isolated rises of AP without concomitant rises in serum bilirubin occur in two major cases: partial biliary obstruction and hepatic masses (benign or malign, primitive or metastatic). Partial biliary obstruction may result from choledocholithiasis or biliary strictures that involve small intrahepatic ducts, as occurs with recurrent pyogenic cholangitis or primary sclerosing cholangitis, or occasionally from malignant obstruction of only the left or right ductal system near the ductal bifurcation (a Klatskin tumour). Normal bilirubin levels are explained by the capacity of hepatocytes from uninvolved areas to secrete the daily bilirubin load. Stones in the common bile duct are frequently nonobstructive and give rise only in AP levels.

Anabolic steroids, estrogens and antipsychotic drugs may cause cholestasis with isolated high AP.

GAMMA GLUTAMYL TRANSPEPTIDASE

Gamma Glutamyl Transpeptidase (GGT) is an enzyme that transfers glutamyl from a peptide to a aminoacid. GGT is found in cellular membranes of different tissues: kidney, seminal vesicles, spleen, pancreas, heart, lung, brain and liver. Hepatic isoenzymes are mainly responsible for seric levels of GGT. GGT is present only in small quantities in bones, and it is thus helpful in confirming the hepatic origin of an elevated AP level.

In the liver, GGT is localised in biliary tree from the hepatocyte to common bile duct. High concentration are found into epithelial cells of small biliary ducts as AP. Seric level of GGT decreases with age and is higher in men than in women.

GGT is a microsomal enzyme and is therefore inducible by alcohol and drugs including most anticonvulsants and warfarin. However, more than one third of habitual consumers of alcohol have normal serum GGT levels, thus the value of GGT for assessing alcohol use is limited.

High seric level of GGT is non-specific for hepatobiliary diseases, it occurs in chronic alcoholism, pancreatic diseases, renal failure, diabetes, chronic obstructive lung diseases.

Levels of GGT and AP correlates in cholestatic conditions.

5'-NUCLEOTIDASE

This enzyme has a role in nucleic acid metabolism. It is found in many tissues, including the liver, cardiac muscle, brain, blood vessels, and pancreas. In the liver it is situated in the canalicular and sinusoid cell membranes, and also in the lisosomes and cytosol.

Despite the presence in different tissues, seric elevations of levels of 5'-Nucleotidase are highly specific for hepatobiliary cholestatic diseases. It is liberated in the blood by biliary salts from cell membranes. The enzyme has a sensitivity comparable to that of AP in detecting biliary obstruction, hepatic infiltration, and cholestasis but may exhibit kinetics that are different from those of both AP and GGT, with levels rising several days after experimental bile duct ligation .

REFERENCES

Friedman LS, Martin P, Munoz SJ. Laboratory evaluation of the patient with liver disease. In:Zakim D, Boyer T (eds). Hepatology. Textbook of liver diseases. 4th edition, Elsevier Science (USA), 2003:661-708.

Penn R, Worthington DJ: Is serum gamma-glutamyl-transferase a misleading test? Br Med J 286:531-535, 1983.

Pratt DS, Kaplan MM: Laboratory tests. In Schiff ER, Sorrell MF, Maddrey WC (eds): Schiff's Diseases of the Liver, Vol 1. Philadelphia, Lippincott-Raven, 1999, pp 205-244.

Reichling JJ, Kaplan MM: Clinical use of serum enzymes in liver disease. Dig Dis Sci 33:1601-1614, 1988.

Seetharam S, Sussman NL, Komoda T, et al: The mechanism of elevated alkaline phosphatase activity after bile duct ligation in the rat. Hepatology 6:374-380, 1986.

The role of US in the diagnosis of obstructive jaundice.
Current advances and perspectives

Leonardou Polytimi, Pappas Paris, Kanematsu Masayuki

INTRODUCTION

During the last two decades a dramatic change has occurred in the development of noninvasive imaging techniques for the biliary tree such as ultrasonography (US), computed tomography (CT) or magnetic resonance imaging (MRI).

Ultrasound is regarded as the best initial imaging procedure for the evaluation of patients presenting with jaundice or a suspected biliary obstruction, because it is accurate, easily accessible, fast and safe.

DEFINITION

Jaundice (icterus) refers to the yellow pigmentation of the skin, sclerae and mucous membranes due to elevated serum bilirubin level. The upper limit of normal total serum bilirubin level is 17 mmol/L. In cases of a mild increase, this can only be detected by biochemical blood analysis. Patients present with clinically evident jaundice when the serum bilirubin level exceeds 30 mmol/L.

Jaundice reflects the presence of cholestasis and can be classified as haemolytic/prehepatic, hepatocellular/hepatic, or obstructive/posthepatic/cholestatic.

Haemolytic jaundice is readily apparent from heamatological and biochemical blood tests, and imaging has little to offer in the diagnosis and management of those patients.

Hepatocellular jaundice is also detected by biochemical or serological blood tests or by liver histological examinations. US imaging detects structural liver changes and the ultrasonographic findings of parenchymal liver disease may suggest the cause. US can also be used to guide a needle for diagnostic aspiration or biopsy.

Obstructive jaundice is the result of an intrahepatic or extrahepatic block in the pathway between the site of bile conjugation in the liver cells and the entry of bile into the duodenum through the ampulla. The extrahepatic block is in the bile ducts and is referred to as "surgical" jaundice, whereas jaundice from all other causes is referred to as "medical".

The three phases of obstruction are:
1. the predilatory phase, when liver function tests and scintigraphy are abnormal but the size of the bile duct remains within the normal limits;
2. the dilatory phase, when a progressive ductal dilatation is manifested; and
3. the icteric phase, when ductal dilatation, bilirubin elevation and clinical jaundice are presented.

Conventional blood tests usually confirm the presence of cholestasis, but provide no reliable information concerning the site of obstruction and its cause.

Dilatation of the biliary tree usually preceds biochemical evidence and therefore ultrasound may be more sensitive than biochemistry in the detection of biliary obstruction. It shall detect biliary dilatation at a total serum bilirubin level of 17-30 mmol/L.

The possibility that jaundice may result from an extrahepatic obstruction is initially suggested by patient's history, physical examination and laboratory studies.

Evaluation of patients with obstructive jaundice is a common clinical problem. The objective in such cases is to determine whether a potentially treatable cause of cholestasis is present without subjecting the patient to potential risk, discomfort or expense.

Although more sophisticated imaging modalities are now available, US still remains the screening method of choice for the evaluation of patients with suspected biliary obstruction and jaundice, because it posses several advantages: high sensitivity in the detection of intra- and /or extrahepatic bile duct dilatation; no ionizing radiation; it works independently of hepatic, biliary or renal function; has no need for contrast material injection; needs short scanning time; examines other abdominal organs as well; is widely available; is widely practiced by radiologists.

The questions that it has to answer to the referring clinicians are mainly:
1. Is there biliary duct dilatation?
2. Where is the level of obstruction?
3. What is the cause of obstruction?
4. Are there any other accompanying related signs in the region, such as ascites, portal vein thrombosis or other?

BILIARY OBSTRUCTION: LEVEL AND CAUSES

Intrahepatic

benign: primary biliary cirrhosis
cholangitis – primary sclerosing
– recurrent pyogenic
– AIDS
primary intrahepatic biliary cystadenoma
Mirizzi's syndrome
hemobilia (bleeding in the biliary tree) – iatrogenic
– spontaneous (due to coagulopathy)
Echinococcal cyst rupture
drug-induced

malignant: primary intrahepatic biliary cystadenocarcinoma
hepatocellular carcinoma
liver metastasis

Porta hepatis

spread of adjacent tumor – gallbladder
– liver
primary cholangiocarcinoma (Klatskin tumor)
hilar lymphadenopathy
surgical stricture

Extrahepatic

benign: congenital   – biliary atresia
                                  – Caroli's disease
                                  – choledochal cyst

cholangitis – primary sclerosing
– recurrent pyogenic
– acquired immunodeficiency (AIDS)

biliary strictures – traumatic
– iatrogenic
– postinflammatory associated with:
    – pancreatitis
    – gallstones
    – infections
    – duodenal ulcer

choledocholithiasis
bile duct mass – papilloma
– cystadenoma
hemobilia
pancreatic pseudocyst
obstruction of the ampulla of Vater – gallstones
– bile plug
– duodenal diverticulum

malignant: primary bile duct cancer (cholangiocarcinoma)
pancreatic carcinoma
tumour of the ampulla of Vater
duodenal carcinoma
gastric carcinoma

ULTRASONOGRAPHIC FINDINGS

Ultrasonographic imaging has primarily the role to determine if biliary dilatation is present. Its sensitivity for biliary dilatation is 68-99% and its specificity is 75-100%. (Figures 1, 2).

Ultrasound has secondary the role to determine the specific level and cause of obstruction. These findings guide the choice of further imaging and possible therapeutic interventions. Ultrasound identifies correctly the level of obstruction in 92% to 95% of the cases while the cause of obstruction in 71% to 88% of the cases can be narrowed to three main categories: neoplastic mass, pancreatitis, and calculi.

Ultrasound is more than 90% accurate in discriminating "medical" versus "surgical" jaundice.

It is able to detect obstructive from non-obstructive jaundice with an accuracy of 95% and if at the porta hepatis it should reach an accuracy of almost 100%.

Ultrasonographic success rates depend on different variables: patient population, equipment, operator/s experience and effort for optimal imaging quality.

A. CONCERNING THE BILLARY SYSTEM

The *intrahepatic ducts* are parallel to the portal vein branches and normally are only visible near the porta hepatis.

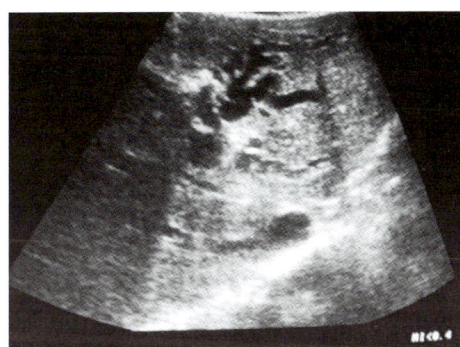

FIGURE 1: Ditaled left lobe biliary tree.

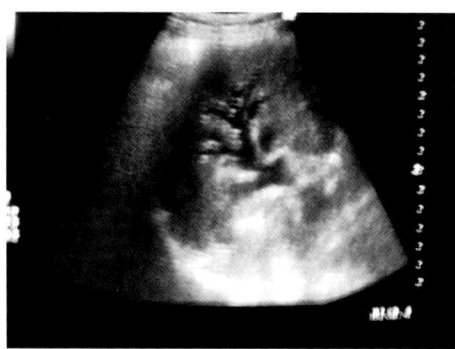

FIGURE 2: Dilated right lobe biliary tree.

Near porta hepatis the intrahepatic ducts normally have a diameter of 5 mm or less or their diameter should not exceed 40% of the adjacent portal vein. At this level dilatation is manifested by a diameter grater than 5 mm or grater than 40% of the portal vein.

Deep intrahepatic ducts are normally not visible. If any bile duct deep within the liver is detected, ductal obstruction should be suggested. (Figure 3).

Bile ducts dilating to become equal to or grater than the diameter of the adjacent portal vein branches are described as "double-burelled shotgun" appearance when viewed in short axis or "parallel-

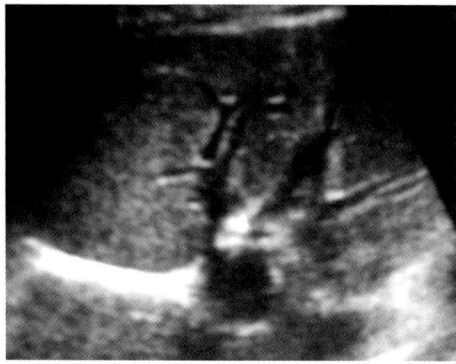

FIGURE 3: Dilated intrahepatic biliary tree compared to the portal vein branches.

channel sign" when scanned along the long axis. In a diffuse fatty liver the outer wall of the ducts merges with the bright hepatic parenchyma and all that is seen is the interface between the vein and the duct, described as "the stylet sign".

Markedly dilated intrahepatic ducts are easily detected by the US as tortuous structures converging to the porta hepatis thus creating "a tangle of worms" and the typical appearance of "too many tubes", which by careful examination do not correspond to arteries or veins and are therefore bile ducts.

Minimal to moderate intrahepatic dilatation can be diagnosed only by exclusion, which is the absence of blood flow inside the ducts and the presence of blood flow in the adjacent blood vessels.

In all circumstances, the use of color Doppler ultrasonography helps identify the absence of blood flow within the bile ducts.

Ultrasound has a relatively poor sensitivity for intrahepatic dilatation, between 50% to 85%, whereas its specificity is high up to 95%.

The **extrahepatic duct** normal caliber varies because of several factors: measurement technique and measurement of different portions of the extrahepatic duct, normal physiologic variation and age-related change in duct caliber. Despite these factors, normal standards have been established concerning the portion measured:

An internal diameter at or near the porta hepatis normally is 6 mm or less. At this level a diameter of 7 mm is considered equivocal, whereas a diameter of 8 mm or grater indicates ductal dilatation.

Below the porta hepatis a diameter ranging between 7 mm to 10 mm is normal.

At any location along the extrahepatic duct a diameter exceeding 10 mm is a manifestation of ductal dilatation.

Extrahepatic dilatation implies obstruction and the probability of obstruction increases with the degree of dilatation.

The ultrasonographic patterns of appearance of the extrahepatic duct are:
- the "sandwich view", where portal vein is seen as the deeper and bile duct as the more superficial parallel tube and in between the right hepatic artery or in some cases a more a tortuous proper hepatic artery.
- the "Mickey Mouse view", where portal vein is considered as the head of Mickey, hepatic artery is represented as the medial ear and bile duct as the lateral ear.

In all cases, the use of color Doppler ultrasonography allows visualization of the blood flow inside the hepatic artery as well as in the portal vein, thus confirming identification of the bile duct. Color Doppler examination is also useful in cases of a replaced right hepatic artery, meaning a right hepatic artery arising from the superior mesenteric artery, because it can trace it to its origin. (Figure 4).

Pitfalls that may cause diagnostic error

Inexperienced sonographer
Ultrasonographic identification of the bile duct may be difficult, especially in the

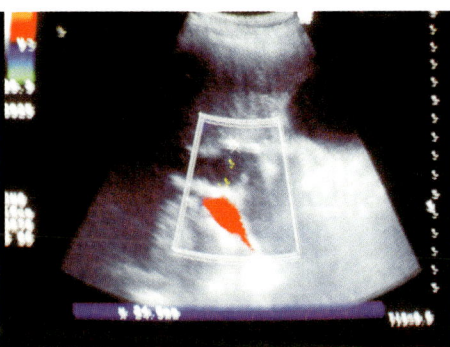

FIGURE 4: Dilated common bile duct compared to the portal vein (red color).

hands of an inexperienced sonographer. Therefore the classic ultrasonographic patterns of the extrahepatic duct as described above should be identified, as well as the use of color Doppler examination may be necessary in some instances.

Ductal obstruction without dilatation
In some circumstances obstruction may occur without duct dilatation related to false negative results that may reach even up to 25% in cases of gallstone jaundice, although recently sensitivity of US for the detection of choledocholithiasis is more than 80%. Obstruction without dilatation is uncommon but may be found in the very early stages of obstruction, during the predilatory phase, that may last a day or two after an abrupt obstruction, because the ducts may not have had the time to dilate despite the complete ductal system obstruction (e.g. bile duct injury or surgical clip placement over the common hepatic duct at cholecystectomy). In such cases that clinical and ultrasonographic findings do not fit, a repeated scanning is recommended after a couple of days to show the proximal dilatation. The finding of obstruction without duct dilatation may be also caused by abnormality in the ducts (e.g. fibrosis in sclerosing cholangitis) or surrounding tissues (e.g. encasement of the common duct by tumor).

Dilatation without ductal obstruction
Biliary dilatation may occur before clinical jaundice is presented and US is able to detect this in cases of chronic incomplete or slowly progressive obstruction (e.g. tumour in the head of pancreas, chronic pancreatitis), or when some intrahepatic ducts are obstructed by a mass and others not. This is also caused by a ball-valve effect of a stone in the common bile duct resulting intermittent relief of the obstruc-

tion, clearance of bile and no development of jaundice. Other causes of non-obstructive dilatation also include loss of ductal elasticity or idiopathic.

Dilatation of the common duct without jaundice must be differentiated by other no pathological causes such as age, post-cholecystectomy or after previous dilatation.

B. Concerning the Underlying Cause

The most common causes of obstructive jaundice are: lithiasis, cholangiocarcinoma, carcinoma of the head of pancreas, carcinoma of the ampulla of Vater, Echinococcal cyst rupture, pancreatitis and neoplastic masses of adjacent organs or systemic diseases such as lymphoma, which cause obstruction due to pressure.

a. Benign

Choledocholithiasis
In the United States of America choledocholithiasis is the most common cause for biliary obstruction. The vast majority of cases of choledocholithiasis include common bile duct stones that originate within the gallbladder. Approximately 15% of the patients with cholelithiasis present also choledocholithiasis. Gallstones are present in the common bile duct in approximately 6% to 12% of all patients undergoing cholecystectomy. Although many patients with choledocholithiasis remain asymptomatic for years, stones within the bile duct may give rise to life-threatening complications such as acute bile obstruction and jaundice, pancreatitis and cholangitis.

Lithiasis of the biliary system is visualized with the typical ultrasonographic appearance of the echogenic structure with the acoustic shadow. Lithiasis may be at the level of the intrahepatic biliary system causing peripheral dilatation or may be at

any level of the bile ducts. The specificity of ultrasound examination for choledocholithiasis exceeds 95%, whereas the sensitivity of the modality for the detection of choledocholithiasis is about 75% to 80%. The difficulties encountered include overlying gas or stones especially at the distal common duct that may not cast an acoustic shadow. Also most of the intraductal calculi are small and obstruction is intermittent, and the ducts are not dilated in 21% to 36% of the cases. In such cases the lack of echo-contrast between the impacted ductal calculus and the surrounding tissues leads to detection rates of the US for intraductal calculi of an average 60%. The visualization of a calculus is easy when it is surrounded by bile in a widely dilated duct. So in cases that a stone is revealed, the diagnosis can be established with certainty on the basis of sonographic evaluation. False positive results present in cases of gas bubbles, surgical clips, parasites or other echogenic material.

Cholangitis
Cholangitis is characterized clinically by Charcot's triad, including swinging fever, jaundice and biliary colic.

There are many different cholangitides that may cause biliary obstruction:

Recurrent pyogenic cholangitis: Recurrent pyogenic cholangitis develops in the presence of bile duct obstruction and infection. It is endemic to areas of Southeast Asia and it is often associated with intrabiliary infections by parasites, especially by Chlonorchis sinensis and less by Ascaris lumbricoides, and by bacteria, mainly Escherichia coli. Gram-negative organisms are the major causative agents with Klebsiella and Escherichia species being present in 54% and 39% of the cases respectively, while Enterococcal and Bacteroides organisms are present in up to 25% of the cases.

Clinical manifestation involves sepsis

and jaundice. The development of strictures as consequence of this condition results dilatation of the intra- and extrahepatic bile ducts. Inside the dilated portions of the ductal system US scans reveal echogenic bile, nonshadowing calculi (present in 25% of the cases) which are soft, mudlike calcium bilirubinate (pigment) calculi, or proteinaceous debris.

Primary sclerosing cholangitis: Primary sclerosing cholangitis is a progressive inflammatory and fibrotic process of unknown origin, recently related to viral infections and alterations in the immune function. It is an uncommon disease which affects more relatively young men with pre-existing condition such as ulcerative colitis or Crohn disease. Both the intra- and extrahepatic bile ducts are affected either in part or all. The intrahepatic ducts present dilated in a nonuniform, segmental way. The suggestive cholangiographic appearance is alternating dilatation and narrowing of the ducts, so-called beading and pruning of the ducts. The extarhepatic biliary tract is also affected in a similar way but with a less severe involvement. The wall of the ducts, which is normally not visible, appears thickened or irregular, with associated gallbladder wall thickening in some cases.

The outcome of this incidious, progressive process is biliary cirrhosis and hepatic failure, with stigmata and portal hypertension presented in cases of long standing disease. In 6% to 9% of the patients with primary sclerosing cholangitis develops a cholangiocarcinoma, which is difficult to be differentiated and the findings that should be noticed and suggest development of malignancy include a single area of obstruction, marked dilatation of the ducts proximal to the tumor, and intraluminal polypoid masses or an extrinsic tumor mass, whereas calculi or debris are uncommon in cases of cholangiocarcinoma.

AIDS cholangitis: AIDS-related cholangitis is an opportunistic infection of the biliary tree. Cytomegalovirus is the causative in two-third of the autopsies. Cryptosporidium is another common cause. Both Cytomegalovirus and Cryptosporidium cholangiopathies may occur at any stage of AIDS presentation, while Mycobacterium tuberculosis usually affects the early to intermediate stage of the disease. AIDS cholangitis may involve the gallbladder and the biliary tree in a focal or a diffuse way and causes typically mural thickening with a stricture of the distal common duct and a mild proximal dilatation.

Primary biliary cirrhosis

Primary biliary cirrhosis is an idiopathic cholangitis affecting the interlobular and septal bile ducts. It affects more middle-aged females than males (9:1).

The ducts are progressively destructed with associated portal fibrosis and regenerative hepatic nodules. Clinically presents with pruritus and jaundice. The sonographic evaluation is not diagnostic in the early stages. In the advanced stages of the disease, portal hypertension signs may be apparent, such as portal vein dilatation, varices, ascites and splenomegaly. Nearly half of the patients have hepatomegaly, whereas almost all patients have perihepatic and portal lymphadenopathy that can be easily visualized by US. The change of caliber of the lymph nodes in the hepatoduodenal ligament may be used as prognostic indicator in cases primary biliary cirrhosis reflecting inflammation and cholestasis.

Parasitic infections

Certain parasites that reside at the gastrointestinal tract may produce symptoms if they traverse the ampulla and enter the biliary tree. This occurs most often with Chlonorchis sinensis and Ascaris lumbricoides.

Chlonorchis sinensis is a liver fluke that typically does not cause radiologic abnormalities. However, occasionally the flukes may be revealed by US examination as echogenic foci or as small filling defects (10-15 mm) within the bile duct. A mild intrahepatic dilatation may also be seen in cases of severe infestation.

Ascaris lumbricoides is a worm grater than 10 cm in length and 3-6 mm in diameter and therefore it is easily recognized radiologically as tubular structure, either straight or coiled, in the extarhepatic duct. It is quite common that this causes biliary obstruction.

Pancreatitis

Biliary obstruction may be the result of pancreatitis due to edema of the head of pancreas, or it may be the cause of it due to distal bile duct calculus.

The normal sonographic appearance of pancreas shows an echogenicity grater than that of the liver. However, with increasing age and its expected atrophy pancreas looks more echogenic and is difficulty differentiated from the retroperitoneal fat tissue.

The average anteroposterior diameters of the pancreas in transverse section are: head 2.5 to 3.5 cm, body 1.75 to 2.5 cm and tail 1.5 to 3.5 cm. The ultrasonographic recognition of the pancreas is based on its anatomic relation to the vessels of the upper abdomen and especially the portal vein, which does not allow diagnostic error when viewed since above it is the caudate lobe of the liver and below the pancreas.

In transverse sections the pancreatic duct is usually difficult visualized and looks as a thin line of no echogenicity with a normal diameter of less than 2 mm. In cases of obstruction, the pancreatic duct is dilated and recognized as an unechoic ductal structure. Pancreatic duct dilatation is a sign of inflammation or neoplasm.

Acute pancreatitis refers to inflammatory changes of the pancreas with activation of pancreatic enzymes and hyper-

amylasemia. In 75% to 80% of all cases acute pancreatitis is related either to gallstones impacted in the distal common bile duct or to alcoholism. The relative prevalence varies according to different patient population. Alcoholism is a more common cause in men, whereas gallstones are a more common cause in women. In the United States the most common cause of acute pancreatitis is alcohol-related, whereas in Europe most cases present due to cholelithiasis. Other factors involved are drugs or idiopathic (15% to 20%).

Clinically presents with midepigastric pain radiating to the back and relieved by sitting, fever and tachycardia. Jaundice is present in 20% to 30% of the cases. Ileus is also a common finding, which whenever is present limits the diagnostic accuracy of US examination, since gas in aperistaltic bowel obscures the pancreas. The diagnostic accuracy of US for pancreatitis is 83-92% when there is no limitation by gas in the abdomen. The role of US imaging in acute pancreatitis is the detection of gallstones, the follow-up of known fluid collections and the guidance of aspiration and drainage.

Independently of the causative factor, acute pancreatitis causes edema of the pancreas and as consequence irregular enlargement and diffuse lowering of the parenchymal echogenicity. Pancreas looks less echogenic and the clear-cut line between the organ and the splenic vein disappears. The use of colour Doppler US examination frequently shows hyperaemia within the hypoechoic regions of acute disease. Although the gland usually keeps its normal contour, a focal interstitial pancreatitis sometimes produces an echo-poor mass that is difficult to differentiate from a tumor mass.

Concerning patients with severe acute pancreatitis, the initial US examination should exclude the presence of gallstone disease. It is important to notice that within the first 24 hours of presentation of acute pancreatitis the sonographic appearance of pancreas may be normal. Therefore a normal pancreatic echogenicity does not exclude the diagnosis, and a repeat US scan should be performed later to identify the echo-poor and bulky gland, and also peripancreatic fluid collections. Extrapancreatic abnormalities that are often more important US findings suggesting the diagnosis include fluid in the lesser sac, in the anterior pararenal spaces, as well as the spread of inflammatory exudates along perivascular spaces. Often the splenic and superior mesenteric veins are involved with a hypoechoic inflammatory reaction creating a phenomenon called perivascular cloaking, leading to thrombosis of any or all portal veins. Ultrasonographic findings may last even after return of serum amylase to the normal levels.

Important *complications of acute pancreatitis* include pseudocyst formation, abscess, biliary obstruction or hemorrhage.

Pseudocysts are the most common complication and occur usually after 2-3 weeks.

They are fluid collections which are not surrounded by epithelial cell lining but only by inflammatory connective tissue. They contain pancreatic fluids and inflammatory excudate with high concentration in amylase. Pseudocysts are localised either inside the pancreatic parenchyma or extend into the abdomen or mediastinum and are usually unilocular. Clinical manifestation involves persistent pain, fever and ileus 2-3 weeks after acute pancreatitis. Ultrasonographically pseudocysts appear as anechoic rounded structures with regular borders, which in certain cases may contain septations or calcifications. Their size may increase or remain unchanged for months, and in most cases they disappear spontaneously by asymptomatic rupture to the intestine or the stomach. Within three weeks 20% of the pseudocysts disappear, while in 75% of the cases they appear with complications after 13-18 weeks. The main complication is intraperitoneal rupture, which appears in US scans as peripancreatic ascites together with the pseudocyst. Other complications include secondary infection, erosion into adjacent organs, bile duct obstruction and hemorrhage into the cyst. In cases of hemorrhage within the pseudocyst, then echogenic material is revealed by US and can be differentiated from an abscess only by percutaneous aspiration.

Abscess is an uncommon complication of acute pancreatitis and demands drainage because it has a high mortality that reaches up to 100%.

Another serious complication related to acute pancreatitis is invasion of the surrounding vessels leading to *gastrointestinal tract hemorrhage.*

A common complication is also the *obstruction of the bile duct,* which presents more often in chronic disease and is easily detected by US. Biliary dilatation is detected either due to pressure from the pseudocyst or due to the primary cause.

In cases of acute pancreatitis the whole upper abdomen should be examined by US in order to identify the cause as well as any possible complications.

Chronic pancreatitis refers usually to changes that result to the pancreas after repeated episodes of acute pancreatitis. Clinical presentation involves continuous or intermittent epigastric/back pain, anorexia and weight loss. Chronic pancreatitis is difficult to be detected only by US. Sonographically pancreas presents abnormal in about 85% of the cases, whereas in the remaining patients the pancreas has normal appearance.

The pancreas is usually normal or even smaller in size due to atrophy, with irregular scarring and poorly defined margins. In the early stages of the disease the gland appears sonographically enlarged and hypoechoic. Later it becomes inhomogeneous with generalized increased e-chogenicity and areas of diffuse or focal enlargement. In the late stages of chronic pancreatitis the gland becomes fibrosed and shrinks, leading to an atrophic, hypoechoic and heterogeneous appearance on US examination.

It is not unusual (20%-40%) to reveal sites of high echogenicity with acoustic shadowing corresponding to calcifications. With advancing disease these become more extensive, especially in an alcoholic background.

A suggestive sign of chronic pancreatitis is the dilated pancreatic duct with a diameter grater than 3 mm and the appearance of an anechoic linear structure along the pancreatic body. In severe chronic pancreatitis the pancreatic duct remains dilated with an irregular or beaded configuration due to multiple strictures.

Biliary dilatation usually occurs in about 30% of the patients.

Chronic pancreatitis is related to fatty degeneration of the pancreas which is probably the main cause of difficulty in the diagnosis of the disease with US and the loss of sonographic contrast between the gland and the surrounding tissues (retroperitoneal fat). Therefore a combination of imaging techniques is required to demonstrate all these features such as pancreatography and CT.

Mirizzi's syndrome

It is an uncommon condition that is characterized by normal sized common bile duct and dilated intrahepatic bile ducts. This occurs when a large calculus is inside the neck of the gallbladder or within the cystic duct, causing extrinsic mechanical compression of the common hepatic duct. Alternatively, post-cholecystectomy an impacted stone inside the cystic duct remnant may cause inflammation or pressure necrosis of the common hepatic duct. Sonography reveals the calculi and the dilated intrahepatic ducts or common hepatic duct.

Caroli's disease

Caroli's disease is an autosomal recessive congenital abnormality, which refers to the communicating cavernous ectasia of the intrahepatic biliary ducts. It has two distinctive forms:
– the "pure" form, which is characterized by saccular communicating intrahepatic ectasia without dilatation of the extrahepatic biliary ducts. It can occur in a focal or diffuse pattern. Frequently it is accompanied by lithiasis. Other complications include pyogenic cholangitis, hepatic abscess, intrahepatic bilary obstruction and development of cholangiocarcinoma (in 7% of the cases). The typical sonographic appearance involves dilatation of the intrahepatic bile ducts with cystic, diverticulum-like outpouchings, which converge toward the porta hepatis. This convergence is sufficient to set the diagnosis. Differentiation of this condition from polycystic liver disease is based on the demonstration of the communication between the sacs and the bile ducts.
– the second form, which appears in childhood and is associated with hepatic fibrosis leading to portal hypertension and end-stage liver failure. Other conditions that may be associated are infantile polycystic kidney disease and choledochal cysts. In cases of hepatic fibrosis involved, sonography reveals less pronounced biliary ductal dilatation, portal hypertension and cystic disease of the kidneys.

Choledochal cyst

Choledochal cyst is a rare congenital dilatation of extrahepatic portion of the biliary tree. It is more common among Asians and predominates in women. Approximately one third of the cases with congenital choledochal cysts are asymptomatic until adulthood. Clinical presentation involves abdominal mass, pain, fever or biliary obstruction and jaundice. It refers to local cystic or aneurysmal dilatation of the bile duct with various subtypes described, including:

Type 1: it is the most common type, characterized by *diffuse* biliary dilatation and by an ectatic appearance proximal to a stenotic or atretic distal common bile duct segment.

Type 2: is a *localized* congenital diverticulum-like outpouching of the common bile duct, which originates from its side wall.

Type 3: it is the *choledochal cyst,* which presents as herniation and dilatation of the common duct within the wall of the duodenum.

Complications associated with choledochal cysts are biliary obstruction and icterus, recurrent bacterial cholangitis, and biliary malignancy which may also involve the gallbladder and the whole biliary tract.

Ultrasound examination can with certainty diagnose the Type 1 cases, because it reveals a cyst-like dilated duct segment which communicates with the remainder of the biliary system. Type 2 is diagnosed by conclusion, because the point of communication between the cyst and the ductal system is not easily demonstrated.

Type 3 presents in 60% of the cases with generalized biliary dilatation.

The diagnosis may be confirmed with scintigraphy and accumulation of technetium (Tc)-99m-labeled iminodiacetic acid radioisotopes within the cyst.

Rupture of echinococcal cyst

Humans are infested by two species of *Echinococcus,* the *E. granulosus* and the *E. multilocularis,* with the granulosus being the more common organism that is classically featured in the literature. The Echinococcal cysts affect predominantly the right lobe (85%) of the liver. They have a three-layered capsule (the outermost layer, called pericyst; the middle, "lami-

nated "layer; and the innermost, one cell thick germinal layer) and a colorless, opalescent content. In many cases "daughter cysts" are generated inside the main cyst as this ages, creating a "cyst-within-a cyst" appearance. Sonographic appearance typically involves visualization of "daughter cysts", a double-line sign at the wall of the cyst due to separation of the layers of the cyst wall, cyst wall calcification suggesting a degenerated echinococcal cyst and the "fallen lily sign" in which the endocyst has fallen away from the fibrous pericyst.

The Echinococcal cysts are usually asymptomatic. They present with early symptoms in case of pressure on adjacent organs and these include pain, tenderness and a palpable mass. Echinococcal cysts may be secondarily infected by biliary bacteria with clinical symptoms of pyogenic abcess. Other complication may be intraperitoneal rupture clinically presenting with anaphylaxis. In 5% to 10% of the cases, they are complicated by intrabiliary rupture which leads to biliary obstruction and clinically presents with colic, jaundice and urticaria. The daughter cysts are visualized within the dilated bile ducts as echogenic structures with no acoustic shadow, while an Echinococcal cyst is also present inside the liver.

Hemobilia

Hemobilia refers to blood within the biliary system either due to trauma, spontaneous or iatrogenic, or due to coagulopathy, congenital (hemophilia) or acquired (anticoagulation therapy, sever liver disease or multiple organ failure). Hemobilia presents with increasing incidence as a result of the increasing number of hepatic and biliary interventions, such as liver biopsy, placement of transjugular intrahepatic portosystemic shunt (TIPS) or percutaneous transhepatic cholangiography (PTC). The radiologic appearance of blood in the biliary tree or in the gallbladder as well depends on the imaging modality and the age of blood products. On ultrasound examination, recently coagulated blood is echogenic, non-shadowing and homogeneous mass-like, while over time the proportion of echogenic components decreases and slight heterogeneity is present. The thrombus may stick to the wall of gallbladder or bile duct and biliary obstruction may occur. As the clot lyses a multiloculated mass appears with or without linear strands, whereas the color Doppler US examination confirms an avascular mass presentation.

Benign biliary tumors

Benign tumors of the bile ducts are extremely rare and include papillomas, adenomas, cystadonomas, hamartomas, lipomas fibromas and granular cell myoblastomas, that all may present with signs of biliary obstruction and jaundice.

Papillomas and adenomas are solid intraluminal masses with low to moderate echogenicity presenting without shadowing.

Cystadenomas manifest mainly in young or middle aged females and are multiloculated cystic lesions with mural nodules.

Granulosa cell tumors present as echogenic masses within the bile ducts that may have shadowing, thus indistinguishable from gallstones.

Strictures

Almost 95% of benign strictures result from surgical injury and more often are associated with cholecystectomy. The common bile duct at the level of the porta hepatis is the most common site of such strictures. During the early postoperative period most bile duct injuries sustained during cholecystectomy are recognized by the manifestation of obstructive jaundice, bile peritonitis or biliary fistula.

Another type of post-operative stricture is the stenosis of a biliojejunal anastomosis months after a major bilio-digestive op-

eration such as a "Whipple" or a partial hepatectomy with portal invasion.

Other benign bile duct strictures occur as a result of inflammation and may be associated with pancreatitis, infections, gallstones or duodenal ulcer disease.

b. Malignant masses

Pancreatic carcinoma

Malignant tumors of the pancreas represent the 4th most frequent type of cancer and usually affect patients 60 years or older. It has a 5 year survival that ranges from 1% to 12% due to insidious development and aggressive nature of the tumor. Diagnostic sensitivity of US for pancreatic carcinoma is between 56% and 94%.

Most cases are detected in the settings of painless jaundice or a palpable mass. In nonjaundiced patients the primary modality to search for an occult pancreatic carcinoma is computed tomography (CT) rather than US. Adenocarcinoma of the pancreas is most commonly (2/3 of the cases) focal, located to the head of the pancreas, whereas only a 6% of the cases are diffuse. In the more advanced stages of the local type of adenocarcinoma, there is a spread of tumor to the whole organ as well as an invasion of the splenic vein with subsequent obstruction.

Pancreatic carcinoma on US examination is usually seen as a focal mass with irregular borders and a relatively low echogenicity. Three types have been described: a. diffuse echogenicity with irregular internal shadowings, b. central echogenicity with anechoic periphery, c. anechoic area with some internal echogenic sites.

Obstructive jaundice is a common sign in cases of pancreatic head carcinoma together with a distended gallbladder. (Figure 5).

Dilatation of the pancreatic duct occurs in 40% of the cases, while dilatation of the common bile duct occurs in 70%

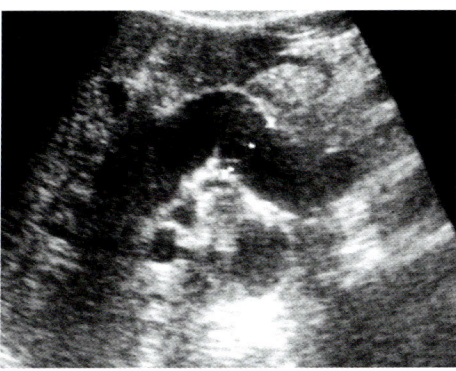

FIGURE 5: Dilated gallbladder (obstruction at a lower level).

of the cases. (Figure 6) The typical "double duct sign" of pancreatic carcinoma refers to simultaneous dilatation of both ducts.

In many cases, cancerous masses although anechoic may be differentiated from cysts by an unclear posterior wall.

Occasionally calcifications are present with the typical strong focal reflections and the acoustic shadows, therefore calcification is not specific for chronic pancreatitis.

A mass of less than 2 cm is usually difficult to be diagnosed by US, however the presence of indirect signs presenting as consequence of the mass are usually

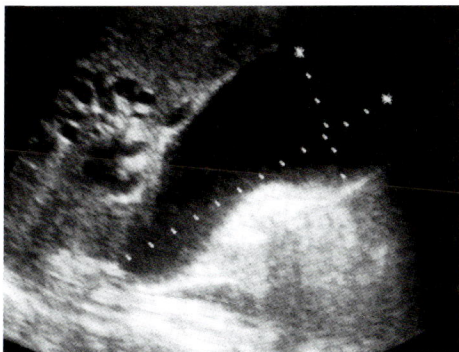

FIGURE 6: Whole length dilated common bile duct.

leading to suspicion and further evaluation towards the correct diagnosis. These signs are: dilatation of the biliary system, lymph node enlargement, metastases. Pancreatic carcinoma gives metastases to the liver, to the peripancreatic tissues, and to the peripancreatic or porta hepatis lymph nodes.

The use of color Doppler ultrasonography is useful in assessing the resectability of pancreatic neoplasms. Curative resection is not possible in the presence of vascular invasion, as well as in the case of extarpancreatic spread of the tumor. Tumor may extend up to invade the splenic and portal veins, while flow within the hepatic and gastroduodenal arteries may also be affected. Portal vein is involved in about 65% of the pancreatic tumor cases. The color Doppler US examination produces a high velocity jet through the narrowed area and a turbulent flow distal to the stenosis. Portal vein occlusion obliterates the Doppler signal, but in some cases collateral vessels may be demonstrated.

Cystadenoma and cystadenocarcinoma are less frequent tumors of the pancreas and are more common in women aged between 50-60 years old. They present with typical ultrasonographic appearance, which is anechoic areas with internal septations. They are frequently related to gallbladder stones, diabetes mellitus or other neoplastic diseases. They are more commonly located in the body and tail of the pancreas and must be differentiated from pseudocyst.

Carcinoma of the ampulla of Vater

Ampullary carcinoma arises from the glandular epithelium of the ampulla of Vater and is better differentiated than other pancreatic carcinomas. It may be associated with Gardner syndrome, familial polyposis coli and colonic carcinoma. Clinically presents earlier than other pancreatic carcinomas due to bile duct obstruction, with signs of intermittent jaundice, epigastric pain and weight loss.

On ultrasound examination, the biliary system is dilated until the level of the head of pancreas, which is visualized normal. (Figure 7)

These tumors are small at presentation and usually not seen on US examination. When seen they usually present as hypoechoic lesions within the lower end of the common bile duct, with or without infiltration of the adjacent pancreatic parenchyma.

Ampullary carcinoma is better visualized by endoscopic ultrasound, which has an accuracy of 87%, and usually reveals a submucosal mass or a prominent papilla or a mass protruding through the orifice.

Cholangiocarcinoma

Primary malignant tumors of the bile ducts occur generally in patients at the 6th and 7th decades and are more common in men than women. Most bile duct tumors are adenocarcinomas that tend to be infiltrative with a gradual obliteration of the bile duct lumen. They may develop at any level of the biliary tree, and when located at the level of the porta hepatis at the confluence of the right and left hepatic ducts primary cholangiocarcinoma is referred as Klatskin tumor. These tumors vary in size from large solid masses to lesions of a few millimeters in thickness infiltrating the submucosa.

Cholangiocarcinoma that involves only one hepatic duct, more frequently the left one, because the left lobe of the liver is usually smaller in size than the right one, may present without signs of obstructive jaundice, which presents only when the other sided bile duct is also obstructed, i.d. the right one.

On US examination, biliary dilatation is revealed down until the level of obstruction. At this level US scan reveals a hyperechoic area and an abrupt cutoff causing proximal dilatation of the intrahepatic bile ducts. This irregular cutoff is highly suggestive of malignancy even if a mass is not evident. An intraluminal mass is occasionally detected, whereas in some cases the only finding may be the thickening of the wall of the bile ducts. Intrahepatic cholangiocarcinoma is not easily diagnosed by US. When located at the extrahepatic duct system, primary cholangiocarcinoma usually causes obstruction at the level of porta hepatis.

The role of ultrasound extends beyond the diagnosis of cholangiocarcinoma to assessment of operability by demonstrating the spread of the mass. Spread of the tumor is a direct invasion to the portal vein, to the hepatic artery, and to the liver, as well as metastatic spread to the regional lymph nodes.

Hepatoma

Hepatocellular carcinoma (HCC) is a malignant neoplasm of the liver that in 30% to 60% of the cases occurs in cirrhotic livers. Hepatitis B viral infection is an important predisposing factor for the development of HCC, while alcohol is also considered as causative agent. The peak incidence of HCC is between the 4th and 6th decades and its 5year survival rate is only 2.4%. HCC presents clinically with weight loss, fatigue and pain, while as

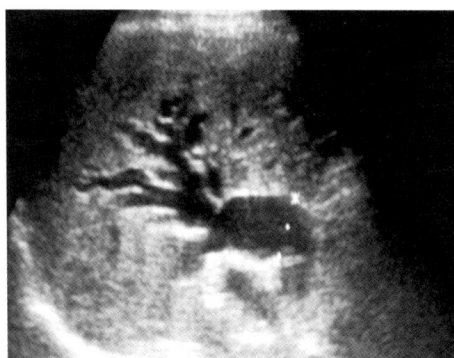

FIGURE 7: Dilated common bile duct at the level of the pancreatic head.

cites is also common. Metastases occur in 48% to 73% of the cases and are more common to the lung and nodes. In 19% to 40% of the cases at the time of diagnosis and usually at the late stages presents jaundice due to diffuse tumor infiltration of the liver, hilar invasion or advanced underlying cirrhosis and progressive liver failure. HCC invades the portal and hepatic veins in 20% to 30% of the cases. Obstructive jaundice is the presenting clinical feature at diagnosis in only 1% to 12% of the HCC patients and these cases have been described as "icteric type hepatoma" or "cholestatic type of HCC". In cases that HCC is located in the left lobe of the liver, a left biliary dilatation may present without obvious obstructive jaundice. Obstructive jaundice then does not present until the right hepatic duct is also involved. The abdominal US in is valuable in the initial investigation and differentiation of patients with presentation of cholestatic HCC.

The ultrasonographic appearance of hepatoma is variable, including in 60% to 65% of the cases a homogeneous mass with an echogenicity higher than the surrounding, often cirrhotic, liver parenchyma, or In the rest 35% to 40% of the patients a hypoechoic and/or heterogeneous mass. The margins of the lesion are either irregular or well defined by a capsule. It is frequent that these masses present mixed characteristics, areas of increased echogenicity and others almost anechoic. The sonographic appearance of HCC is related to the size of the lesions. Large hepatomas tend to present as heterogeneous, hyperechoic masses, often with cystic degeneration, whereas in some cases small calcifications may also be present. Smaller lesions (3 cm or less) demonstrate a tendency to be hypoechoic, homogeneous and better defined.[21]

HCC is known to be hypervascular tumor, and therefore the use of color Doppler sonography is useful in the detection of blood flow inside the tumor mass and hence the differentiation of this from other liver tumors.

Carcinoma of the gallbladder

The normal gallbladder presents by US examination as an oval or round shaped structure with no echogenicity like the cysts. It is located at the edge of the major fissure, which in 70% of the people in transverse section connects the right branch of portal vein with the neck of the gallbladder. The major fissure appears as a highly echogenic line and is an important sign for the identification of the gallbladder, especially in cases of a contracted or small gallbladder. Normally the transverse axis of the gallbladder should not exceed 13 cm and the wall should be less than 3 mm in thickness.

Gallbladder carcinoma is an uncommon and almost always fatal neoplasm of the elderly people, more frequently women. The most common tumors of the gallbladder are malignant adenocarcinomas. Clinical association of gallbladder carcinoma and cholelithiasis has been well described, while a calcified or "porcelain" gallbladder is associated with 20% of the cases. Clinically it is common to present with jaundice due to obstruction of the bile duct. The sonographic appearance is variable and depends on the extent and pattern of tumor growth. It is seen as a moderately echogenic mass projecting within the gallbladder lumen or as nonhomogeneous mass that extends to the adjacent organs. The gallbladder wall is infiltrated with resultant thickening and anomalous contour. Almost all cases of gallbladder carcinoma are related to gallstones, which are present in the residual gallbladder lumen or embedded within the tumor mass and sonographically appear with typical acoustic shadow.

Metastases

Metastases in the liver include the most

common hepatic tumor by a ratio of 20:1. In 25% to 50% of all cancer deaths the cause are liver metastases, which often grow more rapidly than the original tumor and give clinical presentation in 67% of the patients. Clinical manifestations include pain, ascites, jaundice, anorexia and weight loss. Metastases may cause obstructive jaundice by obstruction only of the small peripheral bile ducts without dilatation of the large proximal bile ducts.

Metastases are usually more than two masses within the liver parenchyma and have not a specific sonographic pattern. (Figure 8) They may present with an echogenicity higher or lower than the surrounding normal tissue. Metastases can also present as "target lesions" or anechoic masses. The degree of echogenicity is related to the histology of the lesions. Hypoechoic appearance is related to tissue homogenicity and necrosis, while increased echogenicity is related to tissue heterogenicity, collagen content, microvascularity and calcification. Calcified metastases are related to gastrointestinal tract tumors (especially colon and stomach), thyroid gland carcinoma and malignant carcinoid. The "target lesions" involve 13% of the hepatic metastases with the center of the target hypoechoic and the periphery hyperechoic or vice versa.

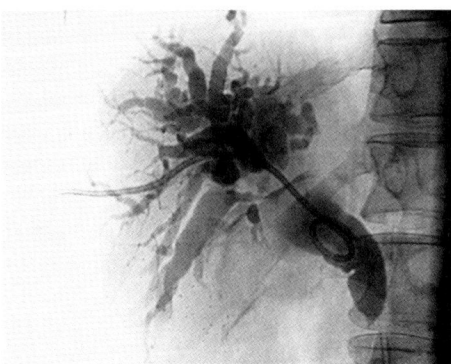

FIGURE 8: Liver metastases and ascites.

In cases of metastatic liver disease, the whole abdomen should be visualized carefully for the identification of the primary site of the tumor or for the staging of the disease by the presence of lymphadenopathy and/or ascites.

Metastatic adenopathy may also cause obstruction either at the level of porta hepatis or between the porta hepatis and the pancreas (suprapancreatic obstruction).

Lymphoma
Obstructive jaundice is a common sign of lymphadenopathy at the hepatoduodenal ligament with accompanying mesenteric and retroperitoneal lymphadenopathy in cases of non-Hodgkin lymphoma.

Hepatic involvement is an autopsy finding in 50% of the lymphoma cases and only 5.2% of those patients are identified with multiple hepatic nodules. The most common ultrasonographic appearance of such hepatic nodules is homogeneous, hypoechoic masses, while parenchymal heterogenicity is not uncommon due to lymphatic infiltration. The non-Hodgkin lymphoma may also present with hyperechoic or target lesions. In all cases, the liver is usually enlarged.

Gastric carcinoma
Gastric carcinoma may cause biliary obstruction by invading the common hepatic duct. Ultrasonographic examination reveals an echogenic mass with irregular margins inside the dilated portion of the common duct.

Patient work-up and relation of US to other imaging modalities

The radiologic imaging evaluation in patients suspected for biliary obstruction is very important, because bile duct dilatation may precede the clinical onset of jaundice.

Plain radiographs of the abdomen are of limited value and routinely not obtained for the assessment of patients with obstructive jaundice. Only up to 20% of the patients have gallstones that are opaque located in the right upper quadrant on plain radiographs.

Ultrasound examination is the initial imaging modality because it is a widely available and also a highly sensitive diagnostic tool, as described above.

Other noninvasive imaging modalities for the evaluation of the biliary tree are:

– **Radionuclide imaging** which refers to the intravenous administration of one of a family of technetium (Tc)-99m-labeled iminodiacetic acid radioisotopes for the hepatobiliary imaging. Complete obstruction is consistent with lack of visualization of the biliary tree while the liver is well seen. When obstruction is incomplete, the tracer is visible until the level of obstruction. This method requires good liver function and has limited usefulness with the advent of high-quality US imaging.

– **CT imaging,** which is done to provide data complementary to a previous US examination, such as to define the precise cause or level of biliary dilatation and to evaluate patients with intrabiliary air that limits the US scan. By using a dynamic contrast-enhancement technique the diagnostic value of CT is optimized, especially in cases of pancreatic mass or metastatic deposits. In cases of choledocholithiasis, their appearance and detection by CT depends on the chemical composition of the calculus. High attenuation calculi are easily detected by CT because of high calcium carbonate and phosphate content, but involve only the 20% of the total calculi. The low attenuation calculi, cholesterol or calcium bicarbonate, need special scanning parameters, such as close intervals (3-5 mm) and thin collimation (3-5 mm) through the transition zone of the distal duct.

With the recent introduction of the three-dimensional CT technique, where images are reconstructed and a helical CT cholangiogram is obtained, the diagnostic ability of CT imaging has improved and can be compared to that of endoscopic retrograde cholangiography, except for the fact that CT is only limited to the detection of a disease, whereas endoscopic retrograde cholangiography has also therapeutic options.

– **MR imaging** has lately gained wide spread acceptance, because of the development of newer pulse sequences and the introduction of paramagnetic compounds directed to hepatobiliary enhancement, which overcome the previous limited spatial resolution, low signal-to-noise ratio and the artifacts caused by normal physiologic motion. MR imaging has become the most challenging imaging modality for the biliary tree due to the development of MR cholangiopancreatography (MRCP), which has a sensitivity of 90%-95% for biliary and pancreatic ductal dilatation and strictures and 72%-95% for choledochlithiasis. Its accuracy is comparable to the endoscopic retrograde cholangiopancreatography (ERCP), although the latter remains necessary in many cases since it combines the ability of diagnostic and therapeutic option. MRCP is a good noninvasive modality that may aid to planning intervention and that is also useful when ERCP is not possible.

Guidelines for the patients who present with jaundice and their liver function tests suggest obstruction include in all cases US examination. Jaundice of unknown etiology by the US scan leads to CT or MR and MRCP, and according to the cause determined biopsy or therapy is performed.

Depending on the US findings, additional imaging examination(s) may be required and the patient managed further as follows:

– If *nondilated ducts* are visualized, then the expectant treatment follows. In certain circumstances, CT or MRCP are decided and also a liver biopsy may be performed.

– If *ductal dilatation* is observed and the etiology is indicated by the US, further patient management is decided according to the location and the cause of obstruction. If the US fails to determine the cause of dilatation, then additional imaging by CT or MRCP is essential.

If a proximal obstruction is present, then percutaneous transhepatic cholangiography (PTC) is suggested, whereas in a distal obstruction ERCP is indicated. (Figure 9, 10) Both of these procedures have therapeutic options with biliary drainage or stenting. (Figure 11) Calculus disease can be diagnosed by MRCP and managed by ERCP or surgery.

Malignant obstruction should be further evaluated by CT or MR for precise localization of the tumor and spread of the disease as well as for guiding a percutaneous biopsy. In cases of a mass disease, curative or palliative surgical intervention is further performed.

Endoscopic ultrasound

Endoscopic ultrasound (EUS) has been described over the last decades as the most significant advance in the upper gastrointestinal tract imaging, allowing structural information about the gastrointestinal

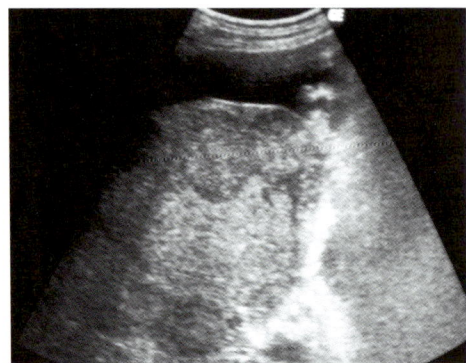

FIGURE 10: Percutaneous transhepatic biliary drainage: radiography (same patient with previous s-lide).

tract and the adjacent organs. The main advantage is that the transducer proximity to the tissues under investigation allows relatively high ultrasound frequencies to be used with consequent improvement of the spatial resolution. The most common frequencies used are from 5 to 20 MHz.

The main indications of EUS in the diagnosis of upper gastrointestinal pathology are the assessment of malignancies and the tumor staging concerning the oesophagus, the stomach, the pancreas, and the extrahepatic bile duct cancer (cholangiocarcinoma). It is also useful in the assessment of recurrence and the evaluation of the submucosal lesions.

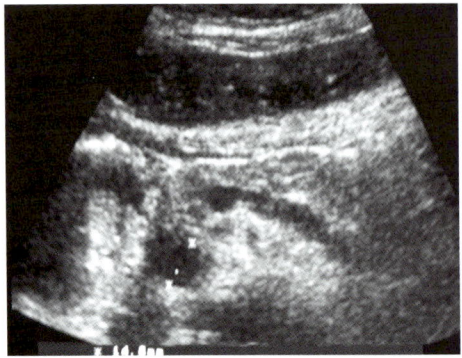

FIGURE 9: Dilated biliary tree and common bile duct.

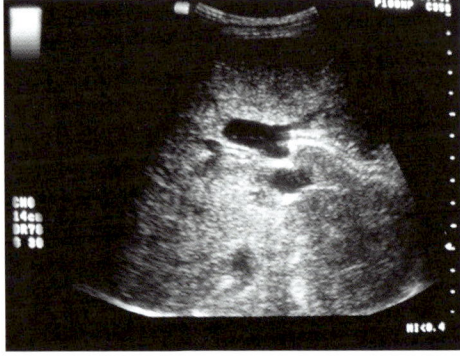

FIGURE 11: Obstructed metallic stent and dilated common bile duct (patient with Ca of the pancreatic head.

EUS has been proven to be superior to other imaging modalities (conventional US, CT, MRI) in terms of sensitivity and specificity in T staging of malignancies of the upper gastrointestinal tract.

EUS can diagnose most of the causes of obstructive jaundice such as pancreatobiliary malignancies and choledocholithiasis.

Pancreatic cancer appears as a hypoechoic lesion which is distinct from the surrounding parenchyma. The smaller masses tend to be roundish, whereas the larger ones appear more nodular and heterogeneous due to necrosis. Difficulties may arise concerning the diagnosis of small masses from inflammatory processes. In these cases general criteria are used for the differentiation, namely lymph node enlargement, vascular involvement or liver meatstases.

EUS is better than the other radiological imaging modalities in the detection of pancreatic head tumors, which are generally not easily detected. Compared to conventional ultrasonography and CT, the EUS has been proven to reach a sensitivity of almost 100% for large pancreatic masses. For smaller lesions measuring less than 3 cm in size, the accuracy in T staging (primary tumor) ranges between 78% and 94% and in N staging (regional lymph node metastasis) between 64% and 82%.

Cholangiocarcinoma appears as hypoechoic, inhomogeneous, intraductal or transductal mass with an associated echogenic rim due to fibrosis. The accuracy of EUS for cholangiocarcinoma is estimated approximately 85%.

However, the full staging of metastases (M staging, remote metastases) is not possible with EUS because of its limited depth of penetration and visualization related to the high frequencies used. Therefore other conventional imaging modalities such as ultrasound, CT or MRI should exclude distant metastases and EUS be limited to the potentially curable/resectable disease.

EUS has not as high specificity rates as sensitivity. However the use of fine needle aspiration during the procedure to obtain also cytological diagnosis increases the sensitivity and therefore the overall diagnostic accuracy. Therefore, EUS together with FNA should always be advocated in cases of painless obstructive jaundice or unexplained weight loss.

Summary

Ultarsound is by far the most common imaging modality used for the diagnosis of the biliary tract and the patients presenting with jaundice and a suspected biliary obstruction.

Despite the evolution of newer imaging modalities, such as CT with the helical CT cholangiogram and MR with the MR cholangiopancreatography, US remains the initial diagnostic approach of those patients due to its reasonably accepted sensitivity, specificity, accuracy in determining the level and cause of obstruction, availability, simplicity, safety and cost.

EUS has been shown to improve local staging of carcinomas and provide useful information in the assessment of most causes of obstructive jaundice such as pancreatic and biliary lesions. However its inability to assess distant metastases still gives conventional US priority in the evaluation of patients presenting with obstructive jaundice.

The site and cause of obstruction determined by US guide the choice of further imaging and possible therapeutic intervention.

REFERENCES

Alpern MB, Sandler MA, Kellman GM, Madrazo BL. Chronic pancreatitis: Ultrasonic features. Radiology 1985, 155:215-219.

Arger PH, Mulhern CB, Bonavita JA, Stauffer DM, Hale J. An analysis of pancreatic sonography in suspected pancreatic disease. J Clin Ultrasound 1979, 7:91-97.

Caroll BA, Oppenheimer DA. Sclerosing cholangitis: Sonographic demonstration of bile duct wall thickening. AJR 1982, 139:1016.

Conrad MR, Landay MJ, Janes JO. Sonographic "parallel channel" sign of biliary tree enlargement in mild to moderate obstructive jaundice. AJR 1978, 130:279.

Deitch EA. The realiability and clinical limitations of sonographic scanning ob the biliary ducts. Ann Surg 1981, 193:167-170

Dong B, Chen M. Improved sonographic visualization of choledocholithiasis. J Clin Ultrasound 1987;15:185-190.

Erickson RA, Garza AA. EUS with EUS-guided fine-needle aspiration as the first endoscopic test for the evaluation of obstructive jaundice. Gastrointest Endosc 2001, 53:475-484.

Federle MP, Cello JP, Laing FC, Jeffrey RB. Recurrent pyogenic cholangitis in Asian immigrants. Radiology 1982, 143:151.

Garber SJ, Donald JJ, Lees WR. Cholangiocarcinoma: ultrasound features and correlation of tumor position with survival. Abdominal Imaging 1993, 18:66-69.

Howard TJ. Pancreatic adenocarcinoma. Curr Probl Cancer 1996, 20:281-328.

Ishizaki Y, Wakayama T, Okada Y, Kobayashi T. Magnetic resonance cholangiography for evaluation of obstructive jaundice. AJR 1993, 12:2072-2077.

Kitamra T, Tanaka S. Evolution of ultrasonographic diagnosis for early cancer. JPN Clin Med 1996, 54:1236-1240.

Laing FC. Jaundice. RSNA Special Course in Ultrasound 1996, pp 59-68.

Laing FC. Ultrasound diagnosis of choledocholithiasis. Semin Ultrasound CT MR 1987, 8:103-113

Lun-Xiu Qin, Zhao-You Tang Hepatocellular carcinoma with obstructive jaundice: diagnosis, treatment, prognosis. World J Gastrocnterol 2003, 9:385-391.

Lyttkens K, Prytz H, Forsberg L. Ultrasound, hepatic lymph nodes and primary biliary cirrhosis. J Hepatol 1992, 15:136-139.

Russel RCG. Carcinoma of the pancreas and the ampulla of Vater. In: Misiewicz JS, Pounder RE, Venebles CW, eds. Diseases of the gut and Pancreas. Oxford: Blackwell Scientific, 1993.

Shawker TH, Garra BS, Hill MC, Doppman JL, Sindelar WF. The spectrum of sonographic findings in pancreatic carcinoma. J Ultrasound Med 1986, 5:169-177.

Shibata T, Kubo S, Itoh K, Sagoh T, Nishimura K, Nakano Y, Yamaoka Y, Ozawa K, Konishi J. Recurrent hepatocellular carcinoma: Usefulness of ultrasonography compared with computed tomography and AFP assay. J Clin Ultrasound 1991, 19:463-469.

Stenberg W, Tenner S. Acute pancreatitis. N Engl J Med 1994, 330:1198-1210.

Taylor KJW, Rosenfield AT, Spiro HM. Diagnostic accuracy of gray scale ultrasonography for the jaundiced patient. Arch Intern Med 1979, 139:60-63.

Trapnell JE, Duncan EHL. Patterns of incidence in acute pancreatitis. Br Med J 1975, 2:179-183.

Weill F, Eisencher A, Zeltner F. Ultrasonic study of the normal and dilated biliary tree: "shot-gun sign". Radiology 1978, 127:221-224

Yim HB, Yap WM, Chong PY. Clinical usefulness of Endoscopic Ultrasonography with or without fine needle aspiration in the diagnosis and staging of pancreatic carcinoma. Ann Acad Med Singapore 2005, 34:124-129.

The role of CT in the diagnosis of obstructive jaundice. Current advances

Triantopoulou Charikleia

INTRODUCTION

Computed Tomography (CT) is traditionally used for the evaluation of patients presenting with obstructive jaundice. The introduction of multidetector CT (MDCT) with increasing numbers of detector channels has also greatly enhanced the capability of CT in the work-up of biliary tract. High-quality multiplanar reconstructions (MPR) can be acquired, which are very helpful for biliary system anatomy assessment. Nowadays CT has become a competitor to Magnetic Resonance Imaging techniques (MRI-MRCP) for the diagnosis of bile ducts obstruction.

We will focus on the general approach of obstructive jaundice by current CT techniques, presenting the imaging appearances of the main liver, biliary, duodenal or pancreatic diseases that can cause biliary tract obstruction. Recent developments in CT cholangiography and virtual cholangioscopy as well as the diagnostic potential of these three-dimensional methods will also be discussed.

CT DETECTION OF BILLARY OBSTRUCTION

CT can accurately predict the presence of bile ducts obstruction, as there is strong correlation between obstruction and the presence of a dilated biliary system. Dilated intrahepatic bile ducts appear as confluent, circular or linear branching structures that enlarge and join together as they approach the porta hepatis. Less frequent patterns of intrahepatic bile duct dilatation include pruning, beading or skip dilatation. When the intrahepatic ducts size exceeds approximately 2 mm in diameter one should consider the presence of biliary obstruction (Figure 1).

The common hepatic duct is nearly always seen coursing through the porta hepatis. It is thin walled and may show mild contrast enhancement. The upper limit of its diameter varies among individuals, but 8-10 mm is generally accepted for common hepatic duct and common bile duct (Figure 2).

It is very important to be aware that there is a time lag from the onset of acute obstruction and the dilatation. So lack of

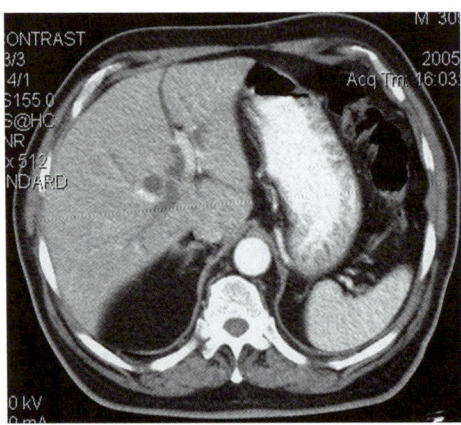

FIGURE 1: Contrast enhanced CT image demonstrates intrahepatic bile ducts dilatation.

biliary dilatation on CT does not preclude the presence of bile ducts obstruction. On the other hand dilated extrahepatic ductal system could be present in the absence of biliary obstruction. This is true for longstanding obstructions, where despite relief from obstruction duct cannot return to its normal diameter. It has also been reported that common bile duct increases in diameter during aging or after cholecystectomy. A predilection for severe bile ducts dilatation to involve left liver lobe more often than right liver lobe, regardless of the point of obstruction, has also been shown.

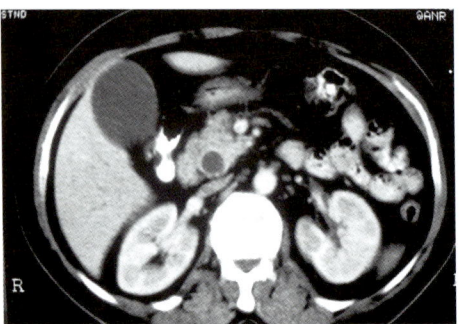

FIGURE 2: Contrast enhanced CT image shows marked common bile duct dilatation.

Determination of obstruction level by imaging is also very important for therapeutic decisions. For CT this level is better appreciated on coronal reformatted images. Nowadays using very thin sections on MDCT scanners we can get excellent reformatted "cholangiographic" views. The evaluation of transition zone from dilated to nondilated or nonvisualized duct can be very helpful in exact localization of obstruction level. Transitional zone appearance can also give a clue as to the cause of obstruction. So abrupt ductal termination with proximal dilatation is more often a result of malignant obstruction, whereas gradually tapering correlates with benign processes.

Concerning wall thickness of extrahepatic bile ducts it has been stated that thickness greater than 1.5 mm should be considered abnormal. There are four patterns of bile duct wall thickening each one associated with a specific group of diseases. Diffuse concentric thickening is found in acute cholangitis while diffuse eccentric pattern is most often seen in recurrent pyogenic cholangitis and primary sclerosing cholangitis. Focal concentric thickening in the distal common bile duct should alert the radiologists to the presence of duct stones, pancreatitis or pancreatic carcinoma. Focal eccentric thickening is a sign suggestive of cholangiocarcinoma. In fact any wall thickness greater than 5 mm should be considered neoplastic.

One of the pitfalls in the diagnosis of intrahepatic duct dilatation is perivascular lymphedema. However lymphedema tends to cause circumferential low attenuation around the veins, while dilated intrahepatic ducts are seen on only one side of the portal vein branches.

LIVER DISEASE

Hepatocellular carcinoma

Obstructive jaundice as the main clinical

feature is uncommon in patients with hepatocellular carcinoma (HCC) presenting in only 1-12% of the cases. Such cases are classified as "cholestatic type of HCC". Identification of this patient group by imaging techniques is very important, as surgical treatment may be beneficial (Figure 3).

HCC may involve the biliary tract in several ways: thrombus formation, hemobilia, compression or infiltration. Jaundice may also result from the external compression on the major bile ducts by metastatic lymphadenopathy at the level of porta hepatis. HCC invasion into bile ducts may be due to one of the following three mechanisms: a. Tumor growth that fills the biliary system, b. Separation of a fragment of necrotic tumor that migrates to the distal common bile duct, c. Hemorrhage that may fill the biliary tract with blood-clots.

Blood raises the attenuation of the bile to a level generally greater than 50 HU. As the blood clots high attenuation material can be shown in the dependent portion of the gallbladder or bile ducts. This appearance can persist for several days. But despite the recent improvements in various imaging modalities hemobilia is still sometimes incorrectly diagnosed as biliary tract carcinoma or stones. Moreover because of the cross-sectional orientation of CT images, anatomy is fragmented and CT alone is not accurate enough in providing detailed information of complex anatomic relationships. On the contrary 3D CT cholangiography with minimum intensity projection has been proven to be very effective in determining the level and cause of intrahepatic biliary obstruction.

Abscesses

Hepatic abscesses may have a pyogenic cause or may result from amebiasis or fungal disease. CT is often nonspecific, but usually shows a round or irregularly shaped hypodense mass, unilocular or

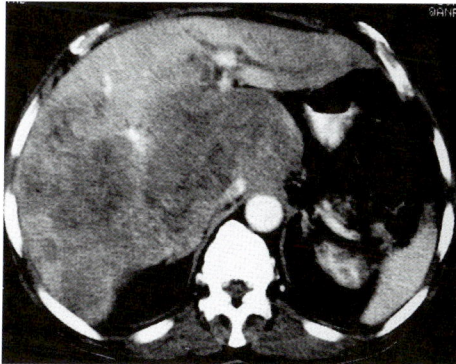

FIGURE 3: Contrast enhanced CT scan, demonstrates a large hepatoma with satellite nodules in right liver lobe, involving biliary tract and producing prominent bile ducts dilatation in left lobe.

multilocular with peripheral rim enhancement (Figure 4).

Obstructive jaundice may be present due to compression or biliary communication. In these cases pus or sludge may be evident in bile ducts. On CT pus measures 30 HU, but these values may be altered due to volume averaging effects.[12]

Pylephlebitis is an extremely rare condition associated with high mortality. It usually occurs secondary to infection in regions drained by the portal system. It is a precursor of liver abscesses that can present

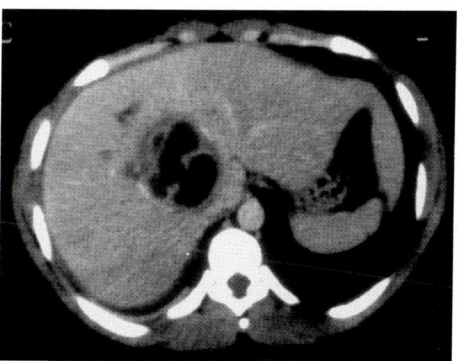

FIGURE 4: Typical CT features of a liver abscess in segment VIII with bile duct dilatation in the periphery.

variable appearances from well-circum-scribed cavities with enhancing rims to het-erogeneous masses indistinguishable from hepatic neoplasms. Rarely pylephlebitis can be complicated by obstructive jaundice.

Hydatic disease

CT appearance of hydatic cysts caused by Echinococcus granulosus depends on the stage of cyst growth. The disease may be complicated by secondary infection and cyst rupture. When the rupture in-volves the biliary system obstructive jaun-dice may be present. The demonstration of a well defined oval or round cystic mass, with multilocular appearance, fluid-density content and enhancement of cyst wall and septa, facilitates the diagnosis on CT imaging (Figure 5). Cyst attenuation contents may have a higher density value approaching 45HU (hydatic sand), while daughter cysts can have lower attenuation than the mother cyst. Dense calcifications indicate non-viability of the lesion.

DISEASES OF THE GALLBLADDER

Acute cholecystitis

Cholelithiasis is the cause of acute chole-cystitis in approximately 95% of the cases. Gallbladder stones can have a variety of appearances on CT depending on their chemical composition and pattern of calci-fication. CT is not indicated in the initial evaluation of patients suffering from acute cholecystitis. However the method is very important in evaluation of patients pre-senting with obstructive jaundice or con-fusing clinical pictures.

The most common CT findings are gallbladder distention (>5 cm in tran-sverse or AP dimension), gallbladder wall thickening (>3 mm), stones in the gall-bladder or cystic duct, poor definition of

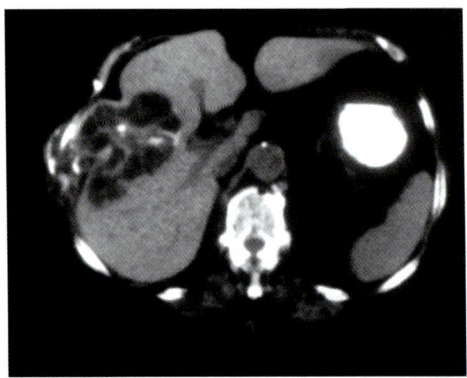

FIGURE 5: A large hydatid cyst on unenhanced CT p-resenting as a multilocular cystic mass with calcifi-cations. Bile duct dilatation at hepatic hilus is also e-vident.

the gallbladder wall at the interface with the liver, pericholecystic fluid, inflammato-ry changes in the pericholecystic fat and increase density of the bile (>20HU) (Fig-ure 6). Marked gallbladder wall enhance-ment is not a specific finding.

In approximately 15-30% of the patients complications may develop such as empyema, gangrene and perforation of the gallbladder leading to abscesses, chole-cystoenteric fistulas or bile peritonitis. CT findings include fluid collections in gallblad-der wall, liver or pericholecystic abscesses, gas in the gallbladder or in the bile ducts and ascites with enhancing peritoneum.

In case of complicated or chronic chole-cystitis a distinction from malignant wall thickening may not always be possible based on CT criteria alone. Diffuse wall thickening and infiltrative changes in peric-holecystic fat are nonspecific. The presence of a low attenuation halo around the gall-bladder is helpful in differentiation, as this is not often seen in gallbladder carcinoma.

Gallbladder carcinoma

Early diagnosis of gallbladder carcinoma is difficult because most patients present

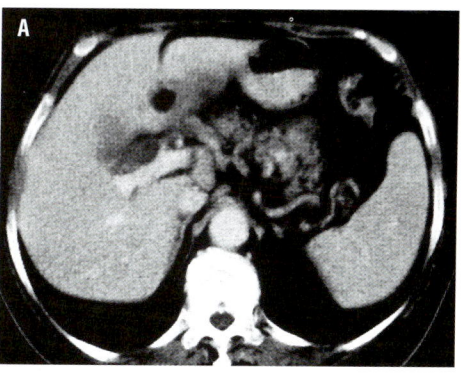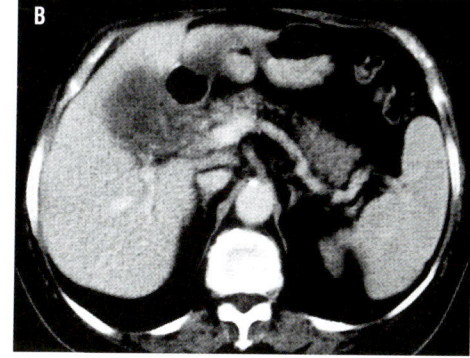

FIGURE 6: Acute cholecystitis: dilatation of common hepatic duct **(A)**, marked gallbladder wall thickening and poor definition of the gallbladder wall-liver interface **(B)**.

with nonspecific findings of right upper quadrant pain, weight loss, jaundice, anorexia or vomiting. CT is very helpful in evaluating local spread and potential resectability.

The most common presentation is a large soft tissue mass, replacing partially or completely the gallbladder. Infiltrative carcinomas show irregular contrast enhancement on CT with regions of internal necrosis. Approximately 25% of gallbladder carcinomas present as intraluminal masses. On CT polypoid cancers enhance homogeneously while adjacent gallbladder wall may be thickened. They usually do not show necrosis or calcification on CT.

The third pattern of presentation (focal or diffuse mural thickening), is the most difficult to diagnose due to the small size of early masses or to the presence of stones that can obscure subtle wall thickening. CT has been proven to be better than ultrasound (US) for evaluating thickness of gallbladder portions that are obscured by gallstones or mural calcifications.

Differential diagnosis of diffuse wall thickening includes cholecystitis, adenomyomatosis, inadequate gallbladder distention, hepatitis or low protein states. Signs helpful in making tumor diagnosis

are the presence of a focal mass associated with gallbladder wall thickening, liver invasion and enlarged lymph nodes in porta hepatis causing bile duct obstruction (Figure 7).

DISEASES OF THE BILE DUCTS

Choledochal cysts

Choledochal cyst is an uncommon cause of obstructive jaundice. The main clinical symptoms (abdominal pain, jaundice and

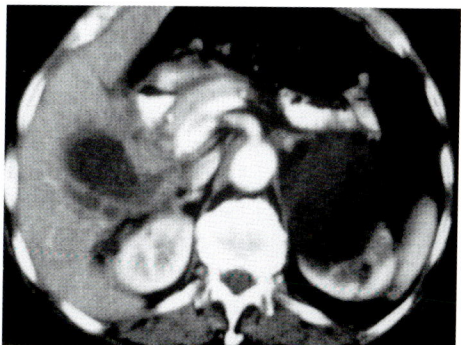

FIGURE 7: Gallbladder carcinoma: heterogeneous peripheral enhancement and liver invasion evident on CT image.

abdominal mass) occur in only one third of the patients. Associated anomalies of biliary system have been reported including double common bile duct, atresia of bile ducts, sclerosing cholangitis, congenital hepatic fibrosis, annular pancreas and finally anomalous junction of the pancreatic and common bile duct.

Todani et al. have expanded and modify the original classification of Alonzo-Lej. Type IA is cystic dilatation of the common bile duct, type IB is focal segmental dilatation of the distal common bile duct and type IC is fusiform dilatation of both the common hepatic duct and the common bile duct. Type II choledochal cysts are true diverticula arising from the common bile duct, while type III cysts are called choledochoceles and are defined as cystic dilatation involving only the intraduodenal portion of the common bile duct. In Type IVA there are multiple intrahepatic and extrahepatic cysts, while in type IVB there are only multiple extrahepatic cysts. Type V or Caroli's disease includes single or multiple intrahepatic cysts.

The role of imaging is to delineate cysts anatomy, determine the relationship of the cysts to intra and extrahepatic biliary tree, evaluate associated biliary tract abnormalities and identify complications including stones, strictures and neoplasms. On CT a choledochal cyst appears as a right upper quadrant fluid-filled structure in contiguity with the extrahepatic bile duct (Figure 8). Differentiation must be done from other cystic lesions that may occur in this region such as pancreatic pseudocysts or enteric duplication cysts. CT defines the anatomy and the extend of ductal dilatation and is very useful for demonstrating a tumor mass, although small wall lesions are better depicted on ultrasound.

Although ultrasound (US) is adequate for the accurate diagnosis of choledochal cysts in most patients, CT can be very

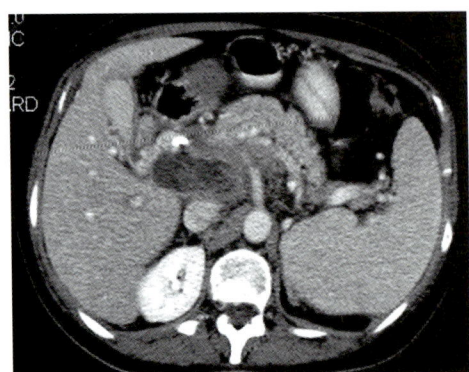

FIGURE 8: Choledochal cyst appearing as a dilated tubular structure that follows the course of common bile duct is shown. High-density material (sludge) in the distal part of the cyst as well as lymph nodes enlargement are also evident.

useful in demonstrating relationships with surrounding structures in cases where US fails to depict entrance of exrahepatic bile ducts into the cyst.

The appearance of a choledochocele on CT differs from that of the other choledochal cysts. This abnormality appears as a fluid-filled mass that protrudes into duodenal wall and can be opacified with the use of an oral biliary contrast agent.

Caroli disease can be diagnosed on CT by the presence of multiple, intrahepatic rounded cystic spaces of varying sizes communicating with the dilated intrahepatic bile ducts. These changes can be observed diffusely throughout the liver or in a single liver segment or lobe. The cystic spaces often contain calculi or debris. Central dot sign is considered as pathognomonic for Caroli disease. This is characterized by the presence of a small dot in the dependent portion of the dilated bile duct that enhances intensely after intravenous contrast administration. This dot is representative of portal venous radicles that are enveloped by the markedly dilated bile ducts.

Caroli disease must be differentiated

from polycystic liver disease and obstructive bile duct dilatation. Cysts in polycystic liver disease are rounder and smoother and they deform bile ducts. Furthermore in obstructive bile duct disease dilatation is most marked centrally, tapers towards the periphery and lacks areas of cystic dilatation.

Multiplanar reformations with or without the use of cholangiographic contrast agent are very helpful in difficult cases. Virtual cholangiography has also been proposed as an alternative imaging technique defining mucosal changes of choledochal cysts suggestive of carcinoma.

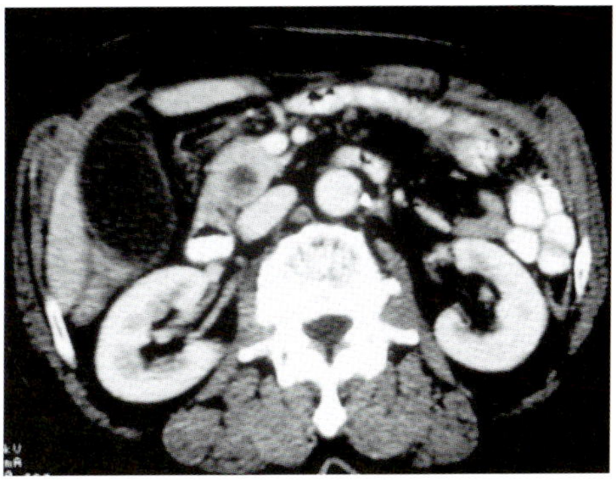

Choledocholithiasis

Detecting stones in the ducts by imaging techniques is easier when biliary dilatation is also present. CT appearances of biliary stones vary with the chemical composition.[27] Detection of stones in common bile duct depends also on the position within the duct and the plane of the stone and the duct relative to the plane of the CT image. 20% of stones are of high attenuation and can easily been identified even in the absence of bile ducts dilatation. Other appearances include soft tissue attenuation, near water attenuation, low attenuation, or a rim of high attenuation.

Visualization of the soft-tissue-density and low attenuation stones depends on the presence of a rim of surrounding water – attenuation bile. This has been considered as the most specific and sensitive sign for the presence of a common bile duct stone known as the target sign. The crescent sign is characterized by a soft-tissue-attenuation stone lying in the dependent portion of the bile duct, with a crescent of lower attenuation bile seen anterior to the stone (Figure 9). Rarely when a soft-tissue-density or low attenuation stone occupies the entire lumen of common bile duct, the dilated duct appears to come to an abrupt termination mimicking a neoplasm.

FIGURE 9: Choledocholithiasis presenting on CT as a soft tissue lesion lying in the dependent portion of the common bile duct.

Proper CT imaging technique is essential to accurate detection of biliary ducts stone and to avoid pitfalls in interpretation. CT best visualizes calculi using the highest kVp technique available. The use of high attenuation oral contrast material should also be avoided. Water can be used instead, providing an excellent enteric contrast medium. Unenhanced CT scan greatly increases the conspicuity of many stones compared with the intravenous contrast enhanced images. On the other hand a clue to the presence of bile duct stones on CT is the visualization of a focally thickened distal common bile duct wall appearing as an enhancing concentric focal thickening (>2 mm).

CT accuracy in bile ducts stones detection is estimated to reach 95%. Main pitfalls are due to pancreatic duct calculi, oral contrast in a duodenal diverticulum or reflux of oral contrast from the duodenum into the common bile duct.

Mirizzi syndrome

The Mirizzi syndrome is an unusual cause of stone disease causing biliary obstruction. The obstruction is caused by the extrinsic compression of the common hepatic duct or the common bile duct from an impacted stone in the gallbladder neck or in the cystic duct. The compression can be caused either by the impacted stone, or by the associated periductal inflammation. Low insertion of the cystic duct into the common hepatic duct has been proposed as the predisposing factor.

The impacted calculus often erodes from the gallbladder neck or cystic duct into the periductal tissues or into the common hepatic duct. This can lead to the formation of a large cavity. CT findings in Mirizzi syndrome include obstruction of the common hepatic duct, widening of the gallbladder neck, an irregular cavity near the gallbladder neck and stones in the periductal or pericholecystic soft tissues[6] (Figure 10).

Mirizzi syndrome must be considered in the differential diagnosis of patients presenting with obstructive jaundice. CT can not only detect the findings of the syndrome but also may help in differentiation from other causes of extrinsic compression of the common hepatic duct like hydrops of the gallbladder, carcinoma of the gallbladder or cystic duct, enlarged lymph nodes in the porta hepatis, pancreatic pseudocysts and an enlarged cystic duct remnant in patients who have had a cholecystectomy.

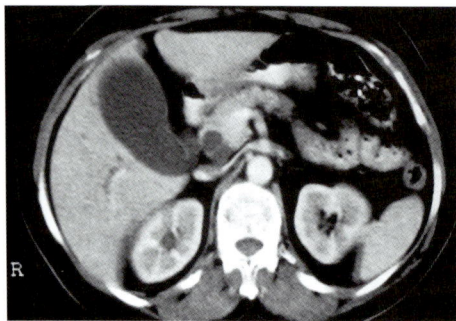

FIGURE 10: Mirizzi syndrome: dilatation of the gallbladder, cystic duct and common bile duct due to lithiasis of the distal cystic duct.

Ascending cholangitis

The classic signs and symptoms of acute ascending cholangitis are right upper quadrant pain, jaundice and sepsis, presenting in only 60-70% of the patients. CT findings include dilatation of intra and extrahepatic bile ducts, increased bile attenuation, diffuse and concentric bile duct wall thickening, gas in the bile ducts or portal vein branches and intrahepatic abscesses. Long-standing and recurrent infections can cause diffuse intrahepatic strictures and duct irregularities.

In fact there is no correlation between the presence and degree of bile duct dilatation and disease severity although the presence of hepatic abscesses, pneumobilia and portal venous gas are indicative of a poor prognosis. In any case the absence of CT findings does not exclude the presence of infection.

Sclerosing cholangitis

Sclerosing cholangitis is either primary or secondary to prior biliary infection. There are many patterns of disease appearance in cholangiography encountered also at CT. Diffuse multifocal strictures, limited duct branching ("pruning"), "beaded" appearance of the bile ducts, diverticular outpouchings and stones are the main possible findings. Abnormalities of the intrahepatic bile ducts have usually an irregular or asymmetric distribution. When there is extrahepatic bile duct involvement wall thickening, bile duct dilatation and enhancing intraluminal mural nodules can be seen.

Long-standing sclerosing cholangitis leads to cirrhosis with characteristic CT findings concerning hepatic morphology. CT or US can not visualize subtle changes of intrahepatic ducts. On the other hand CT is very helpful in the evaluation of the complications of the disease such as bile duct calculi, cirrhosis, portal hypertension or cholangiocarcinoma.

CT findings suggestive of the development of cholangiocarcinoma include a polypoid mass, progressive stricture formation on serial imaging examinations, or the development of large, non segmental areas of marked bile duct dilatation. The advantage of CT over cholangiography is the ability to evaluate the extraductal spread of the disease, including lymph node involvement and distant metastases.

Cholangiocarcinoma

The most common tumor of the bile ducts is cholangiocarcinoma. Cholangiocacinomas generally are classified as intrahepatic (peripheral) lesions, hilar lesions, and distal ductal tumors. Morphologically the tumors can be scirrhous infiltrative neoplasms leading to hepatic lobar atrophy, exophytic bulky masses and rarely polypoid intraluminal ductal lesions. CT appearance depends on their location, morphology and tumor pathology concerning the presence of fibrous stroma and mucin-producing glandular structure.

About 20-30% of cholangiocarcinomas are peripheral intrahepatic masses. On CT tumors are usually of lesser attenuation than liver on unenhanced images and show patchy and peripheral enhancement that becomes more prominent during the portal venous phase (Figure 11). The tumors with a predominant fibrous content demonstrate a characteristic delayed marked retention of the contrast at 6-20 minutes when compared with liver (Figure 12). This delayed enhancement can simulate hemangiomas but can be helpful in differentiating cholangiocarcinoma from metastases. If the tumors produce extensive mucin the appearance on CT can be of low attenuation approaching water and simulating cystic tumors.

A characteristic feature of intrahepatic cholangiocarcinoma is the associated atrophy of liver parenchyma with retraction of the overlying liver capsule. The atrophy can

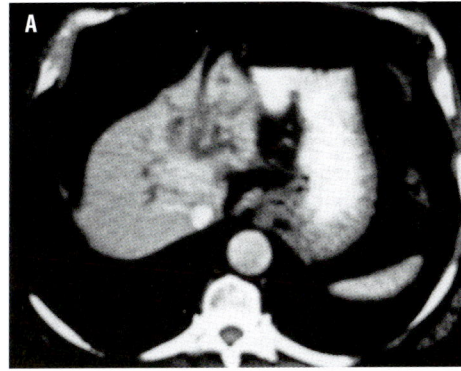

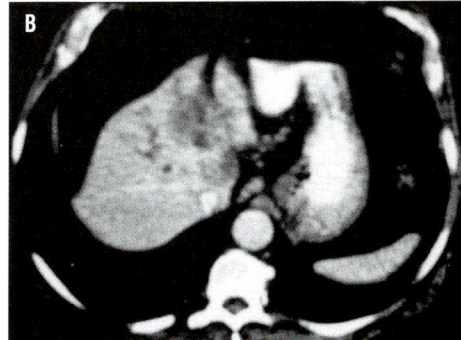

FIGURE 11 A, B: Cholangiocarcinoma presenting on CT images as a poorly defined low attenuating mass with slight peripheral enhancement and dilatation of intrahepatic ducts in left liver lobe.

result from either portal venous obstruction or chronic bile ducts obstruction. These findings may also be seen in other tumors following successful chemotherapy.

The most common location for cholangiocarcinoma is either at the confluence of the right and left hepatic ducts or at the proximal common hepatic duct known as a "Klatskin" tumor. These tumors when small are very difficult to visualize early at cross-sectional imaging. Multi-planar reconstructions of high-resolution images using MDCT scanners are very helpful in defining the level of obstruction and the presence of a mass. Focal eccentric thickening of the bile duct just proximal to complete obstruction by a soft-tissue

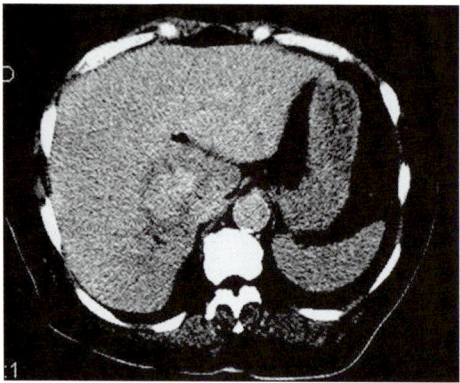

FIGURE 12: Cholangiocarcinoma in liver segment I, on delayed contrast enhanced CT image presenting as a hyperattenuating mass.

mass replacing the bile duct lumen on axial images is the clue for the diagnosis.

If no tumor mass is seen diagnosis of hilar cholangiocarcinoma can be made by the presence of high-grade intrahepatic bile duct dilatation and the absence of right and left hepatic ducts union. If the neoplasm is located at a lower level, at the point of obstuction the duct will terminate abruptly or there may be associated eccentric thickening of bile duct wall.

Hilar cholangiocarcinoma must be differentiating from hilar adenopathy or extrinsic masses causing biliary obstruction due to compression or displacement of the duct. It also important to differentiate hepatocellular carcinoma invading the biliary tree from a primary biliary tumor with liver metastases, because treatment for these tumors is quite different. An additional finding that can be seen in patients with cholangiocarcinoma is segmental or lobar attenuation abnormalities. These are due to obstruction of portal venous flow to the liver that results to a compensatory increase of arterial flow to the affected liver portion.

Three-dimensional CT cholangiography and rotating cine-cholangiography

have been reported to be very helpful in depicting hilar bile ducts anatomy while allowing accurate assessment of tumor extension. Selection of surgical procedure can be influenced by preoperative lesion evaluation with three-dimensional and cine cholangiograms.

The least common location for cholangiocarcinoma is in the distal duct. Small masses are extremely difficult to visualize by CT and differentiation from other periambullary tumors is not always possible. Bile duct wall thickening greater than 5 mm with intense contrast enhancement must be considered as suspicious for the presence of cholangiocarcinoma (Figure 13).

Results of PET-CT in the evaluation of cholangiocarcinomas are controversial. Some authors have found this method valuable for differentiation of benign versus malignant bile duct strictures but others did not found reliable results. However there is consensus that FDG-PET is very helpful in detecting lymph node and distant metastases in hilar cholangiocarcinoma.

Benign bile duct tumors

Bile duct adenoma is the most common benign bile duct tumor. Usually small, in rare cases it can attain a large size and cause biliary obstruction. Distal adenomas often present with obstructive jaundice with or without abdominal pain thus mimicking biliary calculi, cholangitis, choledochal cysts or carcinoma.

The current WHO classification separates all benign tumors within extrahepatic biliary tree into adenomas (papillary, tubular and tubulopapillary), cystadenomas and papillomatosis. Other more rare pathologies include fibromas, lipomas, hamartomas, carcinoid and neuromas. In general there are no specific imaging features of these tumors that allow for differentiation from malignant ones. Neuroen-

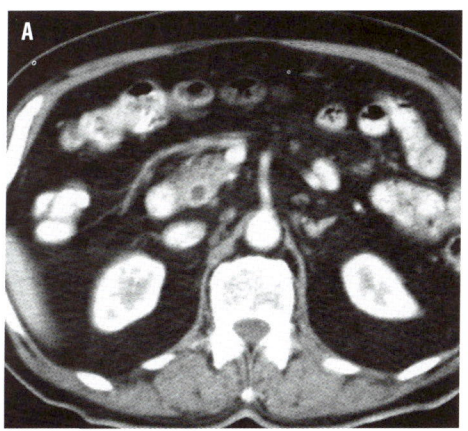 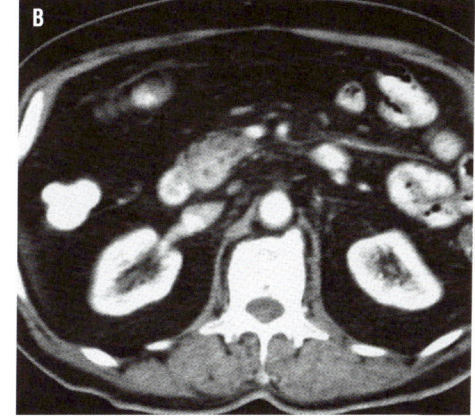

FIGURE 13: Distal cholangiocarcinoma: CT shows thickening of common bile duct wall with marked dilatation **(A)** and contrast enhancement **(B).**

docrine or carcinoid tumors are the exception displaying intense contrast enhancement during the arterial phase.

Postoperative complications

Bile ducts injury can result from a variety of percutaneous and operative hepatobiliary procedures. Main complications are associated with liver transplantation or laparoscopic cholecystectomy. Patients can have non-specific symptoms including obstructive jaundice, abdominal pain or distention and fever.

Biliary complications in liver transplant recipients include bile duct strictures due to ischemia, biliary obstruction, bile duct leaks, bile duct stones, bilomas and cystic duct remnant mucoceles. CT can show bile ducts dilatation, free fluid in abdomen and pelvis, or intrahepatic fluid collections representing bilomas. CT guided FNA is needed in some cases to verify content of fluid collections or possible infection of bilomas.

In cases of cystic duct remnant mucocele, CT can show a well-defined fluid-attenuation mass in the region of the porta hepatis adjacent to the common hepatic duct. These mucoceles may cause bile duct obstruction. Differential diagnosis includes loculated ascites, lymphocele, biloma, abscess or a fluid-filled Roux-en-Y jejunal loop.

Cholecystectomy related complications are retained common bile duct stones, bile duct injury resulting to various degree of stenosis, incomplete gallbladder resection or infection. Bile ducts injuries may result from mistaking the common hepatic duct for the cystic duct. Bile ducts variations that are present in up to 25% of people (like aberrant right hepatic duct) predispose patients to possible postoperative complications. Preoperative knowledge of possible anatomic variations by imagines methods like helical CT cholangiography are very helpful to avoid complications during open or laparoscopic cholecystectomy.

CT findings in patients with bile ducts injuries are nonspecific and differential diagnosis of perihepatic fluid collection includes seromas, lympoceles, hematomas or abscesses. CT may also demonstrate retained stones in the common bile duct or stones dropped into the peritoneal space.

PERIAMPULLARY CARCINOMAS

Periampullary carcinomas arise within 2cm of the major duodenal papilla and comprise carcinomas of distal common bile duct, ampulla, duodenum and pancreas. All these tumors share the same clinical features and therapeutic approach. However their long-term outcomes vary.

Ampullary carcinoma manifests at CT as small mass, periductal thickening or bulging of the duodenal papilla (Figure 14). Dilatation of both biliary and pancreatic ducts are seen in 50% of the cases. Jaundice develops early and precedes other common symptoms. Ampullary carcinomas have a tendency toward intraluminal growth and frequently manifest with a polypoid or papillary form. Extraluminal extension is relatively infrequent.

When the mass is not seen bulging papilla (formed by protrusions of dilated biliary or pancreatic duct) may mimic benign biliary dilatation, pancreatitis or a choledochocele. Double duct sign (dilatation of both the pancreatic and bile ducts) is a common finding also in pancreatic head carcinoma. However the most distal parts of the pancreatic and bile ducts are relatively spared from tumor infiltration. Another clue for the differential diagnosis is that the distance from the duodenal lumen to the stenotic segment is relatively longer in pancreatic carcinoma than in ampullary carcinoma.

In duodenal periampullary tumors variable degrees of pancreatic and biliary duct dilatation can be seen. Primary tumors can be identified as small polypoid masses, fungating masses or scirrhous pattern with eccentric duodenal wall thickening and luminal narrowing (Figures 15, 16).

Patients with ampullary or duodenal carcinoma even with nodal metastases have better 5-year survival rates than those with bile duct or pancreatic carcinoma. Concerning tumor resectabilty it has been proven that CT is the single most useful test providing correct diagnosis and accurate assessment of resectability in a large number of patients. CT reaches the highest sensitivity among other imaging methods in discrimination between benign and malignant tumors. CT is also better in demonstrating locoregional tumor spread. In cases when CT cannot depict the tumor, endoscopic ultrasound (EUS) should be performed. Uncertain venous infiltration can also be verified by magnetic resonance imaging (MRI) or EUS.

PANCREATIC DISEASES

Acute pancreatitis

Acute pancreatitis often creates mass effect on the distal common bile duct with biliary obstruction. CT is the imaging modality of choice for diagnosis and staging of suspected acute pancreatitis, follow-up evaluation and guidance for percutaneous interventions.

The role of CT in establishing patient prognosis has been proven by many studies. Balthazar and colleagues defined a composite CT severity index (CTSI) to assess the severity of parenchymal gland necrosis and the extraglandular inflam-

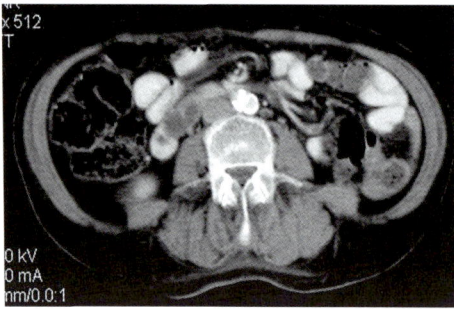

FIGURE 14: Small ampullary carcinoma: contrast enhanced CT shows a dilated common bile duct, and pancreatic duct and a small soft tissue mass into the duodenum.

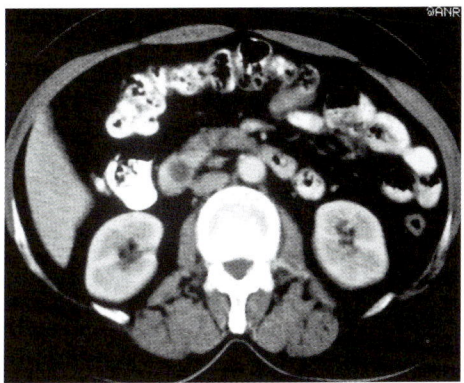

FIGURE 15: A duodenal mass in the region of ampulla is shown on CT in this patient with obstructive jaundice.

matory process. The CTSI ranges from 0-10 and shows excellent correlation with the clinical severity, morbidity and mortality rates.

The mild acute pancreatitis is characterized by swelling of the affected portions or the entire gland. Acute fluid collections, fat necrosis and extrapancreatic inflammatory spread can also be demonstrated on CT imaging. In severe acute pancreatitis the gland is markedly enlarged, no homogeneous and poorly demarcated from surrounding tissues. Necrotic areas in the

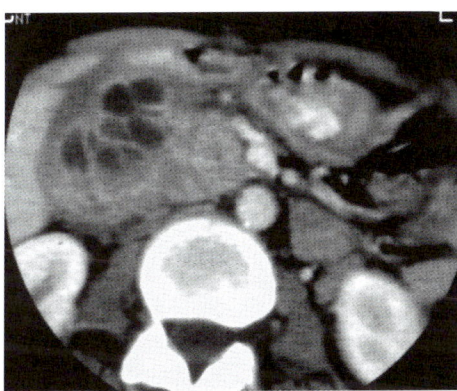

FIGURE 16: A large duodenal mass with multilocular appearance on CT was proven to be a Brunner adenoma.

pancreas appear hypoattenuating with no contrast enhancement. Extrapancreatic exudates and fat necrosis are more extensive and severe than in the mild form of the disease.

The complications of acute pancreatitis include pseudocyst formation, infection, hemorrhage and venous thrombosis or pseudoaneurysms formation. Pseudocysts do not develop until 4-6 weeks after onset of acute pancreatitis. Mostly there are related to acute fluid collections that do not resolve during the course of the disease.

They present as rounded, well-encapsulated fluid collections of varying attenuation (0-25HU). Septations are uncommon while there is often contrast enhancement of the granulation tissue in the cyst wall.[59] Pseudocyst located close to pancreatic head may cause biliary obstruction due to compression of bile ducts (Figure 17). Pseudocysts may also be found in the liver, spleen or mediastinum. A suspected infection (pancreatic abscess) usually requires needle aspiration. Gas bubbles seen on CT are suggestive of abscess formation but they are infrequent while they may also be caused by enteric fistulation or after percutaneous puncture.

Among all imaging methods CT offers several advantages in the evaluation of patients suffering from acute pancreatitis, such as easy accessibility, less cost, more favorable environment to severely ill patients and higher sensitivity in detection of small gas bubbles and calcifications (acute-on-chronic pancreatitis, biliary tract calculi). The wide availability of multidetector CT scanners have improved imaging of inflammatory pancreatic disease mainly due to multiplannar capabilities that lead to better depiction of complex anatomic relationships such as that of pseudocysts and pancreatic or biliary ductal system.

Chronic pancreatitis

Chronic pancreatitis is an irreversible in-

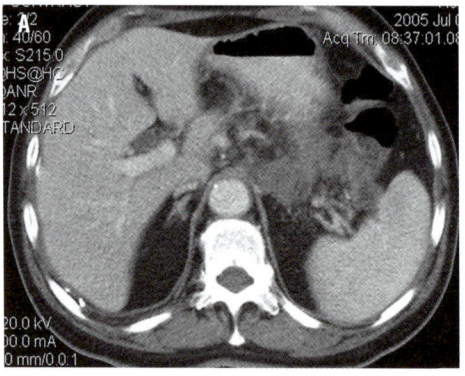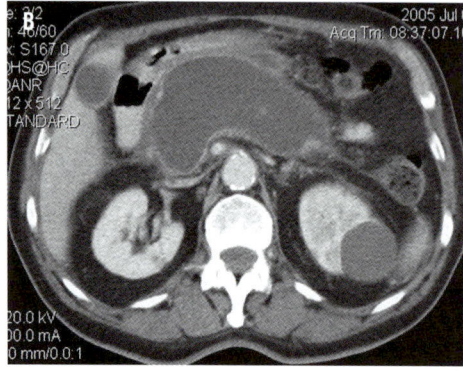

FIGURE 17: During the course of acute pancreatitis, CT scan showed dilatation of common hepatic duct **(A)** due to compression from a large pancreatic pseudocyst **(B)**.

flammatory disease of the pancreas characterized by the replacement of glandular acini, ducts and blood vessels by fibrous tissue causing ductal strictures, obstruction and dilatation leading to parenchymal atrophy and stone formation. Early changes of the disease are very difficult to recognize on CT. On the contrary features of advanced disease are easily recognized and include dilatation of the pancreatic duct and its side branches, focal or diffuse parenchymal atrophy, pancreatic calcifications, focal pancreatic enlargement and biliary ductal dilatation.

Pseudocysts are found in approximately 30% of the cases and may have an intra- or extrapancreatic location (Figure 18).

Widening of the pancreatic duct to more than 4 mm is found in more than 50% of the patients. The duct is more often irregular (beaded) than smooth, in contrast with tumor – related obstruction that is more likely to cause smooth dilatation and abrupt termination of the duct. Calcifications occur in up to 90% of patients with severe pancreatitis and are located adjacent to or within the ductal system.

Goals of CT scanning are to stage disease severity, detect intraductal lithiasis, exclude a pancreatic tumor and detect complications such as inflammatory involvement of the vascular, gastrointestinal and bile duct system causing biliary or duodenal obstruction.

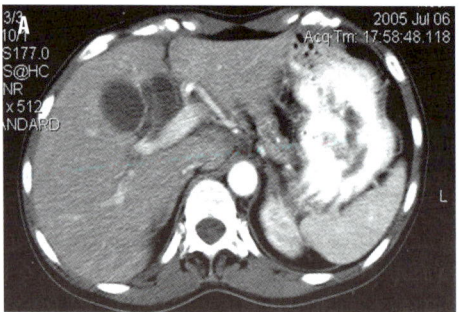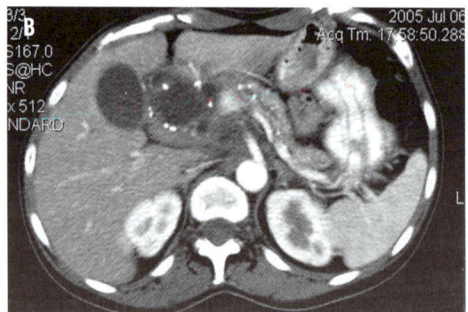

FIGURE 18: Chronic pancreatitis: dilatation of right and left hepatic ducts is evident **(A)**, due to compression from a cystic lesion in pancreatic head. Calcifications and pancreatic duct dilatation are also present **(B)**.

Pancreatic pseudoaneurysm is a rare complication of chronic pancreatitis occurring in less than 10% of the cases. However the evolution is unpredictable and prognosis is severe. The most common arteries involved are the splenic artery, the gastro-duodenal artery, the pancreatico-duodenal artery, as well as other arteries like the superior mesenteric artery, the hepatic artery, the celiac trunk and the left gastric artery. The diagnosis is suggested by the presence of the clinical signs of chronic pancreatitis, obscure upper gastrointestinal bleeding and pulsatile palpable upper abdominal mass.

Pseudoaneurysms may bleed into the gastrointestinal tract, biliary or pancreatic ducts, peritoneal cavity or retroperitoneum. The so-called syndrome of "hemosuccus pancreaticus" is described in the literature as consisting of hemorrhage into duct of Wirsung associated with colicky pain and jaundice.

Only few cases of pancreatic pseudoaneurysms associated with obstructive jaundice are described in the literature. Most of these originate into arteries that are closely related to the bile ducts thus producing extrahepatic cholestasis due to compression of the common bile duct. CT is proposed as an alternative to invasive diagnostic methods showing the origin of the pseudoaneurysms and the anatomic relationship with the bile ducts.

Focal pancreatitis has been reported to occur in 20% of the cases and typically involves the pancreatic head causing occasionally biliary obstruction. It often simulates pancreatic malignancy and differentiation is often difficult due to the overlap of imaging findings. Two different enhancement patterns have been proposed on contrast enhanced two-phase helical CT that may be explained by the difference in the degree of fibrosis. Another clue for the differential diagnosis is that the inflammatory masses are present early in the course of the disease where calcifications or pancreatic atrophy are absent, while pancreatic carcinoma is a late complication of chronic pancreatitis.

Autoimmune pancreatitis is a special form of chronic pancreatitis caused by an autoimmune mechanism or associated with autoimmune or related diseases. CT features include focal or diffuse pancreatic enlargement, absence of any significant pancreatic inflammation, mild or absent parenchymal atrophy and narrowing of main pancreatic duct and common bile duct.

Groove pancreatitis is an uncommon type of focal chronic pancreatitis that affects the "groove" between the head of the pancreas, the duodenum and the common bile duct. The most characteristic CT findings are a sheet like mass between the head of the pancreas and the thickened duodenal wall that shows delayed contrast enhancement on the late-phase, reflecting fibrotic mass.

Pancreatic neoplasms

Pancreatic carcinoma commonly obstructs the distal common bile duct and jaundice is often the first sign of the tumor. Abnormal dilatation of the extrahepatic bile ducts to the level of the tumor and abrupt termination of the bile duct with a short transition from dilated to no visualization is characteristic.

About 90% of pancreatic tumors are ductal adenocarcinomas. On unenhanced CT pancreatic adenocarcinomas generally have attenuation similar to normal pancreatic parenchyma, unless extensive necrosis or cystic change is present. On contrast enhanced CT most adenocarcinomas are hypoenhanced thus aiding detection of small tumors that do not produce visible mass or distortion of the contour. Double duct sign (dilatation of both pancreatic and common bile ducts) is seen in the majority of the cases of pancreatic head cancer (Figure 19).

Goal of imaging is not only to localize precisely a pancreatic tumor but also to distinguish resectable from unresectable tumors. Absolute contraindications for resection include distant metastases to liver, peritoneum, omentum or lungs, as well as arteries encasement. Patients with limited venous involvement may require resection of the portal vein or superior mesenteric vein confluence with reconstruction. The morbidity and technical difficulty of the operation may be diminished by the surgeon's awareness preoperatively of possible vein involvement.

Staging of pancreatic cancer is now more accurate using MDCT scanners and interactive multiplanar reconstructions using advanced post-processing techniques. For unresectable pancreatic adenocarcinoma helical CT has a positive pre-

dictive value of 100%, meaning that if a tumor seems unresectable on CT no further imaging is required. The sensitivity of small vessels involvement was improved with the use of thin – section MDCT and 3D CT angiography.

Islet cell tumors are believed to originate from the neuroendocrine cells of the pancreas. Insulinomas and gastrinomas are the commonest functioning islet cell tumors and are generally small at the time of detection. Non-functioning islet cell tumors frequently are large at the time of diagnosis and often are malignant. Small tumors require meticulous CT imaging technique with multiphase dynamic acquisition and thin slices. These tumors are usually hypervascular and show early but transient enhancement in arterial phase.

Non-functional tumors are also hypervascular and may show calcifications in 22% of the cases. These features are uncommon in pancreatic ductal adenocarcinoma. Furthermore large tumors are less likely to encase adjacent vascular structures and rarely show central necrosis.

The most common types of cystic neoplasms of the pancreas include serous and mucinous tumors. Serous tumors are benign and can be divided into microcystic or macrocystic patterns. Typically microcystic tumors contain many small cysts and have a central stellate scar. Accurate radiologic diagnosis and differentiation from mucinous tumors are crucial to avoid surgical intervention in a case of an asymptomatic serous cystadenoma, which has low malignant potential.

On contrast enhanced CT enhancement of the septations results in a honeycombing appearance, duo to the presence of tiny cysts. The central fibrotic scar may also be appreciated. On the contrary macrocystic tumors present non-specific imaging features and differential diagnosis from congenital cysts or pseudocysts is very difficult.

Mucinous cystic neoplasms appear on

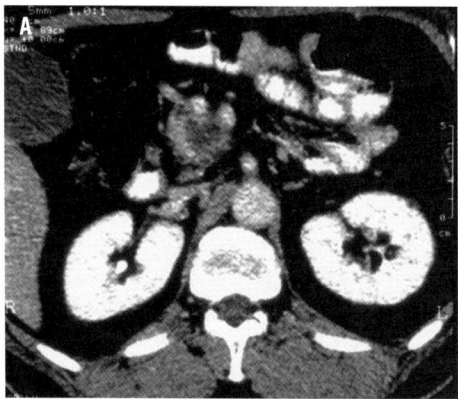

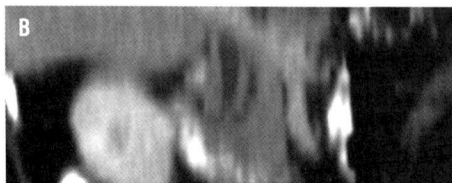

FIGURE 19: Pancreatic carcinoma at uncinate process **(A)** infiltrating both pancreatic duct and common bile duct that appear dilated on the reformatted coronal CT image **(B).**

CT as round to ovoid, externally smooth, near-water-density cystic masses. Amorphous calcifications, septations and solid components may be demonstrated. Enhancement of cystic walls and septations is also evident. Accurate differentiation between serous and mucinous tumors is not always possible based only on CT findings. Peripheral calcifications and wall nodules favor the diagnosis of mucinous tumors.

Intraductal papillary mucinous tumors (IPMT) are recently recognized as a variety of cystic tumors associated with mucin overproduction. These tumors originate from the main pancreatic duct or its collateral branches. CT imaging can show dilated pancreatic duct or branches filled with high-density material or a cluster of cystic spaces usually in pancreatic head (Figure 20).

Pancreatic lymphoma is usually of the non-Hodgkin B-cell type and can produce diffuse pancreatic enlargement, focal pancreatic masses and peripancreatic lymphadenopathy with anterior displacement of the pancreas.

Finally metastases from tumors of the lung, breast, kidney, bowel or melanoma can cause localized, multifocal or diffuse pancreatic enlargement. On CT most metastases are hypodense and show variable contrast enhancement.

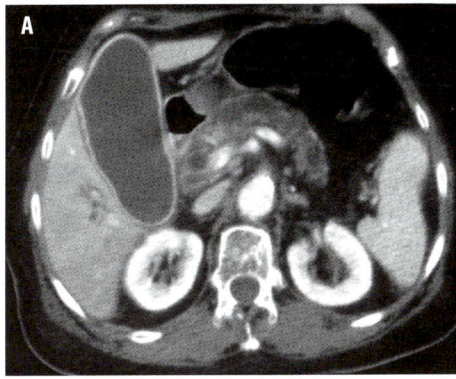

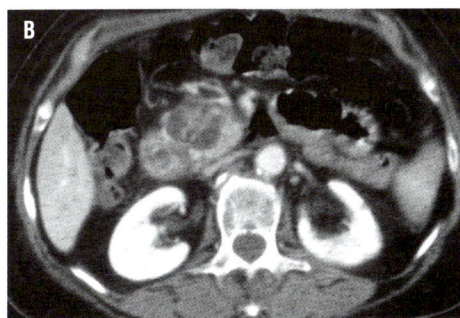

FIGURE 20: IPMT of pancreatic head: there is dilatation of gallbladder, intrahepatic bile ducts and pancreatic duct **(A)**, while the tumor appears on CT as a cluster of "cystic" spaces filled with high density material **(B)**.

CT CHOLANGIOGRAPHY – VIRTUAL CT CHOLANGIOSCOPY

During the last years specific software has been developed for processing data sets obtained from spiral-computed tomography, permiting imaging of inner organ surfaces. This method is known as virtual endoscopy. At first, the method was applied on anatomical structures that contained air and then on various organs, which show a distinct contrast in relation to their environment. It is also known that bile can bo strongly enhanced given that it is supplied with a suitable contrast agent intravenously or orally. So, it has become possible to create intraluminal images of the biliary tree using suitable software. This method is known as Virtual CT Cholangiography (VCTC) or cholangioscopy.

The most reliable method till now for studying the biliary tree, the endoscopic retrograde cholangiography (ERC) is invasive, expensive and accompanied by complications at a rate of 3-10%, while the most reliable noninvasive method the magnetic resonance cholangiography (MRC) is expensive and not always available. Furthermore there are conditions like choledochojejunostomy or duodenal diverticulum located in the ampulla, where ERC may not be feasible. On the other hand as the most common therapeutic approaches to gallbladder and biliary ducts lithiasis are laparoscopic cholecystectomy and ERC it is very helpful to know preoperatively not only the presence of stones or stenoses but the precise anatomy and possible variations as well.

Spiral CT cholangiography with Surface Shaded Display has been proposed as a very effective and accurate alternative method but it is time consuming while intraluminal pathology can be revealed only by axial or MPR images. Recently there have been two reports regarding the application of virtual endoscopy techniques on the biliary tree, with data sets obtained from magnetic resonance imaging. However virtual MR cholangiography has several limitations concerning image quality while another potential disadvantage is the absence of information concerning biliary kinetics as opposed to VCTC. Moreover it is well known that the equipment and procedures of MRI imaging are generally more expensive than CT.

There are also reports from other authors on virtual cholangioscopy, with data sets obtained from spiral computed tomography. Virtual endoscopy of the biliary ducts based on spiral CT data sets, can be performed using two methods. In the first method in order to create a contrast between the ducts and surrounding tissues, the liver and pancreatic parenchyma are enhanced by intravenous infusion of a contrast agent resulting to a relatively hypodense imaging of the biliary tree. The intraluminal images are created afterwards, by selecting the adequate threshold. Main advantages of this method are that the examination does not depend on bilirubin levels and that using the same scanning one can also study liver and pancreas without another contrast agent infusion. A disadvantage of this method is that

the choice of the adequate threshold is difficult, especially in the areas where the biliary tree is not surrounded by enhanced parenchyma, thus resulting in technical errors.

In the second method the fluid in the biliary ducts is enhanced by intravenous infusion of a contrast agent like iotroxindimeglumine. Post processing techniques like maximum intensity projections (MIP) (Figure 21) or virtual endoscopy (Figure 22) can then be used to demonstrate bile ducts. VCTC contributes to the recognition of stones (Figure 23), anatomic variations and stenosis or compression of the bile ducts. VCTC can also provide a high level of confidence in the differential diagnosis of obstructive jaundice thus influencing patient management as far as the choice of the therapeutic intervention is concerned (ERC, laparoscopic cholecystectomy with or without CBD exploration.)

Process time varies according to the specific software tools, the underlying pathology and the experience of the radiologists who conduct the virtual endoscopy. Significant limitations of this method are: a) the demand for bilirubin rates <3 mgr/dL, b) the use of a contrast agent with potential complications, c) the need for additional scanning while using another contrast agent in case of pancreatic or liver pathology, d) the limited region that can be scanned with one breath holding and e) the use of ionizing radiation. Another limitation is that, as there is no density difference between calcified stones and enhanced biliary liquid, these stones may not be identified. However, in these cases, this can be done by using unenhanced axial images.

One of the most common questions that arise concerning virtual endoscopy, is whether this method can add more information from the information provided by the simultaneously interpretation of both axial and reformatted images. It should be

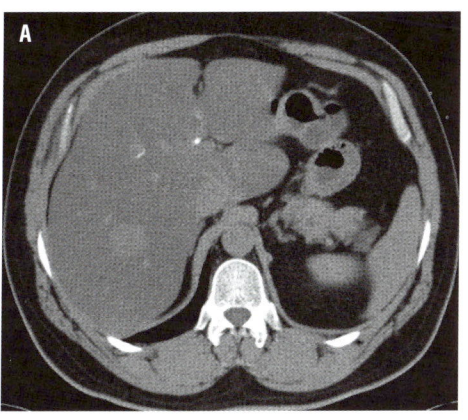

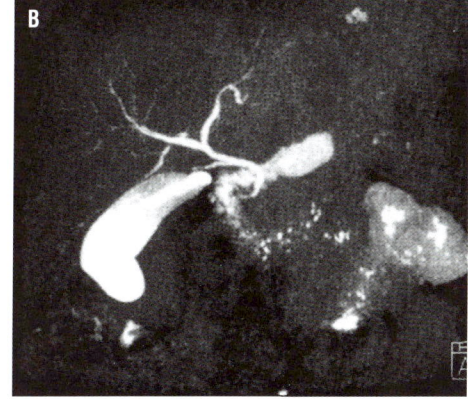

FIGURE 21: CT cholangiography: axial CT image after the administration of cholangiographic contrast material **(A)** and MIP reformatted 3D image showing normal bile ducts **(B)**. *(Courtesy of Dr Ch. Stoupis).*

noted, that navigation through structures such as a biliary tree is a difficult procedure without the aid provided by both axial and MPR images. On the other hand, both axial and MPR images represent a two-dimensional appearance of a three dimensional-reality, with all potential pitfalls included.

It has been shown that intraluminal reconstruction can increase the level of con-

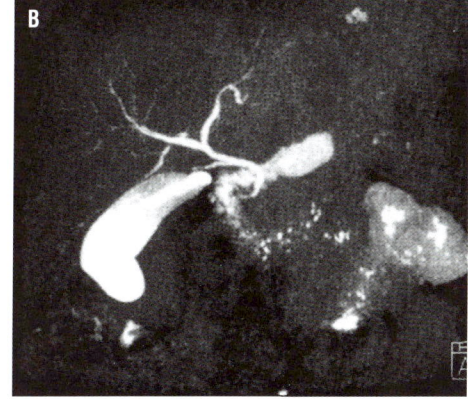

FIGURE 22: Virtual CT cholangioscopy: intraluminal view of non dilated common bile duct.

fidence in diagnosis. So radiologist has now the ability to distinguish, for example, between a partial volume effect and a stone, or prove the presence of bile duct stenosis. It should also be stressed, that the information acquired by the interpretation of numerous axial and MPR images, can be successfully accomplished in a maximum of 4-5 virtual images easily appreciated by non-radiologists.

There are also two more studies presenting the use of VCTC in the evaluation and management of choledochal cyst. Overall it seems that virtual cholangioscopy with intravenous infusion of iotroxindimeglumine can be a feasible clinical tool in cases where the grade of bile ducts obstruction is not prohibitive to its use, in patients unable to undergo MRC or ERC as well as during follow-up.

Alternatively in cases of impaired liver function, the other method of CT cholangiography with minimum intensity projections without biliary contrast agent can be used. It has been shown that thin-slice multislice CT and post processing techniques including miltiplanar reformations and minimum intensity projections can accurate determine the cause and level of biliary obstruction. These results will im-

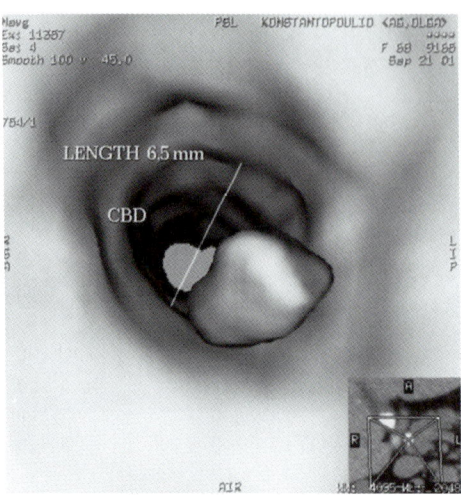

FIGURE 23: Virtual CT cholangioscopy: intraluminal view showing a small stone in the slightly dilated common bile duct.

prove as isotropic voxel imaging becomes possible with 32-slices or 64-slices CT scanners.

Other advantage of this method is the ability to render otherwise imperceptible small caliber ducts visible by reducing the partial volume effect. Theoretically the caliber of ducts could be overestimated with this method, as opposed to maximum intensity projection MR cholangiopancreatography, with which duct caliber or stenosis could be underestimated. However large study findings showed excellent agreement between CT cholangiography and ERCP in duct caliber assessment.

On the other hand it is more important to determine the cause and level of obstruction than to distinguish between complete and incomplete obstruction in the diagnostic procedure. So, in the evaluation of jaundice, duct anatomy can be shown and smooth stricture can be differentiated from abrupt tumor or intraluminal stone obstructions, decreasing the need for additional examinations or serving as a road map for interventional ERCP or other procedures. Furthermore minimum intensity projections are not affected substantially by the presence of stents.

This method has also been proven to be very useful in the evaluation of hilar cholangiocarcinoma while in patients with suspected biliary obstruction it shows important advantages compared with MRC, ERC and percutaneous transhepatic cholangiography (PTC).

Finally it has been reported that 3D-CTC with minimum intensity projection, can correctly determine the level of biliary obstruction and evaluate resectability in patients with gallbladder carcinoma. Clinical relevant information given is comparable with MRC or PTC. Even though 3D-CTC does not provide additional information on top of the source images, the referring physicians find them very useful for conceptualization of the 3D biliary anatomy.

With the advent of faster multislice CT scanners and evolution of advanced post-processing 3D imaging techniques it is possible that VCTC will substitute other imaging methods improving diagnostic accuracy while widening the range of the biliary ducts pathology that can be displayed in the diagnostic workup of obstructive jaundice.

REFERENCES

Akhan O, Demirkazik FB, Ozmen MN, et al. Choledochal cysts: ultrasonographic findings and correlation with other imaging modalities. Abdom Imaging 1994;19:243-247.

Araki T, Itai Y, Tasaka A. CT of choledochal cysts. A-JR 1980; 135: 729-734.

Balthazar EJ, Birnbaum BA, Naidich M. Acute cholangitis: CT evaluation. J Comput Assist Tomogr 1993;17:283-289.

Balthazar EJ, Freeny PC, van Sonnenberg E. Imaging and intervention in acute pancreatitis. Radiology 1994;193:297-306.

Balthazar EJ, Robinson DL, Megibow A,l et al. Acute

pancreatitis: prognostic value of CT in establishing prognosis. Radiology 1990;174:331-336.

Barakos JA, Ralls PW, Lapin SA, et al. Cholelithiasis: evaluation with CT. Radiology 1987;162: 415-418.

Baron RL. Diagnosing choledocholithiasis: how far can we push helical CT? Radiology 1997; 203:601-603.

Baron RL, Rohrmann Jr CA, Lee SP, et al. CT evaluation of gallstones in vitro: correlation with chemical analysis. Am J Roentgenol 1988;26: 216-225.

Baron RL, Tublin ME, Peterson MS, et al. Imaging the spectrum of biliary tract disease. Radiol Clin N Am 2002; 40: 1325-1354.

Baum U, Lell M, Nomaur A, et al. Multiplanar spiral CT in the diagnosis of pancreatic tumors. Radiologe 1999;39:958-964.

Becheur H, Zins M, Levy P, et al. A rare cause of obstructive jaundice: peripancreatic pseudoaneurysm. Gastroenterol Clin Biol 1996;20:1131-1134.

Benz CA, Jakob P, Jakobs R, et al. Hemosuccus pancreaticus: a rare case of gastrointestinal bleeding: diagnostic and interventional radiological therapy. Endoscopy 2000;32:428-431.

Berland LL, Lawson TL, Stanley RJ. CT appearance of Mirizzi syndrome. J Comput Assist Tomogr 1984;8:165-166.

Blomley MJ, Jackson JE. Case report: a gastroduodenal artery pseudoaneurysm presenting with obstructive jaundice and treated by arterial embolization. Clin Radiol 1994;49:715-718.

Bold RJ, Charnsangavej C, Cleary KR, et al. Major vascular resections as part of pancreaticoduodenectomy for cancer: Radiologic, intraoperative, and pathologic analyses. J Gastrointest Surg 1999;3:233-243.

Buck JL, Elsayered AM. Ampullary tumors: radiographic-pathologic correlation. Radiographics 1993;13:193-212.

Buckley JG, Salimi Z. Villous adenoma of the common bile duct. Abdom Imaging 1993;18: 245-246.

Buetow PC, Miller DL, Parrino TV, et al. Islet cell tumors of the pancreas: clinical, radiologic and pathologic correlation in diagnosis and localization. Radiographics 1997;17:453-472.

Buetow PC, Rao P, Thompson LD. Mucinous cystic

neoplasms of the pancreas: radiologic-pathologic correlation. Radiographics 1998;18: 433-449.

Cambell WL, Ferris JV, Holbert BL, et al. Biliary tract carcinoma complicating primary sclerosing cholangitis: evaluation with CT, cholangiography, US and MR imaging. Radiology 1998;207:41-50.

Campell WL, Peterson MS, Federle MP. Using CT and cholangiography to diagnose biliary tract carcinoma complicating primary sclerosing cholangitis. Am J Roentgenol 2001;177:1095-1100.

Caoili EM, Paulson EK, Heyneman LE, Branch MS, Eubanks WS, Nelson RC. Helical CT cholangiography with three-dimensional volume rendering using an oral biliary contrast agent: feasibility of a novel technique. AJR 2000;174(2):487-92.

Carr DH, Hadjis NS, Banks LM, et al. CT of hilar cholangiocarcinoma: a new sigh. AJR 1985;145: 53-56.

Choi BI, Yeon KM, Kim SH, et al. Caroli disease: central dot sign in CT. Radiology 1990;174:161-163.

Co CS, Shea WJ, Goldberg H. Evaluation of common bile duct diameter using high resolution computed tomography. J Comput Assist Tomogr 1986; 10:424-427.

Cohen SA, Siegel JH, Kasmin FE. Complications of diagnostic and therapeutic ERCP. Abdom Imaging 1996;21:385-394.

Cory DA, Don S, West KW. CT cholangiography of a choledochocele. Pediatr Radiol 1990;21:73-74.

Craig DA, MacCarty RL, Wiesner RH, et al. Primary sclerosing cholangitis: value of cholangiography in determining the prognosis. AJR 1991; 157:959-964.

Crittenden SL, McKinley MJ. Choledochal cyst: clinical features and classification. Am J Gastroenterol 1985;80:643-647.

Dodd 3rd GD. Bile duct calculi in patients with primary sclerosing cholangitis. Radiology 1997; 203:443-447.

Dodd 3rd GD. End-stage primary sclerosing cholangitis: CT findings of hepatic morphology in 36 patients. Radiology 1999;211:357-362.

Dubno B, Debatin JF, Luboldt W, Schmidt M, Hany TF, Bauerfeind P. Virtual MR cholangiography. AJR 1998; 171(6):1547-50.

Etemad B, Whitcomb DC. Chronic pancreatitis: diagnosis, classification and new genetic developments. Gastroenterology 2001;120:682-707.

Fenchel S, Boll D, Fleiter T, et al. Multislice helical CT of the pancreas and spleen. European Journal of Radiology 2003;45:S59-S72.

Fishman EK, Horton KM, Urban BA. Multidetector CT angiography in the evaluation of pancreatic carcinoma: preliminary observations. J Comput Assist Tomogr 2000;24:849-853.

Fuhrman GM, Charnsangavej C, Abbruzzese JL, et al. Thin-section contrast enhanced CT accurately predicts the resectability of malignant pancreatic neoplasm. Am J Surg 1994;167:104-113.

Furukawa H, Sano K, Kosuge T, et al. Hilar cholangiocarcinoma evaluated by three-dimensional CT cholangiography and rotating cine cholangiography. Hepatogastroenterology 2000; 47(33):615-620.

Gore RM, Yaghmai V, Newmark GM, et al. Imaging benign and malignant disease of the gallbladder. Radiol Clin N Am 2002; 40: 1307-1323.

Guibaud L, Bret PM, Reinhold C, et al. Diagnosis of c-holedocholithiasis: Value of MR cholangiography. AJR 1994;163:847-850.

Harshfield DL, Teplick SK, Stanton M, et al. Obstructing villous adenoma and papillary adenomatosis of the bile ducts. AJR 1990;154: 1217-1218.

Hoe VL, Gryspeerdt S, Ectors N, et al. Non alcoholic duct-destructive chronic pancreatitis: imaging findings. AJR 1998;170:643-647.

Irie H, Honda H, Baba S, et al. Autoimmune pancreatitis: CT and MR characteristics. AJR 1998; 170:1323-1327.

Jan YY, Che MF. Obstructive jaundice secondary to hepatocellular carcinoma rupture into the common bile duct: choledochoscopic findings. Hepatogastroenterology 1999;46:157-161.

Karakoyunlar O, Sivrel E, Koc O, et al. Mirizzi syndrome must be ruled out in the differential diagnosis of any patients with obstructive jaundice. Hepatogastroenterology 1999;46(28):2178-2182.

Kalra MK, Maher MM, Sahani DV, et al. Current status of imaging in pancreatic diseases. Journal of Computer Assisted Tomography 2002; 26(5): 661-675.

Kawakatsu M, Vilgrain V, Zins M, et al. Radiologic features of papillary adenoma and papillomatosis of the biliary tract. Abdom Imaging 1997;22:87-90.

Kim JH, Kim MJ, Chung JJ, et al. Differential diagnosis of periampullary carcinomas at MR imaging. Radiographics 2002;22(6):1335-1352.

Kim T, Murakami T, Takamura M, et al. Pancreatic mass due to chronic pancreatitis: correlation of CT and MR imaging features with pathologic findings. AJR 2001;177: 367-371.

Klein HM, Wein B, Truong S, Pfingsten FP, Gunther RW. Computed tomographic cholangiography using spiral scanning and 3D image processing. Br J Radiol 1993;66(789):762-7.

Koito K, Namieno T, Hirokawa N, et al. Virtual CT Cholangioscopy: Comparison with fiberoptic cholangioscopy. Endoscopy 2001;33:676-681.

Kossak J, Janik J, Debski J, et al. Pseudoaneurysm of the gastroduodenal artery as a cause of obstructive jaundice. Med Sci Monit 2001;7: 759-761.

Lacomis JM, Baron RL, Oliver 3rd JH et al. Cholangiocarcinoma: delayed CT contrast enhancement patterns. Radiology 1997;203:98-104.

Laokpessi A, Bouillet P, Sautereau D, Cessot F, Desport JC, Le Sidaner A, Pillegand B. Value of magnetic resonance cholangiography in the preoperative diagnosis of common bile duct stones. Am J Gastroenterol 2001;96(8):2354-9.

Lecesne R, Taourel P, Bret PM, et al. Acute pancreatitis: interobserver agreement and correlation of CT and MR cholangiopancreatography with outcome. Radiology 1999;211:727-735.

Lee WJ, Lim HK, Jank KM, et al. Radiologic spectrum of cholangiocarcinoma: emphasis on unusual manifestations and differential diagnoses. Radiographics 2001;21:S97-116.

Levy AD, Murakata LA, Rohrmawn CA. Gallbladder carcinoma: radiologic-pathologic correlation. Radiographics 2001;21:295-314.

Liddell RM, Baron RL, Ekstrom JE, et al. Normal intrahepatic bile ducts: CT depiction. Radiology 1990;176:633-635.

Loyer EM, Chin H, DuBrow RA, et al. Hepatocellular carcinoma and intrahepatic peripheral cholangiocarcinoma: enhancement patterns with quadruple phase helical CT-a comparative study. Radiology 1999;212:866-875.

Lun-Xiu Qin, Zhao-You Tang. Hepatocellular carcinoma with obstructive jaundice: diagnosis, treatment and prognosis. World J Gastroenterol 2003; 9(3): 385-391.

Maniatis P, Triantopoulou C, Sofianou E, et al. Virtual CT cholangiography in patients with choledocholithiasis. Abdom Imaging 2003;28(4): 536-544.

McNulty NJ, Francis IR, Platt JF, et al. Multi-detector row helical CT of the pancreas: effect of contrast enhanced multiplanar imaging on enhancement of the pancreas, peripancreatic vasculature, and pancreatic adenocarcinoma. Radiology 2001;220:97-102.

Memel DS, Balfe DM, Semelka RC. The biliary tract. In: Computed tomography with MRI correlation. Ed J. Lee. Volume 2, 1998.

Merkle EM, Boaz T, Kolokythas O, et al. Metastases to the pancreas. Br J Radiol 1998; 71:1208-1214.

Midwinter MJ, Beveridge CJ, Wilsdon JB, et al. Correlation between spiral computed tomography, endoscopic ultrasonography and findings at operation in pancreatic and ampullary tumors. Br J Surg 1999;86:189-193.

Vining DJ. Virtual endoscopy: is it reality? Radiology 1996;200: 30-31.

M, Chisholm R, Dixon AK. Intrahepatic bile duct dilatation shown by computed tomography-predilection for the left lobe? Br J Radiol 1985;58:499-502.

Narayana DLV Rao, Manpreet Singh Gulati, Shashi Bala Paul, et al. Three-dimensional helical computed tomography cholangiography with minimum intensity projection in gallbladder carcinoma patients with obstructive jaundice: comparison with MRC and PTC. Journal of Gastroenterology and Hepatology 2005;20(2):304-308.

Neff CC, Simeone JF, Wittenberg J, et al. Inflammatory pancreatic masses. Problems in differentiating focal pancreatitis from carcinoma. Radiology 1984;150:35-38.

Neitlich JD, Topazian M, Smith RC, et al. Detection of choledocholithiasis: comparison of unenhanced helical CT and endoscopic retrograde cholangiopancreatography. Radiology 1997;203: 753-757.

Neri E, Boraschi P, Braccini G, et al. MR virtual endoscopy of the pancreaticobiliary tract: a feasible technique? Abdom Imaging 1999;24(3): 289-91.

Nino-Murcia M, Tamm EP, Charnsangavej C, et al. Multidetector-row helical and advanced post processing techniques for the evaluation of pancreatic neoplasms. Abdom Imaging 2003;28: 366-377.

Park SJ, Han JK, Kim TK, et al. Three-dimensional spiral cholangiography with minimum intensity projection in patients with suspected obstructive biliary diseases: comparison with percutaneous transhepatic cholangiography. Abdom Imaging 2001;26:281-286.

Pickleman J, Koelsch M, Chejfec G. Node-positive duodenal carcinoma is curable. Arch Surg 1997;132:241-244.

Prassopoulos P, Raptopoulos V, Chuttani R, McKee JD, McNicholas MMJ, Sheiman RG. Development of Virtual cholangiopancreatoscopy. Radiology 1998;209:570-574.

Procacci C, Graziani R, Bicego E, et al. Serous cystadenoma of the pancreas: report of 30 cases with emphasis on the imaging findings. J Comput Assist Tomogr 1997; 21: 373-382.

Procacci C, Megibow AJ, Carbognin G, et al. Intraductal papillary mucinous tumor of the pancreas: a pictorial essay. Radiographics 1999;19: 1447-1463.

Prokop M, A.J. van der Molen. Liver. In: Computed Tomography of the body. Editors: M. Prokop, M. Galanski. Thieme, N. York, 2003.

Prokop M. Biliary tract. In: Computed Tomography of the body. Editors: M. Prokop, M. Galanski. Thieme, N. York, 2003.

Raptopoulos V, Prassopoulos P, Chuttani R, et al. Multiplanar CT pancreatography and distal cholangiography with minimum intensity projections. Radiology 1998;207:317-324.

Fleischmann D, Ringl H, Schofl R, Potzi R, Kontrus M, Henk C, Bankier AA, Kettenbach J, Mostbeck GH. Three-dimensional spiral CT cholangiography in patients with suspected obstructive biliary disease: comparison with endo-scopic retrograde cholangiography. Radiology 1996;198(3):861-8.

Fletcher ND, Wise PE, Sharp KW. Common bile duct papillary adenoma causing obstructive jaundice: case report and review of the literature. The American Surgeon 2004;70:448-452.

Saftoiu A, Iordache S, Ciurea T, et al. Pancreatic pseudoaneurysm of the superior mesenteric artery complicated with obstructive jaundice. A case report. J Pancreas (online) 2005;6(1):29-35.

Sajjad Z, Oxtoby J, West D, Deakin M. Biliary imaging

by spiral CT cholangiography-a retrospective analysis. Br J Radiol 1999;72:149-152.

Saing H, Chan JK, Lam WW, Chan KL. Virtual intra-luminal endoscopy: a new method for evaluation and management of choledochal cyst. J Pediatr Surg 1998 Nov;33(11):1686-9.

Schaefer - Prokop C. Pancreas. In: Computed Tomography of the body. Editors: M. Prokop, M. Galanski. Thieme, N. York, 2003.

Schulte SJ, Baron RL, Teefy SA, et al. CT of the extrahepatic bile ducts: wall thickness and contrast enhancement in normal and abnormal ducts. AJR 1990;154:79-85.

Schwarz M, Pauls S, Sokiranski R, et al. Is a preoperative multidiagnostic approach to predict surgical resectability of periampullary tumors still effective? The American Journal of Surgery 2001; 182:243-249.

Slanetz PJ, Boland GW, Muller PR. Imaging and interventional radiology in laparoscopic injuries to the gallbladder and biliary system. Radiology 1996;201:595.

Soyer P. Imaging of intrahepatic cholangiocarcinoma: 1. Peripheral cholangiocarcinoma. Am J Roentgenol 1995;165:1427-1431.

Soyer P. Imaging of intrahepatic cholangiocarcinoma: 2. Hilar cholangiocarcinoma. Am J Roentgenol 1995;165:1433-1436.

Soyer P, Laisy JP, Bluemke DA, et al. Bile duct involvement in hepatocellular carcinoma. Abdom Imaging 1995;20:118-121.

Spinzi G, Martegani A, Belloni G, Terruzzi V, Del Favero C, Minoli G. Computed tomography-virtual cholangiography and choledochal cyst. Gastrointest Endosc 1999 Dec;50(6): 857-9.

Spinzi G, Martegani A, Belloni G, et al. Computed tomography-virtual cholangiography and choledochal cyst. Endoscopy 1999;50(6):857-859.

Tabuchi T, Itoh K, Ohshio G, et al. Tumor staging of pancreatic adenocarcinoma using early and late phase helical CT. AJR 1999;173:375-380.

Talamonti M, Denham W. Staging and surgical management of pancreatic and biliary cancer and in-flammation. Radiol Clin N Am 2002;40:1397-1410.

Teefey SA, Baron RL, Rohrmann Jr CA, et al. Sclerosing cholangitis: CT findings. Radiology 1988;169:635-639.

Todani T, Tabuchi K, Watanabe Y, et al. Carcinoma arising in the wall of congenital bile duct cysts. Cancer 1979;44:1134-1141.

Todani T, Watanabe Y, Narusue M, et al. Congenital bile duct cysts: classification, operative procedures and review of 37 cases including cancer arising from choledochal cyst. Am J Surg 1977; 134:263-269.

Triantopoulou C, Komitopoulos N, Polyzou A, et al. Pylephlebitis associated with intrauterine device: CT evaluation. European Journal of Radiology-extra 2005, (in press).

Valette O, Cuilleron M, Cebelle L, et al. Imaging of the intraductal papillary mucinous tumors of the pancreas: literature review. J Radiol 2001; 82: 633-645.

Van Beers BE, Lacrosse M, Trigaux JP, de Canniere L, De Ronde T, Pringot J. Noninvasive imaging of the biliary tree before or after laparoscopic chole-cystectomy: use of three dimensional spiral CT cholangiography. AJR 1994;162: 1331-1335.

VanSonnenberg E, Ferrucci JT. Bile duct obstruction in hepatocellular carcinoma. Clinical and cholan-giographic characteristics. Reports of 6 cases and review of the literature. Radiology 1979; 130:7-13.

Wilbur AC, Sagireddy PB, Aizenstein RI. Carcinoma of the gallbladder: color Doppler ultrasound and CT findings. Abdom Imaging 1997;22:187-189.

Zandrino F, Benzi L, Ferretti ML, et al. Multi-slice CT cholangiography without biliary contrast: technique and initial clinical results in the assessment of patients with biliary obstruction. Eur Radiol 2002;12(5):1155-1161.

Zech C, Schoenberg SO, Reiser M, et al. Cross-sectional imaging of biliary tumors: current clinical status and future developments. Eur Radiol 2004;14:1174-1187.

MRI in obstructive jaundice patients

Liu Terrence, Consorti Eileen

In the adult patient population, calculus disease, strictures, malignancies, pancreatitis, and extrinsic masses are the most common causes of biliary obstruction. Diagnostic imaging and non-operative interventions occupy a major role in the management of these patients with suspected obstructive pathology. Traditionally, abdominal ultrasonography (U/S) is obtained as the initial imaging study, and based on this evluation, those patients with dilated bile ducts and no evidence of cholelithiasis are generally evaluated with computed tomography (CT) to further define the cause and location of obstruction. Whereas, those patients with biliary obstructions related to calculus disease are generally directed toward endoscopic retrograde cholangiopancreatography (ERCP) or direct operative intervention.

Magnetic resonance cholangiopancreatography (MRCP) is a newer MRI technique that has been developed as a noninvasive biliary tract imaging modality. When compared to traditional cholangiographic techniques such as ERCP and percutaneous transhepatic cholangiography (PTC), MRCP has been shown to produce higher success rate, lower cost, lower procedural-related morbidity, and greater patient satisfaction. Over the past several years, expansions in the clinical applications of MRCP and other magnetic resonance imaging (MRI) techniques have led to alternative diagnostic strategies for patients with biliopancreatical diseases. In many centers, MRCP has replaced ERCP as the preferred diagnostic imaging modality for patients with suspected common bile duct pathology. Similarly, MRI are being applied for the evaluation and staging of patients with obstructing biliary tract tumors in many centers. This chapter will discuss the current status of MR imaging and its clinical applications in patients with obstructive jaundice.

MAGNETIC RESONANCE IMAGING TECHNOLOGY

The clinical application of MRCP was initially reported in 1991. MRCP images are created with the application of heavily T2-weighted imaging techniques. Under these conditions, high intensity signals are produced by stationary and slow-moving fluid within the biliary and pancreatic ducts, thereby producing images that permit the visualization of these structures from the surrounding environment. During the early phase of MRCP application there were a number of major technical limitations including motion artifacts and the lengthy time requirement for conventional spin-echo sequence image acquisition that affected its clinical applications. Many of the early technical limitations associated with MRCP have been resolved with the introduction of breath-hold imaging, fat-suppression techniques, and dynamic contrast-enhanced imaging resulting in expanded application of this modality for the diagnosis of pancreatico-biliary pathology.

Many of the technical details of MR imaging are unimportant for MRI clinical applications and are beyond the scope of the current chapter. From the practical standpoint, MRCP involves the use of single-shot fast spin echo sequence, which can be obtained as single-slab acquisition or multiple thin-slice acquisitions. The single-slab approach offers several advantages including rapid acquisition within 2-3 seconds without the need for postprocessing, in addition this technique creates ERCP-like images that provide overviews of the biliary and pancreatic ductal anatomy. A potential limitation of the single-slab approach is the high signal intensity associated with the intraductal fluid often interferes with visualization of fine anatomic details within the biliary system; therefore, to visualize fine intraductal details, multiple-slice thin-collimation sequence is generally applied. In most patients, these acquisition methods are combined to provide complementary data for the evaluation of biliopancreatic pathology.

Technical innovations that will likely result in the broadening application of MRI technology in the near future include the development of MRI compatible therapeutic devices that will permit the expansion of MRI-directed interventions. Similarly, miniature MRI receiver coils are being developed, and it is anticipated that with the placement of these receiver coils within blood vessels and the biliary system, image resolution will lead to improved characterization of disease extension within the hilar and the porta hepatis regions.

CLINICAL APPLICATION OF MR CHOLANGIOPANCREATOGRAPHY

Biliary imaging modalities include trans-abdominal U/S, MRCP, CT, intravenous cholangiography, endoscopic U/S (EUS), ERCP, PTC, intraoperative cholangiography (IOC), intraoperative choledocholscopy, and laparoscopic U/S. (Table 1 lists some of the major characteristics of these modalities)

Many of the initial investigations assessing MRI technologies were focused on the evaluations of MRI diagnostic accuracies; therefore, there were numerous studies that compared the diagnostic accuracy of MRI to existing imaging modalities, such as ERCP, PTC, and EUS. As these investigations have successfully characterize MRI diagnostic accuracies, the current investigational challenges facing the gastroenterologists, radiologists, and surgeons remain in the development of diagnostic and treatment strategies that would produce maximal diagnostic accuracy, patient safety, efficiency, and cost-effectiveness.

MRI OF BILIARY TRACT OBSTRUCTIONS

Evaluation of biliary tract dilatation

The presence of bile duct dilatation often

TABLE 1

SUMMARY OF DIAGNOSTIC MODALITIES FOR COMMON BILE DUCT STONES

Method	Diagnostic Sensitivity (%)	Diagnostic Specificity (%)	Advantages	Disadvantages
ERCP	95-100 (mean 98)	95-100 (mean 98)	Therapeutic capabilities; identifies anatomy and anomalies	Requires sedation and analgesia; associated with patient discomfort and complications
MRCP	57-100 (mean 90) for stones <3 mm	73-100 (mean 96)	Non-invasive; reproducible; identifies anatomy, anomalies, and extra-ductal pathology	Lacks therapeutic capabilities
Transabdominal US	20-38	80-100	Identifies cholelithiasis in 98% of patients; easy to interpret	Limited sensitivity for CBDS identification
CT	Unenhanced CT: 65-90; contrast enhanced CT: 90-96	80-85 95	Widely available; noninvasive	Expertise required for interpretation of unenhanced images
EUS	75-98 (mean 95)	90-100 (mean 96)	Less invasive than ERCP	Equipment, expertise, and sedation requirement; may miss CBDS located in upper biliary tract
Intravenous cholangio-graphy	88-93	97-99	Identifies anatomy and anatomic variations	Adverse reaction reported in 0-12%. With severe reaction reported in 0-9% of patients; not FDA -approvcd in the USA
IOC	75-100 (mean 90) reduced with static cholangiography	70-100 (mean 95)	Identifies anatomy and anatomic variants; special skills and equipment not needed	Success rate varies is limited by inflammation and cjp cholecystitis
Laparoscopic US	90-100 (mean 95)	98-100 (mean 99)	More sensitive than ERCP and MRCP at identifying CBDS <3 mm; may be repeated during the operation	Equipment and expertise requirement
Laparoscopic choledoc-hoscopy	Success rate reported at 67-100 (mean 91)		Therapeutic capabilities	Equipment and expertise requirement; procedur-related pancreatitis, bleeding, and perfo-ration

Adapted with permission from: Liu TH and Organ Jr CH. *Asian J Surg* 2004;27:10

correlates with the presence of mechanical obstruction. Ultrasonography and CT are the imaging modalities most commonly applied for the identification of biliary ductal dilatation. Based on CT imaging, an abnormally dilated intrahepatic duct is defined as a duct diameter that exceeds 40% of the adjacent intrahepatic portal vein diameter. Sonographic measurements of the extrahepatic bile duct are most commonly used for the determination of size, and this is generally measured at a location just distal to the right hepatice artery ain the porta hepatis. At this level, a duct diameter of 6 to 7 mm is generally accepted as the upper size limit; whereas, a diameter of 8-10 mm is generally accepted as the upper limit of normal for CHD and CBD visualized by CT. As valuable as U/S and CT imaging are for the recognition of CBD dilatation, these modalities generally produce insufficient image resolution for the confirmation of pathology. MRCP is a modality that is highly effective for the evaluation of bile duct dilatation. When applied in the evaluation of bile duct obstruction, MRCP has produced accuracy rates of 89-100% for the diagnosis of choledocholiasis[16] and accuracy rate of 98% for identifying the presence and level of biliary tract strictures. Magnuson et al reported their experience with MRCP in the initial evaluation of 143 patients with suspected bile duct obstruction at Johns Hopkins University. During this study, MRCP application identified pathology in 51% of the patient imaged. Based on their observations, the group concluded that the application of MRCP as the initial diagnostic study was not only useful for identifying pathology, but MRCP application could eliminate the need for ERCP in patients without obstructive pathology.

The decision-making value of MRCP was evaluated in 40 patients with suspected biliopancreatic diseases by Sahai et al, and in this patient population, disease processes requiring endoscopic interventions were eventually identified in 97% of the patients. These observations led the investigators to conclude that MRCP contributed very little in the overall patient care decision-making process. These two studies involving highly different patient populations both confirmed MRCP as an accurate diagnostic tool for identifying the causes of biliary obstruction; however, their findings pointed out that the routine application of MRCP in patients requiring therapeutic intervention by ERCP was not beneficial or cost-effective in the overall care of these patients.

Patients with suspected choledocholithiasis

There have been a number of studies conducted to verify the operating characteristics of MRCP for common bile duct stone (CBDS) diagnosis. Cumulatively, these investigations have reported sensitivity of 92% (80-97%), specificity of 96% (90-99%) for CBDS detection, with nearly 100% sensitivity for the visualization of CBDS >3 mm. (Table 2).

Approximately 8-20% of the patients selected to undergo laparoscopic cholecystectomy (LC) may have CBDS present at the time of their operations, and the optimal timing and method of CBDS detection and treatment in these patients remains controversial. As the majority of surgeons continue to prefer to manage CBDS by ERCP and endoscopic sphincterotomy (ES) when patients present with concomitant cholelithiasis and choledocholithiasis, a variety of diagnostic strategies for the preoperative identification of CBDS have been proposed. While ERCP has been the traditional "gold standard" for CBDS diagnosis and treatment, this invasive procedure is associated with patient discomfort and procedural-related complications. The drawbacks associated with diagnostic ERCP have prompted a

TABLE 2

RESULTS OF MRC FOR COMMON BILE DUCT STONES DETECTION

Source	N	Study Design	Patient Disease	CBDS prevalence (%)	Comparison/ study	Sensitivity/ specificity accuracy (%)
Reinhold et al (1998)	110	Prospective	Stones	27	ERCP and IOC	90/100/97
Stiris et al (2000)	50	Prospective	Mixed disease population	56	ERCP	88/94/90
Mendler (1998)	58	Prospective	Mixed disease population	58	ERCP	86/94/90
Laokpessi et al (2001)		Prospective	Stones	76	ERCP and IOC	93/100
Magnuson et al (1999)	143	Prospective	Mixed disease population	58	ERCP and PTC	92/99
Liu et al (1999)	99	Prospective	Stones	30	ERCP and IOC	85/90/89
Soto et al (2000)	49	Prospective	Stones	49	ERCP	92-100/92-100
Scheiman et al (2001)	30	Prospective	Stones and strictures	17	ERCP and EUS	40/96
Holzknecht et al (1998)	61	Prospective	Stones and strictures	40	ERCP	93/96
Zidi et al (1999)	70	Prospective	Mixed disease population	70	ERCP and IOC	57/100
Lomas et al (1999)	69	Prospective	Mixed disease population	13	ERCP	100/97
Soto et al (2000)	51	Prospective	Stones	51	ERCP and CT cholangiography	96/100
Varghese et al (2000)	100	Prospective	Mixed disease population	30	ERCP, PTC, and IOC	93/99/97
Varghese et al (2000)	191	Prospective	Mixed disease population	18	ERCP, PTC, US, and IOC	91/98/97
Chan et al (1996)	47	Prospective	Stones	42	ERCP	95/95/89
Demartines et al (2000)	70	Prospective	Stones	52	ERCP and IOC	100/96
Sugiyama et al (1998)	97	Retrospective	Stones	35	ERCP and US	91/1000/97
Guibaud et al (1995)	126	Retrospective	Mixed disease population	25	ERCP, PTC, and IOC	81/98/94
Fulcher et al (1998)	265	Retrospective	Mixed disease population	5	ERCP, PTC, and IOC	100/100/100
Calvo et al (2002)	116	Prospective	Stones	29	ERCP	91/90

Adapted with Permission from: Liu TH, Organ Jr CH. *Asian J Surg* 2004; 27: 102

number of investigations directed at limiting its application in this setting, and these investigations have uniformly demonstrated MRCP as having similar accuracy as ERCP for CBDS diagnosis. These studies have also shown that the initial application of MRCP was useful for the selection of patient for ERCP and ES. However, given the overall relatively low incidence of CBDS among patients undergoing LC, routine MRCP prior to LC did not appear to be a cost effective strategy for these patients.

The initial results of MRC application have led to the subsequent proposal of strategies to improve MRCP utilization in patients prior to LC. We have developed a triage protocol using a combination of clinical, biochemical, and ultrasonographic criteria, which have helped stratify preoperative patients' probability for CBDS into four levels in our practice. (Table 3) This triage scheme was developed on the basis of our own observations as well as literature reviews. Based on some earlier observations, we recognized that visualization of a dilated CBD by U/S was a non-specific indicator of CBDS, however the presence of a small CBD (<5 mm) was identified as an excellent negative predictor associated with 98% negative-predictive value.[6] The preoperative laboratory evaluations in these patients included serum bilirubin, alkaline phosphatase, AST, and ALT. We considered patients presenting with elevated liver enzymes, CBD >5 mm, and no evidence of cholecystitis or pancreatitis as having very high probability of having CBDS and triaged these patients to undergo ERCP. Since serum biochemical elevations occurred from transient, nonspecific liver injury associated with acute cholecystitis and acute pancreatitis, we considered patients with elevated liver enzymes, CBD >5 mm with clinical presentations of acute chole-

---

TABLE 3

DESIGNATION OF CHOLECOCHOLITHIASIS PROBABILITY

CBDS Probability	Clinical Diagnosis	CBD Measurement by US	Serum Chemistry Results
High	Absence of cholecystitis or pancreatitis	CBD diameter >5 mm	Presence of >2 indicators: total bilirubin >1.5 mg/dL; alkaline phosphatase >150 U/L; AST >100 U/L; ALT >100 U/L
Moderate	Presence of pancratitis, cholecystitis, or resolving choledocholithiasis	CBD diameter >5 mm	Presence of >2 indicators: total bilirubin >1.5 mg/dL; alkaline phosphatase >150 U/L; AST >100 U/L; ALT >100 U/L
Low	Any diagnosis	CBD diameter <5 mm	Presence of >2 indicators: total bilirubin >1.5 mg/dL; alkaline phosphatase >150 U/L; AST >100 U/L; ALT >100 U/L
Very Low	No evidence of jaundice, cholangitis, or pancreatitis	CBD diameter <5 mm	Total bilirubin <1.5 mg/dL; alkaline phophatase <150 U/L; AST <100 U/L; ALT <100 U/L

Adapted With Permission from Liu TH et al. *Ann Surg* 2001;234:36

cytitis or acute pancreatitis as having only moderate probability of having CBDS and triaged these patients to undergo initial screening with MRCP. Patients with elevated liver enzymes, CBD <5 mm and evidence of acute cholecystitis or acute pancreatitis were considered having low probability of having choledocholithiasis and were triage to LC with IOC, and patients with normal liver enzymes and small CBD underwent LC without CBD imaging. (Figure 1).

The application of this triage scheme in 440 patients over a 15 months period resulted in CBDS identification in 92.6%, 32.4%, 3.8%, and 0.9% of patients in each

of the groups. The overall occurrence of choledocholithiasis for the entire study population was 9.8%. This selection process resulted in ERCP application in only 8.9% of the patients and essentially eliminated the occurrence of non-therapeutic ERCP. Similarly, the triage scheme resulted in a dramatic reduction in preoperative MRCP utilization at our institution.

A slightly different CBDS risk-stratification scheme has been developed and tested in a patient population with significantly higher risk for CBDS than those examined by Liu et al. In this study, Kim et al stratified patients into three risk levels for CBDS on the basis of clinical, laborato-

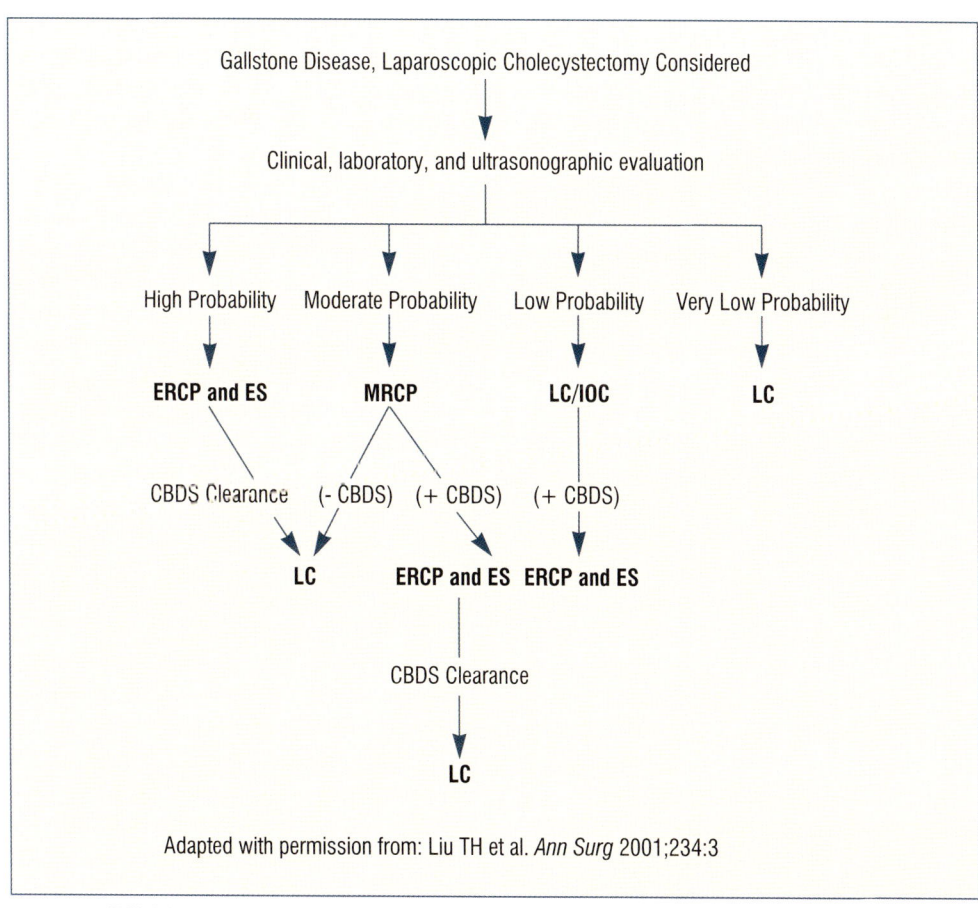

FIGURE 1: Perioperative selective imaging strategy based on choledocholithiasis probability.

ry, and radiographic criteria prior to chole-cystectomy. The application of MRCP for patients in these three groups resulted in excellent diagnostic accuracy for CBDS. Overall, CBDS was identified in 47% of all patients, and this triage scheme identified CBDS in 70%, 32%, and 3% of the patients in the three respective groups.

Hallal et al specifically examined the utility of preoperative MRCP in setting of biliary pancreatitis. In this study, patients with clinically resolved acute biliary pancreatitis were randomized to preoperative MRCP or LC with IOC. The results of the study confirmed the high diagnostic accuracy of MRCP in this patient population and that negative MRCP in these patients eliminated any further need for diagnostic evaluation by ERCP or IOC.

The cost effectiveness of treatment strategies for acute biliary pancreatitis has been the focus of several investigations. Using a decision-tree analysis model, Arguedas et al compared treatment strategies with initial ERCP, endoscopic ultrasonography (EUS), MRCP, and IOC for the diagnosis and treatment of choledocholithiasis in patients with acute biliary pancreatitis. Based on mathematical modeling, it was determined that at probability of CBDS < 15%, observation with IOC was the least expensive treatment strategy; whereas, EUS or MRCP were found to be associated with the greatest cost savings in the moderate risk patients with CBDS probability ranging between 15-58%, while initial ERCP was the least costly strategy in patients with CBDS probability >58%. These findings further support the need for CBDS risk stratification and the selective use of diagnostic strategies for patients undergoing LC.

The role of MRCP imaging after cholecystectomy

Common biliary complications following cholecystectomy include bile leak, bile duct injuries, and retained CBDS. The nature, severity, location, and timing of presentation of injuries are some of the major factors dictating patient therapy. While drainage may be sufficient treatment for selective patients with bile leaks, ensdoscopic, interventional radiologic therapy, and operative therapy are often required. When selecting an imaging modality in this setting, the decision should be based on the level of suspicion and the intended therapy for the suspected complications. An example of this is retained CBDS; in a given patient when the clinical suspicion for this complication is high, ERCP would be the most logical initial diagnostic modality since this approach would also provide immediate access for therapeutic intervention. An example where initial evaluation by ERCP would be less helpful is a patient with bile duct transection and ligation, in whom an ERCP would offer minimal diagnostic and therapeutic benefits.

The Bismuth Classification is most commonly used for the categorization of major biliary tract injuries. In Class I injuries, there is preservation of >2 cm of the common hepatic duct, whereas Class II-IV injuries involve major injuries of the biliary tract proximal to this level. Traditionally, patients with suspected iatrogenic bile duct injuries are managed with initial PTC to help delineate the proximal extent of injury and define the anatomy of the excluded ductal segments. Over the past few years, a number of groups have investigated the role of MRCP in these patients. Coakley et al applied MRCP in a group of patients who were referred to their hepatobiliary surgical practice for the management of suspected postoperative biliary tract complications and found that MRCP accurately differentiated major bile duct injuries, retained CBDS, choledochal cyst, cholangiocarcinoma, and nonspecific biliary dilatation, and based on the

MRCP findings, patients were triaged to appropriate subsequent management. Chaudhary et al compared the image quality, diagnostic accuracy, and information obtained by PTC and MRCP in 26 patients who underwent biliary reconstruction for iatrogenic bile duct injuries; they found that MRCP and PTC images were equally accurate for the visualizing anatomic details needed for the planning of operative reconstructions, and in several patients, MRCP provided valuable additional information such as the presence of extraductal fluid collections and portal hypertension. Yeh et al reported their experience with MRCP evaluations of patients with iatrogenic CBD injuries and concluded that MRCP images were more informative than images produced by PTC and ERCP, since the latter approaches only produced images of the upper or lower biliary systems, rather than the entire biliary system. Vitellas et al reported that contrast-enhanced MRCP produced images that correlated well with standard cholangiograms obtained by PTC and ERCP in patients with bile leaks following cholecystectomy. Park et al and Ragozzino et al applied the combination of conventional T2-weighted and contrast-enhanced MRCP in the evaluation and operative planning of patients with biliary complications following cholecysectomy and reported that the combined imaging approach provided sufficient information for the operative planning of these patients.

Based on result from these observations, it appears that MRCP and MRI techniques produce sufficiently high quality images for the identification of injuries and for the planning of biliary tract reconstruction. However, these limited observations have not helped determine when MRCP, ERCP, or PTC may be the most appropriate initial diagnostic study in the postoperative setting.

Patients with periampullary duodenal diverticulum

Duodenal diverticula are reported in up to 23% of patients undergoing ERCP.

Although the majority of patients with duodenal diverticula remain asymptomatic, symptoms and complications have been reported in approximately 10% of the patients. Due to bacterial overgrowth and diverticula distension leading to partial obstruction of the bile duct, periampullary duodenal diverticula have been reported to cause jaundice, cholangitis, pancreatitis, and CBDS formation. When suspected, ERCP is generally applied for the evaluation of bile duct obstruction and choledocholithiasis in these patients; however, due to altered anatomic orientation and inaccessibility of the ampulla, ERCP in these patients has been reported to be associated with technical difficulties and lower rates of success. MRCP imaging has been applied for the evaluation of duodenal diverticula and has been found to produce low diagnostic sensitivity (34.8%). The low diagnostic sensitivity has been attributed to fasting of the patients prior to imaging resulting in diverticular collapse and the nonvisualization. To improve MRCP visualization of duodenal diverticula, some radiologists have recommended water ingestion or secretin administration to promote diverticula distension prior to MRCP image acquisition. Although it appears that MRCP is associated with low diagnostic sensitivity for duodenal diverticula, MRCP may be a valuable imaging modality for the evaluation of patients with duodenal diverticula and clinical suspicion of diverticula-related biliary obstruction or CBDS. As CBDS is generally identified in approximately half of the patients undergoing ERCP, it would appear that the application of screening MRCP might facilitate CBDS identification and reduce unnecessary ERCP in these patients.

Choledochal cyst evaluation

Choledochal cysts are rare congenital dilatations of the biliary tract, and patients with these abnormalities may present with jaundice, pain, and abdominal mass. The association between choledochal cysts and cholangiocarcinoma is well established and has been postulated to be related to the carcinogenic effects of pancreatic reflux predisposed by anatomic malformation of the pancreaticobiliary junction. Experience with MRCP application for choledochal cysts evaluation has been limited due to disease rarity; however, based on these limited observations, MRCP appears to provide sufficient anatomic information in directing therapy, and when present, MRCP imaging has accurately identified malformations of the pancreaticobiliary junction.

Mirizzi syndrome

Mirizzi syndrome generally develops as the result of acute and chronic gallbladder inflammation, involving the impaction of a single large gallstone or multiple stones within Hartmann's pouch or the cystic duct directly adjacent to the common hepatic duct (CHD). Four types of Mirizzi syndrome have been described; type I disease involves simple external compression of the common hepatic duct by the dilated gallbladder, whereas types II-IV disease describe the formation of fistulas of varying extent between the gallbladder and CHD. Ultrasongraphy and CT have been reported to provide limited value in diagnosing this process. It has been suggested that recognition of Mirizzi's syndrome and the clear delineation of bile duct involvement are beneficial in the planning of operative therapy and the avoidance of iatrogenic biliary tract injuries. The treatment of Type I disease generally require recognition of the process, cholecystectomy, and preservation of adjacent biliary structures. Surgical options for Type II-IV disease include partial cholecytectomy and stone extraction, or excision and biliary reconstruction by hepaticojejunostomy. The application of standard MRCP sequences and T1-weighted sequences have been reported useful for the diagnosis of Mirizzi syndrome, delineation of the level of obstruction, identification of the location of the gallstone, and the differentiation of Mirizzi syndrome from other pathological conditions.

Primary sclerosing cholangitis

Primary sclerosing cholangitis (PSC) is a disease characterized by chronic inflammatory changes and fibrosis of the biliary tract. The diagnosis of PSC is generally established on the basis of cholangiographic features with confirmation by tissue biopsy results. Cholangiographic findings associated with this process most often include diffuse multifocal strictures of the intrahepatic and extrahepatic ducts, and in patients with long-standing PSC, thickening and irregularity of the duct walls may develop. ERCP has been the traditional imaging modality applied for the diagnosis of PSC. The anatomical details provided by CT and U/S are generally inadequate for the diagnosis of PSC, however these imaging tools have been found valuable for the screening and surveillance of cholangiocarcinoma development in patients with PSC. Fulcher et al have assessed the diagnostic accuracy of MRCP and reported diagnostic sensitivity of 85-88% and specificity of 92-97%. Some of the MRCP limitations identified include reduced diagnostic sensitivity in cases of mild PSC and false positive diagnosis in patients with cirrhosis and severe distortion of the intrahepatic ducts. MRCP has been applied with moderate success for the screening of cholangiocarcinoma development in patients with PSC, with reported diagnostic sensitivity of 80%.

MRI diagnosis of cholangiocarcinoma

Cholangiocarcinoma are generally classified by locations as intrahepatic, hilar, and distal. Morphologically, these tumors may present as 1. scirrhous infiltrating tumors leading to narrowing and distortion of the major bile ducts; 2. exophytic and bulky tumor originating from intrahepatic ducts and presenting as space-occupying lesions within the liver; 3. intraluminal polypoid lesions that are generally located in the distal bile ducts.

Intrahepatic cholangiocarcinoma are frequently difficult to differentiate from metastatic carcinoma. Two characteristic findings associated with cholangiocarcinoma that have been found useful for diagnosis incude delayed retention of intravenous contrast during CT and MR imaging and the association of this tumor with liver parenchyma atrophy.[1] Some intrahepatic cholangiocarcinoma are mucin-producing tumors, and when present, these lesions are often difficult to diagnose by CT and MRI. As the result of the high mucin content, these tumors often appear as low attenuation lesions that bear resemblance to hepatic cystic neoplasms.

The confluence of the right and left hepatic ducts and the proximal common hepatic duct are the most common locations for cholangiocarcinoma occurrence. Due to the small size, infiltrative nature, and location of most cholangiocarcinomas, these tumors re generally difficult to identify by traditional CT imaging and ultrasound, therefore PTC and ERCP have been the most common imaging modalities applied for diagnosis.

Recently, helical multi-detector CT and MRI have been applied with greater success for hilar cholangiocarcinoma visualization. As with intrahepatic cholangiocarcinoma, most hilar cholagiocarcinomas exhibit high signal intensity during the delayed phase of gadolinium enhanced T1-weighted imaging. Yeh et al evaluated 40 patients with perihilar biliary obstruction by MRI and reported that this imaging modality effectively differentiated cholangiocarcinoma from other causes of obstruction. With the recent development of intrabiliary MRI, Arepally and colleagues at Johns Hopkins have been able to demonstrate high accuracy for the identification and local staging of small hilar cholangiocarcinomas.

MRI EVALUATIONS OF PANCREATIC DISEASES

MR imaging of the pancreas is usually is generally performed using a combination of T1, T2-weighted, MRCP, and dynamic post-gandolinium fat-suppressed T1-weighted sequences that can be obtained in a single setting. MRCP application in this setting is generally helpful in providing excellent visualization of abnormalities within the distal portion of the biliary tract and the pancreatic ducts. Whereas, T1-weighted fat suppression sequences, delayed post-gandolinium imaging have been found useful for the differentiation and characterization of focal pancreatic mass lesions from the surrounding pancreatic glandular elements. In many case, the combination of these MRI techniques produce images and anatomic information that might otherwise require the use of CT, U/S, and ERCP.

Currently, the most common applications of MRI of the pancreas are: 1. The evaluation of patients with high clinical suspicion of biliopancreatic pathology where CT, U/S, and ERCP have not provided sufficient information. 2. Evaluation of patient with contraindications to ionizing radiation and/or iodinated contrast. 3. Detection and local staging of pancreatic and periampullary tumors. 4. Detection of small intrapancreatic neoplasm and characterization of small parenchymal abnormalities.

Evaluation of the pancreatic duct and pancreas divisum

The normal pancreatic duct has a diameter of 3 mm of less. With the high signal intensity of pancreatic ductal fluid, this structure is generally well visualized by heavily T2-weighted MRCP sequences. In a prospective comparison of the diagnostic capabilities of MRCP and ERCP involving 78 patients with suspected pancreatic pathology, the diagnostic accuracies for normal and abnormal pancreatic ductal anatomy were similar for both imaging modalities. However, the diagnostic values of MRCP was considered superior in two instances, where in one patient, MRCP identified a pancreatic neoplasm in the pancreatic tail as the source of pancreatic ductal abnormality; in another patient, MRCP identified a psuedocyst as the source of pancreatic ductal obstruction.

Pancreas divisum is the most commonly occurring anatomic anomaly of the pancreas and occurs in 5-14% of the general population. Although this entity rarely produces jaundice, it is capable of producing recurrent pancreatitis and chronic abdominal pain. Prior to the introduction of MRCP, ERCP was the most common method of diagnosis for pancreas divisum. Patients with pancreas divisum and functional obstruction of the minor duct are susceptible to the development of recurrent pancreatitis therefore may benefit from papillotomy of the minor papilla. MRCP has been reported as being highly accurate for the diagnosis of pancreas divisum. MRCP has also been investigated as a diagnostic modality for the identification functional obstruction of the minor papilla associated with pancreas divisum. Manfredi et al have reported that the administration of secretin in patients with functional obstruction of the papilla was associated with delayed filling of the duodenum in comparison to those patients with pancreas divisum and no papillary obstruction, therefore suggesting that MRCP with secretin administration may be a promising screening modality in selecting patients who may benefit from papillotomy of the minor papilla.

Pancreatic carcinoma diagnosis

Adenocarcinoma of the pancreas is the most common malignancy in the periampullary region and makes up approximately 75-85% of all pancreatic malignancies. The incidence of this malignancy has increased steadily over the past four decades, where this tumor has become the second most common gastrointestinal malignancy and the fourth leading cause of adult cancer deaths in the United States. Sixty to seventy percent of pancreatic adenocarcinomas are located in the head of the pancreas and are frequently associated with jaundice, weight loss, and nonspecific abdominal pain.

The primary goals during the evaluation of patients with suspected periampullary cancers are early diagnosis and accurate clinical staging to help direct patients toward the most appropriate treatment options. In most centers, the diagnostic approach for jaundiced patients with suspected periampullary tumors begins with abdominal U/S for the confirmation of biliary obstruction. Once biliary obstruction is confirmed, contrast-enhanced CT is generally obtained for tumor detection and staging. Spiral CT is generally considered highly accurate for tumor detection (>90%), with somewhat reduced diagnostic sensitivity for tumors measuring <1 cm.

Obstruction of the main pancreatic duct is a common finding associated with pancreatic adenocarcinoma. When pancreatic ductal obstruction occurs in the setting of carcinoma, the obstruction and ductal abnormality is often segmental, irregular, or eccentric, and based on these characteristics, ERCP have been found useful as a diagnostic tool for pancreatic adenocarcinoma, with reported specificity of 90% for pancreatic carcinoma diagnosis.

The utility of ERCP and MRCP for pancreatic carcinoma diagnosis was assessed in a prospective controlled study involving 124 patients with clinical suspicion of having pancreatic malignancies. During this study, the sensitivity and specificity of MRCP for cancer detection were determined to be superior to those of ERCP. Visualization of a nonobstructive main pancreatic duct by MRCP was identified as a reliable negative predictor for carcinoma, and this finding was found useful in eliminating further evaluation by ERCP in selective patients. ERCP applications produced procedural-related morbidity in 7% of the patients, and it was concluded that MRCP application is potentially valuable in reducing unnecessary diagnostic ERCP and the complications associated with this invasive procedure.

Tumor masses associated with adenocarcinoma generally contain abundant amount of fibrous stroma and interstitial fluid, and as the result of these tumor characteristics, carcinomas generally produce a hypodense appearance during pre-infusion and immediately post-infusion phases of fat-suppressed T1-weighted MRI sequences. With slow contrast diffusion into the tumor after infusion, adenocarcinomas then develop an isodense appearance during the delayed phases of MR imaging. Based on these radiographic features, MRI has been established as an effective diagnostic tool for pancreatic carcinoma, with sensitivity and specificity reported in the ranges of 84-100% and 63-97%, respectively.

One of the most difficult diagnostic dilemmas faced by surgeons, radiologists, and gastroenterologists occurs when a focal pancreatic mass is discovered in the setting of chronic pancreatitis. In these patients, the differentiation between chronic pancreatitis and carcinoma can be highly problematic, since both clinical entities are associated with similar clinical and radiographic features. In many instances, the definitive diagnoses have required tissue diagnosis by percutaneous biopsies or operative resections.

The diagnostic value of MRI for the differentiation of chronic panreatitis and adenocarcinoma has been a focus of several investigations. Experiences with the use of MRCP suggest that this approach is associated high diagnostic specificity when the "duct penetrating sign" or the "double duct sign" is identified. The "duct penetrating sign" refers to a nonobstructed, irregularly dilated main pancreatic penetrating an inflammatory pancreatic mass, which is a finding associated with 85% of patients with chronic pancreatitis and only 4% of patients with pancreatic carcinoma. The "double duct sign" refers to the presence of dilatation and noncommunication of the common bile duct and main pancreatic duct, and this has been described as a finding associated only with pancreatic carcinoma. When present, these MRCP signs have been found useful in differentiating between pancreatitis and carcinoma. However, based on MRCP criteria alone, up to 25% of patients may be misdiagnosed, and for this reason, MRCP is generally obtained with T1-weighted sequence images to improve the diagnostic yield. Even though the use of fat-suppression T1-weighted MRI imaging improves the diagnostic accuracy of MRI, there are diagnostic limitations to this approach. Johnson et al evaluated a group of patients with adenocarcinoma arising from pancreatic glands that are extensively involved with chronic pancreatitis and determined that chronic pancreatitis and adenocarcinoma exhibited similar abnormal appearance by T1-weighted sequences, therefore suggesting that reliable differentiation of these entities by the standard MRI approaches remain problematic.

Magnetic resonance spectroscopy (MRS) is a diagnostic modality that has been developed to provide noninvasive measurement of biochemical information in vivo. This technology has been investigated in experimental models, where MRS has been utilized for the detection and growth monitoring of implanted human pancreatic carcinoma in the pancreas of laboratory animals. Most recently, Cho et al reported their experience with proton-MRS (^{1}H-MRS) for the differentiation of chronic focal pancreatitis and pancreatic carcinoma in 36 patients. Spectroscopic evaluations of the dominant pancreatic mass in these patients revealed significant difference in lipid contents between chronic pancreatitis and adenocarcinoma, where tumor mass associated with chronic pancratitis exhibited significantly lower lipid content than adenocarinoma. Based on ^{1}H-MRS measurements of lipid contents in the tumor mass, the investigators were able to establish a cutoff value that enabled the differentiation of chronic pancreatitis from adenocarcinoma. These preliminary results are encouraging and suggest that this method of imaging may prove to be valuable in the management of these difficult patients in the future.

Pancreatic carcinoma staging and determination of resectability

Overall, only 10-15% of patients with pancreatic carcinoma have disease that is amendable to curative operations, and the selection of patients for operative treatment requires clinical judgment and diagnostic imaging for the determination of clinical stage, tumor locoregional exten-

sion, and resectability. Historically, CT scan is the most frequently used imaging modality for the assessment of tumor resectability, and has remained the mainstay of imaging in most centers. With the recent advances in MRI, PET scan, and endoscopic ultrasonography (EUS), these modalities are being increasing utilized for the staging and preoperative evaluation of patients with pancreatic carcinoma; however, the role of these other imaging modalities has not been clearly determined.

The CT criteria of unresectable disease have traditionally included the presence of ascites, local tumor extension beyond the pancreas, contiguous organ invasion, vascular invasion, and lymph node involvement. Using these criteria, Freeny et al reported in 1988 that CT accurately identified 100% of the patients with unresectable disease; however, 46% of the patients with disease that were determined resectable by CT were found unresectable during abdominal explorations. These early observations suggested that CT had limited value in identifying lymph node metastases, intraperitoneal tumor extension, liver metastases, and vascular invasion. During the past several years, the resectability criteria for periampullary carcinomas have been modified in many centers. With various groups having reported long-term disease-free survival and acceptable postoperative morbidity following pancreaticoduodenectomy (PD) with major vascular reconstructions for locally advanced pancreatic adenocarcinoma, tumor involvement of the superior mesenteric vein (SMV) and portal vein (PV) are currently considered only relative contraindications to PD.

The diagnostic accuracies and utility of CT, MRI, EUS, and angiography have been compared in a recent multicenter investigation from Spain. During this study, the diagnostic accuracies of CT were 74%, 62%, 83%, and 88% for the determination of locoregional tumor extension, regional lymph nodes involvement, vascular invasion, and distant metastases, respectively. Based on their observations, the investigators constructed decision analysis indicating that a strategy involving initial spiral CT and the selective application of EUS was the most reliable and economic approach for preoperative imaging. The combination of preoperative CT and EUS correctly determined tumor resectability in 87% of the patients, and led to 11% of patient undergoing nontherapeutic operations and 2% of patients being excluded from potentially curative surgery.

It should be noted that several groups have specifically compared the diagnostic accuracy and value of CT with MRI and have produce results and conclusions that have differed from those reported by Soriano et al. Shima et al reported MRI as having greater diagnostic accuracy than CT in pancreatic cancer diagnosis and in the identification of small hepatic metasta-

sis. Arslan et al compared diagnostic accuracy of MRI, MR angiography (MRA), and CT for the determination of vascular invasion and concluded that the diagnostic accuracy of MRI with MRA and CT were equal. Based on the various reports, it would appear that accurate diagnosis and staging of patients with pancreatic carcinoma may require combined imaging modalities, and that the diagnostic approach for each patient should be determined on the basis of patient presentation, and the availability of technology and local expertise (Table 4).

SUMMARY

MRI technologic advances have dramatically improved the image resolution for studies performed for the evaluation of biliopancreatic obstructive diseases. MRCP is highly effective for the diagnosis and preoperative evaluation of patients with

TABLE 4

SUMMARY OF MRI DIAGNOSTIC ACCURACIES FOR PANCREATICOBILIARY DISEASES

Disease Condition	MRI Techniques	Sensitivity Mean (range)	Specificity Mean (range)
Common bile duct stones	MRCP	92% (80-97%)	96% (90-99%)
Presence of obstruction	MRCP	97% (91-99%)	98% (91-99%)
Level of obstruction	MRCP	98% (94-99%)	98% (94-100%)
Diagnosis of primary sclerosing cholangitis	MRCP	(85-88%)	(92-97%)
Biliary tract malignancy detection	MRCP + Enhanced T1- weighted MRI	88% (70-96%)	95% (82-99%)
Pancreatic carcinoma diagnosis	MRCP + Enhanced T1- weighted MRI	94% (84-98%)	96% (85-100%)
Detection of pancreatic carcinoma vascular invasion	MRCP + Enhanced T1-weighted MRI + MRA	59% (59-67%)	84% (84-100%)

biliary obstructive processes. The ease of MRCP application may play a future role in the screening and surveillance of selected patient populations, including the screening of cholangocarcinoma in patients with PSC patients, screening and surveillance of patients with Oriental cholangitis and duodenal diverticula for CBDS, and the screening and surveillance of patients for pancreatic adenocarcinoma. MRI appears to be more effective than CT for the identification of small pancreatic adenocarcinoma, however its routine application does not appear to provide any diagnostic advantages over spiral CT.

REFERENCES

Adamek HE, Albert J, Breer H, et al. Pancreatic cancer detection with magnetic resonance cholangiopancreatography and endoscopic retrograde cholangiopancreatography: a prospective controlled study. *Lancet* 2000;356:190-193.

Adamek HE, Schilling D, Weitz M, Riemann JF. C-holedocholcele imaged with magnetic resonance cholagniography. *Am J Gastroenterol* 2000;95: 1082-1083.

Arepally A, Georgiades C, Hofmann LV, et al. Hilar cholangiocarcinoma: staging with intrabiliary MRI. *AJR* 2004;183:1071-1074.

Arguedas MR, Dupont AW, Wilcox CM. Where do ERCP, endoscopic ultrasound, magnetic resonance cholangiopancreatography, and intraoperative cholangiography fit in the management of acute biliary pancreatitis? A decision analysis model. *Am J Gastroenterol* 2001;96:2892-2899.

Aube C, Delorme B, Yzet T, et al. MR cholangiopancreatography versus endoscopic sonography in suspected common bile duct lithiasis, a prospective, comparative study. *AJR;* 2005:55-62.

Balci NC, Semlka RC. Radiologic diagnosis and staging of pancreatic ductal adenocarcinoma. *Eur J Radiol* 2001;38:105-112.

Baron RL, Tublin ME, Peterson MS. Imging the spectrum of biliary tract disease. *Radiol Clin N Am* 2002;40:1325-1354.

Becker CD, Hassler H, Terrier F. Preoperative diagnosis of Mirizzi syndrome: limitations of sonography and computed tomography. *AJR* 1984;143:591-596.

Bortoff GA, Chen MY, Ott DF, et al. Gallbladder stones: imaging and intervention. *Radiographics* 2000;20:751-766.

Bret PM, Reinhold C, Taourel P, et al. Pancreas divism: evaluation with MR cholangiopancreatography. *Radiology* 1996;199:99-103.

Calvo MM, Bujanda L, Calderon A, et al. Comparison between magnetic resonance cholangiopancreatography and ERCP for evaluation of the pancreatic duct. *Am J Gastroenterol* 2002;97:347-353.

Calvo MM, Bujanda L, Calderon A, et al. Comparison between magnetic resonance cholangiopancreatography and ERCP for evaluation of the pancreatic duct. *Am J Gastroenterol* 2002;97:347-353.

Campbell WL, Ferris JV, Holbert BL, et al. Biliary tract carcinoma complicating primary sclerosing cholangitis: evaluation with CT, cholangiography, US, and MR imaging. *Radiology* 1998;207:412-50.

Chaudhary A, Negi SS, Puri SK, Narang P. Comparison of magnetic resonance cholangiography and percutaneous transhepatic cholangiography in the evaluation of bile duct strictures after cholecystectomy. *Br J Surg* 2002;89:433-436.

Cho SG, Lee DH, Lee KY, et al. Differentiation of chronic focal pancreatitis from pancreatic carcinoma by in vivo proton magnetic resonance spectroscopy. *J Comput Assist Tomogr* 2005; 29:163-169.

Coakley FV, Schwartz LH, Blumgart, LH, et al. complex postcholecystectomy disorders: preliminary experience with evaluation by means of breath-hold MR cholangiography. *Radiology* 1998;209:141-146.

DeBacker AI, Van den Abbeele K, DeSchepper AM, Van Baarle A. Choledochocele: diagnosis by magnetic resonance imaging. *Abdom Imaging* 2000;25:508-510.

Fayad LM, Kowalski T, Mitchell DG. MR cholangiopancreatography: evaluation of common pancreatic diseases. *Radiol Clin N Am* 2003;41:97-114.

Fischer U, Vosshenrich R, Horstmann O, et al. Preoperative local MRI-staging of patient with a suspected pancreatic mass. *Eur Radiol* 2002;12: 296-303.

Freeny PC, Marks WM, Ryan JA, Traverso LW. Pancreatic ductal adenocarcinoma: diagnosis and staging with dynamic *CT. Radiology* 1988;166: 125-133.

Fulcher AS. MRCP and ERCP in the diagnosis of common bile duct stones. *Gastrointest Endsoc* 2002;56:S178-S182.

Fulcher AS, Turner MA. MR cholangiopancreatography. *Radiol Clin N Am* 2002;40:1363-1376.

Fulcher AS, Turner MA, Capps GW, Zfass AM, Baker KM. Half-fourier RARE MR cholangiopancreatography: experience in 300 subjects. *Radiol* 1998;207:21-32.

Fulcher AS, Turner MA, Franklin KJ, et al. Primary sclerosing cholangitis: evluation with MR cholangiography-a case-control study. *Radiology* 2000;21:71-80.

Guibaud L, Bret PM, Reinhold, et al. Biel duct obstruction and choledocholithiasis diagnosis with MR cholangiography. *Radiol* 1995;197:109-115.

Hallal AH, Amortegui JD, Jeroukhimov IM, et al. *J Am Coll Surg* 2005;200:869-875.

Hochwald SN, Rofsky NM, Dobryansky M, Shamamian P, Marcus SG. Magnetic resonance imaging with magnetic resonance cholangiopancreatography accurately predicts resectability of pancreatic carcinoma. *J Gastrointest Surg* 1999; 3:506-511.

Holzknecht N, Gauger J, Sackmann, et al. Breath-hold MR cholangiography with snapshot techniques: prospective comparison with endoscopic retrograde cholagiography. *Radiol* 1998;206: 657-664.

Howard TJ, Villanustre N, Moore SA, et al. Efficacy of venous reconstruction in patients with adenocarcinoma of the pancreatic head. *J Gastrointest Surg* 2003;7:1089-1095.

Ichikawa T, Haradome H, Hachiya J, et al. Pancreatic ductal adenocarcinoma: preoperative assessment with helical CT versus dynamic MR imaging. *Radiology* 1997;202:655-662.

Ichikawa T, Sou H, Araki T, et al. Duct-penetrating sign at MRCP: usefulness for differentiating inflammatory pancreatic mass from pancreatic carcinoma. *Radiology* 2001;221:107-116.

Johnson PT, Outwater EK. Pancreatic carcinoma versus chronic pancreatitis: dynamic MR imaging. *Radiology* 1999;212:213-218.

Keogan MT, McDermott VG, Paulson EK, et al. Pancreatic malignancy: effects of dual-phase helical CT in tumor detection and vascular opacification. *Radiology* 1997;205:513-518.

Kim JH, Kim MJ, Park SI, et al. MR cholangiography in symptomatic gallstones: diagnostic accuracy according to clinical risk group. *Radiol* 2002: 224;410-412.

Kim PN, Outwater EK, Mitchell DG. Mirizzi syndrome: evaluation by MR imaging. *Am J Gastroenterol* 1999;94:2546-2550.

Laokpessi A, Bouillet P, Sautereau D, et al. Value of magnetic resonance cholangiography in the preoperative diagnosis of common bile duct stones. *Am J Gastroenterol* 2001;96:2354-2359.

Liu TH, Consorti ET, Kawashima A, et al. The efficacy of magnetic resonance cholangiography in the evaluation of patients with suspected choledocholithiasis before laparoscopic cholecystectomy. *Am J Surg* 1999:178;480-484.

Liu TH, Consorti ET, Kawashima A, et al. Patient evaluation and management with selective use of magnetic resonance cholangiography and endoscopic retrograde cholangiopancreatography before laparoscopic cholecystectomy. *Ann Surg* 2001;234:33-40.

Liu TH, Organ Jr CH. Magnetic resonance cholangiography: applications in patients with calculus disease of the biliary tract. *Asian J Surg* 2004;27: 99-107.

Lobo DN, Balfour TW, Iftikhar SY. Periampullary diverticula: consequences of failed ERCP. *Ann R Coll Surg Engl* 1998;80:326-331.

Lobo DN, Balfour TW, Iftikhar SY, Rowlands BJ. Periampullary diverticula and panreaticobiliary disease. *Br J Surg* 1999;86:588-597.

Loma DJ, Bearcroft WP, Gimson AE. MR cholangiopancreatography: prospective comparison of a breath-hold 2D projection technique with diagnostic ERCP. Eur Radiol 1999;(:1411-1417.

Ly JN, Miller FH. MR imaging of the pancreas: a practical approach. *Radiol Clin N Am* 2002;40: 1289-1306.

Lygidakis NJ, Singh G, Bardaxoglou E, et al. Monobloc total spleno-pancreaticoduodenectomy for pancreatic head carcinoma with portal-mesenteric venous invasion. A prospective randomized study. *Hepatogastroenterology* 2004; 51:427-433.

Magnuson TH, Bender JS, Duncan MD, et al. Utility of magnetic resonance cholangiography in the evaluation of biliary obstruction. *J Am Coll Surg.* 1999;189:63-72.

Manfredi R, Costamagna G, Brizi MG, et al. Pancreas divism and "santorinicele": diagnosis with dynamic MR cholangiopancreatography with secretin stimulation. *Radiology* 2000;217:403-408.

Masci T, Toti A, Mariani S, et al. Complications of diagnostic and therapeutic ERCP: a prospective multicenter study. *Am J. Gastroenterol* 2001;96: 417-423.

Matos C, Nicaise N, Deviere J, et al. Choledochal cysts: comparison of findings at MR cholangiopancreatography and endoscopic retrograde cholangiopancreatography in eight patients. *Radiol* 1998;209:443-448.

Mendler MH, Bouillet P, Sautereau D, et al. *Am J Gastroenterol* 1998;93:2482-2490.

Menon K, Barkun AN, Romagnuolo J, et al. Patient satisfaction after MRCP and ERCP. *Am J of Gastroenterol* 2001;96:2646-2650.

Mortele KJ, Tuncali K, Cantisani V, et al. MRI-guided abdominal intervention. *Abdom Imaging* 2003;28:756-774.

Motohara T, Semelka RC, Bader TR. MR cholangiopancratography. *Radiol Clin N Am* 2003;41:89-96.

Nakagohri T, Kinoshita T, Konishi M, Inoue K, Takahashi S. Survival benefits of portal vein resection for pancreatic cancer. *Am J Surg* 2003; 186:149-153.

Nakano H, Bachellier P, Weber JC, et al. Arterial and vena caval resections combined with pancreaticoduodenectomy in highly selective patients with priampullary malignancies. *Hepatogastroenterology* 2002;49:258-262.

Obuz F, Dicle O, Coker A, Sagol O, Karademir S. Pancreatic adenocarcinoma: detection and staging with dynamic MR imaging. *Eur J Radiol* 2001; 2001:146-150.

Park MS, Kim KW, Yu JS, et al. Early biliary complications of laparoscopic cholecystectomy: evaluation on T2-weighted MR cholangiography in conjunction with mangafodipir trisodium-enhanced 3-d T1-weightly MR cholangiography. *AJR* 2004;183:1559-1566.

Paul A, Millat B, Hothausen U, et al. Diagnosis and treatment of common bile duct stones (CBDS): result of a consensus development conference. *Surg Endosc* 1998;12:856-864.

Pemberton M, Wells AD. The Mirizzi syndrome. *Postgrad Med J* 1997;73:487-490.

Poon RT, Fan ST, Lo CM, et al. Pancreaticoduodenectomy with en bloc portal vein resection for pancreatic carcinoma with suspected portal vein involvement. *World J Surg* 2004;28:602-608.

Ragozzino A, DeRitis R, Mosca A, Iaccarino V, Imbriaco M. Value of MR cholangiography in patients with iatrogenic bile duct injury after cholecystectomy. *AJR* 2004;183:1567-1572.

Reinhold C, Taorel P, Bret PM, et al. Choledocholithiasis: evaluation of MR cholangiography for diagnosis. *Radiol* 1998;209:435-442.

Sahai AV, Devonshire D, Yeoh KG, et al. The decision-making value of magnetic resonance cholangiopancreatography in patients seen in a referral center for suspected biliary and pancreatic diseases. *Am J Gastroenterol* 2001;96:2074-2080.

Saisho H, Yamaguchi T. diagnostic imaging for pancreatic cancer. Computed tomography, magnetic resonance imaging, and positron emission tomography. *Pancreas* 2004;28:273-278.

Salloum RM, Koniaris L. Image of the month. *Arch Surg* 2004;139:449-450.

Sarmiento JM, Sarr MG. *Curr Gastroentrol Rep* 2003;5:117-124.

Sheridan MB, Ward J, Guthrie JA, et al Dynamic contrast-enhanced MR imaging and dual-phase helical CT in the preoperative assessment of suspected pancreatic cancer: a comparative study with receiver operating characteristic analysis. *AJR* 1999;173:583-590.

Shibata C, Kobari M, Tsuchiya T, et al. Pancreatectomy combined with superior mesenteric-portal vein resection for adenocarcinoma in pancreas. *World J Surg* 2001;25:1002-1005.

Shima W, Fugger R, Schober E, et al. Diagnosis and staging of pancreatic cancer: comparison of mangafodipir trisodium-enhanced MR imaging and contrast-enhanced helical hydro-CT. *AJR* 2002; 179:717-724.

Soriano A, Castells A, Ayuso C, et al. Preoperative staging and tumor resectability assessment of pancreatic cancer: prospective study comparing endoscopic ultrasonography, helical computed tomography, magnetic resonance imaging, and angiography. *Am J Gastroenterol* 2004;99: 492-501.

Soyer P. Imaging of intrahepatic cholangiocarcinoma: 1. peripheral cholangiocarcinoma. *AJR* 1995; 165:1427-1431.

Soyer P. Imaging of intrahepatic cholangiocarcinoma: 2. Hilar cholangiocarcinoma. *AJR* 1995;165: 1433-1436.

Stiris MG, Tennoe B, Aadland E, Lunde OC. MR cholangiopancreatography and endsocopic retrograde cholangiopancreatography in patients with suspected common bile duct stones. *Acta Radiologica* 2000;41:269-272.

Tamm E, Charnsangavej C. Pancreatic cancer: current concepts in imaging for diagnosis and staging. *Cancer J* 2001;7:298-311.

Taschieri AM, Elli M, Rovati M, et al. Surgical treatment of pancreatic tumors invading the splenomesenteric-portal vessels. An Italian multicenter survey. *Hepatogastroenterol* 1999;46: 492-497.

Tseng JF, Raut CP, Lee JE, et al. Pancreaticoduodenectomy with vascular resection: margin status and survival duration. *J Gastrointest Surg* 2004; 8:935-949.

Tsitouridis I, Emmanouilidou M, Goutsaridou F, et al. MR cholangiography in the evaluation of patients with duodenal periampullary diverticulum. *Eur J Radiol* 2003;47:154-160.

Varghese JC, Farrell MA, Courtney G, et al. A prospective comparison of magnetic resonance cholangiopancreatography with endoscopic retrograde cholangiopancreatography in the evaluation of patients with suspected biliary tract disease. *Clinical Radiol* 1999;54:513-520.

Varghese JC, Liddell RP, Farrell MA, et al. The diagnostic accuracy of magnetic resonance cholangiopancreatography and ultrasound compared with direct cholangiography in the detection of choledocholithiasis. *Clinical Radiol* 1999;54: 604-614.

Vitellas KM, El-Dieb A, Vaswani KK, et al. Using contrast-enhanced MR cholangiography with iv mangafodipir trisodium (Teslascan) to evaluate bile duct leaks after cholecystectomy. *AJR* 2002; 179:409-416.

Wallner BK, Schumacher KA, Weidenmaier W, Friedrich JM. Dilated biliary tract: evaluation with MR cholangiography with a T2-weighted contrast-enhanced fast sequence. *Radiology* 1991; 181:805-808.

Yeh TS, Jan YY, Tseng JH, et al. Value of magnetic resonance cholangiopancreatography in demonstrating major bile duct injuries following laparoscopic cholecystectomy. *Br J Surg* 1999; 86:181-184.

Yeh TS, Jan YY, Tseng JH, et al. Malignant perihilar biliary obstruction: magnetic resonance cholangiographic findings. *Am J Gastroenterol* 2000;95:432-440.

Yoshimi F, Asato Y, Tanaka R, et al. Reconstruction of the portal vein and the splenic vein in pancreaticoduodenectomy for pancreatic cancer. *Hepatogastroenterology* 2003;50:856-860.

Zhou GW, Wu WD, Xiao WD, Li HW, Peng CH. Pancreatectomy combined with superior mesenteric-portal vein resection: report of 32 cases. *Hepatobiliary Pancreat Dis Int* 2005;4: 130-134.

The role of EUS in the diagnosis and treatment of obstructive jaundice

Maluf-Filho Fauze

INTRODUCTION

Obstructive jaundice is a common clinical problem that can be caused by a variety of disorders. One report, for example, evaluated the principal diagnoses obtained in 702 adults presenting with jaundice to 24 Dutch hospitals over a two-year period. Pancreatic or biliary carcinoma accounted for 20 percent, gallstones for 13 percent and alcoholic cirrhosis for 10 percent.

Differential diagnosis of obstructive jaundice is yet a challenging problem for clinicians, surgeons, endoscopists and radiologists. The diagnostic approach to the jaundiced patient begins with a careful history and physical examination, and screening laboratory studies. A differential diagnosis is formulated and appropriate further testing is performed to narrow the diagnostic possibilities.

The introduction of endoscopic ultrasonography (EUS) as an imaging diagnostic tool brought some expectancies to solve this important dilemma. EUS was incorporated as a diagnostic method in gastroenterology in the 1980's, as a result of some researcher's constant efforts that enabled the improvement of the first prototypes of such equipment.

It soon became clear the high accuracy of EUS for the diagnosis of the two most common causes of obstructive jaundice: periampullary neoplasm, including pancreatic cancer, and choledocholithiasis.

THE ROLE OF EUS IN THE DIAGNOSIS COMMON BILE DUCT (CBD) STONES

There are nine studies which include a total of 601 patients comparing EUS and endoscopic retrograde cholangiography (ERC) to diagnose CBD stones. In eight of these studies, endoscopic exploration of the CBD was used as the reference standard. All of these studies indicate that EUS and ERC have similar sensitivity and specificity in the detection of CBD stones.

Magnetic resonance cholangiography (MRC) is recognized as a highly accurate and noninvasive test for the diagnosis of CBD stones. However, it is also known that the size of the stone has influence on MRC results especially when the diameter of the stone varies from 3 to 5 mm. Sugiyama et al. did the only study that analyzed sensitivity of a test for CBD stone detection according to subgroups of stone size. Sensitivity of MRCP varied from 100% for 11-27 mm stone diameter to 71% for stones sized between 3-5 mm.

Our group performed a study that has compared the diagnostic performance of EUS and ERC for choledocholithiasis according stone size. Two hundred and fifteen patients with symptomatic gallstones were admitted for laparoscopic cholecystectomy. Sixty-eight of them (31.7%) had a dilated common bile duct and/or hepatic biochemical parameter abnormalities. They were submitted to endoscopic ultrassonography and endoscopic retrograde cholangiography. Sphincterotomy and sweeping of the common bile duct were performed if endoscopic ultrassonography or endoscopic retrograde cholangiography were considered positive for choledocholithiasis. After sphincterotomy and common bile duct clearance the largest stone was retrieved for measurement. Endoscopic or surgical explorations of the common bile duct were considered the gold-standard methods for the diagnosis of choledocholithiasis. All 68 patients were submitted to laparoscopic cholecystectomy with intraoperative cholangiography with confirmation of the presence of gallstones. Endoscopic ultrassonography was a more sensitivity test than endoscopic retrograde cholangiography (97 vs. 67%) for the detection of choledocholithiasis. When stones >4.0 mm were analyzed, endoscopic ultrassonography and endoscopic retrograde cholangiography presented similar results (96 vs. 90%). Neither the size of the stone nor the common bile duct diameter had influence on endoscopic ultrasonographic performance (Figures 1 and 2).

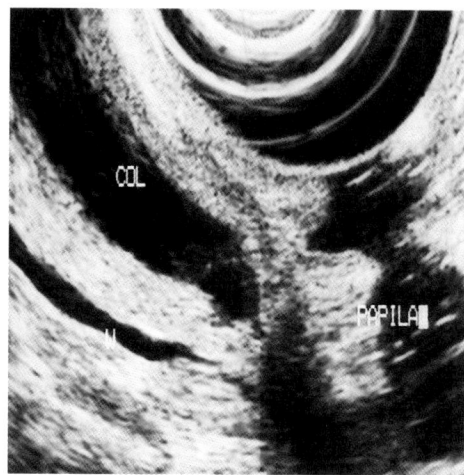

FIGURE 1: Radial echoendoscopic view of the normal biliopancreatic confluence (PAPILA = ampulla; W = main pancreatic duct; COL = common bile duct).

THE ROLE OF EUS IN THE DIAGNOSIS OF PERIAMPULLARY CANCER

Many uncontrolled studies have demonstrated the high accuracy of EUS in detection and staging of the pancreatic (Figure 3) and ampullary adenocarcinoma.

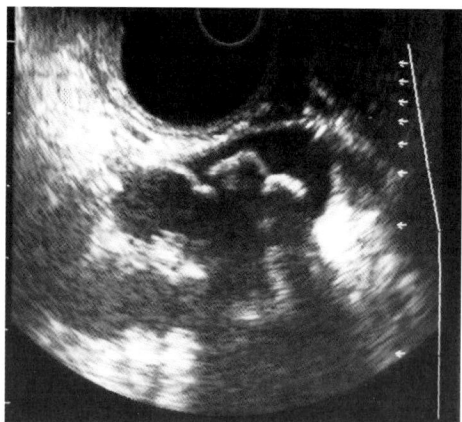

FIGURE 2: Linear echoendoscopic view of small stones floating in a 6mm common bile duct.

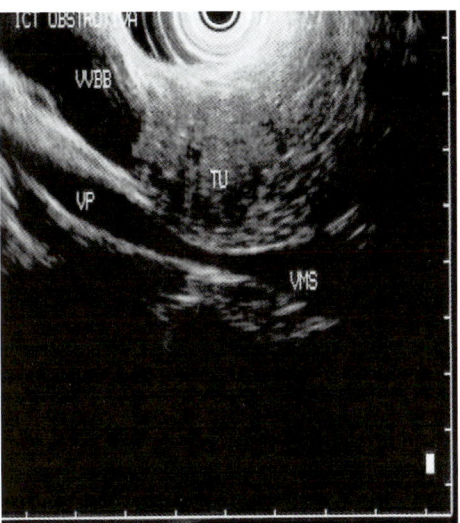

FIGURE 3: Radial echoendoscopic view of pancreatic head tumor compressing the common bile duct. The portal venous axis is free of invasion. TU = tumor; VP = portal vein; VMS = superior mesenteric vein; VVBB = common bile duct.

They have also reported that EUS detected small tumors of 20 mm or less. A major limitation of these studies was the lack of blinded comparisons. These earlier reports also suggested that EUS was superior to conventional computed tomography scanning (CT-scan) in the detection of pancreatic solid tumors. Newer protocols, using spiral and mutidetector CT-scan have reached an accuracy of 95% in detecting pancreatic cancer. In tumors larger than 2 cm, studies using modern staging protocols suggest that EUS and spiral CT have equal accuracy in detecting pancreatic cancer. Muller et al. comparing EUS, spiral CT-scan and magnetic resonance for the evaluation of patients with suspected pancreatic tumor reported a positivity index of 67.3%. They observed a diagnostic accuracy of 96%, 67% and 84%, respectively for EUS, spiral CT-scan and MRI. For tumors sized 20 mm or less the accuracies were, respectively 90%, 40% and 33%. These results

were confirmed by other studies (Figures 4 and 5).

On the other hand, the superiority of EUS over CT in detection of ampullary adenocarcinoma is well known. This observation is related to the fact that up to one third of the cases of ampullary adenocarcinoma remain intra-ampullary, especially the non vegetative forms. The superiority of EUS could also be attributed to the capacity of endoscopic imaging of the ampulla.

Our group compared EUS to spiral CT-scan for the detection and staging of suspected periampullary cancers in sixty-one patients, 46 (75,4 %) of whom presented with obstructive jaundice. Fifty-six (91,8%) patients were surgically explored. Clinical follow-up and/or tissue diagnosis determined the correct diagnosis in the remaining patients. Pancreatic cancer and ampullary cancer were observed in 29 (47, 6%) and 10 (16, 4%) patients, respectively. Both exams were equally effective for detecting pancreatic cancer but EUS predicted more accurately the involvement of portal-mesenteric axis by the tumor (87.0 vs. 67.4% p=0.04). Endoscopic ultrasonography was particularly

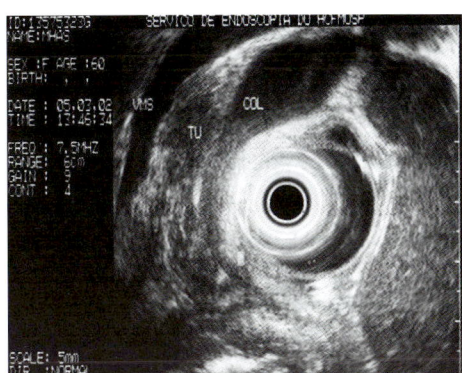

FIGURE 4: Radial echoendoscopic view of a 20 mm pancreatic head tumor compressing the common bile duct. The portal venous axis is free of invasion. TU = tumor; VMS = superior mesenteric vein; COL = common bile duct.

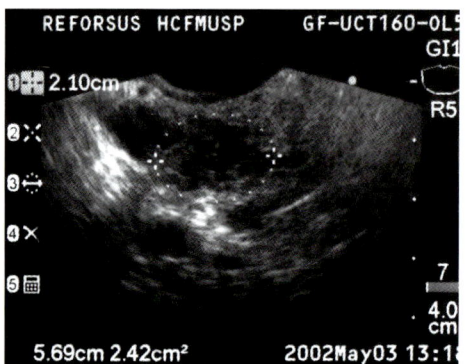

FIGURE 5: Linear echoendoscopic view of a 20 mm pancreatic head tumor (dotted line) compressing the common bile duct. This is the same tumor demonstrated at figure 4.

useful in the diagnosis of cancer of papilla of Vater.

TRIALS COMPARING EUS AND OTHER IMAGING MODALITIES IN THE DIAGNOSIS OF OBSTRUCTIVE JAUNDICE

Three peer-reviewed trials and one trial published as an abstract compared EUS with CT-scan or magnetic resonance imaging for the diagnosis of obstructive jaundice (Table 1).

The high accuracy of radial EUS in all studies could be attributed to the fact that most of the obstructive lesions were located in the extrahepatic biliary tree. It means that radial EUS can not be considered a primary exam for patients with obstructive jaundice. On the other hand, when conventional ultrasonography demonstrates dilation of extrahepatic duct, one might expect the diagnostic accuracy of EUS to achieve more than 90%. It must be also recognized that ampullary tumors, small neoplasms (<20 mm) and small stones (<5 mm) are better identified by EUS when compared with CT-scan or MRI. The possibility of obtaining tissue by EUS-guided fine needle aspiration (EUS-FNA) rendered EUS even more appealing for the patients with extrahepatic cholestasis, especially those in whom a periampullary tumor is suspected (Table 2) (Figures 6 and 7).

On the other hand, EUS-FNA also permits the tissue confirmation of a suspicious metastatic lesion which could change the therapeutic planning. In fact, hepatic metastasis and ascites undetected by CT-scan have been successfully diagnosed and sampled by EUS-FNA.

In summary, EUS and EUS-FNA are indicated for the cholestatic patient with a suspected extrahepatic obstruction in which CT-scan was unable to define the

TABLE 1

EUS COMPARED WITH OTHER IMAGING MODALITIES IN THE DIAGNOSIS OF THE CAUSE OF BILIARY OBSTRUCTION

Author	N	Diagnostic Accuracy (%)			
		US	Radial EUS	CT-Scan	MRI
Amouyal et al.,1989[27]	52	49	97	66*	–
Jellouli et al., 1996†[28]	40	–	95	68**	
Materne et al.,2000[29]	50	–	94	–	92
Maluf-Filho et al.,2004[26]	46	–	87	67**	–

*	conventional CT-scan
**	helical CT-scan
†	published as an abstract

TABLE 2 SENSITIVITY (S) AND NEGATIVE PREDICTIVE VALUE (NPV) OF EUS-FNA IN THE DIAGNOSIS OF PANCREATIC CANCER, INCLUDING PERIAMPULLARY NEOPLASMS

AUTHOR	N	S (%)	NPV (%)
Giovannini et al, 1995[30]	43	75	–
Cahn et al, 1996[31]	24	88	86
Buthani et al, 1997[32]	47	64	16
Chang et al, 1997[33]	44	83	96
Faigel et al, 1997[34]	45	94	82
Gress et al, 1997[35]	121	80	91
Wiersema et al, 1997[36]	124	86	86
Binmoeller et al, 1998[37]	45	70	37
Hunerbein et al, 1998[38]	26	88	–
Williams et al, 1999[39]	144	72	38
Voss et al, 2000[40]	90	75	26
Gress et al., 2001[41]	102	93	91
Ylagan et al., 2002[42]	80	78	78
Fritscher-Ravens et al., 2002[43]	200	85	83
Tada et al., 2002[44]	34	62	67
Harewood & Wiersema, 2002[45]	185	94	63
Eloubeidi et al., 2003[46]	158	84	63
Pellise et al., 2003[47]	57	97	95
Raut et al., 2003[48]	233	91	44
Agarwal et al., 2004[49]	81	89	46
Maluf-Filho et al., 2005[50]	74	82	48
TOTAL	**1941**	**83**	**62**

etiology of the obstruction or when a tissue diagnosis will have impact on clinical management.

THE EUS-GUIDED DRAINAGE OF THE BILIARY TREE

Endoscopic retrograde cholangiography is an established method for palliative treatment of patients with malignant biliary strictures. Duodenal stenosis, papillary stenosis or diverticulum, previous gastrectomy are conditions that may preclude successful endoscopic drainage. For those patients, percutaneous transhepatic biliary drainage and surgery are indicated for biliary decompression. However they are usually related to a higher morbidity and mortality when compared to endoscopic treatment. Recently, endoscopic ultrasound (EUS) guided biliary stent placement has been described in patients with malignant biliary obstruction. That technique was first described by Giovannini et al., in 2001. It is a combined ultrasound and fluoroscopy guided procedure. It consists in a EUS-guided puncture of the common bile duct through the duodenal wall or of the dilated left hepatic duct through the gastric wall. A guidewire is introduced through the needle and passed into the biliary tree under fluoroscopic guidance. The enterobiliary tract is

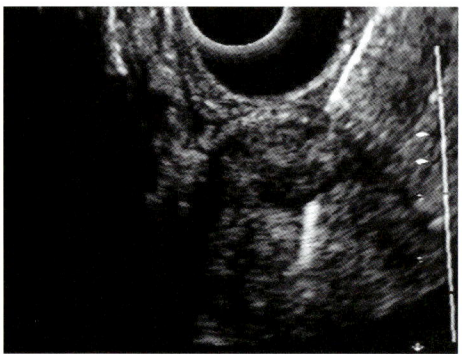

FIGURE 6: Echoendoscopic view of EUS-FNA of a solid mass in the head of the pancreas.

balloon dilated and a stent is inserted. After the left hepatic duct is accessed there are several options to accomplish the biliary drainage: 1- The EUS scope is removed, a duodenoscope is advanced until the duodenum and the guidewire is grasped, allowing a transpapillary insertion of the stent, in a classical rendezvous ERCP procedure; 2- a guidewire is advanced through the stenosis until it reaches the duodenum and a covered metallic stent is placed communicating the left hepatic branch and the stomach; 3 - a guidewire is advanced through the stenosis until it reaches the duodenum and a covered metallic stent is advanced in an antegrade fashion, bridging the biliary stenosis and the duodenal papilla.

At this moment, most of the published articles are case series describing up to six

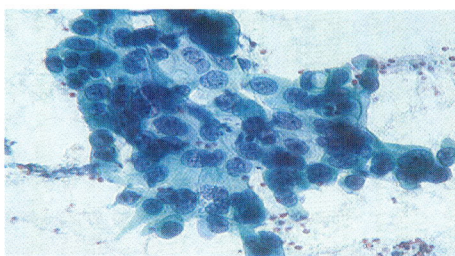

FIGURE 7: Adenocarcinoma of the pancreas (Papanicolau 400x).

patients. They describe a technical success of 80% with no procedure related mortality. Bile leak and bleeding are the most feared complications. Further studies are required to solve pending issues such as the best approach or stent. Randomized trials comparing EUS-interventional cholangiography with percutaneous drainage are needed before the use of these techniques becomes widespread.

REFERENCES

Agarwal B, Abu-Hamda E, Molke KL, Correa AM, Ho L. Endoscopic ultrasound-guided fine needle aspiration and multidetector spiral CT in the diagnosis of pancreatic cancer. Am J Gastroenterol. 2004;99:844-50.

Amouyal P, Palazzo L, Amoyual G, Ponsot P, Mompoint D, Vilgrain V, Gayet B, Flejou JF, Paolaggi JA. Endosonography: promising method for diagnosis of extrahepatic cholestasis. Lancet. 1989;8673:1195-8.

Binmoeller KF, Thul R, Rathod V, Henke P, Brand B, Jabusch HC, Soehendra N. - Endoscopic ultrasound guided, 18-gauge, fine needle aspiration biopsy of the pancreas using a 2,8mm channel convex array echoendoscope. Gastrointestest Endosc. 1998;47:121-7.

Bhutani MS, Hawes RH, Baron PL, Sanders-Cliette A, van Velse A, Osborne JF, Hoffman BJ. Endoscopic ultrasound-guided fine needle aspiration of malignant pancreatic lesions. Endoscopy. 1997;29:854-8.

Bluemke DA, Cameron JL, Hubran RH et al. Potentially resectable pancreatic adenocarcinoma: spiral CT assessment with surgical and pathologic correlation. Radiology 1995;197:381-385.

Burmester E, Niehaus J, Leinewber T, Huetteroth T. EUS-cholangio-drainage of the bile duct: report of 4 cases. Gastrointest Endosc.2003;57: 246-51.

Burtin P, Palazzo L, Canard JM, Person B. Oberti F, Boyer J. Diagnostic strategies for extrahepatic cholestasis of indefinite origin: endoscopic ultrasonography or retrograde cholangiography? Results of a prospective study. Endoscopy 1997;29:349-55.

Cahn M, Chang K, Nguyen P, Bufler J. Impact of endoscopic ultrasound with fine needle aspiration on the surgical management of pancreatic cancer. Am J Surg. 1996; 172:470-2.

Canto MI, Chak A, Stellato T, Sivak MV Jr. Endoscopic ultrasonography versus cholangiography for the diagnosis of choledocholithiasis. Gastrointest Endosc 1998;47:439-48.

Chak A, Hawes RH, Cooper GS, Hoffman B, Catalano MF, Wong RC, et al. Prospective assessment of the utility of EUS in the evaluation of gallstone pancreatitis. Gastrointest Endosc 1999;49: 599-604.

Chang KJ, Nguyen P, Erickson RA Durbin TE, Katz KD. The clinical utility of endoscopic ultrasound-guided fine needle aspiration in the diagnosis and staging of pancreatic carcinoma. Gastrointest Endosc. 1997;45:387-93.

Dancygier H, Nattermann C. The role of endoscopic ultrasonography in biliary tract disease: obstructive jaundice. Endoscopy 1994;26:800-2.

Dufour B, Zins M, Vilgrain V et al. Comparaison de la tomodensitometrie en mode helicoidal et de l'echoendoscopie dans le diagnostic et le bilan des adenocarcinomes du pancreas: etude clinique preliminaire. Gastroenterol Clin Biol 1997;21:124-30.

Eloubeidi MA, Chen VK, Eltoum IA, Jhala D, Chhieng DC, Jhala N, Vickers SM, Wilcox CM. Endoscopic ultrasound-guided fine needle aspiration biopsy of patients with suspected pancreatic cancer: diagnostic accuracy and acute and 30-day complications. Am J Gastroenterol. 2003; 98:2663-8.

Faigel DO, Ginsberg GG, Bentz JS, Gupta PK, Smith DB, Kochman ML. Endoscopic ultrasound-guided real time fine needle aspiration biopsy of the pancreas in patients with pancreatic lesions. J Clin Oncol. 1997;15:1439-43.

Fritscher-Ravens A, brand L, Knofel WT, Bobrowski C, Topalidis, Thonke F, de Werh A, Soehendra N. Comparison of endoscopic ultrasound-guided fine needle aspiration for focal pancreatic lesions in patients with normal parenchyma and chronic pancreatitis. Am J Gastroenterol. 2002; 97:2701-2.

Giovannini M, Moutardier V, Pesenti C, Bories E, Lelong B, Delpero JR. Endoscopic ultrasound-guided bilioduodenal anastomosis: a new technique for biliary drainage. Endoscopy. 2001;33:898-900.

Giovannini M, Seitz JF, Monges G, Perrier H, Rabbia L. Fine needle aspiration cytology guided by endoscopic ultrasound: results in 141 patients. Endoscopy. 1995;27:171-7.

Gress F, Gottlieb K, Sherman S, Lehman G. Endoscopic ultrasonography-guided fine-needle aspiration biopsy of suspected pancreatic cancer. Ann Intern Med. 2001;134:459-64.

Gress FG, Hawes RH, Savides TJ, Ikenberry SO, Cummings O, Kopecky K. Role of EUS in the preoperative staging of pancreatic cancer: a large single-center experience. Gastrointest. Endosc. 1999;50:786-91.

Harewood GC, Wiersema MJ. Endosonography-guided fine needle aspiration biopsy in the evaluation of pancreatic masses. Am J Gastroenterol. 2002;97:1386-91.

Hollerbach S, Willert J, Topalidis T, Reiser M, Schmiegel W. Endoscopic ultrasound-guided fine-needle aspiration biopsy of liver lesions: histological and cytological assessment. Endoscopy. 2003;35:743-9

Hunerbein M, Dohmoto M, Haensch W, Schlag PM. Endosonography-guided biopsy of mediastinal and pancreatic tumors. Endoscopy. 1998;30:32-6.

Imbriaco M, Megibow AJ, Camera L et al. Dual-phase versus single-phase helical CT to detect and assess resectability of pancreatic carcinoma. AJR Am J Roentgenol 2002;178-1473-9.

Jellouli F, Keriven-Souquet O, Henry L, Napoleon B, Pujol B, Valette PJ, Ponchon T, Souqet JC. Endoscopic ultrasound and helical CT scan for biliopancreatic cancer: preliminary study of 40 patients. Endoscopy. 1996; 28:S5.

Kahaleh M, Yoshida C, Kane L, Yeaton P. Interventional EUS cholangiography: a report of five cases. Gastrointest Endosc. 2004;60:138-42.

Kahaleh M, Wang P, Shami VM,Tokar J, Yeaton P. EUS-guided transphepatic cholangiography: report of six cases. Gastrointest Endosc. 2005; 61:307-13.

Legmann P, Vignaux O, Dousset B et al. Pancreatic tumors: comparison of dual-phase helical CT and endoscopic sonography. AJR Am J Roentgenol 1998;170:1315-22.

Maluf-Filho F, Sakai P, Cunha JEM, Garrido T, Rocha M, Machado MCC, Ishioka S. Pancreatology. 2004;4:122-8.

Maluf-Filho F, Kubrusly MS, Cunha JEM, Sakai P, Jukemura J, Montagnini A, Machado MCC, Ishioka S. Gastrointest Endosc. 2004; 59:AB223.

Materne R, Van Beers E, Gigot JF, Jamart J, Geubel A, Pringot J, Deprez P. Extrahepatic biliary obstructions: magnectic resonance imaging compared with endoscopic ultrasonography. Endoscopy. 2000;32:3-9.

Midwinter MJ, Beveridge CJ, Wilsdson JB et al. Correlation between spiral computed tomography, endoscopic ultrasonography and findings at operation in pancreatic and ampullary tumors. Br J Surg 1999;86:189-1993.

Mukai H, Yasuda K, Nakajima M. Tumors of the papilla and distal common bile duct: diagnosis and staging by endoscopic ultra-sonography. Gastrointest Endosc Clin N Am 1995;5:763-72.

Muller MF, Meynberger C, Berstchinger P et al. Pancreatic tumors: evaluation with endoscopic US, CT and MR imaging. Radiology 1994;190: 745-51.

Ney MS, Maluf-Filho F, Zilberstein B, Sakai P, Gama-Rodrigues JJ, Rosa H. Endoscopic ultrasound (EUS) versus endoscopic retrograde cholangiography for the diagnosis of choledocholithiasis: the influence of the size of the stone and diameter of the common bile duct. Arq Gastroent, 2005.

Nguyen PT, Chang KJ, EUS in the detection of ascites and EUS-guided paracentesis. Gastrointest Endosc. 2001;54:336-9.

Norton SA, Aderson D. Prospective comparison of endoscopic ultrasonography and endoscopic retrograde cholangiopancreatography in the detection of bile duct stones. Br J Surg 1997;84: 1366-9.

Pellise M, Castells A, Gines A, Sole M, Mora J, Castellvi-Bel S, Rodriguez-Morata F, Fernandez-E-sparrach G, LLach J, Bordas JM, Navarro S e Pique JM. Clinical usefulness of K-ras mutational analysis in the diagnosis of pancreatic adenocarcinoma by means of endosonography-guided fine-needle aspiration biopsy. Aliment Pharmacol Ther. 2003;17:1299-1307.

Polkowski M, Palucki J, Regula J, Tilszer A, Butruk E. Helical computed tomographic cholangiography versus endosonography for suspected bile duct stones: a prospective blinded study in non-jaundiced patients. Gut 1999;45:744-9.

Prat F, Amouyal P, Pelletier G, Fritsch J, Choury AD, et al. Prospective controlled study of endoscopic ultrasonography and endoscopic retrograde cholangiography in patients with suspected common-bile duct lithiasis. Lancet 1996;347:75-9.

Puspok A, Lomoschitz F, Dejaco C, Hejna M, Sautner T, Gangl A. Endoscopic ultrasound guided therapy of benign and malignant biliary obstruction: a case series. Am J Gastroenterol. 2005;100:1743-7).

Raut CP, Grau AM, Staerke GA, Kaw M, Tamm EP, Wolff RA, Vauthey JN, Lee JE, Pisters PW, Evans DB. Diagnostic accuracy of endoscopic ultrasound-guided fine needle aspiration in patients with presumed pancreatic cancer. J Gastrointest Surg.2003;7:118-26.

Reisman, Y, Gips, CH, Lavelle, SM, Wilson, JH. Clinical presentation of (subclinical) jaundice the Euricterus project in the Netherlands. United Dutch Hospitals and Euricterus Project Management Group. Hepatogastroenterology 1996; 43:1190.

Rösch T, Lorenz R, Braig C et al. Endoscopic ultrasound in pancreatic tumor diagnosis. Gastrointest Endosc 1991;37:347-52, 1991.

Rösch T, Lorenz R, Braig C et al. Endoscopic ultrasonography in diagnosis and staging of pancreatic and biliary tumors. Endoscopy 1992;24:304-8. Supplement 1.

Schwars M, Pauls S, Sokiranski R et al. Is a preoperative multidiagnostic approach to predict surgical resectability of periampullary tumors still effective? Am J Surg 2001;182:243-9.

Sugiyama M, Atomi Y. Endoscopic ultrasonography for diagnosing choledocholithiasis: a prospective comparative study with ultrasonography and computed tomography. Gastrointest Endosc 1997;45:143-6.

Sugiyama M, Atomi, Y. Acute biliary pancreatitis: the roles of endoscopic ultrasonography and endoscopic retrograde cholangiopancreatography. Surgery 1998;124:14-21.

Sugiyama M, Atomi Y, Hachiya J. Magnetic resonance cholangiography using half-Fourier acquisition for diagnosing choledocholithiasis. Am J Gastroenterol, 93:1886-90,1998.

Tada M, Komatsu Y, Kawabe T, Sasahira N, Isayama H, Toda N, Shiratori Y, Omata M. Quantitative analysis of K-ras gene mutation in pancreatic tissue obtained by endoscopic ultrasonography-guided fine needle aspiration: clinical utility for diagnosis of pancreatic tumor. Am J Gastroenterol. 2002;97:2263-70.

Tio TL, Tytgat GN. Endoscopic ultrasonography in analyzing peri-intestinal lymph node abnormality: preliminary results of studies in vitro and in vivo. Scand J Gastroenterol 1986;21:158-63, Supplement 123.

Tio TL, Tytgat GN, Cikot RJ et al. Ampullopancreatic carcinoma: preoperative TNM classification with endosonography. Radiology 1990;175:455-61, 1990.

Valls C, Andia E, Sanchez A, et al. Dual-phase helical CT of pancreatic adenocarcinoma: assessment of resectability before surgery. AJR Am J Roentgenol 2002;178:821-6.

Voss M, Hammel P, Molas G, Palazzo L, Dancour A, O'Toole D, Terris B, Degott C, Bernardes P, Ruszniewiski P. Value of endoscopic ultrasound guided fine needle aspiration biopsy in the diagnosis of solid pancreatic masses. Gut. 2000; 46:244-9.

Wiersema MJ, Vilmann P, Giovannini M, Chang KJ, Wiersema LM. Endosonography-guided fine-needle aspiration biopsy: diagnostic accuracy and complication assessment. Gastroenterogy. 1997;112:1087-95.

Williams DB, Sahai AV, Aabakken L, Penman ID, Velse A, Webb J, Wilson M, Hoffman BJ, Hawes RH. Endoscopic ultrasound-guided fine needle aspiration biopsy: a large single center experience. Gut 1999;44:720-6.

Yasuda K, Mukai H, Fujimoto S et al. The diagnosis of pancreatic cancer by endoscopic ultrasonography. Gastrointest Endosc 1988;34:1-8.

Ylagan LR, Edmundowicz S, Kasal K, Walsh D, Lu DW. Endoscopic ultrasound guided fine-needle aspiration cytology of pancreatic carcinoma: a 3-year experience and review of the literature. Cancer. 2002;96:362-9.

Diagnostic ERCP

Vezakis Antonios, Polydorou Andreas

INTRODUCTION

Duodenoscopy and endoscopic cannulation of the papilla of Vater with visualization of the biliary tree and pancreatic duct was first described in 1968. Many reports on endoscopic retrograde cholangiopancreatography (ERCP) followed, from all over the world in the early 1970s. Within a few years, ERCP became one of the most reliable methods for diagnosing biliary and pancreatic disorders. Endoscopic sphincterotomy, first described in 1973, allowed further advances in endoscopic treatment of biliary and pancreatic diseases. The development of computed tomographic scans (CT), endoscopic ultrasonography (EUS), percutaneous transhepatic cholangiography (PTC) and magnetic resonance imaging (MRI), has not diminished the importance of ERCP.

INSTRUMENTS

ERCP is a combined endoscopic and radiologic method. A high-performance radiographic instrument and video image intensifier is required for optimal radiologic diagnosis and to avoid complications such as inadvertent overfilling of the pancreatic duct. An x-ray room dedicated to ERCP is most convenient.

A side-viewing endoscope with an elevator at the end of the channel is usually used. Cannulation of the papilla of Vater may be easier with a forward-viewing endoscope in patients who have undergone antrectomy and Billroth II gastrojejunostomy. Videoendoscopy is now considered standard for ERCP. A variety of cannulation catheters and guide wires are available to facilitate cannulation of the papilla.

Water-soluble iodinated contrast materials are usually used. The risk of a systemic allergic reaction from the contrast material is low, because there is very little contrast absorption. Patients with history of allergic reaction to iodinated contrast should be premedicated with corticosteroids and antihistamines.

PATIENT PREPARATION

The procedure and its potential benefits and risks should be explained to the patient and consent obtained. The patient is kept fasted for 6 hours prior to the procedure. If therapeutic ERCP may be required, the coagulation status of the patient should be evaluated. This is particularly important in jaundiced patients. Patients with possible biliary obstruction should receive prophylactic antibiotics. A secure intravenous catheter should be placed in the right arm or hand.

SEDATION AND MONITORING

In most centres the procedure is performed under conscious sedation, using midazolam and pethidine. Propofol can also be used, but an anaesthetist or trained nurse is required. Anticholinergic agents such as hyoskine or glucagon can be used before or during the procedure to inhibit duodenal motility. Patients are medicated for the procedure in the left lateral decubitus or in the prone position before passage of the endoscope. Supplementary oxygen should be routinely administered during the procedure.

Continuous patient assessment by a second trained individual is crucial and allows the endoscopist to concentrate on the examination. Continuous monitoring until the patient has fully recovered is essential. Monitoring should include pulse rate and rhythm (usually by electrocardiography), blood pressure (periodic recordings) and pulse oximetry. Resuscitation equipment should be available.

PROCEDURE

The general measures taken for endoscopy must also be taken for ERCP. It involves the use of a side-viewing duodenoscope and special attention should be paid, since the oesophagus is passed blindly. The risk of perforation of an oesophageal diverticulum using this type of endoscope is increased.

The endoscope should be advanced to the second part of the duodenum. The side-viewing endoscope allows en face visualization of the ampulla of Vater. Attempts at cannulation of the papilla begin after the endoscope is in position. In 85% of cases, the pancreatic duct and common bile duct share a common orifice. The first step is to introduce the cannula into the papillary orifice perpendicular to the duodenal wall and directed slightly to the right. This is the optimal direction for cannulation of the pancreatic duct. Cannulation with a small change in direction of the catheter tip should be reattempted if the duct is not immediately opacified. It is better to cannulate many times with frequent changes of catheter direction than to push hard in the same direction. Forceful movements and pushing may create oedema or submucosal injection of contrast, making subsequent cannulation more difficult.

Cannulation of the bile duct requires placement of the catheter in the orifice at the 11-o'clock position. The catheter is further introduced in a direction parallel to the intraduodenal segment of the bile duct. This position is sometimes obtained only by maximal elevator use and by upward deflection of the endoscope tip after the catheter tip is placed just inside the orifice. Slight changes of catheter direction should be tried if the bile duct is not opacified.

The pancreatic duct should be filled with contrast material under fluoroscopic control until the tail and the first-order side branches are visualized. Further filling (acinarization) should be avoided to reduce the risk of acute pancreatitis. Radiographs should be taken at once, while the endoscope and the catheter are still in place, because the pancreatic duct empties rapidly.

The biliary tree is filled with contrast

material until the intrahepatic bile ducts, cystic duct, and gallbladder are opacified, and appropriate films are then taken. The endoscope can be removed after opacification of the biliary tree, and a complete, detailed radiographic examination of biliary anatomy should be made with the patient in various positions. Delayed films should also be taken to detect small gallstones.

Interpretation of the cholangiogram is not always easy. Injection of air with the contrast material should be avoided because air bubbles can be mistaken for gallstones. Air bubbles can be differentiated from gallstones by changing the position of the patient. Air bubbles tend to move proximally and gallstones distally with the patient in the upright position.

The success rate for ERCP is 80-95% but depends on experience. Anatomical causes of failure include a periampullary diverticulum or an ampullary tumour or stricture. Billroth II gastrectomy poses difficulties which may be overcome by an experienced endoscopist, if necessary using a forward-viewing endoscope.

Tissue Sampling at ERCP

An important advantage of ERCP, compared to other imaging modalities, is the fact that the endoscopist can, in most of the cases, take tissue samples or brushing for histology and cytology.

Intraductal bile aspiration cytology

Aspiration of bile is one of the easiest and oldest methods of obtaining a cytologic specimen from a biliary stricture at ERCP. This technique allows collection of bile directly from the biliary tree, thereby avoiding contamination of the specimen by duodenal contents. Aspiration is usually performed by placing a catheter at the level of the stricture and aspirating 10-50 mls of bile. Although specificity is reported to be 100% the sensitivity of bile cytology ranges from 6-32%.

Despite its simplicity and low cost, bile aspiration cytology adds little or nothing to other methods, which have a higher sensitivity for detection of malignancy. Therefore, bile aspiration is recommended only when other sampling techniques cannot be used.

Fine needle aspiration cytology (FNA)

Needle puncture and aspiration of solid tumours is a widely applied method of tissue sampling. Endoscopic FNA of lesions in the head of the pancreas is performed by using 23 or 26 gauge needles passed through the endoscope and then through the gastric or duodenal wall into the pancreatic lesion. If the mass clearly compresses the duodenal or gastric wall, the area of compression is the target of the needle.

Another technique for sampling biliary strictures at ERCP, by endoscopic FNA has been described. This included sphincterotomy and use of a 7 Fr, prebent catheter with a retractable needle. The catheter is inserted into the bile duct to the distal edge of the stricture under fluoroscopy and then the needle is extended into the tumour. Aspiration is performed by using a 20 ml, dry syringe, while moving the needle back and forth within the tumour.

Cannulation of the bile duct with an endoscopic FNA device usually requires prior sphincterotomy because of the stiffness of the catheter. No complications have been reported for endoscopic FNA except those expected for therapeutic ERCP. The overall sensitivity of endoscopic FNA is low (33%) and it is a difficult technique. Thus, it is primarily a supplemental technique

Brush cytology

Brush cytology remains the simplest and safest technique for obtaining tissue samples from biliary strictures at ERCP. It is usually performed by passing a brush with its catheter sheath through the endoscope into the biliary tree under fluoroscopy without use of guidewire, alongside a guidewire or over a guidewire. The brush is advanced from the catheter to a point proximal to the stricture, withdrawn slightly and moved back and forth across the stricture. The brush is then withdrawn into the catheter and catheter and brush are withdrawn from the endoscope as a unit. Usually the tissue on the brush is smeared on a slide immediately upon removal from the endoscope.

Although specificity approaches 100%, the sensitivity of brush cytology for cancer ranges from 30% to 57%. Dilation of the stricture or repeated brushimg have been shown to enhance cancer detection with no increase in risk or technical difficulty.

Endobiliary forceps biopsy

Biopsy specimens can be obtained from biliary strictures at ERCP by using biliary forceps. The forceps is passed through the endoscope into the bile duct under fluoroscopic guidance, opened, and then closed to grasp tissue from the distal rim of the stricture. Sphincterotomy is required in the majority of the cases because of the size and stiffness of the biopsy forceps.

The sensitivity of forceps biopsy ranges from 43% to 81%. Forceps biopsy appears to be the most sensitive of all tissue sampling techniques for biliary strictures. However, because the technique is time consuming and technically dificcult, it is not commonly used.

Pancreatic brush cytology

The majority of patients with malignant bil-

iary strictures have pancreatic cancer. Therefore, obtaining tissue samples from the pancreatic duct may enhance the cancer detection rate. The sensitivity of pancreatic duct brushing ranges from 58% to 73%. However, it has been suggested that it does not enhance the sensitivity of brushing a biliary stricture, when pancreatic cancer is suspected. Brushing the pancreatic duct may be difficult because of disruption of the duct by the cancer, and pancreatitis associated with brushing varies from 0 to 21.5%. The technical difficulty of obtaining cytologic specimens renders the procedure impractical in about half of patients with pancreatic cancer.

Pancreatic juice cytology

The technique requires cannulation of the pancreatic duct and aspiration of pancreatic juice. The sensitivity ranges from 58% to 65%. However, for collection of adequate volume of juice, difficult manoeuvres are required, which may increase intraductal pressure proximal to the stricture, resulting thereby in a higher rate of pancreatitis.

Pancreatic juice cytology is seldom used, as long as other sampling methods are technically easier and faster, and offer equal or better rates of cancer detection.

Multimodal tissue sampling

Tissue sampling of biliary strictures with two or more techniques in a multimodal procedure is the most effective method for obtaining a tissue diagnosis of cancer at ERCP. However, multimodal sampling is more time consuming and more difficult technically, compared with the use of a single technique.

Ancillary techniques

Several ancillary techniques may improve the cancer detection rates of the tissue sampling methods used at ERCP including flow cytometry, digital image analysis, molecular genetic analysis, immunocytochemical techniques and genotyping of specimens. Their role warrants further investigation.

CHOLEDOCHOSCOPY - PANCREATOSCOPY

Direct endoscopic examination of the biliary tree and pancreas has always been an intriguing challenge for endoscopists. The development of the mother-daughter endoscope enabled the performance of peroral choledochoscopy. It consists from two endoscopes, a large one (mother) and a small one (daughter). The baby endoscope is inserted through the working chanel of the mother endoscope into the bile duct, after sphincterotomy. It permits biopsies, stone extraction, insertion of laser fibers or electrohydraulic probe for lithotripsy. Mother-daughter endoscopy requires two light sources and suction units, and two endoscopists are required to perform the procedure.

INTRADUCTAL ALTRASONOGRAPHY (IDUS)

Ultrasound miniprobes have been developed to offer access to narrow intraluminal spaces and to the pancreatobiliary system (Figure 1). The newer models of these probes offer ultraslim diameters, the capability of being inserted over a guidewire, and better acoustic coupling with provision for balloons as a method for maintaining such coupling. The probes used for IDUS can provide high resolution imaging due to the high scanning frequencies used (12-30 MHz). In addition, the small size of the probes used (5-10 Fr) makes it easy to pass them through the

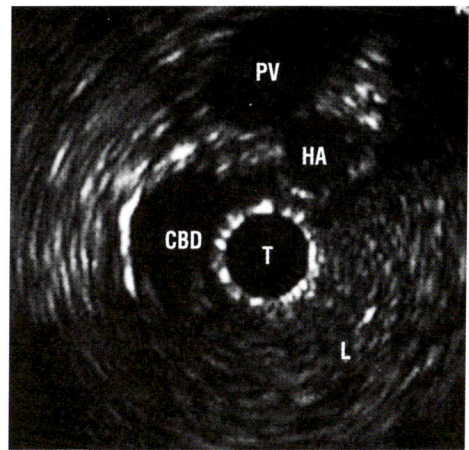

FIGURE 1: IDUS, cholangiocarcinoma obstructing middle common bile duct.

working channel of the endoscope. The probes can be advanced into the bile duct or the main pancreatic duct under fluoroscopic guidance by free cannulation or over a guidewire.

The use of IDUS has a significant impact on management of patients with pancreatobiliary diseases. ERCP supplemented by IDUS gives more reliable and precise information about differentiation of malignant and benign biliary strictures. IDUS has been reported as a reliable method which can be used for a more detailed evaluation of pancreatic tumours, especially intraductal papillary mucinous tumours (IPMT). It permits the differential diagnosis between benign and malignant IPMT and predicts tumour extent. However, IDUS has limited utility in the detection of lesions more than a few millimetres away from the pancreatic duct.

ERCP AND OBSTRUCTIVE JAUNDICE

History, clinical evaluation and blood tests allow the jaundiced patient to be categorised into hepatocellular or extrahepatic biliary obstruction. However, clinical and biochemical evaluation is not infallible. A small proportion of patients with extrahepatic obstruction are incorrectly diagnosed as having intrahepatic cholestasis, whereas a larger proportion of patients with intrahepatic disease are thought to have extrahepatic obstruction. Ultrasound allows the distinction between cholestasis with dilated bile ducts and cholestasis without duct dilatation. If ultrasound shows dilated ducts cholangiography is necessary.

Non invasive imaging of the bile duct using magnetic resonance cholangiopancreatography (MRCP) has a diagnostic accuracy similar to direct cholangiography (ERCP, PTC). MRCP is chosen when the evidence for bile duct disease is equivocal. If direct cholangiography is required then ERCP is the first choice unless access to the papilla is impossible because of duodenal stenosis or previous hepaticojejunostomy. ERCP produces outstanding visualization of the biliary tree in over 95% of patients. Several causes for biliary obstruction and jaundice can be found at ERCP (Table 1).

TABLE 1
CAUSES OF OBSTRUCTIVE JAUNDICE

Stone disease

Inflammatory diseases
    Chronic pancreatitis
    Sclerosing cholangitis

Neoplastic diseases
    Pancreatic tumours
    Cholangiocarcinoma
    Ampullary cancer
    Metastatic disease

Bile duct injuries

Choledochal cysts

STONE DISEASE

Common bile duct stones frequently complicate symptomatic gallstone disease, occurring in up to 15% of patients undergoing cholecystectomy.

ERCP demonstrates common bile duct stones as filling defects after injection of contrast (Figure 2) Although the detection of large or medium size stones is straightforward, problems can arise with the visualization of small stones. They can disappear with overinjection of contrast, or air bubbles can be mistaken for stones. In opacifying the common bile duct, the injection should be made under fluoroscopic control to obtain exposures throughout the injection to provide both early filling and later phases. This facilitates detection of small stones and other

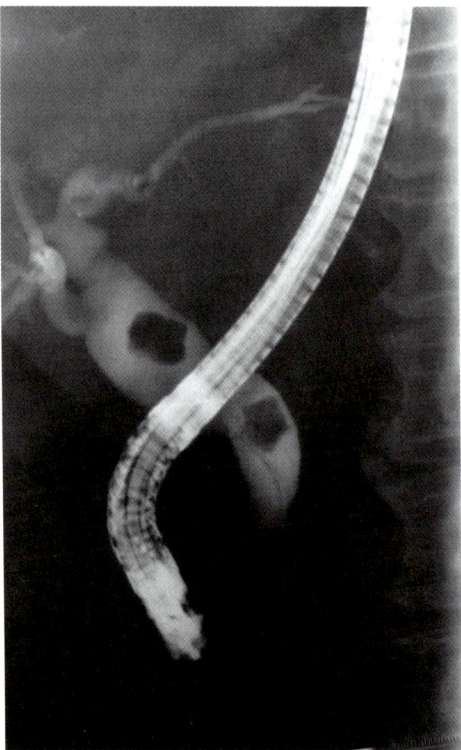

FIGURE 2: A dilated common bile duct with two stones, presenting as filling defects.

more subtle abnormalities. Air bubbles can be differentiated from gallstones by changing the position of the patient.

INFLAMMATORY DISEASES

Primary sclerosing cholangitis

The typical cholangiographic features of primary sclerosing cholangitis include areas of irregular stricturing and dilatation of the intra- and extrahepatic biliary tree. The strictures are short and angular with intervening segments of normal or slightly ectatic ducts. Diverticular outpouchings may be seen along the common bile duct (Figure 3). Cholangiograms may show involvement of intrahepatic ducts alone, extrahepatic ducts alone or even one hepatic duct disease. Small duct disease may appear normal.

Chronic pancreatitis

Bile duct stenosis affects about 8% of patients with chronic alcoholic pancreatitis. The resultant cholestasis may be transient during exacerbations of acute pancreatitis due to oedema and swelling of the pancreas. Persistent jaundice follows encasement of the intrahepatic portion of the common bile duct by a firm fibrotic process. Pseudocysts of the head of the pancreas can also cause biliary obstruction. ERCP shows a smooth narrowing of the lower end of the common bile duct, some times adopting a 'rat tail' appearance. The main pancreatic duct may be tortuous, irregular and dilated with the occasional finding of stones or mucous plugs within the ducts. Pancreatic calcification may be present (Figure 4).

NEOPLASTIC DISEASES

Pancreatic tumours

Although a variety of pancreatic tumours

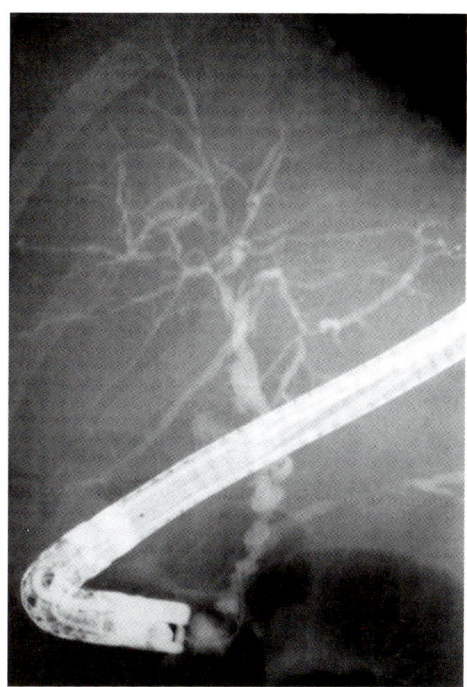

FIGURE 3: Primary sclerosing cholangitis with irregular structuring of the common bile duct and intrahepatic strictures.

exist, the most common is ductal adenocarcinoma, which accounts for well over 90% of all tumours. Pancreatic adenocarcinoma is one of the most aggressive of human malignancies because of its silent course, late clinical manifestation and rapid growth. Eighty per cent occur in the head of the gland.

Pancreatic adenocarcinoma originates from the pancreatic ducts, so a pancreatogram should be abnormal in most of the cases. The most common finding at ERCP is an irregular stricture of the main pancreatic duct with loss of side branches, and proximal dilatation of the duct if contrast can be injected beyond the stricture. Another important finding, which is pathognomonic for carcinoma, is disruption of the duct, due to necrosis and extravasation of contrast especially in an area where side branches are absent. Small

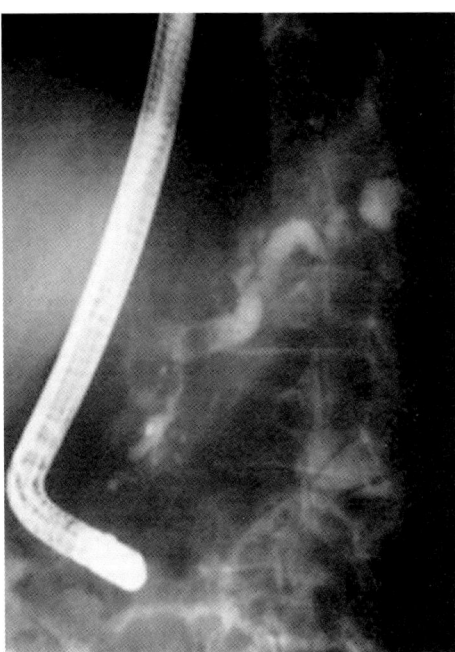

FIGURE 4: A dilated main pancreatic duct with two stones and abnormal secondary branches, findings suggesting chronic pancreatitis.

early cancers and those situated in the uncinate process or tail of the pancreas may be overlooked because of minor ductal changes and a complete pancreatogram with adequate filling of the side branches is mandatory. In a review of 530 examinations in patients with pancreatic cancer, the pancreatogram was normal in only 15 (2.8%).

Tumours of the head of the pancreas usually compress or even invade the distal common bile duct. In these cases the cholangiogram depicts an abrupt stricture of the distal bile duct adjacent to a stricture of the main pancreatic duct, known as the 'double duct sign' (Figure 5).

It can be difficult to distinguish between pancreatic cancer and chronic pancreatitis since the two diseases may share many clinical and radiologic characteristics and the association of chronic pancreatitis and cancer is well known. Careful

evaluation of the pancreatogram will enable the endoscopist to interpret the findings with a high degree of certainty. Dilated secondary branches close to strictures are important findings indicating inflammatory disease, whilst absence of opacification of secondary branches with extravasation of contrast outside the main pancreatic duct suggest malignant disease, if an adequate volume of contrast has been injected to rule out underfilling. It has been also suggested that the presence of a pancreatic duct stricture longer than 10 mm, especially if it is irregular, indicates pancreatic carcinoma instead of chronic pancreatitis, in which the stricture should not exceed 5 mm.

Of course the endoscopist, who is usually a clinician has to consider all the clinical information, scanning data and ERCP findings before rendering an opinion.

Cystic neoplasms account for less than 10% of all pancreatic tumours. They are increasingly being discovered because of the wide use of transabdominal ultrasonography, computed tomography and magnetic resonance imaging for the detection of a variety of conditions. ERCP plays a role in the detection of a communication between the duct and the cystic lesion, indicates the extent of dilatation of the pancreatic duct and the presence and size of mural nodules.

Intraductal papillary mucinous tumours originate from the pancreatic ducts and ERCP was considered the standard for their evaluation and diagnosis. ERCP reveals extreme dilatation along the entire length of the main pancreatic duct with the characteristic finding of mucinous filling defects. There is also an associated cystic dilatation of the side branches in the absence of a pancreatic duct stricture to account for the dilatation. On endoscopy the appearance of a mucin extrusion from a widely patent ampulla is pathognomonic of an IPMT. MRCP is comparable with ERCP for revealing ab-

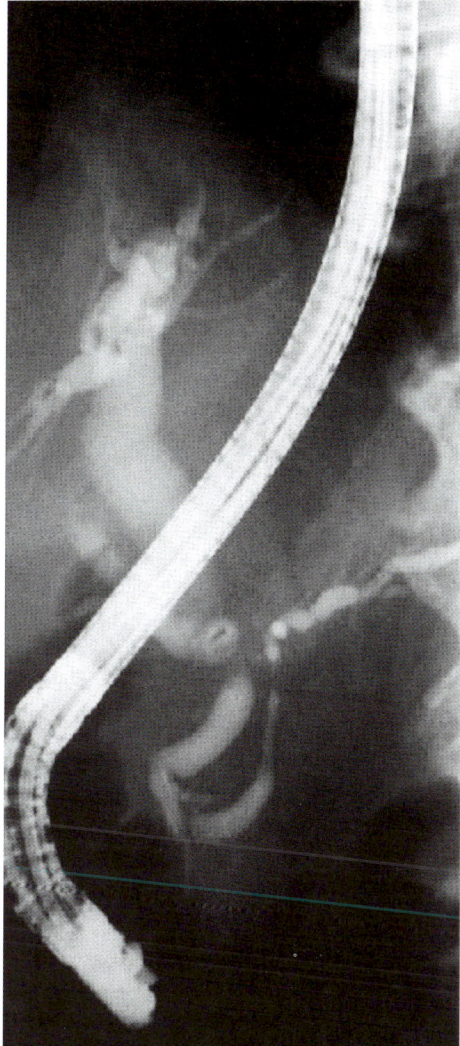

FIGURE 5: A carcinoma of the pancreatic head causing obstruction of the common bile duct and pancreatic duct (double duct sign).

normalities of the main pancreatic duct but is limited with respect to determining the degree of peripheral duct abnormalities. In addition, MRCP is inferior to ERCP for demonstration of a communication between an IPMT and the main duct. MRCP does not afford tissue or cytologic material sampling.

Pancreatic endocrino tumours are mostly located in the pancreatic parenchyma or at the borders of the pancreas within the duodenal wall. ERCP is almost invariably not helpful at all for the diagnosis of these tumours.

Cholangiocarcinoma

Among the extrahepatic bile duct cancers the upper lesions are the most common (50-75%) followed by the middle and distal. Lesions involving the confluence are often called Klatskin tumours. In Klatskin tumours, ERCP shows the normal common bile duct and gallbladder with obstruction at the hilum (Figure 6). Contrast usually passes through the stricture into dilated bile ducts above. The Bismuth classification is used, principally to evaluate resectability of Klatskin tumours:

Type I   Involving the common hepatic duct; confluence is free

Type II   Tumour involving the confluence

Type IIIa   Involving the confluence and the right hepatic duct

b   Involving the confluence and the left hepatic duct

Type IV   Involving the confluence and both right and left hepatic ducts

Middle and lower bile duct tumours are presented as strictures with dilated bile duct above (Figure 7).

With the newer non-invasive imaging modalities the role of ERCP and direct cholangiography for the diagnosis of cholangiocarcinoma has changed. Modern CT techniques and MRI with MR cholangiography allow a high degree of non-invasive evaluation. However, ERCP still has a role. ERCP allows bile sampling, brush cytology and forceps biopsy for histological diagnosis of the tumours. Negative endoscopy or biopsy does not exclude malignancy.

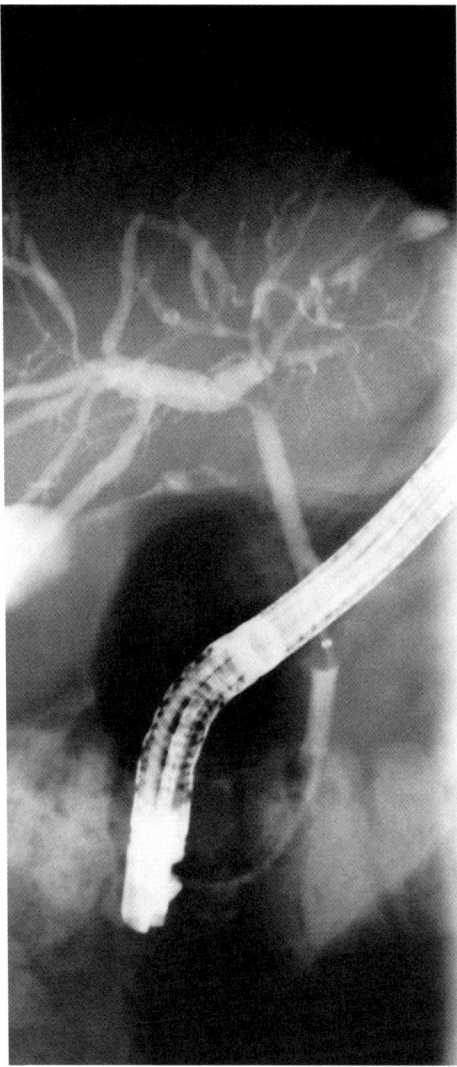

FIGURE 6: Klatskin tumour involving the confluence (type II).

Ampullary tumours

Adenocarcinoma is by far the most common malignant ampullary neoplasm. Carcinoid tumours, neuroendocrine neoplasms and sarcomas may arise from the ampulla, but these are exceedingly rare. More common are benign neoplasms such as villous adenomas.

The major advantage of ERCP over M-RCP and PTC is the direct visualization of the ampulla and surrounding duodenum. The endoscopic appearance of ampullary cancer varies widely. Small intra-ampullary lesions may cause almost imperceptible changes to the ampulla. Intraduodenal lesions may appear polypoid (potentially benign), while infiltrating or ulcerated lesions are clearly malignant (Figure 8). Multiple biopsies should be obtained to establish the diagnosis. Biopsy of the tumor surface or brush cytology may be negative in up to 30% of carcinomas; therefore a negative biopsy does not exclude invasive carcinoma. Although a greater risk of bleeding exists with endoscopic snare biopsy, its use for polypoid or papillary lesions may reduce the incidence of false negative and thus aid in the diagnosis of cancer.

Ampullary carcinoma often produces obstruction to the bile duct and occasional-

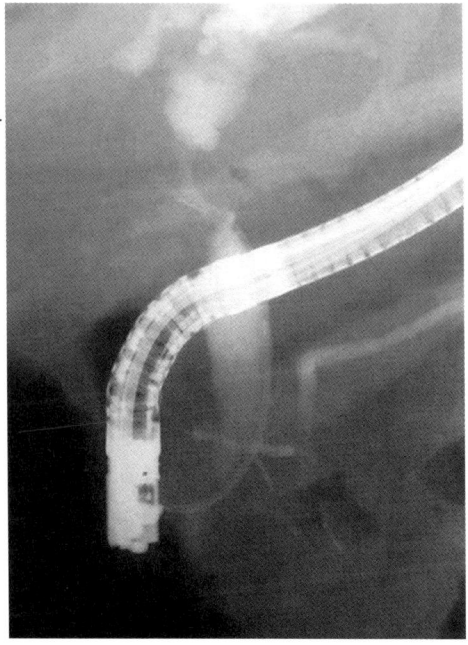

FIGURE 7: A cholangiocarcinoma causing stricture of the middle common bile duct.

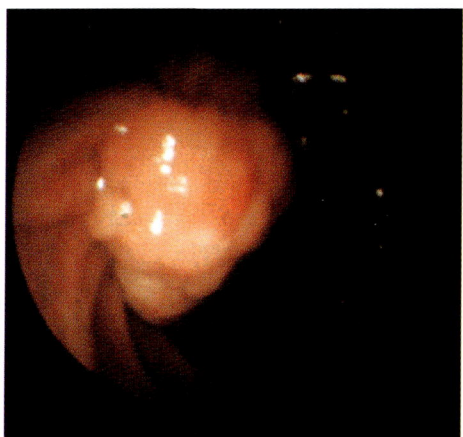

FIGURE 8: Endoscopic appearance of an ampullary carcinoma.

ly the pancreatic duct. Therefore, ERCP demonstrates dilatation of the entire biliary tree emanating from the ampulla with or without an associated dilatation of the entire pancreatic duct. When common bile duct dilatation exists without an obvious ampullary tumour, the judicious use of sphincterotomy with biopsy of the interior of the ampulla can establish the diagnosis. Resampling 7 to 10 days after sphincterotomy, to allow for resolution of cautery artifact and inflammation, improves sensitivity.

Metastatic tumours

Cholestatic jaundice developing following the diagnosis of carcinoma elsewere (colon, breast), in the absence of liver metastases, may be due to bile duct obstruction by nodes at the hepatoduodenal ligament. ERCP usually demonstrates irregularity of the common hepatic or bile duct, with indentations due to lymphadenopathy and a normal pancreatic duct. Differential diagnosis from cholangiocarcinoma, by means of ERCP only, is difficult. History and other imaging modalities (IDUS, US, CT, MRI) will contribute to establish the diagnosis.

BILE DUCT INJURIES

Biliary strictures develop in 0.2% to 0.5% of patients after cholecystectomy. Results of audits, national syrveys and the large number of patients with iatrogenic biliary injuries referred to tertiary centres, suggest that laparoscopic cholecystectomy is associated with more risk of bile duct injury than open cholecystectomy. Biliary strictures can also complicate liver transplantation.

The postoperative biliary stricture is often the result of partial or complete transection by clipping or ligation of the bile duct. Occasionally the stricture is caused by ischaemia resulting from dissection or a thermal injury. Biliary injury may be recognised during surgery or the postoperative period. Symptoms include jaundice, cholangitis, abdominal discomfort and biliary fistula. The presentation may also be delayed with cholestasis and recurrent cholangitis.

The gold standard for diagnosing a bile duct stricture is cholangiography. Either PTC or ERC can confirm the site of the injury or stricture. ERC is most often the initial route of cholangiography for early bile duct injuries, in that the biliary tree may often not be dilated, making PTC technically more difficult. ERC may often demonstrate a normal sized distal bile duct up to the site of the stricture without visualization of the proximal biliary system. This is frequently the case in patients with injury sustained during laparoscopic cholecystectomy, where the distal bile duct is often clipped and divided (Figure 9). PTC is more useful in that it defines the anatomy of the proximal biliary tree, that is to be used in the surgical reconstruction. The Bismuth classification is used to describe the level of the stricture:

Type 1: low common hepatic (>2 cm from hilum) or common bile duct

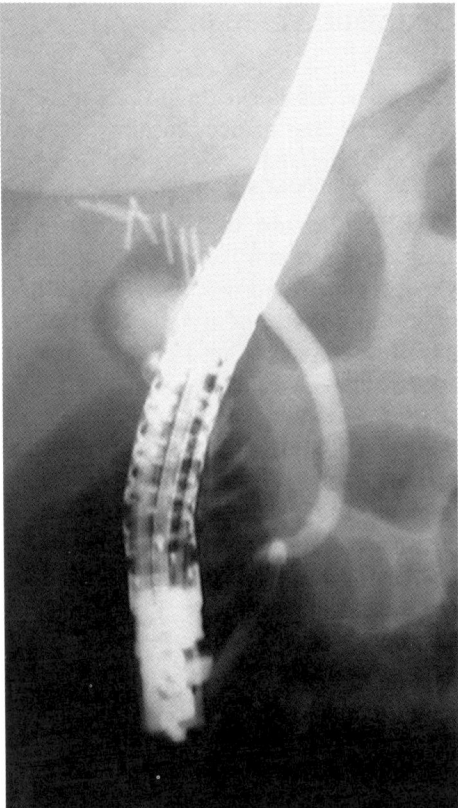

FIGURE 9: Common bile duct injury after laparoscopic cholecystectomy. The common bile duct is clipped not allowing visualization of the proximal biliary system.

Type 2: mid common hepatic duct (<2 cm from hilum)

Type 3: hilar stricture

Type 4: destruction of hilar confluence

Type 5: involvement of the right hepatic duct alone or with the bile duct

Most post-cholecystectomy strictures are type 2 or 3.

MRCP is a non invasive technique and is suggested to have a diagnostic value similar to ERCP and PTC. It can demonstrate the proximal and distal to the injury biliary tree and display the anatomy completely and accurately.

CHOLEDOCHAL CYSTS

Choledochal cysts include a wide spectrum of diseases that involve isolated or combined intrahepatic or extrahepatic cysts. Choledochal cysts may account for jaundice owing to mechanical obstruction by the cyst or stones and by debris or a neoplasm. Choledochal cysts are classified as following:

Type I: cystic (Ia), segmental (Ib) or fusiform (Ic) dilatation of the extrahepatic biliary tree

Type II: saccular diverticulum of the extrahepatic biliary tree.

Type III: cystic dilatation of the distal common bile duct, lying mostly within the duodenal wall (choledochocele).

Type IV: type I anatomy together with intrahepatic bile duct cysts. It has been proposed that IVa, IVb and IVc describe this picture with cystic, segmental or fusiform change of the extrahepatic biliary tree.

Type V: intrahepatic cysts only, also known as Caroli' s disease.

The commonest types are I and IV accounting for more than 80% of cysts (Figure 10).

MRCP is the first choice imaging technique for examining these cysts. It does not however, remove the need for other approaches including ERCP. ERCP provides accurate information on the presence and type of a choledochal cyst. It has the advantage of being able to define the lower anatomy of the duct and the junction of the pancreatic and bile ducts. However, many of the cysts are quite large and the proximal extent of the cyst cannot be evaluated without injecting a large volume of contrast. Overaggresive distention of a choledochal cyst with contrast can be associated with cholangitis. Differentiation between the fusiform type (Ic) and dilatation of the bile duct secondary to obstruction is based on a common bile duct diameter greater than 30 mm and the presence of an anomalous bile duct junction, shown at cholangiography.

The duodenoscopic appearance of a choledochocele is variable, but characteristically includes a smooth, soft, compressible periampullary protrusion into the lumen with an eccentric papillary orifice. Injection of contrast reveals a bulging distal common bile duct and further protrusion of the intraluminal component into the duodenum. It is important to differentiate from inflammatory and neoplastic disorders of the papilla and duodenal duplication cysts. Biopsy and brushing of the papilla help identify the former, whereas the latter characteristically fail to opacify when contrast is injected into the biliary tree.

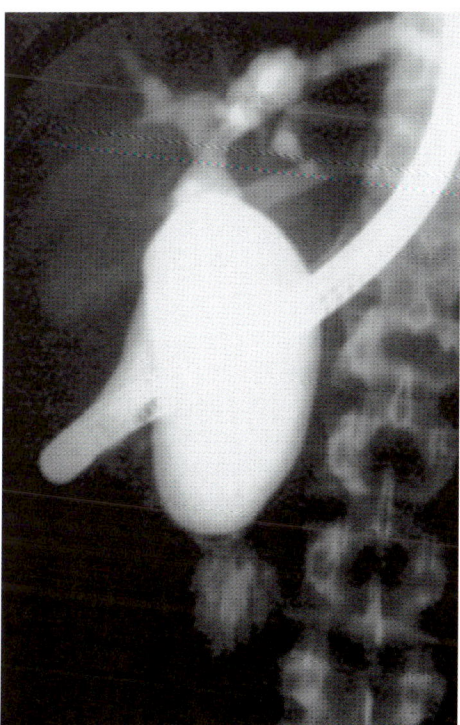

FIGURE 10. Fusiform dilatation of the extrahepatic biliary tree (choledochal cyst type Ic).

COMPLICATIONS OF ERCP

The evolution of ERCP has occurred simultaneously with that of other diagnostic and therapeutic modalities, most notably MRCP, laparoscopic cholecystectomy (with or without intraoperative cholangiography) and EUS. As such, the appropriate use of ERCP changes constantly. In order for endoscopists to accurately assess the clinical appropriateness of ERCP, it is important to have a thorough understanding of the potential complications of this procedure. Reported complication rates vary widely. To some extent this is the result of study design, with retrospective studies being prone to under-reporting adverse events. In addition, reported rates can vary depending upon the case mix (including the proportion of patients undergoing sphincterotomy or evaluation of suspected sphincter of Oddi dysfunction). Finally complication rates are critically affected by the definitions used for each complication.

ERCP with or without associated therapeutic interventions, can cause a variety of short term complications including pancreatitis, haemorrhage, perforation, cardiopulmonary problems and others. These complications can range from minor with 1 or 2 days extra hospitalization and full recovery, to severe and devastating with permanent disability and death. Complications are listed in Table 2.

Pancreatitis

Pancreatitis is the most common ERCP complication. Although transient elevation of serum pancreatic enzymes is extremely common, such an elevation does not necessarily constitute pancreatitis. The consensus definition for ERCP pancreatitis is as follows: new or worsened abdominal pain and a serum amylase that is 3 or more times the upper limit of normal 24 hours after the procedure that requires at

TABLE 2	
COMPLICATIONS OF ERCP	
Pancreatitis	0.7-5.2%
Haemorrhage	
Perforation	
Cholangitis	
Cholecystitis	
Cardiopulmonary	
Miscellaneous	

least 2 days of hospitalization. Reported rates after diagnostic ERCP vary from 0.74% to 5.2%.

Numerous factors have been found to correlate with the development of pancreatitis. In order to identify these factors a meta-analysis of 15 prospective clinical factors was conducted. With regard to patient related risk factors, sphincter of Oddi dysfunction was associated with a relative risk of 4.09, female sex with 2.23, and previous pancreatitis with a relative risk of 2.46. With regard to endoscopy related risk factors, precut sphincterotomy (relative risk 2.71) and injection of contrast media into the pancreatic duct (relative risk 2.2) led to an increased risk for developing post-ERCP pancreatitis. However, several potential risk factors, such as the difficulty of cannulation, could not be analysed due to the heterogenicity of the studies.

Careful patient selection is probably the most important method for reducing unnecessary pancreatitis, especially with the existence of other imaging modalities for the diagnosis of choledocholithiasis and pancreatobiliary malignancy. Many of the factors identified in the previous meta-analysis can be assessed before the examination and should be accounted for when considering ERCP. In general, alternatives to ERCP should be considered when multiple risk factors are present and the likelihood of therapeutic intervention is

low. For example the risk of pancreatitis in a female with normal bilirubin and suspected sphincter of Oddi dysfunction is 18% compared with 1.1% for a typical low risk patient.

MRCP and EUS both have negligible risk of pancreatitis and similar sensitivity to ERCP for the detection of common bile duct stones. These modalities should be considered reasonable alternatives to ERCP. Intraoperative cholangiography should be considered as an alternative to ERCP in patients undergoing cholecystectomy with low to intermediate likelihood of common bile duct stones. EUS is highly accurate for the diagnosis and staging of pancreaticobiliary malignancies and can identify patients who may proceed directly to surgery without ERCP. ERCP should be reserved for those patients with a reasonable likelihood of requiring therapeutic intervention, either based on clinical criteria or abnormalities identified by other imaging modalities.

The highest rate of complications appears to occur in a group of patients that is less likely to benefit from standard ERCP. The most effective method of reducing post-ERCP pancreatitis is to avoid unnecessary ERCP.

Several methods of pharmacologic prophylaxis of post-ERCP pancreatitis have been proposed. Somatostatin and octreotide reduce pancreatic secretion and therefore may limit pancreatic duct hypertension. The effectiveness of somatostatin has been a matter of controversy. A previous metaanalysis did not show any benefit but a new one is required since the last trials are in favour of the administration of somatostatin. Octreotide, unlike somatostatin, increases basal pressure in the sphincter of Oddi and does not prevent pancreatitis. Interleukin-10 has been postulated to prevent pancreatitis by means of its anti-inflammatory activities. Published studies have conflicting results. Nitrates have been shown to prevent pancreatitis by decreasing sphincter of Oddi pressure, but their use is limited by their hypotensive effect and should be used cautiously, if at all, in patients on antihypertensives or those with vascular disease. Gabexate inhibits proteolytic activity and it has been shown to reduce the rate of post-ERCP pancreatitis. Agents shown not to be effective include corticosteroids, allopurinol, platelet-activating factor inhibitors and use of non-ionic contrast.

Treatment of post-ERCP pancreatitis is like that for any other pancreatitis. Early recognition of impending post-ERCP pancreatitis can be facilitated by checking serum amylase within a few hours after the procedure in patients who are at high risk or have abdominbal pain. If serum amylase is normal, the probability of developing pancreatitis is very low and the patient can be considered for same day discharge if otherwise reasonable. On the other hand if the pancreatic enzymes are significantly elevated, premature same day discharge may be avoided and pre-emptive hospitalization for observation, fasting, and intravenous hydration initiated.

Haemorrhage

Haemorrhage is primarily a complication related to sphincterotomy rather than diagnostic ERCP. The incidence varies widely depending on definitions, detection of delayed bleeding, patient factors and endoscopic technique, and is reported to range from 0.76% to 2%.

Perforation

Reported perforation rates for ERCP are 0.3% to 0.6%. Three distinct types of perforation have been described: intraperitoneal as a result of perforation of the bowel wall by the endoscope, guidewire or other catheter induced perforation, and retroperitonoal because of extension of a sphincterotomy incision beyond the intramural portion of the bile duct. Diagnostic ERCP is associated with the first two types of perforation. Management of perforations depends on the location and severity; bowel wall perforations usually require surgery, whereas contained retroperitoneal leaks at the site of a sphincterotomy can often be managed conservatively.

Cholangitis

The rate of cholangitis is 1% or less. Risk factors for cholangitis after ERCP (with or without sphincterotomy) consist primarily of failed or incomplete biliary drainage and use of combined percutaneous - endoscopic procedures. Routine prophylactic use of antibiotics is not supported by currently available data. Prevention and treatment of cholangitis centers about obtaining adequate biliary drainage. Prophylaxis continues to be recommended for patients with biliary obstruction and prosthetic heart valves, a prior history of endocarditis, systemic pulmonary shunt, or recent (<1 year) synthetic graft placement.

Cholecystitis

Cholecystitis complicates approximately 0.2% to 0.5% of ERCPs. It may be difficult to distinguish from cholangitis on clinical grounds. It appears to be correlated with the presence of stones in the gallbladder and possible filling of the gallbladder with contrast during the examination. There is no way of preventing post-ERCP cholecystitis other than cholecystectomy.

Cardiopulmonary complications

Significant cardiopulmonary complications may arise because of cardiac arrhythmia, hypoventilation or aspiration.

These may be due to underlying disease or problems related to medication used for sedation and analgesia. The incidence of these complications is low (<1%), but they constitute a leading cause of death from ERCP. Such complications might be reduced by careful pre-operative evaluation, intraoperative monitoring and collaboration with anaesthesiologists.

Mortality

The overall mortality rate after diagnostic ERCP is roughly 0.2% whereas it is twice as high after therapeutic ERCP. Death may occur from any of the complications described above.

Training in ERCP

The teaching of ERCP has been an area of lively and controversial debate in recent years. Many issues regarding the number of endoscopists needed to perform ERCP, the adequacy of training, and the numbers of ERCPs performed have been raised. It has been shown that in excess of 200 ERCPs are required for trainees to achieve a minimum goal of 80% success rate at selective biliary cannulation. The minimum volume of cases required in order to maintain proficiency in practice is probably in excess of 100 ERCPs per year. The available data suggest that outcomes will be optimal if fewer endoscopists perform more ERCPs. Adequate training during fellowship is essential for all those intending to perform ERCP and advanced training programs should be available.

Further Reading

Adverse outcomes of ERCP. ML Freeman. Gastrointet Endosc 2002; 56(6) (Suppl): S273-S282.

Bailliere's Clinical gastroenterology. The biliary tract. HA Pitt. Volume 11/Number 4, Dec 1997.

Biliary tree and cholecyst: post surgery imaging. V Valek, Z Kala, P Kysela. Eur J Radiology 2005 (53): 433-440.

Complications of ERCP. American Society For Gastrointestinal Endoscopy. Gastrointest Endosc 2003; 57(6): 633-638.

Cystic neoplasms of the pancreas. WR Brugge, GY Lauwers, D Sahani, C Fernandez-del Castillo, AL Warshaw. NEJM 2004; 351(12): 1218-1226.

Diagnostic endoscopic retrograde cholangiopancreatography. M Hafner, R Schofl. Endoscopy 2005; 37(2):133-138.

Diseases of the liver and biliary system. Sheila Sherlock & James Dooley. Blackwell Publishing 2002.

Endoscopic Retrograde Cholangio-Pancreatography. Technique, diagnosis, and therapy. Jerome H Siegel. Raven Press 1992.

Endosonographic evaluation of intraductal papillary mucinous tumors of the pancreas. A Soweid, C Azar, B Labban. J Pancreas 2004; 5(4): 258-265.

Evidence-based assessment of diagnostic modalities for common bile duct stones. DH Mark, CR Flamm, NAronson. Gastrointest Endosc 2002; 56(6) Suppl: S190-S194.

Guidelines for the diagnosis and treatment of cholangiocarcinoma: consensus document. SA Khan, BR Davidson, R Goldin, SP Pereira, WMC Rosenberg, SD Taylor-Robinson, AV Thillainayagam, HC Thomas, MR Thursz, H Wasan. Gut 2002; 51(Suppl VI): vi1-vi9.

Hepatobiliary and pancreatic disease. The team approach to management. HA Pitt, DL Carr-Locke, JT Ferrucci. Little, Brown and company 1995.

Intraductal ultrasound for the evaluation of patients with biliary strictures and no abdominal mass on computed tomography. Stavropoulos S, Larghi A, Verna E, Battezzati P, Stevens P. Endoscopy. 2005 Aug;37(8):715-21.

Pancreatic carcinoma. AL Warshaw, C Fernandez-del Castillo. NEJM 1992; 326(7): 455-465.

Pancreatic tumors. Achievements and prospective. CG Dervenis, C Bassi. Thieme 2000.

The SAGES manual. Fundamentals of laparoscopy and GI endoscopy. Carol EH Scott-Conner. Springer 1998.

Tissue sampling at ERCP in suspected malignant biliary strictures (Part 1). M de Bellis, S Sherman, EL Fogel, H Cramer, J Chappo, BS, CT (ASCP), L McHenry, JL Watkins, GA Lehman. Gastrointest Endosc 2002; 56(4): 552-561.

Tissue sampling at ERCP in suspected malignant biliary strictures (Part 2). M de Bellis, S Sherman, EL Fogel, H Cramer, J Chappo, BS, CT (ASCP), L McHenry, JL Watkins, GA Lehman. Gastrointest Endosc 2002; 56(5): 720-730.

Percutaneous cholangioplasty: minimally invasive techniques and laparoscopy

Tarun P. Jain, Gurpreet S. Gulati, Manpreet S. Gulati

INTRODUCTION

Nonsurgical intervention in the biliary tract was introduced in the early 1970s when the procedure of percutaneous transhepatic biliary drainage (PTBD) was introduced by Molnar and Stockum. Percutaneous transhepatic cholangiography (PTC) had been performed for several years prior to this, but therapeutic biliary interventions had been outside the radiologists' domain. In the last 30 years, improved diagnostic imaging techniques and interventional hardware, developments in endoscopy and experience gained by clinical trials have revolutionized and clearly defined the role of percutaneous biliary interventions.

The role of PTC has progressively diminished in the face of noninvasive imaging techniques such as ultrasonography (US), magnetic resonance cholangiography (MRC), three-dimensional computed tomographic cholangiography (3D CTC) and the recently available 3D CT cholangiography with minimum intensity projection (3D CTC with minIP). Endoscopic retrograde cholangiography, has further reduced its diagnostic role In the recent years. PTC is now reserved only for problematic cases and as an evaluation immediately prior to percutaneous intervention.

PTBD, which was initially proposed as a routine preoperative measure for those with severe obstructive jaundice, is now more of a palliative procedure in patients with inoperable malignant obstruction. This has been brought about by improved preoperative patient preparation, good antibiotic therapy, improved surgical techniques and easy availability of endoscopic biliary drainage expertise. One of the most important recent advances has been the introduction of self expanding metallic stents for use in malignant obstructions. The use of covered metallic stents, removable metallic stents and the biodegradable stents being developed currently might be good strategies for the management of benign strictures. PTBD also continues to play a very important role in the management of suppurative cholangitis, postoperative obstructions, and in select patients with cholelithiasis. Percutaneous access to the biliary system is also possible via the T-tube tract in the postoperative (cholecystectomy) situation giving the opportunity to perform percutaneous stone extraction from the biliary tract.

In this chapter we would be discussing all of the aforementioned percutaneous interventional radiological techniques, their indications and the other issues involved.

Palliative biliary drainage for malignant strictures

Malignant biliary obstruction is a not uncommonly encountered clinical problem in routine gastrointestinal medical and surgical practice. Carcinoma of the gallbladder, which frequently involves the bile ducts at the hepatic hilum, carcinoma of the head of the pancreas and ampulla, cholangiocarcinoma, metastatic hilar and peripancreatic adenopathy and carcinoma of duodenum are the most important causes of malignant biliary obstruction.

Biliary obstruction is potentially fatal because of the adverse pathological effects including depressed immunity, impaired phagocytic activity, reduced kupffer cell function and paucity of bile salts reaching the gut, with consequent endotoxemia, septicaemia and renal failure. There is, therefore, a need to decompress the biliary system. The majority of malignant hepatic tumours such as carcinoma of the gallbladder, carcinoma of the pancreas and cholangiocarcinoma are unresectable and only 20%-30% of these tumours are resectable at the time of diagnosis. Palliation of the malignant obstruction relieves the patient of itching and jaundice, reduces the risk of infection and septicaemia and generally improves the quality of life. Surgical, endoscopic and percutaneous interventional radiologic techniques are available for palliation. Non-surgical techniques are preferred because they are associated with lower morbidity and mortality.

Endoscopic stenting, in general, is preferred over the percutaneous techniques because of a higher success rate, shorter hospital stay, lower complication rate and a lower 30-day mortality and also the fact that this is a tool that provides direct access to the treating gastroenterologist. The percutaneous approach is required only in situations in which endoscopic drainage has failed, or is not possible, such as a previous Billroth-II surgery, duodenal obstruction by a tumour, high hilar obstruction not negotiable by transpapillary route, periampullary diverticulum and a large, papillary, fungating growth making cannulation difficult. Hilar malignant strictures are particularly difficult to traverse via the endoscopic approach. Since carcinoma of the gallbladder commonly invades the hilar structures and is the commonest cause of malignant biliary obstruction, percutaneous drainage is a very important palliative option that has not been fully utilized. In clinical practice, a cohesive team consisting of a gastroenterologist, a surgeon and a radiologist should participate in a multidisciplinary approach to the management of the patient before treatment is initiated.

Role of imaging before palliative biliary drainage

Management of malignant biliary obstruction depends on the resectability of the underlying tumour, therefore, patients should undergo accurate staging following the diagnosis. One of the important goals of preoperative imaging is to identify vascular invasion by the tumour at the hepatic hilum. Hitherto, angiography was used to identify the vascular anatomy prior to surgery in carcinoma gall bladder and hilar cholangiocarcinoma. Recently dual phase helical CT has been used to evaluate vascular invasion in hilar tumours. As a single modality, it can not only detect the malignancy, but also has the potential of comprehensively evaluating each patient for criteria of unresectability. In a study by Kumaran et al vascular invasion was diagnosed whenever the mass was in close contact with the artery/vein and there was loss of the intervening fat plane. The presence of irregularity of the luminal outline, narrowing of the calibre of the blood vessel in serial images and the presence of a tumour on both sides of the vessel were considered definite evidences of invasion.

High quality three dimensional (3D) reconstruction images made possible by helical CT are uniquely suited for the depiction of the complex anatomy of the biliary tract. Van Beers et al evaluated 3D CTC which was done by 3D-reconstructions following slow intravenous infusion of the cholangiographic agent iodipamide. Kwon and colleagues utilized combined oral and intravenous cholangiographic agents prior to helical CT. Zeman et al devised a protocol extending the application of 3D CT to preoperative planning for patients with obstructing pancreatic or biliary neoplasms in whom oral and intravenous cholangiographic agents have limited efficacy due to impaired biliary excretion. 3D reconstructions can be produced successfully by taking advantage of the negative contrast effect of low-attenuation bile in the dilated ducts relative to the adjacent enhanced liver. 3D CTC with minimum intensity projection can determine the level and cause of biliary obstruction. It can be obtained from regular thin section helical CT data and may be a strong competitor against MRCP because of the additional information on adjacent soft tissues, such as contiguous organ involvement, regional metastasis, vascular invasion and the ductal involvement itself. In a study by Park et al, the diagnostic potential of 3D CTC with minimum intensity projection (3D CTC minIP) was considered in 9 patients with percutaneous transhepatic cholangiography as the gold standard. 3D CTC minIP demonstrated dilated intrahepatic ducts up to tertiary branches and correctly diagnosed the lev-

el of biliary obstruction in all patients. We have been using this modality for the last two years in all hilar malignant lesions. Not only is the resectability of the tumour better defined, but also, the identification of variant ductal anatomy is possible. Additionally, it helps in choosing the appropriate duct for drainage.

MRI performs as well as CT for direct spread of the tumour to the liver and hepatic metastases. Visualization of intra hepatic bile ducts on MRI depends on the size of the ducts, concentration of bile, pulse sequence used, motion artifact and periportal high signal. CT and US are more sensitive than MRI for detecting intra hepatic bile duct dilatation. Advent of Magnetic Resonance Cholangio Pancreaticography (MRCP) has been a very useful development for imaging of biliary disease. In this technique, solid organs and moving fluid appear as low signal intensity as against stationary fluid (bile), which appears as high intensity. Either gradient echo or fast spin echo (FSE) sequences are obtained and 3D maximum intensity projection is used to reconstruct the projectional images. Otherwise, direct thick slab T2 weighted images in various coronal planes can be used to achieve images similar to PTC. MRCP can thus combine the advantages of projectional and sectional imaging methods. Half fourier turbo spin echo or HASTE sequence is currently favored and some newer sequences such as SMASH and SENSE are also on the horizon. MRCP has the advantages of being non invasive & free of complications. MRCP is highly accurate for defining extent of ductal involvement in patients with malignant hilar and perihilar obstruction. Ductal dilatation, strictures and anatomical variation are well depicted by this technique and this ability makes this modality well suited for planning the optimal therapeutic approach for patients with biliary obstruction.

Invasive percutaneous cholangiography (PTC) is thus only indicated when:
- Above mentioned imaging modalities are not available
- As a first step in the therapeutic percutaneous biliary intervention.

Percutaneous intervention in malignant billiary obstruction

All patients with potentially resectable tumours should undergo surgery. Biliary drainage is required in the preoperative stage in patients with high bilirubin levels or cholangitis and a potentially resectable tumour. In patients with unresectable tumour, palliative drainage can be offered as the only definitive treatment.

Preoperative percutaneous transhepatic biliary drainage

Although the practice of PTBD prior to surgery is controversial, it is advocated by many surgeons before curative resection, to correct metabolic derangements produced by biliary obstruction and decrease the complications of biliary surgery in the jaundiced patient. Either internal/external biliary drainage catheters or more preferably plastic stents are inserted 2-6 weeks prior to elective surgery. Many surgeons advise preoperative P-TBD because the biliary catheters are easy to locate at surgery particularly during difficult dissections of lesions at the hepatic hilum.

Palliation of malignant biliary obstruction using PTBD

PTBD is now standard management for patients with incurable malignant biliary obstruction, particularly in certain specific situations.
The indications for PTBD are:
- To treat cholangitis secondary to obstruction.
- To treat symptomatic obstructive jaundice when an endoscopic retrograde approach fails or is not possible (as discussed earlier).
- To gain access to the biliary system to perform transhepatic brachytherapy for cholangiocarcinoma.
- Preoperative decompression and stent placement to assist in surgical manipulation (controversial).

Relative Contraindications for PTBD are:
- Incorrectable bleeding diathesis
- Large volume of ascites (relative; procedure may be difficult with potential for bile peritonitis. Consider a left-sided approach)
- Segmental isolated intrahepatic obstructions that do not cause significant symptoms should not be drained. Bacterial contamination usually occurs when an isolated ductal system is accessed. As a consequence of this contamination, it is often impossible to withdraw drainage even if the drainage is not required clinically. Thus a patient could be left with a permanent, unwanted, and potentially problematic drainage catheter.
- Totally uncooperative patient (may require general anaesthesia or heavy conscious sedation).

Preparation for PTBD involves:

Blood tests:
Coagulation profile: The International normalized ratio (INR) should be less than 1.5. Vitamin K, fresh frozen plasma, and platelets (as needed) should be administered to correct any coagulopathy.
Liver function tests: Serum bilirubin and alkaline phosphatase levels should be checked. (an elevated alkaline phosphatase level, even in the setting of a near-normal bilirubin indicates a low grade obstruction).
Baseline renal function: Blood urea and creatinine should be checked, espe-

cially before administering preprocedure nephrotoxic antibiotics.

Informed consent:

The procedure should be explained completely to the patient, outlining the risks with specific attention to sepsis and bleeding.

Prophylactic antibiotics

Appropriate antibiotics are administered 1-2 hours before the procedure to avoid biliary sepsis. The spectrum of antibiotic coverage must include both Gram positive and Gram negative organisms. In our set-up, a combination of third generation cephalosporins, amikacin and metronidazole is administered in appropriate dosages. The antibiotics should be continued for 24-72 hrs following the procedure. A regular appraisal should be done to identify the prevalent infectious organisms and their drug resistance pattern in the local setting.

Sedation/Analgesia:

The patient should be placed on a clear liquid diet several hours prior to the procedure (for conscious sedation) with a well functioning intravenous line and adequate hydration. Preprocedural sedation is helpful but not mandatory. It is performed under conscious sedation (midazolam and Fentanyl) with liberal infiltration of local anesthetic at the site of puncture and upto the capsule of the liver.

Skin preparation:

It is best to prepare a wide area, which will permit access to the biliary system from the left and right sides, as needed.

Procedure

Technical approach: entry from right or left side

We use the Bismuth Corlette classification to initially categorize the biliary obstruction. According to this classification system - a type 1 obstruction occurs distal to the confluence of the right and left hepatic ducts (primary confluence); type 2 involves the primary confluence but not the secondary confluence; type 3 involves the primary confluence and, additionally, either right (3a) or left (3b) secondary confluence, and type 4 involves the secondary confluence of both the right and left hepatic ducts. Whether to use a right- or left-sided approach must be decided on a case-by-case basis. Extensive right-side disease with sparing of the left side makes the decision easy (left-approach), as does a patient with an atrophic left lobe (right approach).

It is worth mentioning some broad guidelines that we use in our own setup. In the case of a type 1 lesion, there are two advantages in approaching from the right side (especially right anterior): the angle of approach to the point of obstruction is 90° or greater, making for easy catheter insertion; and the radiologist's hands are well away from the primary X-ray beam. The advantage of using the left sided approach is that US can be utilized for the initial puncture, avoids the accidental breach of pleural space and, also, the patient has less catheter related discomfort (the right intercostal approach being more painful). This approach is also preferable when there is ascites.

When the obstruction is at the confluence, the situation is more complex. It is important to be aware of the anatomy of the right and left hepatic ducts. The right hepatic duct is short, unlike the left which is 2-3 cm long until its bifurcation into the segmental ducts. Thus a catheter placed in the right system initially drains a greater part of the liver because of the size difference between the lobes. However, once the tumour grows, the situation reverses. The catheter placed in the right side now drains only one segment, whereas the left sided catheter drains all of the left lobe. Thus, for type 2 lesions either right anterior system or the left system is chosen (left is chosen if the left lobe of the liver is of good size). For type 3a lesions, if there is extensive involvement of the right secondary confluence, we do either a single left sided drainage or ideally combine it with right anterior or posterior drainage (keeping in mind the cost of the procedure, life expectancy and the subjective assessment of the amount of liver to be drained as seen on CT). It has been shown that drainage of 25% of the liver volume using a single catheter/endoprosthesis may be sufficient. For type 3b lesions the approach is similar. For type 4 lesions one should use at least two drains. Lobes and segments that are atrophic are excluded from the proposed drainage plan. A duct suspected to be already infected or contaminated due to the procedure is always drained. Another approach in type 4 lesions is to perform Chi-configuration stenting, which allows drainage of the entire major segmental ducts. One stent extends from the left duct through the hilar stricture to right anterior duct; the other stent is placed across the right posterior segmental duct through the hilar stricture into the common bile duct or transpapillary duodenum. Stent deployment should be performed simultaneously. Ultimately the two stents form a chi-shaped configuration.

Technique

After opacification of the ducts by PTC, the study is reviewed to select the best bile duct to puncture. The duct should be punctured at a peripheral location to gain a sufficient length of duct above the obstructing lesion, to avoid injury to the large portal venous and arterial structures present at the hilum of liver, and to reduce the length of the transhepatic tract. The left ducts are catheterized via an anterior subxiphoid approach. US guidance can often be helpful for dilated left ducts. For the right lateral approach, the point of skin entry should be intercostal and lower than the costophrenic angle. The entry point should be chosen to allow the shortest path to the target duct. A well chosen path will facilitate

subsequent maneouvers by minimizing any sharp angles along its course.

In some cases, the duct punctured at the time of original diagnostic PTC provides a suitable site for cannulation. In that case, a conversion system (see below) can be used. However, it is important to resist the temptation to convert a suboptimal PTC entry site. One should keep switching between anteroposterior and lateral views to see the progress of the needle toward the target duct. Intermediate oblique views are also of great help. A variety of needle systems can be successfully used to gain access to the bile ducts. These systems are of two main types: (i) those using a fine 21- or 22- gauge needle for the initial puncture followed by insertion of a 0.018" wire (Seldinger technique) and subsequent conversion using a Neff, Cope or similar set, and (ii) those in which the puncture is performed using an 18-19 gauge needle covered by a flexible 4.8 F sheath. Once the needle is removed, the sheath will accept an 0.038 inch guidewire and the sheath can then be advanced over the guidewire into the bile duct. Once the duct is catheterized, the next step is to cross the lesion/obstruction and gain access to the duodenum (Figure 1). This often requires the use of an angiographic or a biliary manipulation catheter, and a hydrophilic guidewire (such as Terumo). In the case of difficult to traverse obstruction, finer guidewires and microcatheters can be used. Additionally, it may be necessary to establish peripheral drainage for a short time and then bring the patient back for a subsequent, or very rarely, a third attempt. With the obstruction crossed, the angiographic catheter should be advanced over the hydrophilic guidewire into the bowel. The guidewire is then removed and a stiff wire such as Amplatz super stiff, Ultrastiff or Lunderquist is used. With the stiff wire in place, the transhepatic tract can be dilated using serial dilators to accommodate the large-bore drainage catheter. A variety

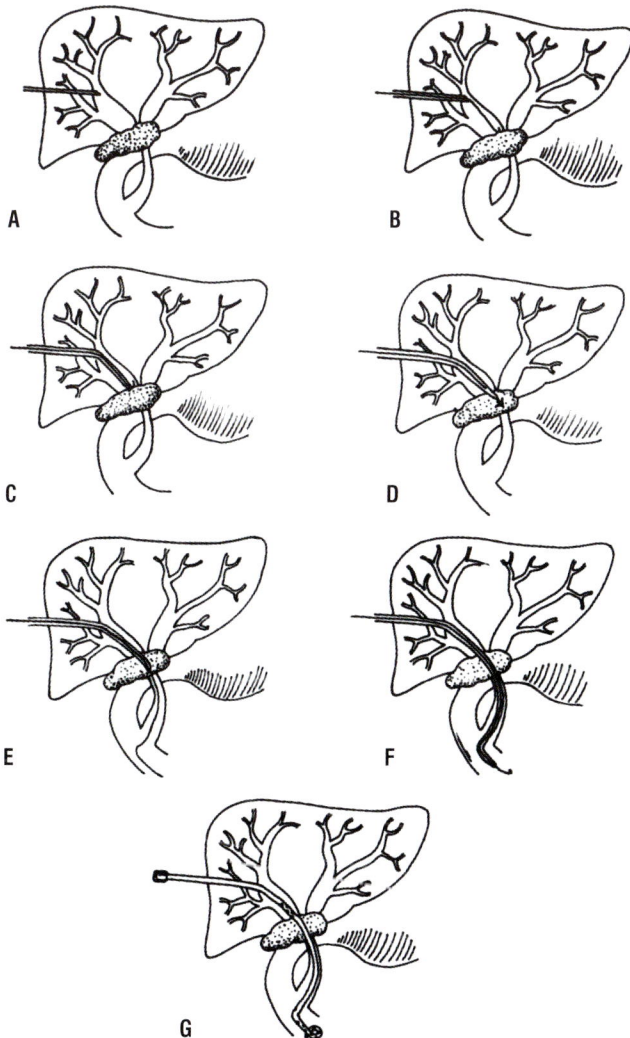

FIGURE 1: The technique of placing a Ring Biliary Catheter. **(A).** A needle is placed under ultrasound or fluoroscopy control (following PTC). The duct to be punctured is carefully chosen as outlined in the text. Bile is aspirated and some contrast is injected to confirm correct positioning. **(B).** An extra-stiff guidewire is passed through the needle into the system. While keeping the guidewire steady, the needle is withdrawn over the guidewire and is replaced by a 4-5 F angiographic or biliary manipulation catheter. **(C).** The stiff guidewire is replaced by a hydrophilic guidewire and the catheter guidewire assembly is brought close to the tumour. **(D).** The guidewire is slightly withdrawn so that it comes to lie within the catheter, and the catheter is "dug" into the tumour. **(E).** The guidewire is again pushed and this will usually cross the obstruction into the distal duct and the duodenum. Sometimes repetitive forward and backward movement of the guidewire may be required. **(F).** The catheter is moved over the wire into the duodenum. The hydrophilic guidewire is now again exchanged for an extra-stiff guidewire. The transhepatic tract and the obstruction are dilated by serial dilators. **(G).** A ring biliary catheter is finally pushed over the guidewire, with its end lying in the duodenum, facilitating internal and external drainage because of the multiple side holes in its distal part.

of drainage catheters are available with different characteristics suited for specific clinical situations.

Biliary drainage can be established in three ways:

(i) External biliary drainage: The percutaneous catheter is positioned within the biliary tree and is attached to a collection bag outside the body to allow external drainage of bile. As an initial step, this allows the patient to recover from an acute septic state due to cholangitis. Indeed, an attempt to traverse the obstruction should not made in such situations to avoid any extra manipulation as it can lead to cholangio-venous reflux into the blood stream and cause septicaemia/toxaemia which can develop over a very short period of time. External drainage also gives time for clot or debris to clear and the percutaneous tract to mature but is not suitable in the long term because of large fluid and electrolyte losses. The diversion of bile salts from the gut adversely affects the general state of well-being. The patient may be advised to regularly drink the drained out bile. The bile can be mixed with an aerated drink for this purpose or given through a nasogastric tube. Sepsis and pericatheter leakage are other problems. The catheter is also a grim reminder to the patient of his malignancy.

(ii) Internal external drainage: This involves positioning the PTBD catheter across the obstruction and down into the duodenum (Figure 2). There are multiple side holes in the distal part of the catheter shaft (ring biliary drainage catheter available from Cook, Bard, etc.). If a standard catheter is not available, one can also punch several side holes into an ordinary drainage catheter over a distance of 10-12 cm in the distal part of the catheter, which can satisfactorily function as a ring biliary drainage catheter. Because of the multiple side holes, which come to lie both above and below the obstruction, the catheter not only drains the bile out into the bag connected externally but, when capped outside, serves to drain the bile internally across the obstruction. Although it is generally preferable to replace this tube with an endoprosthesis or stent within 48-72 hours, the cost and other considerations may dictate that long term drainage be allowed to continue via such a catheter. The advantages of internal external drainage are that fluid loss is eliminated and bile drains into the bowel. Such catheters are easily exchanged over a guidewire on an outpatient basis so that the problem of catheter obstruction can be easily managed. Pain, infection and bile leakage at the skin site may be the problems encountered with this technique.

(iii) Implanted endoprosthesis: This provides all the advantages of internal drainage without the problems associated with the percutaneous catheter exiting from the skin. In most situations the stenting is done in the second sitting (especially for plastic stents), after having placed an external or preferably a ring biliary catheter which has been draining for 24-72 hours. This is to avoid the discomfort of dilatation of up to 10-12 F of the transhepatic tract in one session.

Initially, a careful cholangiogram should be performed to delineate the exact extent of obstruction and to determine where the stent is to be positioned. Malignant obstructions should be overstented, with the stent extending well past the borders of the stricture to maintain patency as the tumour enlarges. After a stiff wire is placed across the stricture, a vascular introducer sheath of an appropriate size (usually 8 or 9 F) is placed. In most situations, it is advantageous to balloon-dilate the stricture (using a balloon 8-10 mm diameter) prior to stent placement, particularly for self-expanding metallic stents, to facilitate rapid expansion of the device. This leads to more efficient bile drainage, minimizing the chances of cholangitis and bile leakage.

There are a number of plastic and me-

FIGURE 2: A ring biliary catheter inserted percutaneously from the right side with proximal part in the right ducts and the distal part in the duodenum. Note the side-holes present in the entire distal length of the catheter (see text).

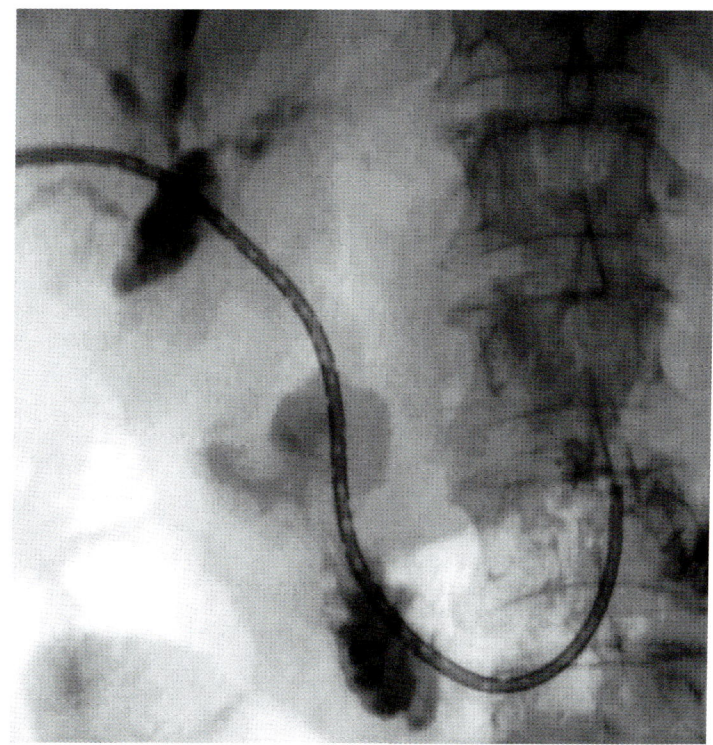

tallic biliary endoprostheses. The more commonly used plastic endoprostheses, which are far cheaper than the metallic ones, include the Carey Coons Percuflex (Meditech), Ring Kerlan, Lunderquist Owman Teflon (Cook), Lammer polyurethane (Cook) stents etc. The Carey Coons stent is a 19 cm long, 12 F or 14 F tube with multiple side holes and a gradual 90° bend in its most distal part. A 3-0-nylon suture is attached to the proximal shaft, extending to a silastic button, which acts as a subcutaneous anchor preventing distal migration of the stent. The Ring Kerlan stent is 12 F in diameter. It is made from Percuflex, with its length varying from 8 cm to 10 cm and is perforated throughout its shaft. A Mallecot mushroom tip is present at the trailing end for stabilization. A loop suture for repositioning is present proximal to the Mallecot. The Lunderquist Owman Teflon catheter is available in various sizes from 8 F to 12 F and is tapered at both ends. We normally place a loop of suture around the proximal side hole emerging from the proximal end hole while pushing the stent, so that the stent can be pulled back in case it gets pushed further inside than necessary. We have occasionally had to use a vascular snare to reposition a distally migrated stent at the time of deployment. These and other routinely used and easily available endoscopic stents (even those with flaps) can be easily pushed through a large 10 F-12 F sheath (after placing it across the obstruction) using any appropriate blunt head catheter which can serve as a pusher. Once the stent is accurately in place, the suture can be removed, followed by withdrawal of the sheath over the stent till it is just proximal to the stent. The guidewire is then withdrawn from within the stent, finally releasing it. During all 3 steps, the pusher is kept steady with its head firm a-gainst the proximal end of the stent. The pusher is then removed over the guide-wire. An external drainage catheter can be left inside with its tip just proximal to the stent, which can be used for flushing of the system for 24-48 hours, when it can be removed after a check cholangiogram.

Metallic stents of various types are used with the intent of achieving a higher patency rate and better bile flow. These are positioned in a compressed state (7 F-12 F) but expand to achieve a diameter of 8-12 mm. This yields the advantage of placing a large diameter stent with minimal trauma. The newer stents with a 7 F deliv-ery system can be positioned in a single sitting because the tract has to be dilated only up to 8 F and hence avoids the mor-bidity of multiple procedures. Metallic sten-ts include the balloon-expandable stents (Palmaz, Johnson & Johnson and Tan-talum Strecker, Boston Scientific Corp.). These stents are positioned over a balloon angioplasty catheter and are deployed by inflating the balloon. These are not pre-ferred because of their poor radial force and inflexibility. Self-expanding stents with very good radial force, such as the Gi-anturco Rosch Z stents (Cook), Wallstents (Cook), Nitinol Strecker (Boston Scientific Corp.), Memotherm (Bard), and Zilver stents (Cook) are available. The Z stent is made of stainless steel wire (0.016-0.018 inch diameter) and has 6 zigzag bends. It is available in a number of lengths (1.5-9 cm) and diameters (6-12 mm) and is de-ployed through a 10 F-12 F introducer/sheath system, with a method of delivery very similar to that used for the plastic stent. The problem with Z stents is that of tumour ingrowth through the relatively wide mesh holes. The most widely used Wallstent endoprosthesis is deployed via a 7 F-8 F delivery catheter, which is very flexible and allows for easy sheath-free passage through hard malignancies. It can vary from a length of 20-94 mm and is

available in pre-determined diameters of 8 mm, 10 mm and 12 mm. Its chief disad-vantage is longitudinal shortening (up to 40%), which has to be taken into account for precise positioning. The newer nitinol stents, such as the Memotherm and Zilver, have virtually no shortening when com-pared to the Wallstent, and these are also relatively more flexible and very kink-re-sistant. For deployment, the delivery sy-stem is introduced over an extra-stiff gui-dewire and the stent is positioned across the obstruction. The stent is then released by retraction of the outer membrane cover-ing it (which makes the stent lie in the con-strained state prior to release) (Figure 3).

Covered stents represent an evolution of bare stents and are aimed mainly to prevent obstruction caused by tumor in-growth within the stent lumen. The first clinical studies of polyurethane-covered Wallstents showed that these stents can be safely implanted. However, the 6-mon-th patency rate was found to be inferior to that of noncovered Wallstents (46.8% vs 67%), partly because of a breach in the covering membrane that allowed tumor in-growth. It was concluded that such a type of covered stent had no significant advan-tages versus bare stents. Now polyte-trafluoroethylene and fluorinated ethylene propylene (ePTFE/FEP)–covered metallic stents have been introduced. The stent consists of an inner ePTFE/FEP lining and an outer supporting structure of nitinol wire. Multiple wire sections elevated from the external surface provide anchoring. Stents are available in two versions, with or without holes in the proximal stent lin-ing. Holes should provide drainage of the cystic duct or biliary side branches when covered by the proximal stent end. They are more effective than polyurethane-cov-ered Wallstents.

It is generally advisable to have the distal end of the stent project through the ampulla into the duodenum. This is be-cause the rigid nature of the stent can

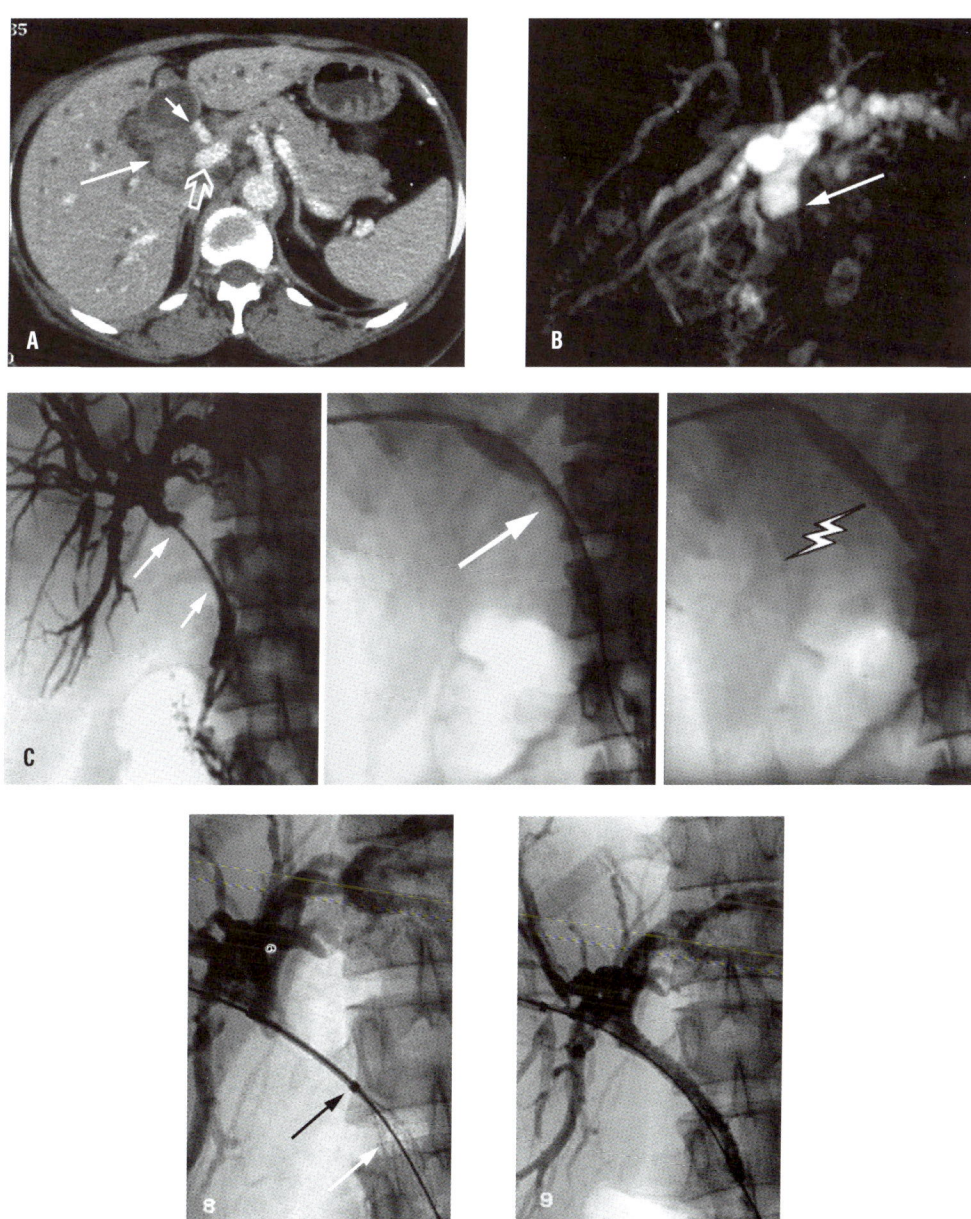

FIGURE 3: Metallic stent placement in a patient with unresectable carcinoma of gallbladder. **(A).** Contrast enhanced axial CT image showing a mass (large arrow) arising from the gallbladder and encasing the main portal vein (open arrow) and proper hepatic artery (small arrow). Intrahepatic biliary ducts are also dilated. **(B).** MRC frontal projection showing the block of common hepatic duct 2 cm beyond the confluence (arrow). **(C).** A ring biliary drainage catheter was placed and the cholangiogram shows the extent of the stricture (small arrows). This was dilated using a balloon catheter which initially shows a waist (large arrow) at the site of the stricture and later disappears (wavy arrow) indicating adequate dilatation. **(D).** A nitinol stent (Memotherm) is being deployed at the site of the stricture. A partially open stent mesh (white arrow) is seen being released by the withdrawal of the covering membrane (black arrow). **(E).** Following deployment, cholangiogram done from the access catheter shows good patency of the stent.

sometimes cause kinking of the lower part of the common bile duct, which may cause obstruction (with the newer flexible nitinol stents, this may probably be unnecessary). Additionally, it is easier to cannulate them endoscopically for clearance or for additional endoprosthesis insertion. If the stent projects too far into the duodenum, it can cause erosion of the opposite wall. So-called overstenting of the obstruction by at least 3 cm was recommended by Kanasaki et al, to minimize tumour overgrowth, while avoiding placement of the proximal end in the liver track. Side branches covered by the uncovered stents during placement are not associated with branch occlusion.

Once the stent is in position, a cholangiogram is done through the side arm of the introducer sheath to determine if contrast flows freely across the obstruction (Figure 3e). If the system is being adequately drained, a drainage catheter replaces the introducer sheath, its tip positioned proximal to the stent, to facilitate 4-6 hourly flushing of the system and to perform a cholangiogram 24-48 hours later, to assess stent patency. If all is well, the drainage catheter can be removed.

Hilar strictures

Stenting of hilar strictures present the most challenging problem for biliary interventionists. Hilar strictures can be treated by using a single stent if there is a free communication between the right and left duct systems. If at PTC, no opacification of the left-sided system is seen and there is adequate opacification of the right-sided system, then again a single stent may be used on the right side. The same is true of the left side, provided that the left lobe is hypertrophied and will provide adequate biliary drainage. If, however, there is opacification of the system of the opposite side, and the drainage will be inadequate with a single stent then, through a unilateral or bilateral, transhepatic route,

double stenting should be done. In the former, two stents are placed from a single track, one passing from the right to the left hepatic duct and the second from the right hepatic duct to the common bile duct (or an equivalent arrangement from the left side) in a T-shaped configuration (Figure 4). The duct expands to accommodate both stents without any problem. In the latter, one stent each is placed from the right and the left side tracts with the distal ends of both stents placed in the common bile duct in a Y-shaped configuration. For Bismuth type 4 lesions, Chi configuration stenting, as described above, can be done.

Combined transhepatic endoscopic approach (Rendezvous procedure)

Transhepatic placement of a catheter of small diameter across the obstructed duct and into the duodenum offers a second chance for the endoscopist. This arrangement is very useful when the endoscopist has initially failed to negotiate the obstruction at an earlier attempt, and it is not advisable to create a large transhepatic track because of the risk of bile leakage into the peritoneum, or in patients with coagulopathy. With a transhepatically inserted 4 or 5 F catheter negotiated across the obstruction into the duodenum, a 450 cm exchange guidewire such as Zebra (Microvasive) is inserted into the catheter. The patient is placed in the prone oblique position for the insertion of the endoscope. The endoscopist grasps the lower end of the guidewire with a snare or biopsy forceps and brings it out of the proximal end of the endoscope biopsy channel, while the radiologist keeps feeding the wire at the skin entry site. The transhepatic catheter is now withdrawn so that its tip lies in the intrahepatic portion of the biliary tree above the malignant stricture. The endoscopist now proceeds with the placement

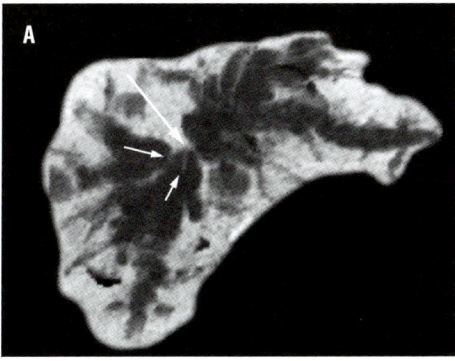

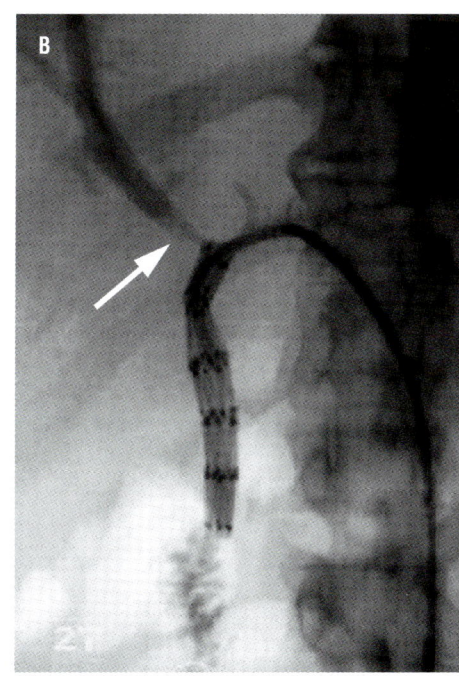

FIGURE 4: Malignant hilar biliary obstruction. Hilar reconstruction. **(A).** CT cholangiogram axial minimum intensity projection (as seen from below) shows blocked primary confluence (large arrow) and right secondary confluence (small arrows) **(B).** Hilar reconstruction done from the left transhepatic access. An indigenous plastic stent (arrow) has been placed connecting the right and the left ducts and a metallic Z stent has been placed between the left duct and the common duct.

of a large-bore biliary endoprosthesis in the standard fashion, while the guidewire is held taut between the endoscopic and percutaneous ends (Figure 5). When the endoprosthesis is in position and free ogress of bile is documented, the transhepatic catheter can be removed. However, if the patency of the endoprosthesis or adequacy of decompression is questionable, the transhepatic catheter may be retained for observation and re-intervention, if required.

Post procedure management following biliary drainage

- Patients should be hospitalized for at least 24 hours following biliary drainage and monitored for sepsis and vitals signs.
- An appropriate antibiotic combination should be continued after drainage is established.
- The internal external biliary drainage catheter should be used for external

drainage for the first 12-24 hrs. If the catheter permits drainage of bile into the bowel, then the drainage catheter can be capped to allow internal drainage. If the patient is able to tolerate internal drainage for 8-12 hours, then he/she can be discharged. If internal drainage is not possible, then external bag drainage must be maintained. Bile output can range from 400 to 800 ml/day. With external drainage, dehydration can occur, unless adequate steps are taken to replace the lost fluids.

- Biliary drainage catheters should be forward flushed with normal saline every 48 hours. This helps prevent debris from accumulating in the catheter and causing it to occlude.
- The dressing around the drainage catheter should be changed at least every 48 hours and bathing avoided. Also, the biliary drainage catheters should be changed every 3-4 months.
- Pericatheter leakage is the result of catheter occlusion or displacement. Flu-

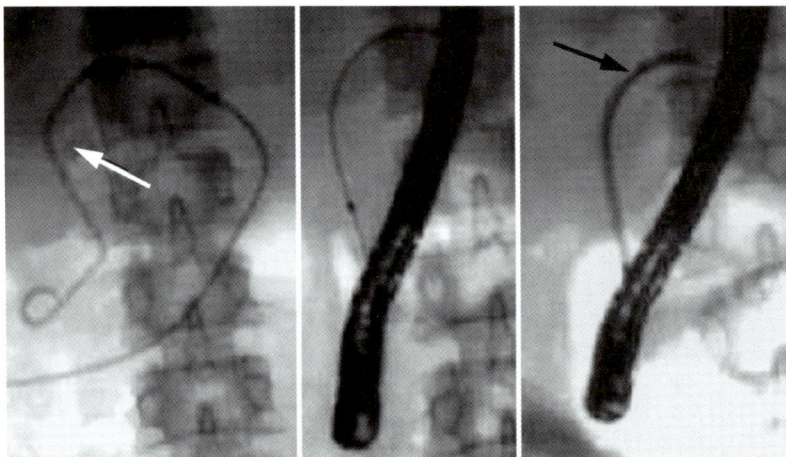

FIGURE 5: Rendezvous procedure. An 8 F ring biliary catheter (straight arrow) had been placed earlier by the left-sided transhepatic route in a patient who had a hilar stricture. The patient had developed ascites and plastic stent placement was planned. A 450 cm zebra guidewire was introduced through the catheter, which was snared by an endoscope placed in the duodenum and was brought out through the endoscope. By keeping the guidewire taut at the cutaneous entry site and the proximal end of the endoscope, a 10 F plastic stent (curved arrow) was deployed via the endoscope.

oroscopic evaluation is essential for determining and correcting this problem. Serum bilirubin values may be followed as an indicator of adequate drainage. Depending on the size and type of drain, it takes, on an average, 10-15 days for the bilirubin levels to drop by 50%. If the bilirubin level starts rising, catheter occlusion should be suspected.

- After adequate drainage, biliary sepsis should be relieved. If sepsis remains a problem, then additional studies should be performed to determine the cause, which can be catheter occlusion or undrained biliary ducts. A thorough cholangiogram with special attention to the ductal anatomy can sometimes identify a missing ductal segment, indicating an isolated undrained system. Alternatively, a MRCP or CT cholangiogram can be performed.
- Late sepsis, manifesting as fever several days or weeks after the patient has been adequately drained, is usually indicative of obstruction of the drainage catheter. If the patient has a capped biliary catheter, the tube should be uncapped to allow the bile to drain externally. If externalizing the drainage catheter resolves the infection, then fluoroscopic evaluation of the catheter can be performed electively. However, if fever persists after externalization, then an emergency catheter evaluation should be performed. If catheter obstruction is not the source of sepsis, then the patient should be evaluated for undrained ductal segments.

Complications

Complications of percutaneous biliary interventions can be divided into early, that is, procedural complications and late complications. Most procedural complications are related to the initial biliary drainage with mortality ranging from 0-2.8% and major complications occurring in 3.5%-9.5%. Also, higher procedure-related deaths have been reported for malignant diseases (3%) compared to benign diseases (0%). This is also true of procedure-related complications (7% Vs 2%). Minor complications such as mild self-limiting haemobilia, fever, and transient bacteremia occur in upto 66% of patients.

Immediate complications

These may be:

1. *Sedation:* Problems may occur if care is not taken to constantly monitor patients during and after the procedure for complications of cardiorespiratory depression. Pulse oximetry should be used for monitoring all patients undergoing procedures involving conscious sedation.

2. *Haemorrhage:* Mild haemobilia is common, occurring in upto 16% of cases. More severe bleeding requiring transfusion occurs in approximately 3% of patients. Haemorrhage is minimized by the correction of coagulation defects and avoidance of percutaneous intervention in patients with severe incorrectable coagulopathies. It is usually self-limited and seldom requires treatment. If bleeding is mild and venous in origin, repositioning the catheter so that the trailing side holes are located within the biliary tree and not within the hepatic parenchyma and upsizing the catheter to tamponade the bleeding point usually suffice. The catheter should be regularly irrigated with saline to maintain its patency and to clear any thrombus from the bile ducts. If haemobilia does not resolve with these measures or is severe, vascular embolization should be performed through the transhepatic track or by hepatic arteriography.

3. *Sepsis:* Manipulation of catheters and guidewires within an infected biliary tract can produce rapid bacteremia, which may progress to septicaemic shock if antibiotic coverage is not administered prior to the procedure. Intravenous antibiotics should be continued following biliary drainage until the catheter is removed.

4. *Pericatheter leak* in approximately 15% of the patients

5. *Pancreatitis* (0%-4%)

6. *Pneumothorax, haemothorax, bilothorax* (<1%)

7. *Contrast reaction* (<2%)

Delayed complications

These include the following:

1. *Cholangitis:* Approximately 50% of bile cultures will be positive when obtained at initial puncture. When an internal-external drainage is performed with an 8 F catheter, recurrent cholangitis secondary to inadequate drainage is possible. The rate of sepsis will decrease if this is replaced by a 10-12 Fr drain.

2. *Catheter dislodgment* (approximately 15%-20%)

3. *Peritonitis* (1%-3%)

4. *Hypersecretion of bile* (0%-5%): This can cause significant fluid and electrolyte imbalance and is usually seen within several days of drainage.

5. *Cholecystitis* – due to blockage of the cystic duct by covered stents. To address this complication, holes in the proximal stent lining are made, which should hypothetically allow for drainage of cystic or branch biliary ducts when their orifice is covered by the stent. But still, this complication may be seen, for which percutaneous cystic duct stent placement, percutaneous cholecystostomy or cholecystectomy may be required.

6. *Bilio-pleural fistula*

7. *Skin infection, irritation*

8. *Intrahepatic/perihepatic abscess*

9. *Metastatic seeding* of the serosa or tract with cholangiocarcinoma and pancreatic carcinoma has been reported.

Some routine precautions that help in significantly reducing the incidence of complications are provided in Table 1.

Plastic versus metallic stent placement

Short-term complications are similar to those related to PTBD, such as cholangi-

TABLE 1

METHODS OF REDUCING FREQUENCY OF COMMON COMPLICATIONS

Sepsis	Antibiotic prophylaxis Minimal manipulation Restrict volume of contrast injected and aspirate bile prior to contrast injection
Hemorrhage	Normalize coagulation factors Fine-needle coaxial technique Peripheral duct puncture Careful positioning of side holes to avoid communication with an intrahepatic vessel Avoid puncture of extra hepatic ducts Single puncture site in liver capsule
Bile leak	Ensure adequate drainage by careful positioning of side holes
Cholangitis	Irrigation of catheter with sterile saline Large diameter catheters (12 F) for long drainage Routine tube exchange every 2-3 months
Catheter dislodgement	Safety stitch method Self-retaining (pigtail) catheter

tis, haemorrhage and bile leakage. Metallic stent placement is associated with a lower incidence of cholangitis than with plastic stents. Stents are prone to obstruction, but over the long term expandable metallic stents have a better patency rate than plastic stents: 272 Vs 96 days in a randomized trial by Lammer et al. Obstruction of the plastic stent is caused by bile decomposition, deposition and encrustation, usually following bacterial contamination. This would require replacement either by endoscopic or percutaneous means. Metallic stents, on the other hand, get obstructed due to tumour overgrowth and/or impaction of food debris. Unblocking metallic stents involves a repeat intervention, such as the introduction of a plastic or metallic stent within the obstructed lumen of the stent. Kanasaki et al recommended "overstenting" of the obstruction by at least 3 cm, to minimize tumour overgrowth. Plastic stents are prone to migration (early or late), which occurs in 3%-6% of cases. Although metallic stents may get dislodged by balloon dilatation immediately after deployment, long-term spontaneous migration is very unusual. Fully or partially covered stents seem to be prone to migration, which has been observed in 3%-11% of cases. However, metallic stents (ePTFE/FEP) with anchoring fins at each end do not show migration.

Patients should be followed up by clinical criteria, liver function tests and US to look for early signs of stent occlusion.

Clinical results

PTBD

The results of various series are tabulated in Table 2. In general, the technical success rate has varied from 86% to 100% with successful drainage rates of 81%-96%. The 30-day mortality rate has been 1%-49% and complication rate of 6%-58%. This marked variation in results is proba-

TABLE 2

RESULTS OF PTBD IN MALIGNANT OBSTRUCTION

Author	Number of Patients	Technical Success (%)	Drainage Success (%)	30-Day Mortality (%)	Complication rate (%)
Pereiras et al	12	100	83	–	58
Voegeli et al	76	97	92	27	20
Joseph et al	39	90	–	49	53
Lammer & Neumayer	162	100	96	15	9
Schild et al	220	–	92	1	22
Gazzaniga et al	362	97	81	–	15
Murai et al	92	86	–	–	–
Schoder et al	42	100	100	20	5
Bezzi et al	26	100	100	11.5	19

bly due to differences in the criteria for patient selection, the experience and expertise of different operators, and the criteria used to define success and complications.

Plastic and metallic stenting

Evaluation of patency rates for stents in malignant biliary obstruction is difficult because some patients may die with patent stents and others may die with occult stent occlusion, making data collection and analysis difficult. Additionally, because stents occlude over time, patient groups with a short mean survival have improved stent patency rates compared to those with longer mean survival times. Therefore retrospective analysis of stent patency is difficult and not so useful. Only well-designed, prospective, randomized control trials with stent occlusion as a measurable end point can provide the necessary information (Table 3). One by Lammer et al, which compared transhepatic placement of metallic and plastic stents, showed that the occlusion rates for metallic stents were significantly lower than those for plastic

stents (19% vs. 27%), the median duration of patency for metallic stents is longer (272 days vs. 96 days) and the 30-day mortality was significantly lower for metallic stents (10% vs. 24%). Finally, placement of a metallic stent was associated with a significantly shorter hospital stay (10 vs. 21 days) and lower overall costs per patient. Hilar strictures have been reported to have lower patency rates than common bile duct obstructions, although these reports have been contradicted. Lee et al explained that when one of the two stents is occluded in a hilar obstruction, jaundice develops later because the second stent is patent. In contrast if a stent is occluded in the common bile duct, jaundice will develop immediately.

Patient survival
Although the possibility of patient survival after metallic stent placement is difficult to estimate and compare between various reports, patients receiving this treatment have been reported to live 93 to 420 days longer. In patients with hilar obstruction, longer survival rates have been observed after both lobes have been drained as

Authors	Number of Patients	Obstruction rate: Plastic Stent (%)	Obstruction Rate: Metal Stent (%)	Median Duration of Plastic Stent Patency (days)	Median Duration of Metallic Stent Patency (days)
Davids et al	105	54	33	126	273
Knyrim et al	62	43	22	-	-
Lammer et al	101	27	19	96	272

compared to those who had one lobe drained.

Rationalizing biliary drainage and stenting in malignant obstruction

PTBD should be done only in those patients with malignant obstruction who are clearly symptomatic, such as those with intense pruritis and acute cholangitis, to improve the quality of life, if curative resection is not possible. In patients with unresectable disease who do not have any of these indications, one should consciously decide not to do the procedure to avoid complications. The decision to perform PTBD should be taken after close consultation and discussion among the physician, surgeon and radiologist, as emphasized earlier.

Cost considerations should also be borne in mind. Since the patency of plastic and metallic stents is similar during the first 3 months after stent insertion, only patients with a life expectancy of more than 3 months should be offered expandable metallic stents. Plastic stents can also be easily exchanged by endoscopic or percutaneous means. If plastic stents occlude rapidly and repeatedly, metallic stents should be used. Patients who are in good health with a life expectancy of more than 3 months, and those from remote areas with no facility for stent exchange are good candidates for metallic stents. Rationalizing the procedure by carefully choosing the patients, the nature of the procedure and cost-effective materials, can go a long way in giving the maximum benefit to patients with malignant biliary obstruction.

Other interventions in malignant biliary obstruction

Biliary cytology and biopsy procedures

In suspected malignant biliary obstructions, the percutaneous tract can be used for cytologic or histologic confirmation. Bile collected from the external drainage bag is more likely to yield positive cytology than fluid obtained at PTC alone. Cytologic study is positive in roughly 50% of the patients with cholangiocarcinoma, although the reported sensitivity varies widely. The positive cytology rate is lower for primary pancreatic tumours.

If cytology is negative, percutaneous biopsy can be done by cholangiographic or US guidance. Alternatively the cholangiographic tract could also be used to obtain brushings or biopsy using forceps, bioptome, myocardial biopsy needle, or a needle biopsy through a transhepatic sheath.

Endoluminal irradiation

Inoperable malignant biliary obstructive lesions can be subjected to endoluminal radiotherapy after insertion of catheters and stents through the obstructive lesion. This method is particularly useful in patients with cholangiocarcinomas because some of these patients may live for years and the combination of stenting and radiotherapy provides a much better and longer-lasting palliation than stenting alone. Very high doses of local radiation can be administered by means of iridium-192 seeds with little exposure of liver beyond the tumour. In a study by Golfieri et al, mean survival of patients with unresectable hilar cholangiocarcinoma undergoing multi-modality treatment with percutaneous and intraluminal plus external radiotherapy was 10.5 months, similar to surgical results and higher than the control group treated with percutaneous stenting (2.75 months) or biliary drainage alone (1.75 months), with an average hospital stay of 10-15 days and no procedure-related mortality. Unfortunately patients treated with endoluminal radiotherapy are subject to episodes of severe cholangitis, periductal abscess and haemobilia.

Percutaneous intervention in benign biliary obstruction

The majority of benign strictures are a result of upper abdominal surgery, particularly cholecystectomy. Bile ductal injuries are seen in 0-4% of open procedures, including cholecystectomies. The other most common cause of iatrogenic stricture is anastomotic stricture following biliary-enteric anastomosis. Most anastomotic strictures are extrahepatic and can present several years following surgery. Multiple intrahepatic strictures are usually a manifestation of sclerosing cholangitis or bile duct ischaemia. The latter can occur due to hepatic artery occlusion following liver transplantation, cholecystectomy or hepatic chemoembolization. Multiple intrahepatic benign strictures are the ones that are most difficult to treat.

Patients with benign strictures present with recurrent jaundice, cholangitis and pain. Intrahepatic calculi are commonly found above benign strictures. These also contribute to intermittent obstruction. If the underlying cause is not treated, chronic biliary sepsis and obstruction may result in chronic liver insufficiency and may progress to biliary cirrhosis.

Imaging assessment
The principles of noninvasive radiologic evaluation remain the same as those for malignant obstruction. For more direct evaluation ERC is usually employed, to define the exact location, length and character of the biliary stricture. However, for patients with very tight strictures and hilar strictures, PTC is usually required due to insufficient opacification of proximal ducts by ERC method. Additionally, PTBD can be performed immediately following PTC.

Management options
Benign strictures have a tendency to restenose following treatment and hence are difficult to treat. The main treatment options available are surgery and radiological dilatation.

Surgery
This treatment essentially involves resection of the strictured segment of the duct and primary anastomosis of the duct, or the formation of biliary-enteric anastomosis (hepatico-, choledocho-duodenostomy or-jejunostomy). Surgery is challenging for strictures close to the liver hilum, especially for those involving the hepatic ducts. For multiple intrahepatic strictures, liver transplantation is the only surgical option. The reported recurrence rate of surgical treatment for strictures is 7%-30%. The surgical treatment of recurrent stricture is even more difficult and the recurrence rate is 22% and the mortality is 10%. Concurrent hepatobiliary disease, portal hypertension and scarring of the liver hilum

from previous surgery can contribute to the increase in the surgical procedure time, morbidity and mortality.

Radiological balloon stricturoplasty

This method involves securing an access to the biliary system in the same manner as described for PTBD. Since benign structures require repeat treatments because of frequent restenosis, surgeons should actively consider creating access jejunal loops, which may be placed at the time of formation of the biloenteric anastomosis as a prelude to the programme of balloon dilatation. The access point of this loop is fixed to the anterior abdominal wall and is identified by a radiopaque marker such as a ring of metallic sutures or surgical staples (Figure 6). It is usually easy to puncture the access loop and then gain retrograde access to the anastomosis for repeat interventions without the need for PTBD.

Once access is gained to the anastomosis via the biliary tract or the access loop, the stricture is crossed with a wire and a catheter. A balloon catheter is then placed across the stricture and inflated to dilate the stricture (Figure 6). There are no clear guidelines available in literature as to the length of time for the balloon to be kept in the inflated state. In our center we usually dilate the stricture for 10 minutes and look for recoil or "waist" formation in the balloon on repeat inflation to consider longer period of inflation at a higher pressure. A large diameter catheter is left across the anastomosis to prevent restenosis during the initial period of healing by fibrosis, and to provide ready access to the system. This catheter is removed after 6 weeks after ensuring a satisfactory cholangiogram and asymptomatic clinical status of the patient.

Complications are similar to those seen in PTBD. Success rates range from 70%-93%. Balloon dilatation for sclerosing cholangitis has a much lower success rate of 42%-59%. However, this subgroup of patients are poor surgical candidates and balloon stricturoplasty is a good temporizing measure in candidates for liver transplantation.

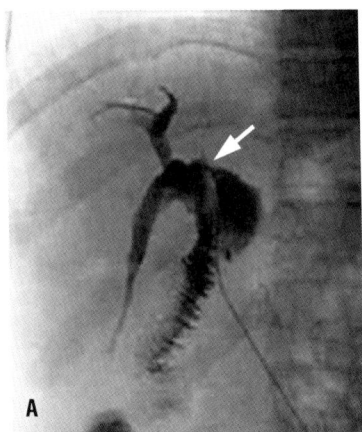 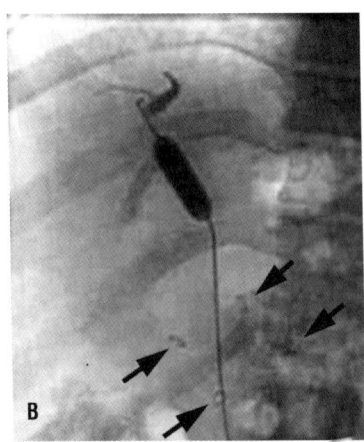

FIGURE 6: A patient operated for cholecystectomy also underwent biliary enteric anastomosis and presented with repeated attacks of cholangitis. **(A).** A cholangiogram done by placing a catheter in the intrahepatic biliary ducts via the access loop (multiple black arrows), shows an anastomotic stricture (white arrow). **(B).** A balloon catheter has been used to dilate the stricture.

Radiological endoprosthesis placement

Most patients with benign biliary strictures are relatively young and are expected to lead near normal lives once the obstruction is relieved. Therefore, the treatment provided should be durable and without significant long-term complications. There is no role for plastic endoprostheses placement in the management of benign biliary strictures, mainly due to their early occlusion. Metallic endoprostheses should be placed only as a last resort in these patients (patients unfit or unsuitable for surgery, failed repeated balloon dilatations), due to stent related problems such as recurrent cholangitis, stent occlusion, and stone formation. Three-year patency rates for benign strictures following insertion of Gianturco stents are 68.7%. Biodegradable and drug-eluting (which prevent obstruction) stents, which are experimental at present, might be useful options in the future.

ACKNOWLEDGEMENT

The authors wish to thank Prof SK Acharya, Editor of the jounal "Tropical Gastroenterology"; and co-editor of the book 'Clinical Approach to Jaundice', for kindly consenting to reproduce part of the text and the figures from the article and chapter in the same journal and book respectively.

REFERENCES

Abramson AF, Javit DJ, Mitty HA, Train JS, Dan SJ. Wallstent migration following deployment in right and left hepatic ducts. JVIR 1992; 3: 463-465.

Adamck HE, Albert J, Lietz M, Breer H, Schilling D, Riemann JF. A prospective evaluation of Magnetic Resonance cholangiography in patients with suspected bile duct obstruction. Gut 1998; 43: 680-683.

Asch MR, Jaffer NM, Baron DL. Migration of a biliary wallstent into the duodenum. JVIR 1993; 4: 381-383.

Becker CD, Glattli A, Maibach R et al. Percutaneous palliation of malignant obstructive jaundice with the wallstent endoprosthesis: follow-up and reintervention in patients with hilar and non-hilar obstruction. J Vasc Interv Radiol 1993;4:441-447

Berquist TH, May GR, Johnson CM Adson MA, Thistle JL. Percutaneous biliary decompression: internal and external drainage in 50 patients. AJR 1981; 136: 901-906.

Bezzi M, Zolovkins A, Cantisani V, Salvatori FM, Rossi M, Fanelli F, Rossi P. New ePTFE/FEP–covered stent in the palliative treatment of malignant biliary obstruction. JVIR 2002;13: 581-589

Bismuth H, Corlette MB. Intrahepatic cholangioenteric anastomosis in carcinoma of the hilus of the liver. Surg Gynecol Obstetr 1975; 140: 170-178.

Bismuth H. Postoperative strictures of the bile duct. In Blumgart LH (Ed): The biliary tract: clinical surgery international. Edinburgh: Churchill Livingstone 1982;5:209-218.

Blumgart LH. Cholangiocarcinoma, In: Blumgart LH ed. Surgery of the liver and biliary tract. Edinburgh: Churchill Livingstone 1998; 1: 721-753.

Born P, Neuhaus H, Rosch T, et al. Initial experience with a new, partially covered Wallstent for malignant biliary obstruction. Endoscopy 1996; 28:699-702

Carrasco CH, Zornoza J, Bechtel WJ. Malignant biliary obstruction: Complications of percutaneous biliary drainage. Radiology 1984; 152: 343-346.

Cha JH, Han JK, Kim TK, Kim AY, Park SJ, Choi BI, Suh KS, Kim SW, Han MC. Preoperative evaluation of Klatskin tumour: accuracy of spiral CT in determining vascular invasion as a sign of unresectability. Abdom Imaging 2000;25:500-507.

Choi BI, Lee JH, Han MC, Kim SH, Yi JG, Kim CW. Hilar cholangiocarcinoma: comparative study with sonography and CT. Radiology 1989; 172:689-692.

Clark RA, Mitchell SE, Colley DP Alexander E. Percutaneous catheter biliary decompression. AJR 1981; 137: 503-509.

Cowling MG, Adam AN. Internal stenting in malignant biliary obstruction. World J Surg 2001;25: 355-361

Cutherell L, Wanebo HJ, Tegtmeyer CJ. Catheter tract seeding after percutaneous biliary drainage for pancreatic cancer. Cancer 1986; 57:2057-2060.

Davids PH, Groen AK, Rauws EA, Tytgat GN, Huibregtse K. Randomised trial of self expanding metallic stents versus polyethylene stents for distal malignant biliary obstruction. Lancet 1992; 340: 1488-1492.

Davids PH, Groen AK, Rauws EA, Tytgat GN, Huibregtse K. Randomised trial of self expanding metallic stents versus polyethylene stents for distal malignant biliary obstruction. Lancet 1992; 340: 1488-1492.

Dawson SL, Neff CC, Mueller PR, Ferrucci JT Jr. Fatal hemothorax after inadvertent transpleural biliary drainage. Am J Roentgenol 1983; 141: 33-34

de Aretxabala X, Roa I, Burgos L, Araya JC, Fonseca L, Wistuba I, Flores P. Gallbladder cancer in Chile. A report on 54 potentially resectable tumours. Cancer 1992;69:60-65.

Denning DA, Ellison EC, Carey LC. Preoperative percutaneous transhepatic biliary decompression lowers operative morbidity in patients with obstructive jaundice. Am J Surg 1991; 141: 61-65.

Deviere J, Baize M, de Toeuf J et al. Long-term follow-up of patients with hilar malignant stricture treated by endoscopic internal biliary drainage. Gastrointest Endosc 1988;34:95-101

Dhil V, Huibregtse K. Endoscopic placement of expandable biliary stents: current applicability. Indian J Gastroenterol 1996; 15: 142-146.

Ede RJ, Williams SJ, Hatfield ARW, McIntyre S, Mair G. Endoscopic management of inoperable cholangiocarcinoma using iridium-192. Br J Surg 1988;76:867-869.

Ferrucci JT Jr, Mueller PR, Harbim WP. Percutaneous transhepatic biliary drainage: technique, results and applications. Radiology 1980; 135: 1-13.

Feydy A, Vilgrain V, Denys A, Sibert A, Belghiti J, Vullierme MP, Menu Y. Helical CT assessment in hilar cholangiocarcinoma: correlation with surgical and pathologic findings. AJR 1999;172:73-77.

Garg PK, Tandon RK. Nonsurgical drainage for biliary obstruction. Indian J Gastroenterol 1994; 13: 118-127.

Gazzaniga GM, Faggioni A, Bondanza G et al. Percutaneous transhepatic biliary drainage- twelve years experience. Hepatogastroenterology 1991; 38: 154-159.

Golfieri R, Giampalma E, Fusco F, Galuppi A, Faccioli L, Galaverni C, Frezza G. Unresectable hilar cholangiocarcinoma: multimodality treatment with percutaneous and intraluminal plus external radiotherapy. J Chemother. 2004 Nov;16 Suppl 5:55-7

Gulliver DJ, Baker ME, Cheng CA, Meyers WC, Papas TN. Malignant biliary obstruction: efficacy of thin section dynamic CT in determining resectability. AJR 1992;159:503-507.

Gulati MS, Paul SB. Radiological management of the Jaundiced Patient. In: Tandon RK, Acharya SK, eds (on Behalf of the Indian College of Physicians). Clinical Approach to Jaundice. New Delhi: Byword Viva Publishers Private Limited, 2005; 16-45

Gulati MS, Srinivasan A, Agarwal PP, Paul SB, Garg P, Rao NDLV. Percutaneous management of malignant biliary obstruction: the Indian perspective. Trop Gastroenterol 2003;24:47-58.

Gunther RW, Schild H, Thelen M. Percutaneous transhepatic biliary drainage: Experience with 311 procedures. Caediovascular Intervent Radiol 1988;11:65-71.

Hamlin JA, Friedman M, Stein MG Bray JF.. Percutaneous biliary drainage: complications of 118 consecutive catheterizations. Radiology 1986; 158: 199-202.

Harell GS, Anderson MF, Berry PF. Cytologic bile examination in the diagnosis of biliary duct neoplastic strictures. Am J Roentgenol 1981;137: 1123-1126.

Hausegger KA, Thurnher S, Bodendorfer G, et al. Treatment of malignant biliary obstruction with polyurethane-covered Wallstents. AJR Am J Roentgenol 1998; 170:403-408

Joseph PK, Bizer LS, Sprayregan SS, Gliedman ML. Percutaneous transhepatic biliary drainage. Results and complications in 81 patients. JAMA 1986; 255: 2763-2767.

Kanasaki S, Furukawa A, Kane T, Murata K. Polyurethane-covered nitinol Strecker stents as primary palliative treatment of malignant biliary obstruction. Cardiovasc Intervent Radiol 2000,23: 114-120

Kersjes W, Koster O, Heuer M, Schneider B. A comparison of imaging procedures in the diagnosis of gallbladder and bile duct carcinomas. Rofo Fortschr Geb Rontgenstr Neuen Bildgeb Verfahr 1990;153:174-180.

Knyrim K, Wagner HJ, Pausch J, Vakil N. A prospective, randomized, controlled trial of metal stents for malignant obstruction of the common bile duct Endoscopy 1993 Mar;25(3):207-12

Kumaran V, Gulati MS, Paul SB, Pande GK, Sahni P, Chattopadhyay TK. The role of dual phase helical CT in assessing resectability of carcinoma of the gallbladder. European Radiology 2002;12: 1993-1999.

Kwon AH, Uetsuji S, Yamada O, Inoue T, Kamiyama Y, Boku T. Three dimensional reconstruction of the biliary tract using spiral computed tomography. Br J Surg 1995; 82: 260-263.

Lamaris JS, Stoker J, Dees J Nix GA, Van Blankenstein M, Jeekel J. Nonsurgical palliative treatment of patients wirh malignant biliary obstruction-the place of endoscopic and percutaneous drainage. Clin Radiology 1987; 38: 603-608.

Lammer JL. Biliary endoprostheses: Plastic versus metal stents. Radiol Clin N Am 1990; 28: 1211-1222.

Lammer J, Hausegger KA, Fluckiger F, Winkelbauer FW, Wildling R, Klein GE, Thurnher SA, Havelec L. Common bile duct obstruction due to malignancy: Treatment with plastic versus metal stents. Radiology 1996; 201: 167-172.

Lammer J, Neurager K. Biliary drainage ondoprosthesis: experience with 201 patients. Radiology 1986; 159: 625-629.

Lee BH, Cohe DH, Lee JH et al. Metallic stents in malignant biliary obstruction: prospective long-term clinical results. AJR 1997;168:741-745

Lee KH, Lee DY, Kim KW. Biliary intervention for cholangiocarcinoma. Abdom Imaging 2004;29: 581-589

Lopera JE, Soto JA, Mïnera F. Malignant hilar and perihilar biliary obstruction: Use of MR Cholangiography to define the extent of biliary ductal involvement and plan percutaneous interventions. Radiology 2001;220:90-96

Maccioni F, Rossi M, Salvatori FM. Metallic stents in benign biliary strictures: three years follow-up. Cardiovasc Intervent Radiol 1992;15;360-366.

Meyers WC, Jones RS. Internal radiation for the bile duct cancer. World J Surg 1988;35:213-214.

Morgan RA, Adam A. Percutaneous management of biliary obstruction. In Gazelle GS, Saini S, Mueller PR (eds): Hepatobiliary and pancreatic radiology Imaging and Intervention. Thieme,1998, pp 677-709.

Motte S, Deviere J, Dumonceau JM et al. Risk factors for septicemia following endoscopic biliary stent. Gastroenterology 1991;101:1374-1381

Mueller PR, Ferrucci JT Jr, Teplick SK, vanSonnenberg E, Haskin PH, Butch RJ, Papanicolaou N. Biliary stent endoprosthesis: analysis of complications in 113 patients. Radiology 1985; 156: 637-639.

Mueller PR, vanSonnenberg E, Ferrucci JT Jr. Percutaneous biliary drainage: Technical and catheter related problems in 200 procedures. AJR 1982; 138: 17-23.

Mueller PR, Van Sonnenberg E, Ferrucci JT. Biliary stricture dilatation: multicenter review of clinical management in 73 patients. Radiology 1986;160:57-22.

Murai R, Hashiguchi F, Kusuyama A Yoshimi M, Watanabe K, Okui S, Ando H, Itsubo K. Percutaneous stenting for malignant biliary stenosis. Surg Endosc 1991; 5: 140-142

Miyayama S, Matsui O, Terayama N, Tatsu H, Yamamoto T, Takashima T. Covered Gianturco stents for malignant biliary obstruction: preliminary clinical evaluation. J Vasc Interv Radiol 1997;8:641-648

Nicholson DA, Cheety N, Jackson J. Patency of side branches after peripheral placement of metallic biliary endoprosthesis. JVIR 1992; 3: 127-130.

Okuda K, Ohto M, Tsuhiya Y. The role of ultrasound, percutaneous transhepatic cholangiography, computed tomographic scanning and magnetic resonance imaging in the preoperative assessment of bile duct cancer. World J surg 1988;12:18-26.

Park SJ, Han JK, Kim TK, Choi BI. Three-dimensional spiral CT cholangiography with minimum intensity projection in patients with suspected obstructive biliary disease: comparison with percutaneous transhepatic cholangiography. Abdom Imaging 2001; 26 (3): 281-86

Pellagrini CA, Thomas MJ, Way LW. Recurrent biliary stricture: pattern of recurrence and outcome of surgical therapy. Am J Surg 1984;14: 175-180.

Pereiras RV Jr, Rheingold OJ, Huston D, Mejia J, Viamonte M, Chiprut RO, Schiff ER. Relief of malignant obstructive jaundice by percutaneous insertion of a permanent prosthesis. Ann Intern Med 1978;89:589-93

Pillai VAK, Shreekumar KP, Prabhu NK, Moorthy S. Utility of MR cholangiography in planning transhepatic biliary interventions in malignant hilar obstructions. IJRI 2002; 12: 37-42.

Pitt HA, Miyamoto T, Parapatis SK. Factors influencing outcome in patients with postoperative biliary strictures. Am J Surg 1988;144:14-19.

Polydorou AA, Chisholm EM, Romanos AA, Dowsett JF, Cotton PB, Hatfield AR, Russell RC.. A comparison of right versus left hepatic duct endoprosthesis insertion in malignant hilar biliary obstruction. Endoscopy 1989; 21: 266-271.

Rieber A, Brambs HJ. Metallic stents in malignant biliary obstruction. Cardiovasc Intervent Radiol 1997;20:43-49

Rosenblatt M, Aruny JE, Kandarpa K. Transhepatic cholangiography, Biliary decompression, Endobiliary stenting, and Cholecystostomy. In Kandarpa K, Aruny JE (eds): Handbook of Interventional radiology procedures. Philadelphia: Lippincott Williams & Wilkins; 2002: pp 302-331

Rossi P, Bezzi M, Rossi M et al. Metallic stents in malignant biliary obstruction: results of a multicenter European study of 24 patients; J Vasc Interv Radiol 1994;5:279-285

Rossi P, Bezzi M, Salvatori FM, Panzetti C, Rossi M, Pavia G. Clinical experience with covered Wallstents for biliary malignancies: 23-month follow-up. Cardiovasc Intervent Radiol 1997;20: 441-447.

Rossi P. Salvotri FM, Bezzi M. Percutaneous management of benign biliary strictures with balloon dilatation and self expanding metallic stents. Cardiovasc Intervent Radiol 1990;13:231-239.

Schild H, Klose KJ, Staritz M, Borner N, Nagel K, Gunther R, Ruckert K, Junginger T, Thelen M. The results and complications of 616 percutaneous transhepatic biliary drainages. Rofo Fortschr Geb Rontgenstr Neuen Bildgeb Verfahr 1989 Sep;151 (3):289-93

Schoder M, Rossi P, Uflacker R, Bezzi M, Stadler A, Funovics MA, Cejna M, Lammer J. Malignant biliary obstruction: treatment with ePTFE-FEP– covered endoprostheses — initial technical and clinical experiences in a multicenter trial. Radiology 2002;225:35-42

Sheiman RG, Stuart K. Percutaneous cystic duct stent placement for the treatment of acute cholecystitis resulting from common bile duct stent placement for malignant obstruction. JVIR 2004; 15:999-1001

Shim CS, Lee JH, Cho JD, et al. Preliminary results of a new covered biliary metal stent for malignant biliary obstruction. Endoscopy 1998; 30: 345–350

Speer AG, Russel CG, Hatfield ARW. Randomised trial of endoscopic versus percutaneous stent insertion in malignant obstructive jaundice. Lancet 1987; 11: 57-62.

Strange C, Allen ML, Freedland PN Cunningham J, Sahn SA. Biliopleural fistula as a complication of percutaneous biliary drainage: experimental evidence for pleural inflammation. Am Rev Respir Dis 1988; 137: 959-961

Thurnher SA, Lammer J, Thurnher MM, Wilkenbauer F, Graf O, Wildling R. Covered self-expanding transhepatic biliary stents: clinical pilot study. Cardiovasc Intervent Radiol 1996; 19: 10–14.

Van Beers BE, Lacrosse M, Trigaux JP, de Canniere L, De Ronde T, Pringot J. non invasive imaging of the biliary tree before or after laparoscopic cholecystectomy: use of three dimensional spiral CT cholangiography. AJR 1994; 162: 1331-1335.

Vorgeli DR, Gummy AB, Weese JL. Percutaneous transhepatic cholangiography, drainage and biopsy in patients with malignant biliary obstruction. An alternate to surgery. Am J Surg 1985; 150: 243-247.

Williams HJ, Bender CE, May GR. Benign postoperative biliary strictures: dilatation with fluoroscopic guidance. Radiology 1987;163:629-634.

Wittich GR, VanSonnertberg E, Simeone JF.Results and complications of percutaneous drainage. Seminars in Interventonal Radiology 1985; 2: 39-49

Yee AC, Ho CS. Complications of transhepatic biliary drainage: benign vs malignant diseases. AJR Am J Roentgenol 1987; 148: 1207-1209.

Zeman RK, Berman PM, Silverman PM, Cooper C, Garra BS, Patt RH, Ascher SM. Biliary tract: Three dimensional helical CT without cholangiographic contrast material. Radiology 1995; 196: 865-867.

Future perspectives in the diagnosis and management of obstructive jaundice

Zingg Tobias, Filippou Dimitrios, Krähenbühl Lukas

MALIGNANT DISEASES

In the previous chapters the distinguished invited authors have described the malignant disorders that cause obstructive jaundice, as well as diagnostic and therapeutic developments for managing these diseases. In the past ten years, significant technological developments have changed the diagnostic and therapeutic approach to these patients dramatically. In spite of the great progress during this time, the long-term results are not satisfactory in most cases and the survival of these patients remains limited. What can we expect in the future? In this last chapter, we aim to summarise possible future perspectives in the diagnostic and therapeutic approach to patients with malignancy associated with obstructive jaundice.

Pancreatic cancer is a relatively common malignancy usually associated with a poor prognosis. It is estimated that only 13-33% of patients have resectable tumours at diagnosis and the best 5-year survival is really expected in patients with small tumours (<2 cm) and without metastases to the regional lymph nodes.

Surgery is considered the treatment of choice if it is applicable, and neither chemotherapy nor radiation offers curative options.

In the past decade, descriptions of the key molecular events that mainly contribute to the processes of tumour genesis and development have been published. Development of malignancy requires at least two disorders in fundamental processes. The first process is the functional loss by mutation or deletion of one or more tumour-suppressor genes. This genetic transformation results in the loss of control over critical aspects of the cell cycle. The second process that results in tumourgenesis is the mutation of genes involved in the cell signal transduction process, which are called oncogenes. The oncogenes also play an important role as secondary signal messengers. These cellular and molecular processes also play an important role in the genesis and development of pancreatic cancer. Knowledge of these events may improve our understanding of pancreatic cancer and contribute to the development of better and more effective diagnostic and therapeutic tools.

In the past decade, molecular biology has also contributed to the development of more accurate prognostic and diagnostic markers and modalities, such as gene *p53*. However, confirmation is still needed on whether determination of genetic parameters such as *p53* offers the possibility of predicting response to several chemotherapeutic agents, including 5-fluorouracil, which could provide more selective and more effective chemotherapy even in advanced disease. Other than the recently developed classical chemotherapy, it is still very early to extract definitive conclusions concerning the efficacy of the therapeutic strategies that have appeared employing gene therapy.

The introduction of the *RB1* gene into cancer cells with deletions in the *RB1* locus using retroviral vectors resulted in suppressed tumourgenicity of these cells. A similar reversion of transformed cells was obtained by restoring *p53* function in vitro and in vivo. Another approach is based on the exogenous administration of short, single-stranded oligonucleotide sequences that act by blocking the mRNA translation. The preliminary results suggest that this method will be useful in blocking dominant gene expression, but further studies are required to evaluate the prognostic value of alterations defined by molecular techniques. We are only now beginning to evaluate the usefulness of various cellular or genomic markers for their diagnostic, prognostic, and even therapeutic value. A better understanding of the molecular genetics of this tumour type is the main challenge for further investigations of pancreatic cancer.

In recent years, several cancer-related genes, implicating pancreatic, hepatocellular and periampulary carcinoma, have been identified, mostly by conventional methods. However, considering the complexity of the genome, many of the molecular changes causing pancreatic cancer still need to be elucidated and the four - omes (genome, transcriptome, proteome and glycome) of the cell need to be analysed.

Current research is focusing on detecting new sequence polymorphisms, defining the specific phenotypes using DNA micro arrays in the analysis of signalling pathways.

Several studies using this technique with various methods have elucidated gene expression changes in pancreatic cancer and generated large sets of new class II cancer genes, revealing deregulation at the level of gene expression. These genes seem to be differently expressed in normal and neoplastic pancreatic cells. Future studies are required to establish any possible diagnostic or therapeutic uses of these molecular biology techniques.

Pancreatic cancer is usually suspected on US findings and confirmed by CT scan, which is the most commonly used diagnostic modality, with a predictive value for non-resectability of 90% and accuracy varying from 85-95% in various series.

Unfortunately, in spite of the significant technological advances in CT technology (spiral CT, cholangio-CT, minimisation of radiation exposure), interpreting the results is sometimes difficult. Magnetic resonance imaging (MRI, MRCP and MRA), despite technological improvements, presents the same results as CT, while EUS, which offers the possibility of tissue diagnosis with FNA, is of limited value.

FDG-PET imaging combined with a CT scan seems to be a sensitive and useful adjunct to CT alone in the preoperative diagnosis of pancreatic carcinoma, particularly in cases with highly suspicious lesions where CT fails to define a tumour mass and FNA is non-diagnostic. FDG-PET can also differentiate post-therapy changes from recurrence and in the future will probably become the gold standard for monitoring neo-adjuvant chemo-radiation therapy in patients with pancreatic cancer.

Diagnostic laparoscopy seems to posses a significant role in evaluating and staging patients with pancreatic cancer. Most authors suggest that a laparoscopy should always be performed at the beginning of the operation. Between 20% and 30% of the patients with tumours that are preoperatively considered respectable, have local lymph node involvement or distant metastases revealed during diagnostic laparoscopy. These patients should receive only palliative treatment, preferably laparoscopically to avoid an unnecessary laparotomy.

Curative resections are generally problematic due to the location of the tumour near large upper abdominal vessels such as the mesenteric artery and portal vein and to its ability to spread even at small tumour sizes into regional lymph nodes and distant organs. This very aggressive tumour behaviour reduces pancreatic cancer treatment to largely palliative options.

It is already well known that surgery presents the best therapeutic results, although in the vast majority of the cases the prognosis is extremely poor, and the morbidity and mortality are high. In most patients with pancreatic cancer, the operations are palliative; only in very few are they therapeutic. As far adjuvant chemotherapy is concerned, most authors agree that it does not increase survival; they also doubt if it improves the quality of life. Classical radiotherapy presents a small therapeutic advantage and it generally appears that although preceding chemo-radiotherapy with a modest radiation dose does not significantly increase the surgical morbidity or mortality, neither does it increase total survival.

Various chemotherapeutic agents have been used to treat patients with pancreatic cancer. The efficacy of these agents is being evaluated in controlled trials, but the primary results do not indicate that they contribute to better prognosis. The discovery of new and more efficient agents is a future target for pancreatic oncology.

Many clinical trials focus on the role of neo-adjuvant preoperative chemo-radiation therapy in locally advanced pancreatic cancer. A phase II clinical study from the USA that evaluates a combination of cisplatin, cytarabine, caffeine and continuous infusion of 5-FU followed by external beam radiotherapy presented promising results without severe toxicity. Modification with newer less toxic drugs may provide better results and further reduce the toxicity. In a second study from Europe, the feasibility of neo-adjuvant chemo-radiotherapy for treating primarily non resectable pancreatic carcinoma focusing on tumour regression was examined, as was the possibility of subsequent resection and tolerability. The authors refer to a feasible protocol with tolerable acute toxicity, and although the survival rate remained the same, the resectability rate was increased. Additional intra-arterial or intraportal application of drugs such as mitomycin C or cisplatin seems to be more promising.

Research into discovering an effective therapy for pancreatic cancer that can inhibit the development of the disease and improve the quality of life has led to the development of new therapeutic approaches derived from hormone manipulation. Various factors and hormones appear to stimulate pancreatic carcinoma, such as Epidermal Growth Factor (EGF), the Insulin-like Growth Factor I (IGF-I), the androgens and cholecystokinin. Several studies on animal models indicate a possible anti-tumour effect of anti-hormonal drugs and hormones or hormonal analogues. Although the results of these studies are promising, further investigations and clinical trials need to prove their therapeutic efficacy.

A recent study on an interferon-α based adjuvant chemo-radiation therapy following pancreaticoduodenectomy published by Traverso et al., suggests that overall survival may be improved for patients with pancreatic adenocarcinoma who follow a specific protocol. These results are preliminary and further evaluation of this regime in a multi-centre setting is needed.

Several novel promising approaches to radiotherapy, including the combination of radiotherapy with celecoxib (a cyclooxygenase-2 inhibitor) and amifostine (WR-2721) are currently under investigation. Some other large clinical trials are evaluating the efficacy of novel radiotherapy techniques, including intensity-modulated radiotherapy (IMRT) and stereo-tactic radio-surgery.

In the near future, many questions concerning radiotherapy in pancreatic cancer, including the optimal dose-fractionation of radiotherapy, the radiation treatment volume, the combined chemotherapy regimen and even whether chemo-radiotherapy is better than systemic chemotherapy alone, must be answered.

Considering the poor prognosis of the patients with pancreatic cancer, minimising the overall treatment time and improving the patients' quality of life after treatment are necessary. The optimal therapeutic strategy should combine minimal morbidity and mortality, longer survival and better quality of life.

Cholangiocarcinoma is a malignancy with poor prognosis but with worldwide increasing incidence and high mortality. The majority of affected patients seek treatment with advanced disease, and only a small percentage of them (about 30%) are suitable for surgical treatment. Complete surgical resection of the tumour is the only chance for long-term survival. Conventional treatments do not present respectable results and the long-term survival is poor. Conventional chemotherapy and radiotherapy have not been

shown to be effective in extending the long-term survival. Several new therapeutic approaches have also been developed. Photodynamic therapy combined with biliary stenting was promising and effective as a palliative treatment but not as a curative one. We need to develop novel and more effective therapeutic strategies that mainly focus on selected molecular targets.

Recent studies suggest that selective targeting of up-regulated iNOS and COX-2, together with altering the composition of the hydrophobic bile acid pool decreases the possibility of carcinogenesis and may provide a rational strategy for the chemo-prevention of cholangiocarcinoma in high-risk patients. Selective iNOS inhibitors also have been shown to exhibit chemo-preventive effects in rodent models of several cancers but their chemo-preventive effects have not been evaluated in preclinical *in vivo* models. Well-planned studies are now needed to evaluate the chemo-preventive factors and targets as well as to assess the safety and translational relevance of such treatments for patients with a high-risk of developing cholangiocarcinoma.

Other preclinical studies suggest several potential therapeutic selected-targeting strategies for gallbladder cancer and cholangiocarcinoma based on molecular biology advances. These therapeutic approaches are mainly based on experimental in vitro and in vivo models, which validate MUC4, hTERT, catenin, VEGF/VEGF-R and TGF-signalling pathways as promising molecular therapeutic approaches to treating cholangiocarcinoma.

The combined targeting of selected RTK pathways with other molecular targets (for example, combining ErbB-2/EGFR with COX-2) may present a more effective anti-tumour and therapeutic alternative, possessing synergistic and stronger anti-cancer effect for cholangiocarcinomas that over-express these gene products.

The role of classical chemotherapy and radiotherapy is limited in cholangio-carcinoma. Large clinical trials performed in recent years have failed to demonstrate a possible therapeutic advantage of these conservative treatment modalities in patients with cholangiocarcinoma. It is possible that the efficacy of the various chemotherapeutic agents will alter dramatically with the progress in the molecular biology of cholangiocarcinoma. Molecular and immunochemical marker expression has been evaluated in identifying selected targets for novel therapeutic approaches. COX-2 and selected RTK inhibitors are being evaluated as radio-sensitisers. The existing data suggest that they may enhance the anti-cancer effects of conventional chemotherapeutic agents, such as gemcitabine, and the effect of the phototherapy applied in cholangiocarcinomas as palliative treatment.

The efficacy and the clinical value of these novel therapies against cancer of the biliary tract that are based on selective molecular targets, such as neutralising antibodies, RTK inhibitors, anti-senso vectors and RNA therapies, should be evaluated in future experimental studies. Recently, COX-2 up-regulation and the over-expression of various genes such as c-erb-2 and c-met have been studied in cholangiocarcinoma in animal models. Such animal models are suitable for testing molecular therapeutic and chemo-prevention strategies that may posses a significant clinical advantage in humans.

We believe that in the near future the development of novel orthotopic cell transplantation models using animal and human cholangiocarcinoma cell lines, such as the rat C611B cholangiocarcinoma cell line, will contribute to the development of experimental therapeutic strategies for cholangiocarcinoma and the other biliary tract malignancies.

Cholangiocarcinoma is difficult to diagnose with the existing conventional imaging examinations such as US, CT and MRI. PET-FDG and/or in combination with CT scan seems to present a good and efficient alternative diagnostic modality, although the cost-effectiveness for cholangiocarcinoma has yet to be evaluated. Development of novel diagnostic techniques with higher accuracy, specificity and sensitivity or modification of the existing modalities may be another possible future target in the diagnosis of biliary tract malignancies.

BENIGN DISEASE

Choledocholithiasis. More than a century after the Swiss surgeon Ludwig Courvoisier performed the first gallstone removal while exploring the common bile duct through a choledochotomy in 1889, optimal diagnosis and management of choledocholithiasis remain highly controversial and debated issues. No procedure has so far been identified as the gold standard for detecting and treating common bile duct stones. In an era where laparoscopic cholecystectomy (LC) is being accepted as the standard of care for treating symptomatic cholecystolithiasis, the incidence of common bile duct stones varies between 7% and 20% in most series. Certain authors recommend and have demonstrated the feasibility and effectiveness of laparoscopic common bile duct exploration and stone clearance. Nevertheless, due to a lack of expertise and the need for special equipment, laparoscopic common bile duct exploration (LSCBDE) is still reserved for specialised centres and the classical 2-stage procedure (ERCP, ES & LC) remains the strategy of choice in most surgical units. While LSCBDE is not widely available, one of the aims of undergoing studies is to optimise the current management of patients with possible CBD stones and to lower the morbidity and mortality associated with diagnosis and treatment. The first difficulty in managing patients with cholelithiasis is to correctly diagnose the presence of common bile duct stones, meaning adequately employ or avoid available technologies that may themselves be associated with significant morbidity and mortality.

As has been previously mentioned, about 7-20% of symptomatic cholecystolithiasis cases harbour common bile duct stones. Which of these stones actually need to be removed in one way or another cannot be predicted. Collins et al. have found spontaneous passage in more than one third of stones after six weeks in patients diagnosed with common bile duct lithiasis by intraoperative cholangiography (IOC) during LC. Another study by Tranter estimates that up to 73% of all CBD stones will eventually pass spontaneously. Jaundice and acute cholangitis seem to be more frequently associated with complicated CBD stones. This data implies a high degree of unnecessary morbidity and mortality induced by diagnostic manoeuvres that potentially could be avoided. A panel of international experts stated that every patient with symptomatic gallstone disease should be assessed for the presence of CBD stones and if diagnosed, should be treated. Strategies to diminish the number of purely diagnostic invasive procedures associated with a non-negligible degree of morbidity and mortality have been developed. Biological markers combined with abdominal US have been proposed as a reliable screening tool for the presence of CBD stones to avoid unnecessary diagnostic tests.

If performed routinely in patients prior to cholecystectomy, negative ERCP results in 20-60% of patients, and severe morbidity may result as a consequence of the procedure. A review by Tranter & al. has found an overall success rate of cannulation of the papilla of Vater of 94%. In the presence of gallstone disease, the common bile duct can be cleared by this technique in more than 90% of cases. The success rate of the procedure is strongly operator dependent and ERCP is impossible to perform in certain situations due to anatomical considerations, i.e. post-gastric surgery states or in the presence of a periampullary diverticulum. Sphincterotomy-related complications occur in about 8% of patients. The most frequent complication, especially in younger patients, is pancreatitis, which is self-limited in 3% and occurs in about 1% as a severe disease. Other less frequent complications are bleeding in 1-6%, sepsis (up to 4%) and perforation (1-2%). Medium and long-term problems associated with ERCP and ES are cholangitis with recurrent stone formation (2-16%), biliary strictures (1-7%) and a high risk of bile duct malignancy. Stone recurrence rate ten years after endoscopic sphincterotomy has been cited as being as high as 19%, compared to 2% after open bile duct clearance. Recurrent duct stones are often soft brown stones, which are a result of chronic bacterbilia from duodenobiliary reflux. Another consequence of bacterbilia is chronic cholangitis, which may be associated with a higher risk of cholangiocarcinoma. More long-term data about the incidence of cholangiocarcinoma after ES should be gathered in the future, but it already seems clear that preservation of the sphincter of Oddi is important, especially in young patients. As an alternative to sphincterotomy, endoscopic balloon sphincteroplasty has been used, without any effect on the incidence of pancreatitis or bacterbilia. Mortality from ERCP is less than 1%, mostly due to perforation or severe necrotising pancreatitis. As it is the commonest complication, several groups have been working on ways to prevent ERCP-associated pancreatitis. Topically employed lidocaine on the papilla of Vater, with the aim of diminishing post-interventional pancreatitis, in a randomised study by Schwarz et al. was not shown to diminish the incidence of pancreatitis or improve the success rate of cannulation of the papilla of Vater. In another randomised, multi-centric series of 448 patients, the prophylactic administration of low molecular heparin did not prove to be beneficial to the incidence or severity of pancreatitis, but augmented the risk of bleeding compared to the placebo-group. Another randomised controlled trial examined the effect of prophylactically administered somatostatin prior to performing ERCP. The results showed that the incidence of pancreatitis was smaller in the somatostatin group than in the control group. A meta-analysis by Andriulli et al. did not previously show any significant advantages of somatostatin prior to ERCP. Regarding the problem of post-ERCP pancreatitis seeming to be related to the difficulty of CBD cannulation and concomitant periampullary trauma, one recent randomised trial has shown that using a Teflon tracer with a soft tip can diminish the incidence of post-ERCP pancreatitis. When performed routinely in patients with cholecystolithiasis, up to 86% of ERC will be normal, and, considering its potentially devastating complications, it should only be employed if indicated. As long as ERC with ES followed by LC remains a widely used strategy for treating choledocholithiasis, studies that emphasise refining those indications and diminishing the incidence of ERCP-related complications will be needed.

IOC performed during laparoscopic cholecystectomy is associated with a success rate of more than 95%. It is the method of choice for diagnosis in patients with suspected CBD stones who undergo LC in centres with the expertise and equipment necessary for LSCBDE. Stones not manageable this way undergo postoperative ES during ERCP or open CBD exploration.

Recent studies have found the sensitivity of magnetic resonance cholangiography (MRC) for detecting common bile duct stones to lie between 92% and 100%, which is about the same as for direct cholangiography. By obtaining 3-D reconstructions of the standard MRC, its sensitivity and specificity have been reported to be even higher. No consensus has been found as for the indications for the use of MRC. For selective use of MRC, patients have been classified into risk groups according to history, laboratory results and transabdominal US. Such a strategy has been shown to reduce the rate of purely diagnostic ERCP significantly. Future efforts should be directed towards refining such strategies for optimising patient care.

Endoscopic ultrasound has been shown to be even more accurate than MRC in diagnosing common bile duct stones. The main drawbacks are that it is strongly operator dependent and is less well tolerated by patients. The future will show if there is a place for intraoperative laparoscopic ultrasound and whether it could replace intraoperative cholangiography.

When confronted with common bile duct stones (before, during or after LC), surgeons try to avoid open exploration of the common bile duct to avoid adverse long-term effects such as bile duct strictures. A wide range of management options exist and no single strategy has so far been proven to be clearly superior to another. In the future, further prospective randomised studies are needed to compare the outcome of the two main strategies, i.e. 1-step (LSCBDE) versus 2-step (ES & LC) approach, and to decide which can be accepted as the standard of care. Nevertheless, it is unlikely that such a study can give a definitive answer, because of the many important variables between the different strategies (ES before, after, during LC, LSCBDE through transcystic versus transductal route, size of stones, diagnostic technique etc.).

Success rates of CBD clearance during open cholecystectomy in the pre-laparoscopic era were well above 90%. Since the introduction of LC as the standard for cholecystectomy, endoscopic stone removal has become more frequent. The associated morbidity, mortality and costs led to the development of new techniques and strategies for laparoscopic exploration of the biliary tract. Laparoscopic common bile duct exploration started in the early 1990s. Since then, several authors have demonstrated the feasibility of 1-session treatment of biliary stone disease through laparoscopic cholecystectomy (LC) and laparoscopic common bile duct exploration and clearance (LCBDE) with success rates of more than 90%. Claimed advantages of the entirely laparoscopic approach are the need for only one anaesthesia, significantly shorter hospital stay, associated cost savings and the importance of preservation of the duodenal papilla. Disadvantages are the need for advanced laparoscopic skills as well as expensive and sophisticated equipment. Trials in which the 1-stage LC & LSCBDE was compared to the 2-stage preoperative endoscopic CBD clearance (ERCP & ES) followed by LC have found no differences in stone clearance rates, similar morbidity and mortality, but a significantly reduced length of hospital stay in the 1-stage procedure group, especially if LSCBDE was performed through a transcystic approach. Other studies have shown the 1-stage procedure to be more cost-effective than the 2-stage procedure. In a review by Tranter the median rate of bile duct clearance was over 90%, with a median retained stone rate of 5%. Rate of conversion was 4%, mortality 1% and the complication rate 8%. In one study by Petelin, it has been shown that in the hands of an experienced operator, LCBDE was

successful in clearing the CBD in more than 95% of cases. Approaches into the CBD are described through either the cystic duct (transcystic) or through a transverse or longitudinal choledochotomy (transductal), according to stone characteristics and ductal anatomy. It has been shown that in patients undergoing choledochotomy, selective placement of T-tube drainage as an alternative to routine drainage seems to be a safe option. The transcystic approach, when feasible, has been shown to carry a lower morbidity and mortality than the transductal approach and is successful in clearing the CBD in about two thirds of patients. The postoperative course of these patients is comparable to that of a simple laparoscopic cholecystectomy. A recent randomised, controlled trial by Nathanson has compared laparoscopic transductal CBDE with postoperative ERCP for the one third of patients in which laparoscopic transcystic CBDE failed. There were no differences in significant morbidity, hospital stay and need for reoperation between the two groups. In the future, more trials will be needed to clarify the strategy for the one third of patients who fail laparoscopic transcystic CBD clearance. A recent trial with a mean follow-up of 72 months by Paganini et al. found laparoscopic transverse transductal stone clearance to be a safe option. In the future, laparoscopic transcystic CBDE might become accepted as the therapeutic strategy of choice in case of choledocholithiasis, with the advantage of avoiding trauma to the sphincter, which seems to be a major source of medium and long-term complications. The best strategy in cases of failed transcystic exploration is currently under investigation.

ERCP with sphincterotomy has been shown to be successful in clearing the CBD in more than 90% of cases. Its value is obvious in patients with CBD stones who are unfit for general anaesthesia, in whom it is acceptable to leave the gallbladder in situ. To avoid unnecessary ERCP, diagnostic algorithms and scoring systems for the probability of presence of CBD stones have been proposed, which will reduce the rate of unnecessary ERCP. In a large series by Sarli et al., the combined morbidity of such a strategy (ES & LC) can be as low as 4.5% (mainly due to self-limited post-ERCP pancreatitis) with mortality as low as 0.1%. To avoid two sedations, ERCP can be performed during the same anaesthesia as for LC, but this option is obviously limited by the coordinated availability of a gastroenterologist to perform the ERCP and ES.

REFERENCES

Al-Sukhun S, Zalupski M, Ben-Josef E, Vaitkevicious V et al. Chemoradiotherapy in the treatment of regional pancreatic carcinoma :a phase II study. Am J Clin Oncol 2003, 26:543-9.

Andriulli A, Solmi L, Loperfide S, Leo P, Festa V, Belmonte A, Spirito F, Silla M, Forte G, Terruzi V, Marenco G, Ciliberto E, Sabatino A, Monica F, Mognolia MR, Perri F: Prophylaxis of ERCP-related pancreatitis: A randomized controlled trial of somatostatin and gabexate mesylate: Clin Gastroenterol Hepatol 2 (2004) 713-718.

Aregui M, Davis CJ, Arkush AM, Nagan RF: Laparoscopic cholecystectomy combined with endoscopic sphincterotomy and stone extraction or laparoscopic choledochoscopy and electrohydraulic lithotripsy for management of cholelithiasis with choledocholithiasis. Surg Endosc (1992) 10-15.

Arvanitis D, Anagnostopoulos GK, Giannopoulos D, Pantes A, Agaritsi R, Margantinis G, Tsiakos S, Sakorafas G, Kostopoulos P : Can somatostatine prevent post-ERCP pancreatitis? Results of a randomized controlled trial : J Gastroenterol Hepatol 19 (2004) 278-282.

Bai YR, Wu GH, Guo WJ, et al. (2003) Intensity modulated radiation therapy and chemotherapy for locally advanced pancreatic cancer: results of feasibility study. World J Gastroenterol 9:2561- 2564.

Baker SJ, Markowitz S, Fearon ER, Willson JKV, Vogelstein B (1990) Suppression of human colorec-tal carcinoma cell growth by wild-type p53. Science 249:912-915.

Bardeesy N, DePinho RA, Pancreatic cancer biology and genetics. Nat Rev Cancer 2002, 2:897-909.

Beger HG, Buchler M, Friess H (1994) Chirurgische Ergebnisse und Indikation zu adjuvanten Maßnahmen beim Pankreaskarzinom. Chirurg 65:246-252.

Bergman JJGHM, Rauws EAJ, Tytgat GNJ, Huibregtse K: A prospective randomised trial comparing endoscopic sphincterotomy with endoscopic balloon dilatation for removal of common bile duct stones; initial report. Gastrointest Endosc (1994); 40: 99 (Abstract).

Berthiaume EP, Wands J. The molecular pathogenesis of cholangiocarcinoma. Semin Liver Dis 2004;24:127-137.

Bluemke DA, Fishman EK, CT and MR evaluation of pancreatic cancer. Surg Oncol Clin North Am 1998, 7:103-124.

Bockhorn M, Tsuzuki Y, Xu L, Frilling A, Broelsch CE, Fukumura D. Differential vascular and transcriptional responses to anti-vascular endothelial growth factor antibody in orthotopic human pancreatic cancer xenografts. Clin Cancer Res 2003;9:4221- 4226.

Bookstein R, Shew JY, Chen PL, Scully P, Lee WH (1990) Suppression of tumorigenicity of human prostate carcinoma cells by replacing a mutated RB gene. Science 247:712-715.

Carr-Locke DL: Acute gallstone pancreatitis and endoscopic therapy. Endoscopy (1990) 180-183.

Carroll BJ, Phillips EH, Daykhovsky L, Grundfest WS, Gersham A, Fallas M, Chandra M: Laparoscopic c-holedochoscopy: an effective approach to the common duct. J Laparoendosc Surg (1992) 15-21.

Carter G, Lemoine NR (1993) Antisense technology for cancer therapy: does it make sense? Br J Cancer 67:869-876.

Catalano C, Pavone P, Laghi A, et al., Pancreatic adenocarcinoma: combination of MR angiography and MR cholangiopancreatography for the diagnosis and assessment of resectability. Eur Radiol 1998, 8:428-434.

Collins C, Maguire D, Ireland A, Fitzgerald E, O'Sullivan GC: A prospective study of common bile duct calculi in patients undergoing laparoscopic cholecystectomy: Natural history of choledocholithiasis revisited: Ann Surg; 239 (2004) 28-33.

Cotton PB: Endoscopic management of bile duct stones (apples and oranges). Gut (1984) 587-597.

Courvoisier L: Casuistisch: Statistische Beitrage zur Pathologie und Chirurgie der Gallenwege. (1890) Leipzig: Vogel; 387: 57-58.

Crane CH, Antolak JA, Rosen II, et al. (2001) Phase I study of concomitant gemcitabine and IMRT for patients with unresectable adenocarcinoma of the pancreatic head. Int J Gastrointest Cancer 30:123-132.

Crane CH, Mason K, Janjan NA, et al. (2003) Initial experience combining cyclooxygenase-2 inhibition with chemoradiation for locally advanced pancreatic cancer. Am J Clin Oncol 26:S81-84.

Crnogorac-Jurcevic T, Missiaglia E, Blaveri E, Gangeswaran R, Jones M, Terris B, Costello E, Neoptolemos JP, Lemoine NR, Molecular alterations in pancreatic carcinoma: expression profiling shows that dysregulated expression of S100 genes is highly prevalent. J Pathol 2003, 201:63-74.

Cushieri A, Croce E, Faggioni A Jakimwicz J, Lacy A, Lezoche E, Morino M, Ribeiro VM, Toouli J, Visa J, Wayand W: EAES ductal stone study. Preliminary findings of multi-center prospective randomized trial comparing two-stage versus single stage management. Surg Endosc (1996) 1130-1135.

Cushieri A, Lezoche E, Morino M, Croce E, Lacy A, Toouli J, Ribeiro VM, Jakimovicz J, Visa J, Hanna GB: E.A.E.S. multicenter prospective randomized trial comparing two-stage vs single-stage management of patients with gallstone disease and ductal calculi. Surg Endosc (1999) 952-957.

Deans GT, Sedman P, Martin DF, Royston CMS, Leow CK, Thomas WEG: Are complications of endoscopic sphincterotomy age-related? Gut (1997); 41: 545-548.

De Ledinghen V, Lecesne R, Raymond JM, Gense V, Amouretti M, Drouillard J, Couzigou P, Silvain C: Diagnosis of choledocholithiasis: EUS or magnetic resonance cholangiography? A prospective controlled study. Gastrointest Endosc (1999);49(1):26-31.

Diederichs CG, Staib L, Vogel J, et al, Values and limitations of FDG PET with preoperative evaluations of patients with pancreatic masses. Pancreas 2000, 20:109-116.

Diehl SJ, Lehman KJ, Sadick M, Lachman R, Georgi M, Pancreatic cancer: value of dual-phase helical CT in assessing resectability. Radiology 1998, 206:373-378.

Dion YM, Ratelle R, Morin J:Common bile duct exploration. Surg Endosc (1994) 1168-1175.

Endo K, Yoon B, Pairojkul C, Demetris AJ, Sirica AE. ERBB-2 overexpression and cyclooxygenase-2 up-regulation in human cholangiocarcinoma and risk conditions. Hepatology 2002;36:439-450.

Endo K, Yoon B, Pairojkul C, Demetris AJ, Sirica AE. ERBB-2 overexpression and cyclooxygenase-2 up-regulation in human cholangiocarcinoma and risk conditions. Hepatology 2002;36:439-450.

Enochson L, Lindberg B, Swahn F, Arnelo U: Intraoperative endoscopic retrograde cholangiopancreatography (ERCP) to remove common bile duct stones during routine laparoscopic cholecystectomy does not prolong hospitalization. Surg Endosc (2004); 18: 367-371.

Fambrough D, McClure K, Kazlauskas A, Lander ES, Diverse signalling pathways activated by growth factor receptors induce broadly overlapping, rather than independent, sets of genes. Cell 1999, 97:727-741.

Franklin ME, Pharand D: Laparoscopic common bile duct exploration. Surg Laparosc Endosc (1994) 119-124.

Friess H, Yamanaka Y, Buchler M, Ebert M, Beger HG, Gold LI, Korc M (1993) Enhanced expression of transforming growth factor beta isoforms in pancreatic cancer correlates with decreased survival. Gastroenterology 105:1846-1856.

Fulcher AS, Turner MA, Capps GW, Zfass AM, Baker KM: Half-Fourier RARE MR cholangiopancreatography: experience in 300 subjects. Radiology (1998); 207: 21-32.

Gansauge S, Gansauge F, Beger H, Molecular oncology in pancreatic cancer. J Mol Med 1996, 74:313-320.

Gansauge S, Gansauge F, Beger H, Molecular oncology in pancreatic cancer.J Mol Med 1996, 74:313-320.

Gores GJ. Cholangiocarcinoma: current concepts and insights. Hepatology 2003;37:961-969.

Gregg JA, De Girolami P, Carr Locke DL: Effects of sphincteroplasty and endoscopic sphincterotomy on the bacteriologic characteristics of the common bile duct. Am J Surg (1985); 149: 668-671.

Grieco A, Miele L, Giorgi A, Civello IM, Gasbarrini G. Acute cholestatic hepatitis associated with celecoxib. Ann Pharmacother 2002;36:1887-1889.

Gudjonsson B (1987) Cancer of the pancreas: 50 years of surgery. Cancer 60:2284-2303.

Hamy A, Hennekinne S, Pessaux P, Lada P, Randria-mananajo S, Lermite E, Boyer J, Arnaud JP: Endoscopic sphincterotomy prior to laparoscopic cholecystectomy for the treatment of cholelithiasis. Surg Endosc (2003) 872-875.

Han H, Bearss DJ, Browne LW, Calaluce R, Nagle RB, Von Hoff DD, Identification of differentially expressed genes in pancreatic cancer cells using cDNA microarray. Cancer Res 2002, 62:2890-2896.

Hayashi N, Yamamoto H, Hiraoka N, Dono K, Ito Y, Okami J, et al. Differential expression of cyclooxygenase-2 (COX-2) in human bile duct epithelial cells and bile duct neoplasm. Hepatology 2001;34:638-650.

Hayashi N, Yamamoto H, Hiraoka N, Dono K, Ito Y, Okami J, et al. Differential expression of cyclooxygenase-2 (COX-2) in human bile duct epithelial cells and bile duct neoplasm. Hepatology 2001;34:638-650.

Hruban RH, Offerhaus GJ, Kern SE, Goggins M, Wilentz RE, Yeo CJ, Tumor-suppressor genes in pancreatic cancer. J Hepatobiliary Pancreat Surg 1998,5:383-391.

Huang HJ, Yee JK, Shew JY, Chen PL, Bookstein R, Friedmann T, Lee EY, Lee WH (1988) Suppression of the neoplastic phenotype by replacement of the RB gene in human cancer cells. Science 242: 1563-1566.

Hunter J: Laparoscopic transcystic common bile duct exploration. Am J Surg (1992) 53-58.

Huster D, Schubert C, Berr F, Mossner J, Caca K. Rofecoxib-induced cholestatic hepatitis: treatment with molecular adsorbent recycling system. J Hepatol 2002;37:423- 414.

Iacobuzio-Donahue CA, Maitra A, Shen-Ong GL, van Heek T, Ashfaq R, Meyer R, Walter K, Berg K, Hollingsworth MA, Cameron JL, Yeo CJ, Kern SE, Goggins M, Hruban RH, Discovery of novel tumor markers of pancreatic cancer using global gene expression technology. Am J Pathol 2002, 160: 1239-1249.

Iacobuzio-Donahue CA, Maitra A, Olsen M, Lowe AW, Van Heek NT, Rosty C, Walter K, Sato N, Parker A, Ashfaq R, Jaffee E, Ryu B, Jones J, Eshleman JR, Yeo CJ, Cameron JL, Kern SE, Hruban RH, Brown PO, Goggins M, Exploration of global gene expression patterns in pancreatic adenocarcinoma using cDNA microarrays. Am J Pathol 2003, 162:1151-1162.

Irie H, Honda H, Kaneko K, et al., Comparison of helical CT and MR imaging in detecting and staging small pancreatic adenocarcinoma. Abdom Imag 1998, 22:429-433.

Johnson PT, Outwater EK, Pancreatic carcinoma versus chronic pancreatitis: dynamic MR imaging. Radiology 1999, 212:213-218.

Kastl S, Bruner T, Hermann O, Riepl M et al. Neo-adjuvant radio-chemotherapy in advanced primarily non-resectable carcinomas of the pancreas. Eur J Surg Oncol 2000, 26:578-82.

Khan SA, Taylor-Robinson SD, Toledano MB, Beck A, Elliott P,Thomas HC. Changing international trends in mortality rates for liver,biliary and pancreatic tumours. J Hepatol 2002;37:806-813.

Kiguchi K, Carbajal S, Chan K, Beltrán L, Ruffino L, Shen J, et al. Constitutive expression of ErbB-2 in gallbladder epithelium results in development of adenocarcinoma. Cancer Res 2001;61:6971-6976.

Kim JH, Kim MJ, Park SI: MR cholangiography in symptomatic gallstones: diagnostic accuracy according to clinical risk group. Radiology (2002); 224: 410-416.

Kim YJ, Kim MJ, Kim KW, Chung JB, Lee WJ, Kim JH, Oh YT, Lim JS, Choi JY: Preoperative evaluation of common bile duct stones in patients with gallstone disease. AJR (2005) 1846-1854.

Kluge R, Schmidt F, Caca K et al. Positron emission tomography with [(18)F]fluoro-2-deoxy-D-glucose for diagnosis and staging of bile duct cancer. Hepatology 2001;33:1029-1035.

Kwong KY, Zou Y, Day C-P, Hung M-C. The suppression of colon cancer cell growth in nude mice by targeting _-catenin/TCF pathway. Oncogene 2002;21:8340-8346.

Lai G-H, Radaeva S, Nakamura T, Sirica AE. Unique epithelial cell production of hepatocyte growth factor/scatter factor by putative precancerous intestinal metaplasias and associated "intestinal-type" biliary cancer chemically induced in rat liver. Hepatology 2000;31:1257-1265.

Lammer J, Herlinger H, Zalaudek G, Hofler H, Pseudotumorous pancreatitis. Gastrointest Radiol 1995, 10:59-67.

Legmann P, Vignaux O, Dousset B, et al, Pancreatic tumors: comparison of dual-phase helical CT and endoscopic sonography. AJR Am J Roentgenol 1998, 170:1315-1322.

Lella F, Bagnolo F, Colombo E, Bonassi U: A simple way of avoiding post-ERCP pancreatitis: Gastrointest Endosc 59 (2004) 830-834.

Lemoine NR (1994) Genetic intervention for therapy and prevention of pancreatic cancer Dig Surg I 1: 170-177.

Liberman MA, Philipps EH, Carroll BJ, Fallas MJ, Rosenthal R, Hiatt J: Cost-effective management of complicated choledocholithiasis: laparoscopic transcystic duct exploration or endoscopic sphincterotomy. J Am Coll Surg (1996); 182: 488-494.

Liu TH, Consorti ET, Kawashima A: Patient evaluation and management with selective use of magnetic resonance cholangiography and endoscopic retrograde cholangiopancreatography before laparoscopic cholecystectomy. Ann Surg (2001); 234: 33-40.

Logsdon CD, Simeone DM, Binkley C, Arumugam T, Greenson JK, Giordano TJ, Misek DE, Hanash S, Molecular profiling of pancreatic adenocarcinoma and chronic pancreatitis identifies multiple genes differentially regulated in pancreatic cancer. Cancer Res 2003, 63:2649-2657.

Lu DSK, Reber HA, Krasny RM, Sayre J, Local staging of pancreatic cancer: criteria for unresectability of major vessels as revealed by pancreatic-phase, thin section helical CT. Am J Radiol 1997, 168:1439-1444.

MacMathuna P, White P, Clarke E, Merriman R, Lennon JR, Crowe J: Endoscopic balloon sphincteroplasty (papillary dilatation) for bile duct stones: efficacy, safety, and follow up in 100 patients. Gastrointest Endosc (1995); 42: 468-474.

Maisey NR, Webb A, Flux GD, Padhani A, Cunningham DC, Ott RJ, Norman A, FDG PET in the prediction of survival of patients with cancer of the pancreas: a pilot study. Br J Cancer 2000, 83:287-293.

Mann M, Sheng H, Shao J, Williams CS, Pisacane PI, Sliwkowski MX, et al. Targeting cyclooxygenase 2 and HER-2/neu pathways inhibits colorectal carcinoma growth. Gastroenterology 2001;120:1713-1719.

Mertz HR, Sechopoulos P, Delbeke D, Leach SD, EUS, PET, and CT scanning for evaluation of pancreatic adenocarcinoma. Gastrointest Endosc 2000, 52:367-371.

Milano MT, Chmura SJ, Garofalo MC, et al. (2004) Intensity modulated radiotherapy in treatment of pancreatic and bile duct malignancies: toxicity and clinical outcome. Int J Radiat Oncol Biol Phys 59:445-453.

Nathanson LK, O'Rourke NA, Martin IJ, Fielding GA, Cowen AE, Roberts RK, Kendall BJ, Kerlin P, Devereux BM: Postoperative ERCP versus laparoscopic choledochotomy for clearance of selected bile duct calaculi. Ann Surg (2005); 242: 188-192.

Nellen W, Lichtenstein C (1993) What makes an mRNA antisenseitive? Trends Biol Sci 18:419-423.

Ortner MEJ, Caca K, Berr F, Liebetruth J, Mansmann U, Huster D, et al. Successful photodynamic therapy for nonresectable cholangiocarcinoma: a randomized prospective study. Gastroenterology 2003;125:1355-1363.

Paganini AM, Guerrieri M, Sarnari J, De Sanctis A, D'Ambrosio G, Lezoche G, Lezoche E: Long-term results after laparoscopic transverse choledochotomy for common bile duct stones. Sur Endosc (2005); 19: 705-709.

Pardi DS, Loftus Jr EV, Kremers WK, Keach J, Lindor KD. Ursodeoxycholic acid as a chemopreventive agent in patients with ulcerative colitis and primary sclerosing cholangitis. Gastroenterology 2003;124:889-893.

Paul A, Millat B, Holthausen U: Diagnosis and treatment of common bile duct stones. Results of a consensus development conference. Scientific Committee of the European Association for Endoscopic Surgery (E.A.E.S.). Surg Endosc (1998) 856.

Peppelenbosch AG, Naber AHJ, van Goor H: Recurrence rate of common bile duct stones is higher after endoscopic sphincterotomy than after common bile duct exploration in patients below 60 years of age: a long term follow-up study. Br J Surg (1998); 85: 54 (Abstract).

Perilli D, Mansi C, Savarino V, Cele G. Hormonal therapy of pancreatic carcinoma. Rationale and perspectives. Int J Pancreatol 1993, 13:159-68.

Petelin J: Laparoscopic approach to common duct pathology. Am J Surg (1993) 487-491.

Petelin J: Laparoscopic common bile duct exploration. Surg Endosc (2003) 1705-1715.

Petelin J, Laparoscopic common bile duct exploration: evolution of a protocol which minimizes the need for ERCP. Presented at the annual meeting of the SAGES, Mashville, TM, USA, 18. April 1994.

Phillips E, Carroll BJ, Pearlstein R, Daykhovsky L, Fallas MJ: Laparoscopic choledochoscopy and extraction of common bile duct stones. World J Surg (1993) 22-28.

Picozzi VJ, Kzarek RA, Traverso LW. Interferon-based adjuvant chemoradiation therapy after pancreaticoduodenectomy for pancreatic cancer. Am J surg 2003, 185:476-80.

Pitt HA: Role of open choledochotomy in the treatment of choledocholithiasis. Am J Surg (1993) 483-486.

Prat F, Malak NA, Pelletier G, Buffet C, Fritsch J, Choury AD: Biliary symptoms and complications more than 8 years after endoscopic sphincterotomy for choledocholithiasis. Gastroenterology (1996); 110: 894-899.

Prins J, DeVries E, Mulder N (1993) Antisense of oligonucleotides and the inhibition of oncogene expression. Clin Oncol 5:245-252.

Rabenstein T, Fischer B, Wiessner V, Schmidt H, Radespiel-Toger M, Hochberger J, Muhldorfer S, Nusko G, Messmann H, Scholmerich J, Schultz HJ, Schonekas H, Hahn EG, Schneider HAT: Low-molecular-weight heparin does not prevent acute post-ERCP pancreatitis : Gastrointest Endosc 59 (2004) 606-613.

Raval B, Kramer LA: Advances in the imaging of common duct stones using magnetic resonance cholangiography, endoscopic ultrasonography, and laparoscopic ultrasonography. Semin Laparosc Surg (2000);7(4):232-6.

Regan F, Fradin J, Khazan R, Bohlman M, Magnuson T: Choledocholithiasis: evaluation with MR cholangiography. AJR (1996); 167: 1441-1445.

Rhodes M, Sussman L, Cohen L, Lewis MP: Randomised trial of laparoscopic exploration of common bile duct versus postoperative endoscopic retrograde cholangiography for common bile duct stones. Lancet (1998); 351: 159-161.

Rossleand AR, Solhaug JH: Primary endoscopic papillotomy in patients with stones in the common bile duct and the gallbladder in situ: a 5 -8 year follow-up study. World J Surg (1988); 12: 111-116.

Sarli L, Costi R, Gobbi S, Iusco D, Sgobba G, Roncoroni L: Scoring system to predict asymptomatic choledocholithiasis before laparoscopic cholecystectomy. Surg Endosc (2003) 1396-1403.

Sarli L, Iusco DR, Roncoroni L: Preoperative endoscopic sphincterotomy and laparoscopic cholecystectomy for the management of cholecystolithiasis : 10-Year experience. World J Surg (2003) 180-186.

Schwartz JJ, Lew RJ, Ahmad NA, Shah JN, Ginsberg GG, Kochmann ML, Brensinger CM, Long WB : The effect of lidocaine sprayed on the major duodenal papilla on the frequency of post-ERCP pancreatitis: Gastrointest Endosc 59 (2004) 179-184.

Sgourakis G, Dedemadi G, Stamatelopoulos A, Leandros E, Voros D, Karaliotas K: Predictors of common bile duct lithiasis in laparoscopic era. World J Gastroenterol (2005) 3267-3272.

Shammas MA, Koley H, Beer DG, Li C, Goyal RK, Munshi NC. Growth arrest, apoptosis, and telomere shortening of Barrett's-associated adenocarcinoma cells by a telomerase inhibitor. Gastroenterology 2004;126:1337-1346.

Simone M, Mutter D, Rubino F, Dutson E, Roy C, Soler L, Marescaux J: Three-dimensional virtual cholangioscopy: a reliable tool for the diagnosis of common bile duct stones. Ann Surg (2004); 240: 82-88.

Singh AP, Moniaux N, Chauhan SC, Meza JL, Batra SK. Inhibition of MUC4 expression suppresses pancreatic tumor cell growth and metastasis. Cancer Res 2004;64:622- 630.

Sirica AE, Lai G-H, Zhang Z. Biliary cancer growth factor pathways, cyclo-oxygenase-2 and potential therapeutic strategies. J Gastroenterol Hepatol 2001;16:363-372.

Slebos RJ, Hoppin JA, Tolbert PE, Holly EA, Brock JW, Zhang RH, Bracci PM, Foley J, Stockton P, McGregor LM, Flake GP, Taylor JA, K-ras and p53 in pancreatic cancer: association with medical history, histopathology, and environmental exposures in a population-based study. Cancer Epidemiol Biomarkers Prev 2000, 9:1223-1232.

Subramanian G, Schwarz RE, Higgins L, Mc Enroe G, Chakravarty S, Dugar S, et al. Targeting endogenous transforming growth factor receptor signaling in SMAD4-deficient human pancreatic carcinoma cells inhibits their invasive phenotype. Cancer Res 2004;64:5200 -5211.

Suissa A, Yassin K, Lavy A, Lachter J, Chermech I, Karban A, Tamir A, Eliakim R: Outcome and early complications of ERCP: A prospective single center study. Hepatogastroenterology (2005) 352-355.

Tanaka K, Oshimura M, Kikuchi R, Seki M, Hayashi T, Miyaki M (1991) Suppression of tumorigenicity in human colon carcinoma cells by introduction of normal chromosome 5 or 18. Nature 349:340-342.

Tanaka M, Takahata S, Konomi H, Matsanuga H, Yokohata K, Takeda T: Long term consequences of endoscopic sphincterotomy for bile duct stones. Gastrointest Endosc (1998); 48: 465-469.

Tan ZJ, Hu XG, Cao GS, Tang Y, Analysis of gene expression profile of pancreatic carcinoma using cDNA microarray. World J Gastroenterol 2003, 9:818-823.

Torok NJ, Higuchi H, Bronk S, Gores GJ. Nitric oxide inhibits apoptosis downstream of cytochrome C release by nitrosylating caspase 9. Cancer Res 2002;62:1648 -1653.

Tortora G, Caputo R, Damiano V, Melisi D, Bianco R, Fontanini, G, et al. Combination of a selective cyclooxygenase-2 inhibitor with epidermal growth factor receptor tyrosine kinase inhibitor ZD 1839 and protein kinase A antisense causes cooperative antitumor and antiangiogenic effect. Clin Cancer Res 2003;9:1566 -1572.

Tranter SE, Thompson MH: Spontaneous passage of bile duct stones: Frequency of occurrence and relation to clinical presentation. Ann R Coll Surg Engl (2003) 174-177.

Tranter SE, Thompson MH: Comparison of endoscopic sphincterotomy and laparoscopic exploration of the common bile duct. BJS (2002); 89: 1495-1504.

Trede M, Rumstadt B, Wendl, et al, Ultrafast magnet-ic resonance imaging improves the staging of pancreatic tumors. Ann Surg 1997, 226:393-405.

Urbach DR, Khajanchee YS, Jobe BA, Standage BA, Hansen PD, Swanstrom LL: Cost-effective management of common bile duct stones: a decision analysis of the use of endoscopic retrograde cholangiopancreatography (ERCP), intraoperative cholangiography, and laparoscopic bile duct exploration. Surg Endosc (2001); 15: 4-13.

Valls C, Guma A, Puig I et al. Intrahepatic peripheral cholangiocarcinoma: CT evaluation. Abdom Imaging 2000;25:490-496.

Vitale GC, Larson GM, Wieman TJ, Cheadle WG, Miller FB: The use of ERCP in the management of common bile duct stonesin patients undergoing laparoscopic cholecystectomy. Surg Endosc (1993) 9-11.

Wang J, Torbenson M, Wang Q, Ro JY, Becich M. Expression of inducible nitric oxide synthase in paired neoplastic and non-neoplastic primary prostate cell cultures and prostatectomy specimen. Urol Oncol 2003;21:117-122.

Wiedmann M, Berr F, Schiefke I, Witzigmann H, Kohlhaw K, Mossner J, et al. Photodynamic therapy in patients with non-resectable hilar cholangiocarcinoma: 5-year follow-up of a prospective phase II study. Gastrointest Endosc 2004;60:68 -75.

Wright BE, Freeman ML, Cumming JK, Quickel RR, Mandal AK: Current management of common bile duct stones: is there a role for laparoscopic cholecystectomy and intraoperative endoscopic retrograde cholangiopancreatography as a single-stage procedure? Surgery (2002); 132: 729-735.

Yavuz AA, Aydin F, Yavuz MN, et al. (2001) Radiation therapy and concurrent fixed dose amifostine with escalating doses of twice weekly gemcitabine in advanced pancreatic cancer. Int J Radiat Oncol Biol Phys 51:974-981.

Yeh TS, Jan YY, Tseng JH et al. Malignant perihilar biliary obstruction: magnetic resonance cholangiopancreatographic findings. Am J Gastroenterol 2000;95:432-440.

Zhang Z, Lai G-H, Sirica AE. Celecoxib-induced apoptosis in rat cholangiocarcinoma cells mediated by Akt inactivation and Bax translocation. Hepatology 2004;39:1028 -1037.

Index